Comprehensive Healthcare Simulation

Series Editors

Adam I. Levine, Department of Anesthesiology
Mount Sinai Medical Center
New York, USA
Samuel DeMaria Jr., Department of Anesthesiology
Mount Sinai Medical Center
New York, USA

This series focuses on the use of simulation in healthcare education, one of the most exciting and significant innovations in healthcare teaching since Halsted put forth the paradigm of "see one, do one, teach one." Each volume focuses either on the use of simulation in teaching in a specific specialty or on a cross-cutting topic of broad interest, such as the development of a simulation center. The volumes stand alone and are also designed to complement Levine, DeMaria, Schwartz, and Sim, eds., THE COMPREHENSIVE TEXTBOOK OF HEALTHCARE SIMULATION by providing detailed and practical guidance beyond the scope of the larger book and presenting the most up-to-date information available. Series Editors Drs. Adam I. Levine and Samuel DeMaria Jr. are affiliated with the Icahn School of Medicine at Mount Sinai, New York, New York, USA, home to one of the foremost simulation centers in healthcare education. Dr. Levine is widely regarded as a pioneer in the use of simulation in healthcare education. Editors of individual series volumes and their contributors are all recognized leaders in simulation-based healthcare education.

Jared M. Kutzin • KT Waxman
Connie M. Lopez • Debra Kiegaldie
Editors

Comprehensive Healthcare Simulation: Nursing

Springer

Editors
Jared M. Kutzin
Emergency Medicine
Icahn School of Medicine at Mount Sinai
Director of Emergency Medicine Simulation
Mount Sinai Hospital
New York, NY, USA

Connie M. Lopez
Perinatal Patient Safety
Kaiser Permanente
Pleasanton, CA, USA

KT Waxman
School of Nursing
University of California San Francisco
San Francisco, CA, USA

Debra Kiegaldie
Eastern Health Clinical School, Faculty of
Medicine, Nursing & Health Sciences
Monash University
Melbourne, VIC, Australia

ISSN 2366-4479 ISSN 2366-4487 (electronic)
Comprehensive Healthcare Simulation
ISBN 978-3-031-31089-8 ISBN 978-3-031-31090-4 (eBook)
https://doi.org/10.1007/978-3-031-31090-4

This Springer imprint is published by the registered company Springer Nature Switzerland AG
The registered company address is: Gewerbestrasse 11, 6330 Cham, Switzerland

This book is dedicated to my family, friends, and mentors without whom it would not have been possible. Thank you to Jenny Rudolph for indulging a graduate student's question and shedding light on "how the way we talk, changes the way we work." Thank you to Chuck Pozner for opening the doors of STRATUS many years ago. To my loving and supportive wife, Melissa, without whom the late nights would not have been possible. And to my children, Sylvie and Eli, who provide me with endless hours of practice in advocacy, inquiry, and debriefing.

Jared M. Kutzin

I would like to dedicate this book to all of those educators who believe in simulation, advocate for it, and are passionate about the outcomes. For those of us who have seen the "lightbulb come on" in debriefing, it makes what we do worth it. I would like to thank my family for supporting me all of these years as I traveled the world to spread the word about simulation! Thank you Steve, Ashley, Sam, Brian, Tom, and the grands: Olive, Meyer, and Bette.

KT Waxman

Simulation is a wonderful teaching strategy that has transformed the way we deliver education in the nursing profession. I dedicate this book to the simulation champions in nursing. I would like to thank my family for their unwavering support throughout my academic and simulation journey—this is for you Farnel, Aaron, Ashleigh, and Brittany.

Debra Kiegaldie

I extend my heartfelt gratitude to my fellow editors, whose unwavering support and dedication have been invaluable throughout the creation of this textbook. I deeply appreciate my family and friends' endless encouragement and understanding, which have been instrumental in navigating this professional endeavor. Thank you for your support, and I hope you enjoy this read!

Connie M. Lopez

A special thank you to the inspiring authors and dedicated healthcare simulation teams around the world. Your commitment to patient safety and innovation through simulation has reshaped the learning, training, and patient care landscape.

To the authors who weaved expertise and insight onto pages, your words serve as bridges connecting theory to practice, fostering a deeper understanding of simulation, and drive the evolution of healthcare education.

To the healthcare simulation teams who bring scenarios to life, your creativity and efforts in crafting realistic simulations empower healthcare professionals to hone their skills, refine their approaches, and ultimately deliver safer, more effective patient care.

Thank you for your passion and collaborative spirit, which continues to elevate the standards of healthcare education and practice. Your contributions resonate profoundly, shaping the future of healthcare for generations to come.

Foreword

One cold Nebraska January day, our college president stopped in my office and asked if I would go to a conference in Florida. Of course, I said yes. Later, I asked her what she wanted me to do there, and she said, "check out this patient simulator and let me know if I should buy it." She already had the money due to years of fundraising. My response: "What's a patient simulator?" This was in 2003 and thus began my career in simulation. Upon my return with an enthusiastic "Yes!" she placed me in charge of simulation because I was now the expert—being as I was the only one that knew what a simulator was. Her gift to me was allowing me to replace my clinical responsibilities with simulation and giving me the time and freedom to figure it out on my own. Of course, in those days there were no books, journals, courses, or organizations. On weekends, I played with the technology until I learned the nuances of the programming, but then also purposefully did things incorrectly so I could figure out how the machines worked. After a year, I moved to industry, designing curriculum for nursing schools to use with simulation. I returned to academia after 2 years and have since worked with nursing, medicine, and allied health both in academia and clinical environments.

Nurse simulationists were supported by the early work of the National League for Nursing (NLN) which began studying simulation in the early 2000s. The NLN partnered with Medical Education Technologies, Inc. (METI, now known as CAE Healthcare) to provide research grants to support nurses to learn how to best teach with the Human Patient Simulator. A partnership with Laerdal to develop and test simulation models to promote learning, led by Dr. Pamela Jeffries, continues to provide support for nursing educators through the development of a theoretical framework to guide decisions related to all aspects of simulation education (Forneris et al. 2017). These early collaborations between academia and vendors were crucial to the progress of nursing's use of simulation, helping to elevate simulation to a viable pedagogy, and providing resources to support nurse educators to learn a new teaching role. In 2011, the International Nursing Association of Clinical Simulation and Learning (INACSL) published the first standards of best practice for simulation educators (Leighton 2011). These efforts helped to support early adopters when promoting simulation to their leadership.

The use of simulation has grown significantly over the years; however, cost has always been a factor. Nursing education is expensive due to the need for small clinical groups with low student-to-faculty ratios. We had been teaching this way for decades; however, the cost of simulation was a major barrier. The vendors realized that nursing education could not bear the expense of the simulators (our first one cost $216,000!) and worked hard over the ensuing years to lower the price point. In addition, grant funding and major donations helped many schools to overcome the cost of the equipment. However, money continues to be scarce for faculty development. Numerous programs have been developed over the years from 1-day courses to doctoral programs; however, the cost of these opportunities often falls to the simulationist rather than the employer. Anecdotally, annual conferences are heavily attended by novices, indicating that the field is still new enough that people are hired into their positions without adequate knowledge or experience. This is supported by social media posts from people asking for help in learning their new job role. There is work to do in order to help employers understand that simulation is a unique pedagogy with evidence-based standards of best practice that can lead to excellent learning outcomes when facilitated by qualified educators. Support for education and training of the facilitators, as well as the operations personnel continues to be substandard.

We are at a point in time where we need to carefully consider the role of simulation in nursing education and training. During the pandemic, many faculty converted in-person training to online platforms but often without support and training for how to teach online. Some State Boards of Nursing agreed for online simulation to replace traditional clinical hours; however, without the rigor of a multi-site study such as the one that compared outcomes of traditional clinical and in-person simulation (Hayden et al. 2014). Early research indicates that learning needs are met differently in the traditional clinical, in-person simulation, and screen-based simulation environments (Leighton et al. 2021), and it is imperative that outcomes are thoroughly evaluated before online simulation becomes a viable substitution.

I have believed for a while that manikin-based simulation will be replaced to a great extent by virtual reality due to the ability to create immersive, realistic, and less costly learning experiences. However, as a result of the pandemic, I suspect that the timeline will shorten as we had to learn (although under duress and stress) how to drastically change how we teach with simulation. There is a lot to learn yet, but we do know that some of the ways we accomplished simulation virtually worked very well and should be continued. Others didn't work and need to be refined. It is exciting to see the volume of research being produced that shows favorable learning outcomes that will inform future best practices in this area. We have an opportunity to take what has been learned while researching various aspects of simulation and use these results to better inform traditional clinical practice.

We have made tremendous progress with simulation pedagogy in the past two decades and I'm excited to see what comes next. The early efforts in nursing education were fueled by the excitement of intuitively knowing that simulation was an important modality to add to our teaching arsenal. We learned a lot by trial and error, but isn't that the same thing we are asking of our learners? I am forever grateful to be on this exciting, innovative, challenging, and rewarding career path and look forward to seeing where the future takes us.

References

- Forneris SG, Tagliareni ME, Jeffries PR, Rizzolo MA. National league for nursing and simulation innovation resource center. In: Foisy-Doll C, Leighton K, editors. Simulation champions: courage, caring and connections. Wolters Kluwer; 2017. p. 61–69.
- Hayden JK, Smiley RA, Alexander M, Kardong-Edgren S, Jeffries PR. The NCSBN national simulation study: a longitudinal, randomized, controlled study replacing clinical hours with simulation in prelicensure nursing education. J Nurs Regul. 2014;5(2):S3–40. https://doi.org/10.1016/S2155-8256(15)30062-4.
- Leighton K. President's message. Clin Simul Nurs. 2011;7(Suppl):S2. https://doi.org/10.1016/j.ecns.2011.05.004.
- Leighton K, Kardong-Edgren S, Schneidereith T, Foisy-Doll C, Wuestney K. Meeting nursing students' clinical needs: traditional, simulation, and screen-based simulation environments. Nurse Educ. 2021;46(6):349–54.

Kim Leighton
Executive Director, Itqan Clinical Simulation
and Innovation Center, Hamad Medical Corporation

My earliest days in manikin-based sim were with Mindi Anderson at UT Arlington around 2004–2006. I was one of the faculty assigned to help in her physical assessment class. She started using a METI Man that the graduate school had purchased with a grant but decided that they did not have time to learn how to use. She dug him out of the crate and fired him up. We used him to help our students listen and learn lung and bowel sounds and some heart sounds. We also wrote little vignettes for practicing the assessment of various body systems, for example, skin–hair–nails. Hours were spent finding images of skin cancer on Google and transferring them to clear overheads, then cutting and pasting them down to stick on the manikin for a 15-min experience each week in our physical assessment class. There were few scenarios available then, so we made things up as we went along and invented our own ways to use this $250,000 resource. Our course was the first one to start using simulation, if I recall correctly.

Our nursing school leadership came to see this manikin in action, and they all "got it" at first glance. So much so that they wrote for and received a large grant for the building of a Smart Hospital that was designed for 20 Laerdal manikins. And it happened quickly, towards the end of a spring semester. The manikins arrived and were stacked like cordwood in the school hallways, on racks. It looked like a morgue. The "adoption" of simulation was eased by the vision of the leadership.

Many (and I use the word many deliberately) faculty were threatened by the "rise of the machines." Many said the words "you are trying to take my job" with little understanding or desire to learn what might be possible. When we say it takes 17 years on average for a new practice to become accepted, it has been about 17 years since manikins like SimMan 3G and the CAE manikins came on the nursing scene. To have the pandemic hit and have to move to screen-based simulation and widespread adoption of vendor or individually developed screen-based scenarios or virtual reality simulation is ironic. The same things may now be said by those who became skilled at running a manikin, "you're trying to take my job." Manikins were going to be one stop on the way to Star Trek Holodeck. If you paid attention, you could see this. Manikins were too big, too expensive, and too finicky, for the average nursing program to deal with. The great thing we learned was that it was not about the manikin. It was about how to teach more effectively. So as the manikins begin to disappear to a certain extent and are replaced with screen-based simulation and VR, we are better educators overall. We have figured out that the skills we developed in simulation apply to traditional clinical situations, i.e., pre-briefing, debriefing, and Socratic questioning.

Barriers to simulation and whether or not they have been broken down-Through death and retirement, the last simulation naysayers will finally disappear. In reality, simulation and the knowledge of simulation pedagogy saved the spring class of 2020 nursing students by providing a way (for many, the *only* way) to complete requirements for graduation, to get them out into the working population, to help with the pandemic. What would we have done without this highly developed understanding of how to teach using this pedagogy? The real barriers to simulation adoption continue to be: the costs, the need to understand technology on a level that most of us do not, and the continued lack of education on how to use simulation in so many nursing graduate educator programs. It is astonishing to me that after 17–20 years of simulation use by all health professions education, multiple journals devoted to healthcare simulation, multiple societies and associations, and conferences worldwide on this topic, there are still nursing MS educator programs with cursory mention of simulation.

Suzie Kardong-Edgren
Associate Professor at the MGH Institute of
Health Professions in Boston

I was fortunate to be appointed the NLN program director in the early 2003 work with program coordinators across ten different schools including associate degree, diploma, and baccalaureate programs. Using simulation pedagogy was just beginning and my charge from the NLN was to conduct simulation research—does it work? Working with the program coordinators, we embarked on a literature review/systematic analysis just like we would start any new research program of study. We found very little in the literature regarding simulations. Many of the studies conducted talked about how the participants liked being immersed in simulations, but there were gaps in the findings on what a simulation looked like, how to implement a high-quality simulation and how to evaluate the outcomes of this new emerging pedagogy. As a group, we conducted our first study in simulation research but realized that we had more to offer to nurse educators and that was creating a "cookbook" on how to develop, implement, and evaluate simulations. This conclusion led me to the first NLN book called *Simulation in*

Nursing Education: From Conceptualization to Evaluation published in 2007. Since then, we have two other editions (2012, 2021). This book was written for nurse educators who were beginning to embrace simulation pedagogy; the content provided direction and strategies on getting started with simulations, setting up early simulation centers, and overall, provided the NLN Jeffries framework which served as a model to guide the development, implementation, and evaluation of simulations. In 2015, working with many nurse researchers in INACSL and the NLN and nursing theorist, Dr. Beth Rodgers and nurse scientist Dr. Katie Haerling, the NLN Jeffries Simulation Framework was deemed to be a mid-range theory now called The NLN Jeffries Simulation Theory. A monograph was published in 2016 highlighting this theory, the components, and utilization of the important work.

In the early 2000s, the use of clinical simulation in nursing education was embryonic; many were just beginning to explore with few embracing the technology. Within 5 years, the notion of clinical simulations exploded, more schools of nursing were adopting the use of simulations although at times, faculty were not developed in knowing how to use simulations in their teaching, however, many of the schools' leaders were purchasing manikins for the educators, but not providing faculty development in this area. There was a great need at this time for more faculty development. Continuing to work with the NLN, a new project was created and this was to develop the Simulation Innovation Resource Center (SIRC) that served as a one-stop-shop for simulation information and provided a mechanism to build an online community with other educators who were asking questions and embarking on clinical simulations. In addition, I worked with several different authors to create online courses in faculty development in simulation so we had a convenient, accessible, cost-effective mechanism to develop faculty in using this pedagogy. The SIRC site still exists today and more courses have been added throughout the years.

In addition to providing faculty development opportunities to those educators who wanted to embrace the simulation pedagogy, the rise of simulations became more prevalent as more evidence was obtained and disseminated across the health professions. In 2014, I had the privilege along with Dr. Suzie Kardong-Edgren, to serve as a consultant on the national, landmark National Council of State Boards of Nursing (NCSBN) study. This study recruited leaders from ten, pre-licensure schools of nursing to invest if simulations worked—there were three arms of the study that included a control group, substitution of simulations at 25 and 50% across the curriculum. This landmark study provided strong evidence and robust results that substituting simulations for clinical hours did not affect the learner's knowledge, skills, or transition to practice therefore recommendations stated that simulations could be used up to 50% to substitute for clinical education in schools of nursing if best practices used in the study were implemented. The national study had policy implications across the 50 states and internationally; state boards of nursing heeded the evidence and began to make policy changes based on the evidence. In addition, a blue-ribbon panel of researchers, educators, and leaders from prominent nursing organizations met and wrote a paper on providing guiding principles when using the simulation pedagogy based on the study findings.

I always saw the use of clinical simulations as a "clinical redesign" in helping to improve nursing and other health professions education. The way we have been doing clinical education (the gold standard of sending students to clinical with one instructor taking care of one patient during the day) leaves many gaps when graduates transition to practice. I believed in "experiential learning" which the use of simulation pedagogy provides. Using simulations, the students actually get to "practice" his/her role they are preparing for, for example, the RN and the NP. Faculty members observing simulations provide direct feedback during debriefing when using this pedagogy. The student learns what he/she did right or wrong. A good faculty facilitator in debriefing will help the student to "connect the dots" from theory to practice. The value of simulations can't be underestimated! The evolution and quick adoption of simulations, I believe, is because of the value in our educational arena's faculty see when incorporating clinical simulations into the curriculum. Students want more simulations; they definitely learn from clinical simulations when done in a high-quality manner. We now have more evidence from the health professions providing "best practices" in using clinical simulation pedagogy and outcome data that demonstrate using simulations can make a difference in the knowledge and understanding of clinical practice. Of course, I am a believer of clinical simulations, an early pioneer, an early adopter, and will continue to support and disseminate the value of clinical simulations across health professions education.

The biggest barrier of using and incorporating clinical simulations into a nursing program/curriculum is the lack of faculty development. The simulation pedagogy requires training education on how to use this pedagogy, how to create simulations, implement, and debrief. During the past year in the pandemic, many nursing faculty/educators had to pivot quickly; even if they were not using simulations, one ended up using simulation, specifically virtual or screen-based simulations in order to provide instructional continuity at the school level so students could progress and graduate. Faculty development even became more important during this time since clinical simulations were the "go to" to provide the needed, required clinical education.

Were barriers broken down? I am not sure about that, but I do know faculty were immersed in using different teaching pedagogies they were not used to using whether it was online teaching or providing clinical education via virtual simulations. Other barriers pre-COVID and still existing today include the need for evidence and best practices. The evidence has emerged in these areas but more is still needed. There are many gaps in the use of simulations not only for pre-licensure students, but also for NPs and graduate clinical education. We have much more work to do to develop nursing and other health professions' faculty members to teach using simulation pedagogy, but we have grown tremendously in this area and looking ahead, the future looks very promising.

Pam Jeffries
Dean, Vanderbilt School of Nursing
Valere Potter Distinguished Professor of Nursing

Preface

I have been in simulation since 2004. I was fortunate to receive grant funding from the Gordon and Betty Moore Foundation to create the Bay Area Simulation Collaborative which eventually evolved into the California Simulation Alliance. The impact that simulation has had on nursing education and practice in California has been significant. We were well prepared for the pandemic in terms of moving to online learning using simulation. We are at a point now that we are advocating for regulatory changes at the Board of Nursing level.

Simulation has grown into a profession evidenced by the Society for Simulation in Healthcare's certification process, new jobs opening up, and employers taking notice of how important educated and experienced simulationists are to the growth of their programs and their return on investment. In the late 2000s, it was all about the technology, the manikin. Now, simulation encompasses a wide range of methodologies such as task trainers, role-play, standardized patients, computer-based, min/mid/high-fidelity simulators, and virtual reality. The evolution of simulation has been exciting to watch. With schools being the early adopters, hospitals followed suit and now, the next step is to build academic/service relationships to maximize the utilization of the equipment and space to train both students and staff together. I envision orientation times in hospitals to go down if students are able to learn in a simulated environment in the hospital before touching patients on the units. I envision more VR being used in both hospitals and schools.

There are many barriers to simulation, and I believe these are because administrators, staff, and faculty naysayers do not understand the value proposition for simulation. As simulationists, we need to continue to advocate for simulation at all levels in our organizations. We need to be able to articulate the value of simulation as it relates to patient safety. Simulation is here to stay; we cannot go back to old mental models of education!

KT Waxman
San Francisco, CA, USA

Nursing is a complex and specialized field of study with many nuances between specialties, areas of practice, and environments of care. Similarly, education, especially adult education, is equally complex. Creating rich learning opportunities that engage multigenerational learners with complex learning styles is a challenge that must be met every day by nurse educators in academia and clinical practice. Simulation-based education has emerged as a tool to bridge the gap between theory and practice often cited as a cause for poor outcomes, inefficient/unsafe care, high turnover of nursing staff, and an underprepared nursing workforce. The need for expertise and continuing professional development to correctly utilize simulation has never been greater. Simulation has taken a prolific role in replacing clinical sites as part of undergraduate nursing education programs, has filled gaps in the graduate nursing programs, and is utilized by nurse educators with clinical staff daily in hospitals across the globe. From resource-limited environments to top academic medical centers, simulation has a place to improve education, clinical practice, and the care provided to patients.

We have tried to take a practical approach in this textbook with many examples for specific educational environments and specialties. We want to provide a resource for nurse educators on how part-task trainers, high-technology full-body simulators, standardized patients, virtual reality, and distance simulation techniques can be used to help prepare the current and future generations of nurses.

This textbook opens with an introduction and foundational simulation concepts. It then branches into three core sections, focused on specific learner groups (undergraduate, graduate, and continuing professional development). It concludes with a section on operations and administration of simulation programs and a look into the future of simulation with examples of unique and forward-thinking simulation programs from other specialties.

We hope that you find this book filled with exemplars that you can use to broaden your understanding and use of simulation. We recognize that many nurse educators have spent years developing their specialized clinical (and educational) practice. Simulation is still novel to many in nursing education, and it is a wonderful tool to help break down silos, build comradery, and expand your mindset. We see this text as a nurse educators' handy reference when developing or collaborating on a program that may fall slightly out of their comfort zone.

Thank you to all our authors for sharing their expertise, their tireless effort in putting their knowledge onto paper, their patience, and their dedication to enhancing simulation education for nurses across the globe!

New York, NY, USA — Jared M. Kutzin
San Francisco, CA, USA — K.T. Waxman
Pleasanton, CA, USA — Connie M. Lopez
Moorabbin, VIC, Australia — Debra Kiegaldie

Contents

Part I

Fundamentals of Simulation in Nursing

1 History of Simulation in Nursing: An Overview

Elizabeth Horsley and Judy Bornais

Nurse educators have historically been extremely creative in their teaching methods. In fact, nurses of a certain age will remember injecting oranges to practice psychomotor skills. Others may remember practicing bed baths and positioning on classmates, and although we did not have the terminology at the time, those were forms of simulation. These creative approaches to teaching have given rise to simulation-based education. However, modern-day simulation education has evolved into a specialized discipline with its own established theories, frameworks, and best practices [1]. Nurse educators in academic and clinical practice have embraced the pedagogy, and as such, there has been an astounding trajectory of the integration of simulation-based education (SBE) into nursing curricula. Not only has simulation pedagogy evolved, but simulation technologies have also developed over the years. Ranging from full-body patient simulators to highly realistic task trainers to virtual reality experiences being integrated into curriculums. Simulation has grown to encompass professional designations, advanced education, and a robust body of scholarship.

Health professionals education has undergone radical changes in recent decades. Historically, medical education traditionally relied on an apprenticeship-type model where skills were learned from a combination of textbooks and observation and then practiced on patients [2]. The training was deemed satisfactory if the learner had "seen one, done one, and taught one" [3], or it was declared that a learner had accumulated enough time or exposure to a particular skill or specific type of case. This traditional approach to training and teaching was fairly well entrenched across health professions for decades and remained unchallenged. The rise of educational research into how learning happens and the most effective types of teaching strategies has debunked these traditional models. For example, teams at Northwestern University in Chicago researched medical residents' level of competence with a number of procedural skills and concluded that simply having accumulated hours of clinical experience did not correlate with technical competence in performing the skills [4]. A similar observation could be made about traditional nursing clinical practicums, in that total hours spent on a clinical unit -which has been lauded as the gold standard of practicum education—does not translate to competence [5]. These factors have made it necessary to explore innovative and alternative ways of teaching and training and have helped simulation-based education to emerge as an effective teaching strategy for both student learners and practicing health professionals.

Simulation is an experiential learning approach that can "… replace or amplify real experience along with guided experiences that evoke or replicate substantial aspects of the real world in a fully interactive manner" ([6]: i2). Well-constructed simulation activities allow a learner or teams of learners to participate in realistic situations, then reflect on the experience, whether at intermittent points during the scenario or at the end, through a guided debriefing. Simulation provides learners with the opportunity to experience the complexity of a clinical environment without the risk to patients or the possible hazards of an actual adverse patient event. A simulation activity that has been planned, developed, and implemented according to established best practice standards can facilitate the simultaneous evaluation of knowledge, clinical reasoning, and teamwork [7]. Simulation-based education is not restricted to undergraduate education or novice practitioners but can provide seasoned staff and clinicians with an opportunity to learn in a safe environment without the risk of harming patients or fear of judgment or punishment if they make mistakes [8].

E. Horsley (✉)
The Brooklyn Hospital Centre, New York, NY, USA

J. Bornais
Office of Experiential Learning, Faculty of Nursing, University of Windsor, Windsor, ON, Canada

Adjunct Faculty, Schulich School of Medicine & Dentistry, Western University, London, ON, Canada

J. M. Kutzin et al. (eds.), *Comprehensive Healthcare Simulation: Nursing*, Comprehensive Healthcare Simulation,
https://doi.org/10.1007/978-3-031-31090-4_1

This chapter begins with the evolution of simulation and the societal factors that made it possible for simulation to become an accepted teaching strategy within nursing and healthcare. We then outline the background and development of simulation equipment and technology as well as contextualize the development of simulation as a teaching strategy within nursing education and practice.

Establishing Simulation as a Teaching Strategy

It is important to explore the roots of simulation in order to fully understand and appreciate its trajectory in nursing education. Simulation in nursing education has drawn upon the experiences of the military, aviation, and other health professions, such as medicine and, more specifically, anesthesia, who were early adopters of simulation within healthcare. The earliest evidence of simulation models is the documented remains from antiquity which appears to be models of patients made from clay and stone [9]. It is presumed that these were used to illustrate features of the disease. These simulators would have been used by male physicians to diagnose women during a time when modesty rules precluded full exposure of the body [9]. An obstetrical trainer, “the phantom,” was made from a human pelvis and a deceased baby in eighteenth-century Paris and used to teach delivery techniques to obstetricians [10].

Some of the earliest recorded immersive simulations come in the form of war games [11, 12]. The game of chess, developed in the tenth century, represents a form of simulation whereby the game was played with the objective of testing out potential battle strategies [13]. In 1664, jousting, a recreational activity of medieval knights, allowed for the development of battlefield skills [12]. Simulation, as we know it, in the nursing field has more closely modeled itself on the initiatives of the aviation industry [14]. The aviation industry is arguably one of the most substantial adopters of simulation and an industry that sets the standards for both technical and team training. The earliest flight simulator can be attributed to Edwin Link, who built and patented the “Link Trainer” in 1929 [15]. The Link Trainer allowed for the simulation of poor weather conditions, and pilots were able to hone their skills in instrument flying. This trainer was slow to gain traction; however, in 1934, after numerous postal carriers were involved in fatal crashes in bad weather, the potential for Link Box training was realized [14]. All pilots were expected to engage in this simulated training as the value of simulation to prevent catastrophic events was realized [10]. Flight simulators gained popularity for many of the same reasons simulation in healthcare education gained popularity—it provided a safe, standardized environment for learners at various levels of expertise. Aviation, much like healthcare, is an arena where waiting to test and train in real situations would be too dangerous and cost prohibitive [12]. Much like aviation, early nursing simulation focused on the technical skills nurses need to learn, especially those which occurred infrequently but which were critical to patient outcomes.

While aviation training was initially focused on the technical skills of the pilot, World War II created a need for team training within the newer and larger aircraft. Simulation now had to include the pilot, the navigator, and the bomber. While each had tasks and responsibilities which required role-specific training, the crew also needed team training so they would have the best chance of being successful on their mission [11]. The shift now was for entire flight crews to become to be educated in team training. As such, aviation not only set the standard for the technical training of pilots but is often credited as the originator of Crew Resource Management (CRM), a team-based training program that was introduced in the 1980s in an effort to flatten the hierarchy among flight crews and enhance communication amongst members of the flight team. In an examination of airline disasters in the 1970s, it appeared that failures in communication were causal factors. It was hypothesized and hoped that training such as CRM could potentially alleviate the hesitation junior crew members felt in speaking to superiors [11].

The importance of simulation in communication and team training expanded beyond just aviation to health care education. A team from Stanford began to incorporate the aviation industry’s principles of crew resource management into anesthesia crisis resource management [13]. This type of training adapted CRM principles of teamwork and communication and was renamed Crisis Resource Management to focus on situations faced by anesthesia professionals, whether they happened in the operating room, intensive care unit, or emergency department. CRM has grown beyond just anesthesia to a method of team training focusing on communication patterns, crisis management, and giving all team members the confidence to assert themselves and speak up. CRM can be woven into a plethora of healthcare simulation activities ranging from cardiac arrest to trauma team training. Along this line, in 2005, the Agency for Healthcare Research and Quality collaborated with the U.S. Department of Defense (in the United States) to develop “Team Strategies and Tools to Enhance Performance and Patient Safety, more commonly known as TeamSTEPPS®. TeamSTEPPS® consists of a number of evidence-based teamwork tools geared towards optimizing patient outcomes through effective communication and teamwork skills among the healthcare team. Simulation has proven to be an ideal platform for team training to develop and solidify CRM and/or TeamSTEPPS® skills. Interestingly, the TeamSTEPPS® curriculum now has a designated section on how to incorporate simulation into this training.

The idea of using simulation, whether it be an orange or a link box, has a long history, but it was arguably the patient safety movement that brought simulation to the forefront. One of the pivotal moments which shifted so much of how healthcare professionals practice, and subsequently health professions education, was the release of the Institute of Medicine Report "To Err is Human" in 1999, which concluded that up to 98,000 deaths each year could be the result of a preventable error. These findings shocked and reverberated through healthcare and the health professions education communities. The landmark report by the Institute of Medicine around safety and quality in healthcare is still often referred to in the simulation literature as one of the drivers towards the proliferation of the use of simulation [16].

Simulators and Simulated Patients

While there is a lengthy history of using replications of anatomical structures for education, what we commonly think of as simulation started evolving in the early twentieth century [12]. Most notably, and arguably the most often referred to, early instance of using simulation in nursing education was recorded in 1911 with the life-sized doll known as "Mrs. Chase." Mrs. Chase was developed when the principal of the Harford Hospital (CT) Training School, Ms. Lauder Sutherland (a nursing graduate of the Toronto General Hospital), hypothesized that if students could practice skills on some type of doll, patients could be spared some discomfort [17]. In 1910, Ms. Sutherland contacted a doll maker, the M. J. Chase Company (named for real-life dollmaker Martha Jenkins Chase) of Pawtucket, Rhode Island, USA. The real "Mrs. Chase" and her husband Julian designed and crafted the first prototype [18]. By 1911, the first Mrs. Chase was ready to be put into service as the first patient for generations of nursing students to come as a means to teach and refine psychomotor skills, such as dressing and transferring. The prototype doll was tested at Memorial Hospital in Pawtucket. She had injection sites and was able to have numerous genito-urinary skills completed on her. Much like today, not every school could afford to acquire its own Mrs. Chase, so by 1914, do-it-yourself patterns were available from Columbia University. Over time, Mrs. Chase's appearance was refined, and her body functions upgraded. She remained a constant in many nursing programs until the early '80s [17, 19]. The incredibly and increasingly diverse range of realistic patient simulators we see today can trace their lineage back to the venerable Mrs. Chase.

Next to Mrs. Chase, one of the most well-recognized names in simulation is "Resusci Anne." Anne evolved from the imagination and skill of Asmund Laerdal, a Norwegian toy maker who was encouraged by a Norwegian anesthetist to develop a "doll" that could be used for teaching and practicing mouth-to-mouth resuscitation skills [20]. His creation was Resusci Anne, whose face was modeled after a young unidentified French girl who had drowned and was found floating in the River Seine in the 1890s. Anne was more than simply a doll, as she had a degree of physical fidelity in her neck that allowed for hyperextension in order for there to be adequate ventilation. Laerdal, acting on the recommendations from the medical community, also built a spring mechanism into the chest wall so that cardiac compressions could be simulated, and Anne became one of the first mass-produced manikins [20]. This unit gave rise to the subsequent iterations of full-body simulators that followed, and the Laerdal Company evolved into a major manufacturer of simulators and task trainers. Resusci-Anne continues to be used to teach basic cardiopulmonary resuscitation skills, albeit in a much more modernized and technologically enhanced form [21].

By the end of the 1960s more computer-driven, mechanical patient simulators, like we are familiar with today, were in the early design and development phases. Sim One was developed by Dr. Stephen Abrahamson, an engineer, and Dr. Judson Denson, a physician from the University of Southern California. The model, which began as a teaching tool for anesthesia, evolved into a simulated human form that had a full panel of vital signs and was able to respond physiologically to the treatments administered. The inventors saw the potential for a much safer way of training novice clinicians in skills, such as intubation, as opposed to the then-common method of allowing novices to practice on real patients. Although this looked like a potential breakthrough for medical education, it did not garner enough traction to gain widespread popularity. The unit was costly to produce and maintain, the apprenticeship model of medical education was still prevailing, and no one was actively looking for any radical changes in medical education [12].

In 1968 "Harvey," the cardiac assessment simulator developed by Dr. Michael Gordon at the University of Miami, was unveiled. Clinicians could assess Harvey (named for Dr. Gordon's mentor at Georgetown University, Dr. W. Proctor Harvey) by auscultation and palpation of some pulse points, and he was able to replicate a wide variety of cardiac conditions. Harvey underwent rigorous testing and vetting for educational efficacy [20]. He continues to thrive and have an enduring presence and popularity in the simulation community because of his ability to help learners develop their cardiac assessment skills and knowledge of cardiac abnormalities.

The concept of full-body simulators came to the forefront again in the 1980s. Two separate groups, one at the University of Florida led by Dr. Michael Good, Dr. J. S. Gravenstein, and Dr. Samsun Lampotang, and the other at Stanford University led by Dr. David Gaba, experimented and produced prototypes of the full body simulators we are familiar with today. Medical Education Technologies Inc. (METI, now CAE) and MedSim, respectively [20]. From these developments emerged the movement in the 2000s of units that solely represented the airway and/or allowed for cardiac arrest practice to life-like humans replicating pediatrics, geriatric, maternal, and other conditions. This allowed for a broad application among healthcare professions. Manufacturers also expanded their offerings to support simulation-based education beyond simply producing manikins and task trainers. METI produced ready-made curricula to be used alongside their patient simulators. Similarly, Laerdal developed its own scenario packages, ready for full integration with their manikins.

Simulation as a Teaching Strategy Within Nursing Education and Practice

Describing the full history of nursing practice and education is beyond the scope of this chapter, but we will provide a brief overview to contextualize how simulations use was developed. Early nursing practice in North America has its roots in religious orders. Of note, the first hospital in North America, the Hotel Dieu in Montreal, was opened by Sister Jeanne Mance in 1645 [22]. Prior to the evolution of formal institutions to care for the ill or infirm, families assumed responsibility for their own. Following the Civil War in the United States (1861–1865) and the rise of industrialization in the US, public institutions began to open and provide care. Hospitals thus evolved, but they fell prey to the societal problems of the times and were often unsanitary, overcrowded, and a source of outbreaks [23].

Florence Nightingale, who is by and large most credited with the origination of what we know as nursing today, heralded a new age of nursing care in a secular age. She established the first nursing school, St. Thomas, in London in 1860. The three overarching objectives of the school were: to train matrons who could organize and train future nurses; train nurses who could supervise and educate in indigent care in the community. The school's objectives were to train matrons in both the theoretical and practical (hands-on) content of nursing; train them to organize and train future nurses and educate them in indigent care in the community. Nightingale's apprenticeship training model solidified nursing as a respectable occupation for women. Before this model was implemented, hospital care was carried out by a range of available ward attendants—"male and female, religious and lay, paid and unpaid, skilled and unskilled" caregivers ([22]: 74). Following the Nightingale Model, the first nursing school in the US, the Bellevue Hospital School of Nursing in New York City, and the first nursing school in Canada, the Mack School of Nursing in St. Catharines, Ontario, were opened in 1873 and 1874, respectively.

As hospital and scientific medicine advanced in the late 1800s, hospital care became focused on treatment and therapy ([22]: 74). Over this time, the practice of nursing and the requisite education began to take shape. Apprenticeship training became popular as a way to elevate the status of nursing and attract middle-class paying patients as trained nurses boosted the status of a hospital. This model provided the necessary knowledge, skills, and attitudes to care for the ill, indigent, and infirmed with a central focus on mastering technical skills and became the primary method of training nurses for nearly a century. Over time, this evolved into a more concerted effort to integrate theoretical and clinical knowledge, incorporating the scientific and humanistic basis for practice as nursing education was incorporated into universities and community colleges. As the twentieth century progressed, there was a gradual incorporation of sciences with defined competencies in the cognitive, psychomotor, and affective domains.

In order to help nurses develop their psychomotor skills, nursing labs started to emerge with the first iterations of a simulation lab in a school of nursing in the 1930s. The Indiana University Training School for Nurses was described as having manikins for the purpose of teaching students to give injections [8]. By the 1960s, like other forms of professional education, nursing was demanding higher standards of preparation in order to practice. Nurses need to be prepared for more complex and diverse roles. There was a proliferation of specialized intensive care units, while at the same time, the intensity of care required on a general duty unit increased. Nursing roles were expanding into the community, and advanced practice roles for nurses, such as Certified Registered Nurse Anesthetists (CRNAs), Nurse Practitioners (NPs), and Clinical Nurse Specialists (CNS), were expanding. In order to provide the necessary skills training for their learners, nursing programs across the continent began the process of designing and outfitting their own versions of a skills practice lab or learning resource centers.

In the earliest days of the adoption of simulation in nursing programs, the commonly referred to reasons for its implementation was the lack of clinical placement sites and the changing demographics of patients in hospitals. Hospital stays were becoming increasingly shorter and the patients were more acute and complex. These factors made it imperative to explore innovative and alternative ways of teaching and training. "With increasing numbers of nursing students and decreasing numbers of available clinical sites and nursing faculty, the use of simulation has become an integral part of nursing education" ([24]: 528). The traditional ideas around clinical practicums were that with sufficient hours in a clinical placement, regardless of whether a student was actively engaged or was merely observing, it was reasonable to assume the student somehow gained the knowledge and skill necessary to progress. The reality, however, is that students are often at the mercy of patient census and random happenstance. There really is no way for any clinical instructor to standardize the experiences of a clinical group. Literature began to explore the student clinical experience, and a thorough examination of the clinical day revealed students had significant amounts of downtime and were often "looking for something to do" [24].

As simulation was becoming more and more commonplace in nursing education, nursing leaders in the United States, in 2008, began to entertain the idea of simulation being a reasonable replacement for clinical time. To contextualize the societal changes that were influencing this decision, it is important to note that in 1995 the first National Conference on Nursing Skills Labs occurred to help educators share ideas and research findings on how best to engage and teach nursing skills. By 1999–2000 a group of nursing educators "identified the need for a professional organization to meet the growing needs of nurse educators using simulation" [25]. In 2002 the INACSL (International Association for Clinical Simulation and Learning) organization was founded, which examined simulation research and advocating of simulation evidence and best practice. In 2011 INACSL published the first edition of the Standards of Best Practice in simulation. The most recent iteration of these standards renamed the Healthcare Simulation Standards of Best Practice™, was published in 2021. This rebranding reflects an effort to broader the applicability of these standards beyond just nursing.

In 2014 simulation in undergraduate nursing education was advanced with the landmark 2014 NCSBN (National Council of State Boards of Nursing) multi-site study, which concluded that up to 50% of the clinical time could be substituted with high-quality simulation activities [26]. With a robust simulation program in place, a clinical educator could make deliberate and meaningful choices for educational experiences for students, as opposed to the uncertainty and lack of standardization of the clinical placement. By 2015, using the data gathered from the NCSBN study as well as previous simulation research studies, an expert panel convened by NCSBN used the simulation data along with the International Nursing Association for Clinical and Simulation and Learning (INACSL) Standards of Best Practice: Simulation℠ to develop simulation guidelines for nursing programs [27]. Today, many state boards of nursing and state legislatures in the United States have started to explore adopting specific standards and requirements to allow nursing schools to replace clinical hours with simulation. The early work by INACSL and the Society for Simulation in Healthcare (SSH) has provided the foundation for this evolution in nursing education.

Simulation Modalities

Well into the third decade of the 2000s, simulation for nursing education came in a variety of formats. For many nurse educators in the early 2000s, training was provided by the manufacturers, and many believed that higher levels of technology made for a better learning experience. While many of the current simulation tools have become sophisticated and incorporate technology, it is important to recognize that technology is not needed for a simulation to be effective. As simulation has developed, so too has our understanding of what makes for a quality simulation-based educational experience. A study by Levett-Jones et al. [28] suggests that students highly value simulation regardless of the level of sophistication and fidelity, suggesting that expensive simulation equipment is not required to achieve the learning benefits that occur from the immersive education design.

In light of that, it is still important to discuss the various iterations of patient simulators. Mrs. Chase, the life-sized model discussed earlier, is an example of a low-fidelity basic simulator. In addition to life-sized static manikins, simulators include part(ial) task trainers—plastic or gelatinous models of body parts or manikins which allow learners to focus on developing specific psychomotor skills such as urinary catheterization or central line care. Other examples of low-technology simulators include simulated wound sites and homemade trainers. Low-technology simulators, which tend to be less complex than their mid- and high-technology counterparts, are ideal for use when the objective is to learn and develop competency in a specific psychomotor skill. But, this category of simulation tool can be used for much more than just repetitive practice and skill development; it all depends on how they are utilized. As an example, when detailed patient information and different participant roles are integrated along with low-technology simulators into a simulated learning scenario, the development of critical thinking and integration of theory with practice can occur.

Medium-Fidelity Simulators

Medium-fidelity simulators offer a higher level of interactivity with the learner and are more realistic than their low-technology counterparts. Often these simulators have some programming capabilities and can respond to learners' actions but are limited in their physiological responses and verbal noises [29]. Examples of medium-fidelity simulators include CAE JUNO Nursing Skills Manikin and Laerdal's Megacode Kelly™ with VitalSim capability. Medium-Fidelity manikins, like their high-fidelity counterparts, are often integrated into full-scale simulations with props, make-up, and replicated environments to create a level of realism that allows learners to integrate their assessment, psychomotor, and critical thinking skills to make clinical judgments and see the outcome of their decisions.

High-Fidelity Simulators

High-fidelity human simulators were introduced in the 1980s. The two early models were the CASE (Comprehensive

Anesthesia Simulation Environment) 1.2 model and the Gainesville Anesthesia Simulator (GAS), which were developed primarily for anesthesia training [20]. These early models have since evolved into sophisticated full-body computerized high-fidelity simulators that "have the ability to mimic, at a very high level, human body functions" ([30]: 14). With embedded software, current models may be programmed to allow the learner to experience different clinical presentations, and simulationists can control the manikin's response to the learners' actions and their clinical decisions. These full-body computerized simulators typically come equipped with a functioning mouth and airway that allow for intubation and ventilation. They contain a chest wall that expands and relaxes with respirations and which can be programmed with various lung sounds. In addition, these sophisticated mannikins also contain programmable heart and bowel sounds that can be auscultated using a stethoscope just as they would on a real patient. Included with these mannikins is the ability to project real-time displays of an electrocardiogram, arterial pressures, pulse oximetry, temperature, and the respiratory cycle. Designed with physiological modeling, these manikins are capable of realistic verbal and physiological responses. Typical features also include the ability for endotracheal tube insertion, bilateral chest tube insertion, intravenous lines which allow for running IV and "blood" flashback, and urinary catheters which, when inserted, can drain yellow fluid, simulating "urine". As a result of their realistic features, these manikins are often most useful in full-scale, also referred to as full-mission, simulations. Full mission simulation requires a realistic environment and the use of actual medical supplies and equipment [31]. When the focus is on obtaining a health history, incorporating psychomotor skills and clinical judgment and decision-making, along with providing effective communication, the human-patient simulator is a great option.

Simulated Patients and Simulated Participants

An SP, also known as a simulated or standardized patient, the two terms are used interchangeably, is an individual who is "trained to portray a patient in realistic and repeatable ways" ([32]: 2). The use of SPs dates back to 1963 when neurologist and medical educator Howard Burrows created the first documented simulated patient who provided the same symptoms to allow clerkship students to practice and receive feedback. Despite the widespread use of SPs in medical education [33], it took until the early 2000s for SPs to be noted in the nursing literature [34]. The majority of the literature reporting the use of SPs is with graduate or post-degree nursing programs such as NP programs [35] though more recent studies have incorporated SPs to facilitate effective communication skills by nursing students [36] and have shown that SPs can improve health assessment skills among first-year nursing students [34]. SPs have not only been used to portray a patient, but they have also been used as family members in hybrid simulations. Because of this increased role of SPs, the terminology has also evolved, and the term "simulated participant" is now more commonly used. The more inclusive term, simulated participant, refers to all human role players involved in any simulation context [32]. An ideal time to incorporate simulated participants into a simulation is when the learning objective is focused on communication, developing health history-taking skills, or health teaching. Using simulated participants as the simulation modality allows for face-to-face human interactions with both verbal and nonverbal cues, facial expressions, and emotions.

Computer-Based and Virtual Reality Simulation

Screen-based simulations have evolved significantly over the last 10 years. From programs in the early 2000s that allowed participants to observe blood flow and listen to heart sounds based on where the computer-based stethoscope was placed to highly interactive immersive simulation environments whereby learners use avatars to make clinical decisions and see the outcomes of their decisions, the use of computer-based simulation continues to evolve in nursing education [37]. Computer simulation games, as well as three-dimensional projections, whereby learners can manipulate images that appear suspended before them, are helping to provide safe environments for learners. Virtual reality (VR) simulations have also progressed in the last two decades, with social network platforms providing opportunities for students and nursing faculty to interface to create safe learning experiences [38]. In addition, technology has advanced to allow for haptic feedback whereby the learner receives feedback not only on the clinical decisions they made but on the technique they used. The virtual reality IV simulator is an example commonly used for nursing students to develop their phlebotomy skills, whereby the student can palpate and "feel" for a vein prior to inserting the IV cannula into a touchpad. The virtual reality program incorporates input from the touchpad and registers the depth of the needle as well as the angle and insertion technique. Haptic systems are ideal for use when the learning goal is to develop a specific skill where feedback is helpful or to evaluate specific skills with real-time tracking of the learner's performance [31].

Augmented reality (AR) or mixed reality (MR), on the other hand, involves a blending of interactive digital-based elements, sometimes through specialized viewing headgear or digital apps, with aspects of the real world. In simulations where the learning objective is to help students understand the interconnectedness of the human body, use of a

Hololens, a headworn AR device, allows students to display, enlarge, rotate, and manipulate anatomy within a manikin. This is far more effective in meeting the desired outcome than plastic models. VR/AR/MR, collectively known as Extended Reality (XR) is only beginning to see its place in nursing education, and its use will increase in the future as clinical placements continue to become more limited.

Simulation has a long and storied history, even though many may not be familiar with how it has been translated from the military and aviation into healthcare and from straw-stuffed dolls to highly complex computer and virtual reality simulators. The advent of simulation in nursing education (both academic and clinical) has led to an enhanced ability to educate and assess learners and improve the systems of care provided to patients by nurses globally. The future of simulation in nursing education is endless.

References

1. Bell R, Friedland N. The use of theoretical frameworks guiding interprofessional simulation: an integrative review. Nurs Educ Perspect. 2020;41(3):141–5.
2. Pietersen PI, Laursen CB, Petersen RH, Konge L. Structured and evidence-based training of technical skills in respiratory medicine and thoracic surgery. J Thorac Dis. 2021;13(3):2058–67.
3. Albert BD, Burns JP. Is "See one, do one, teach one" still relevant in the 21st century? Pediatr Crit Care Med. 2018;19(7):678–9.
4. Barsuk JH, Cohen ER, Feinglass J, McGaghie WC, Wayne DB. Residents' procedural experience does not ensure competence: a research synthesis. J Grad Med Educ. 2017;9(2):201–8.
5. Leighton K, Kardong-Edgren S, McNelis AM, Foisy-Doll C, Sullo E. Traditional clinical outcomes in prelicensure nursing education: an empty systematic review. J Nurs Educ. 2021;60(3):136–42.
6. Gaba DM. The future vision of simulation in health care. BMJ Qual Saf. 2004;13(suppl 1):i2–i10.
7. Hall AK, Pickett W, Dagnone JD. Development and evaluation of a simulation-based resuscitation scenario assessment tool for emergency medicine residents. Can J Emerg Med. 2012;14(3):139–46.
8. Sanko JS. Simulation as a teaching technology. Q Rev Distance Educ. 2017;18(2):77–85.
9. Saud Alshafi N, Alduais W. History of simulation. In: Alaraj A, editor. Comprehensive healthcare simulation: neurosurgery. Springer International Publishing; 2018.
10. Jones F, Passos-Neto CE, Braghiroli OF. Simulation in medical education: brief history and methodology. Prin Pract Clin Res. 2015;1(2):56–63.
11. Aebersold M. The history of simulation and its impact on the future. AACN Adv Crit Care. 2016;27(1):56–61.
12. Bradley P. The history of simulation in medical education and possible future directions. Med Educ. 2006;40(3):254–62.
13. Rosen KR. The history of medical simulation. J Crit Care. 2008;23(2):157–66.
14. Singh H, Kalani M, Acosta-Torres S, El Ahmadieh TY, Loya J, Ganju A. History of simulation in medicine: from Resusci Annie to the Ann Myers Medical Center. Neurosurgery. 2013;73(suppl_1):S9–S14.
15. Scherer YK, Bruce SA, Graves BT, Erdley WS. Acute care nurse practitioner education: enhancing performance through the use of clinical simulation. AACN Adv Crit Care. 2003;14(3):331–41.
16. Phrampus PE. A historical perspective of simulation in emergency medicine. In: Comprehensive healthcare simulation: emergency medicine. Cham: Springer; 2021. p. 3–11.
17. Herrmann EK. Mrs. Chase: a noble and enduring figure. Am J Nurs. 1981;81(10):1836.
18. Grypma S. Regarding Mrs. Chase. J Chris Nurs. 2012;29(3):181.
19. Nehring WM, Lashley FR. Nursing simulation: a review of the past 40 years. Simul Gaming. 2009;40(4):528–52.
20. Cooper JB, Taqueti V. A brief history of the development of mannequin simulators for clinical education and training. Postgrad Med J. 2008;84(997):563–70.
21. Schiavenato M. Reevaluating simulation in nursing education: beyond the human patient simulator. J Nurs Educ. 2009;48(7):388–94.
22. McPherson K The Nightingale's influence and the rise of the modern hospital. In: On all frontiers: four centuries of Canadian nursing. 2005. p. 73–88.
23. Baer ED. Key ideas in nursing's first century. Am J Nurs. 2012;112(5):48–55.
24. Ironside PM, McNelis AM, Ebright P. Clinical education in nursing: rethinking learning in practice settings. Nurs Outlook. 2014;62(3):185–91.
25. https://www.inacsl.org/index.php?option=com_content&view=article&id=101:healthcare-simulation-standards-history&catid=20:site-content
26. Hayden J. Use of simulation in nursing education: national survey results. J Nurs Regul. 2010;1(3):52–7.
27. Alexander M, Durham CF, Hooper JI, Jeffries PR, Goldman N, Kesten KS, Spector N, Tagliareni E, Radtke B, Tillman C. NCSBN simulation guidelines for prelicensure nursing programs. J Nurs Regul. 2015;6(3):39–42.
28. Levett-Jones T, McCoy M, Lapkin S, Noble D, Hoffman K, Dempsey J, Arthur C, Roche J. The development and psychometric testing of the satisfaction with simulation experience scale. Nurse Educ Today. 2011;31(7):705–10.
29. Lapkin S, Levett-Jones T. A cost–utility analysis of medium vs. high-fidelity human patient simulation manikins in nursing education. J Clin Nurs. 2011;20(23–24):3543–52.
30. Lopreiato, J. O., Downing, D., Gammon, W., Lioce, L., Sittner, B., Slot, V., Spain, A. E., and the Terminology & Concepts Working Group. (2016). Healthcare Simulation DictionaryTM. Retrieved from http://www.ssih.org/dictionary
31. Decker S, Sportsman S, Puetz L, Billings L. The evolution of simulation and its contribution to competency. J Contin Educ Nurs. 2008;39(2):74–80.
32. Lewis KL, Bohnert CA, Gammon WL, Hölzer H, Lyman L, Smith C, Thompson TM, Wallace A, Gliva-McConvey G. The association of standardized patient educators (ASPE) standards of best practice (SOBP). Adv Simul. 2017;2(1):1–8.
33. Williams RG. Have standardized patient examinations stood the test of time and experience? Teach Learn Med. 2004;16(2):215–22.
34. Bornais JA, Raiger JE, Krahn RE, El-Masri MM. Evaluating undergraduate nursing students' learning using standardized patients. J Prof Nurs. 2012;28(5):291–6.
35. Gibbons SW, Adamo G, Padden D, Ricciardi R, Graziano M, Levine E, Hawkins R. Clinical evaluation in advanced practice nursing education: Using standardized patients in health assessment. J Nurs Educ. 2002;41(5):215–21. Retrieved from http://www.journalofnursingeducation.com/
36. Yoo MS, Yoo IY. The effectiveness of standardized patients as a teaching method for nursing fundamentals. J Nurs Educ. 2003;42(10):444–8. Retrieved from http://www.journalofnursingeducation.com/
37. Waxman KT, Bowler F, Forneris SG, Kardong-Edgren S, Rizzolo MA. Simulation as a nursing education disrupter. Nurs Adm Q. 2019;43(4):300–5.
38. Campbell SH, Daley K, editors. Simulation scenarios for nursing educators: making it real. Springer Publishing Company. 2017.

Simulation Modalities

2

Jaclyn Conelius, Nancy Spear Owen, and Susan Reynolds

Introduction

This chapter will discuss definitions and types of modalities for simulations. It will also give some helpful tips regarding each of the modalities as well as examples for use in a nursing undergraduate or graduate curriculum. However, the learning objectives and resources will always drive the choice of simulation modality.

Modality: Manikin-Based Simulation

Definition: Manikins are full-body simulators used to educate students and healthcare professionals by simulating the structure and function of the human body (ssh.org). They can be found in sizes and simulated ages that extend across the lifespan.

Scope: There is a wide range of complexity to manikins with varying levels of fidelity and physiologic function. General guidelines are described below, but please read the manufacturer's instructions for details of available functions on specific manikins.

Low-fidelity manikins have the basic structure of a human body without internal electronics to mimic sounds such as voice or lung, heart, and bowel sounds. They are relatively inexpensive, tolerant of water, and can be good choices for learning and practicing nursing procedural skills such as enema administration, nasogastric tube insertion, and tracheal suctioning. A low-fidelity manikin gives students the ability to integrate patient safety skills like patient identification using a wristband with the procedural skill they are practicing.

Mid-fidelity manikins have internal electronics. They typically have assorted heart, lung, and bowel sounds which can be programmed for students to practice identification and treatment. Further options across this modality often include static pupil variation, chest rise, and voice options. Scenario programming is also usually available.

High-fidelity human patient simulators can simulate more complex scenarios. These manikins typically have the abilities of a well-equipped mid-fidelity manikin with chest rise, voice, and body sound, plus additional functions such as adjustable pulse strength, airway compliance, and seizures. More dynamic changes intra-scenario are often possible such as pupillary changes and the use of radio frequency identification (RFID) technology to elicit physiologic responses to medications. Due to internal electronics, the installation of fluids may be more limited. Some high-fidelity models fit a certain professional specialty, such as trauma or midwifery, which give the opportunity for even more specialized functions.

Tips: When designing simulation experiences, developing objectives early in the process is key to ensuring a proper educational program and selecting the right simulation modality. The facilities and resources that are available will also dictate the simulation modality that can be used. Most nursing programs have a need for variety in their fleet of manikins. When using mid and high-fidelity manikins, users have the choice of running scenarios on the fly or pre-programming them to run in automatic mode. Examples of manikin-based simulations for undergraduate and graduate nursing students are presented in Table 2.1.

Modality-Task Trainer/Partial Task Trainer

Definition: Task trainers or partial task trainers are the choice when the goal of the simulation is to focus on a psychomotor skill in isolation. They allow learners to repetitively practice one specific task, which develops muscle memory and ultimately competency. Part-task trainers do not usually incorporate patient feedback. Instead, they offers

J. Conelius · S. Reynolds
Fairfield University, Fairfield, CT, USA

N. S. Owen (✉)
Columbia University School of Nursing, New York, NY, USA
e-mail: nso2108@cumc.columbia.edu

J. M. Kutzin et al. (eds.), *Comprehensive Healthcare Simulation: Nursing*, Comprehensive Healthcare Simulation,
https://doi.org/10.1007/978-3-031-31090-4_2

Table 2.1 Examples of use of manikin-based simulations in undergraduate and graduate nursing

	Undergraduate nursing students	Graduate nursing students
Human patient simulators	Use when simulation objectives entail high-risk procedures or when accurate assessment findings are critical to meeting them	
Low fidelity	Practice labs to learn how to change the linens of an occupied bed A scenario in a nursing skills lab entails placing an indwelling urinary catheter or nasogastric tube	Practice CPR skills
Mid fidelity	A scenario that requires a student to identify adventitious breath sounds and provide appropriate interventions	A scenario that involves a primary care or neonatal nurse practitioner student identifying a murmur in a neonate
High fidelity	A scenario that involves a student identifying that their patient is having a seizure and intervening appropriately	A scenario that involves a midwifery student attending the birth of an infant complicated by shoulder dystocia A scenario that involves a CRNA student managing an airway during surgery A scenario that involves an acute care practitioner caring for a critical care patient with ARDS

faculty a way to provide immediate directive feedback and to verify skill competency prior to performing on a real person.

Scope: Some examples of skills in which partial task trainers can be used are venipuncture of the arms, ultrasound-compatible central line trainers, pelvic exam trainers, and prostate exam trainers.

Tips: Task trainers allow for focused, repetitive skills practice and consistency in experiences among learners. Some aspects of task trainers that may be a barrier are the time required to train faculty to use the trainers, the cost of the trainers themselves, space for implementing them into a simulation program, and upkeep and storage of equipment.

Modality: Role Play

Definition: Role Play is a simulation modality that capitalizes on the importance of the social context of learning. It is the interaction of two or more players to simulate communication [1].

Table 2.2 Examples of use of role play simulations in undergraduate and graduate nursing

	Undergraduate students	Graduate students
Role play	These examples can be adjusted for all types of students	
	During a health assessment lab, give student partners symptoms to verbalize during the exam	During an advanced health assessment lab, give student partners symptoms to verbalize during the exam
	Practice conflict management skills	In a leadership class, practice interviewing skills
	Practice SBAR communication	With a scripted role-play, demonstrate good and inadequate practices around the use of interpreters

Scope: Role play can be used in a variety of scenarios. Students can role-play a patient, the nurse, or another scenario role. The level of the script can vary from fully scripted, partially scripted, and unscripted [1]. In an unscripted patient/ nurse role play, the nurse can be provided a task that they need to accomplish while the patient is provided a character and emotional context to the situation at hand.

Tips: Students who play the role of a patient can often gain invaluable empathy for the vulnerable position that their patients occupy. When the objective of the exercise is to build effective communication techniques, role-play simulation experiences are experiential activities that can have a positive starting point for student learning. Examples of role-play simulations for undergraduate and graduate nursing students are presented in Table 2.2.

Modality: Unfolding Case

Definition: An unfolding case is a patient experience that evolves over time. The experiences involve one patient or a family unit. Changes in the patient's condition develop with each encounter (NLN.org).

Scope: Unfolding cases are useful for all levels of students. The timing of the unfolding case can vary from one class period to an entire semester to an entire program. They can simulate a patient across one admission, one life event, a lifetime, or anything in between. Unfolding cases span two or more encounters with the patient but have no other limiting conditions.

Tips: Unfolding cases can help students build relationships with their patients over time and offer students the opportunity to practice transfers of care across providers. Examples of unfolding case simulations for undergraduate and graduate nursing students are presented in Table 2.3.

Table 2.3 Examples of use of unfolding case simulations in undergraduate and graduate nursing

	Undergraduate students	Graduate students
Unfolding case		
	Students care for a patient across admission, surgical procedure, post-op management, and discharge Students care for elderly patients at home with complications that arise in each visit, such as wounds, memory loss, and depression	Primary care FNP students care for a patient through healthy yearly visits, diagnosis of chronic illness, and end-of-life situations Midwifery students care for patients through well-woman visits, 9 months of prenatal visits, labor and birth, and postpartum care CRNA students care for patients during pre-operative consent, operative anesthesia, and post-op complications or pain control

Modality: Standardized or Simulated Patients (SPs)

Definition: The terminology involved with standardized or simulated patients can be confusing. Both terms are referred to as SPs and refer to a person specially trained to play the role of a *patient* in a simulation. If a person is in the role of someone other than a patient, such as a family member or healthcare worker, they are referred to as a standardized or simulated *participant*. The Healthcare Simulation Dictionary, Ed 2.1, defines a *standardized patient* as "an individual who is trained to portray a real patient to simulate a set of symptoms or problems used for healthcare education, evaluation, and research ([2]: 49). Other terms used to refer to SPs are actor, simulated person, or role player, but should be avoided as they fail to capture important components of the role. SPs in any role interact with learners to facilitate learning objectives. They are coached by a standardized patient educator (SPE) to perform in the same way for each new learner, which is the reason for the term *standardized*. SPs may provide learners with feedback on their interactions which is a unique feature of this modality.

Standardized refers to the ability to bring conformity with a standard and repeat in a consistent way. The term *standardized patient* is used when every learner needs to experience the same patient interaction, such as with competency testing or objective structured clinical exams/encounters (OSCE). *Simulated* refers to making something appear genuine or real. The term *simulated patient* can have more variability in the portrayal of the patient and is a term used for formative assessments. Although standardized and simulated are often used interchangeably, it is crucial to distinguish the purpose of the SP role to match learner assessments during the design phase of a scenario. The Human Simulation Continuum Model developed by Gliva-McConvey et al. describes how the degree of SP standardization ranges from low to high in six different applications. The six applications of SPs from low standardization to high standardization are role player, structured role player, embedded participant, simulated patient, standardized patient, and standardized patient for high stakes assessment (HSA) ([3]: 32).

Scope: Standardized patient programs have been developed around the world. SPs are used across a continuum of less structured simulations, such as role play to strict standardization for high-stakes exams [3]. SPs have historically been used for teaching and learning the following: health assessment and physical examinations; communication skills; emergency preparedness and disaster drills; and culture and diversity. Most recently, the standardized patient methodology has expanded use to distance learning with telepresence web conferencing software. Ballman and colleagues reported that using standardized patients in distance learning in graduate nurse practitioner programs facilitates confidence, clinical reasoning, and problem-solving skills.

Preparing students with SP simulation before attending mental health clinical helps to ease anxiety and build confidence. Standardized patients have also been brought into the classroom to work through an unfolding case study with larger groups of students. Therapeutic communication between patient and nurse, as well as professional communication between a nurse and other healthcare providers, are effective uses of standardized patients.

SPs are often used for an objective structured clinical exam/encounter (OSCE) which is "a station or series of stations designed to assess performance competency in individual clinical or other professional skills". Learners are evaluated via direct observation, checklists, learner presentations, or written follow-up exercises. The examinations may be formative and offer feedback or summative and be used for making high-stakes educational decisions ([2]: 34).

A specialized group of standardized patients used for NP programs are male urogenital teaching associates (MUTA) and gynecological or genitourinary teaching associates (GTA). A MUTA is a male and a GTA is a female, "specifically trained to teach, assess, and provide feedback to learners about accurate urogenital and rectal examination techniques" ([2]: 20). MUTA's and GTA's also "address the communication skills needed to provide a comfortable exam in a standardized manner, while using their bodies as teaching tools in a supportive, non-threatening environment (ASPE)" ([2]: 20).

Tips: The Association of Standardized Patient Educators (ASPE) is a global interprofessional organization that provides ASPE Standards of Best Practice, resources, mentoring, a case development template, and professional development [2]. If a simulation program is new to the use of SPs, it may help to start small with only one or two simulations and to find a mentor through ASPE. The expansion of remote simulations offers an opportunity to build diversity in SP programs. Many programs hire SPs through a staffing agency, and this may help eliminate onboarding and staff costs, especially as the cost of SPs varies considerably, based on experience and location. When developing a new SP program, the *Comprehensive Healthcare Simulation: Implementing Best Practices in Standardized Patient Methodology*, 2019, book would provide additional valuable resources. Examples of standardized patient simulations for undergraduate and graduate nursing students are presented in Table 2.4.

Table 2.4 Examples for use of standardized patient simulations in undergraduate and graduate nursing

	Undergraduate students	Graduate students
Standardized patients		
	Students care for homebound patients following hospital discharge to address safety during transitions in care Competency checkout for medication administration, including patient education Mental health issues include hearing voices, substance use disorders De-escalation Students practice communication techniques for handoffs and situation-background-assessment-recommendation (SBAR) reports SP plays the role of a family member in pediatric simulation	Objective structured clinical exams (OSCE) Primary care FNP students in telehealth conduct remote patient monitoring to assess EKG, vital signs, and cardiac output for management of cardiovascular disease Acute care NP assessment of chest pain in ER setting Oncology sub-specialty practices difficult conversation of starting a chemotherapy regime Psych mental health NP suicidal ideation screening and plan of care CRNA students conduct a pre-operative physical assessment with a health history for co-morbidities

Modality: Virtual Reality

Definition: Virtual reality simulation "use a variety of immersive, highly visual, 3D characteristics to replicate real-life situations and /or health care procedures; virtual reality is distinguished from computer-based simulation in that it generally incorporates physical or other interfaces such as a computer keyboard, mouse, speech and voice recognition, motion sensors, or haptic devices" ([2]: 41).

Additional terms to include when choosing immersive technologies and virtual reality are headgear and haptics. Headgear can also be referred to as a head-mounted device, HMD, or headset. Haptics refers to "devices that provide tactile feedback to the user. Haptics can simulate touching, palpating an organ, or body part, and the cutting, tearing, or traction on a tissue" ([2]: 15).

Scope: The newer simulation modality that is expanding in use for both undergraduate and graduate nursing students is immersive VR. Immersive virtual reality modality follows a continuum of low to high immersion and includes a growing number of different types of VR. Immersion "describes the level to which the learner becomes involved in the simulation; a high degree of immersion indicates that the learner is treating the simulation as if it was a real-life (or close to real-life) event" ([2]: 17). A form of virtual reality that is less immersive but highly interactive is computer-generated environments involving a screen-based, three-dimensional program, a computer mouse, keyboard, or joystick. There is less sensory involvement than in other forms of VR, but it can be highly interactive as students play in the first person. In these virtual reality games, students can participate in clinical situations as an avatar to assess clinical situations, make clinical decisions, and practice skills. Some VR games offer learners a single patient or a multi-patient scenario to develop prioritization skills and clinical judgement. Other technologies are live muti player VR games which allow development of teamwork, interdisciplinary collaboration, communication skills, and real-time instructor feedback.

Tips: Virtual reality is an area that is rapidly changing as the technology develops. This modality is being used in healthcare to improve patient outcomes, such as decreasing pain and improving relaxation. VR in nursing education has been found to improve learners in cognitive, psychomotor, and affective domains but additional research is needed to determine best practices [4]. Head-mounted device or display (HMD) is used for viewing images for viewing and comes in many styles with different qualities and price ranges. HMDs can be as simple as a Google cardboard or a low-cost plastic device to a highly sophisticated and more expensive one. Examples of virtual reality simulations for undergraduate and graduate nursing students are presented in Table 2.5.

Table 2.5 Examples for use of virtual reality simulations in undergraduate and graduate nursing

	Undergraduate students	Graduate students
Virtual reality		
	Donning and doffing PPE Urinary catheterization Decontamination Mass casualty event BLS & Resuscitation Cultural empathy development	IV insertion Advanced health assessment Ultrasound skills Neonatal resuscitation Emergency responses Advanced cardiac life support Interprofessional training

Table 2.6 Examples of use of computer-based simulations in undergraduate and graduate nursing

	Undergraduate students	Graduate students
Computer simulation		
	Communication skills Head-to-toe assessments Pharmacology Med-Surg Community Pediatrics Maternal child health	Clinical case studies Differential diagnosis Prescribing medications Health assessment

Modality: Screen Based or Computer Simulations

Definition: A simulation is presented on a computer screen using graphical images and text, like popular gaming formats, where the operator interacts with the interface using a keyboard, mouse, joystick, or other input device.

Scope: These computer-based products are expanding and offer options for first-semester pre-licensure through graduate nursing programs. Computer software can measure clinical judgment, clinical reasoning, and learning outcomes [5, 4]. Computer-based simulation programs often align with textbooks which makes the scenarios easy to connect clinical with didactic content. High-quality computer simulation programs are mapped to nursing accreditation standards. A computerized simulation offers standardized content and can be repeated as many times as needed, which benefits students who learn best with repetition. Since the computer simulations can be done for remote learning, there is flexibility with students completing them on their own time. This modality helps to limit scheduling conflicts and can be useful for clinical make-ups. The American Heart Association (AHA) and other publishers offer several computer-based options for learning about resuscitation, cardiac care, and first aid.

Tips: Internet connections are often needed. It is helpful to have a designated simulation educator or faculty member be the person to implement a new software program to help students, simulation team members, faculty, or administration with understanding how to implement, sustain the product use, assess student learning, and evaluate the effectiveness of the program. Some programs provide feedback directly to the student, but it is still best practice to ensure students are given a chance to debrief the scenario and ask questions. Examples of computer-based simulations for undergraduate and graduate nursing students are presented in Table 2.6.

Modality: Augmented Reality/Mixed Reality

Definition: Augmented reality (AR) is when "stimuli are superimposed on real-world objects (overlays digital computer-generated information on objects or places in the real world)" for enhancing the user experience. "A technology that overlays digital computer-generated information on objects or places in the real world for the purpose of enhancing the user experience" ([2]: 9). Mixed reality simulation combines both physically real and computer generated content to create a learning environment ([2]: 30).

Scope: AR in nursing is a newer concept. Only certain simulation centers have investing in the technology and space for AR. There is not much of a demand for this type of simulation in undergraduate or graduate nursing curriculums to date and there is limited literature regarding the evaluation of this type of simulation [6]. Mixed reality use in nursing is growing as computer and technology engineering improves. One example of the use of mixed reality would be immersion spaces where 360 video images are projected on walls to create a computer generated hospital unit, community setting, or global view, combined with a real manikin that is brought into the space for a scenario. In mixed reality, sound, odor, or other interactive components can be added to improve the immersive experience.

Tips: There are multiple pros to using AR in nursing, such as time-saving by not needing all the expensive equipment during a simulation, easy information retrieval from the program, and the facilitator and the students being able to see different perspectives during a simulation. Some ways to utilize AR in the undergraduate nursing curriculum would be simulating the birth of a patient and showing the cardinal movements in the AR headset as the baby descends in the manikins abdomen. Another way would be augmenting the simulation environment so it feels more like an ICU or operating room environment through an AR device. Furthermore, in an advanced graduate practice curriculum, AR may be used for special tasks, such as identifying latent safety threats in a patient environment and allowing multiple students to participate in this experience independently, simultanesouly, and repeatedly. Mixed reality immersion spaces are beneficial for teamwork training, interprofessional education, and learning in the affective domain as the sensory aspects stimulate emotions during clinical situations.

Distance (Telepresence) Simulation

Definition: "Telesimulation (TS) is a novel concept that uses the internet to link simulators between an instructor and a trainee in different locations" ([7]: 417). Lioce [8], expanded definitions related to distance simulation due to the shift to remote simulation during the COVID-19 pandemic and presents the terms in the Healthcare Simulation Dictionary V2.0 Addendum.

Scope: Tele simulation uses video technology to link the remote learner with their instructors. This type of simulation may limit hands-on skills. However, if part-task trainers are sent to each student and they all log-in, a synchronous session, focusing on basic skills can be achieved. For example, sending a suture pads and sutures to students houses during the pandemic allowed them to practice skills remotely. However, for many distant simulation programs, learners will not be able to improve their skills through tactile deliberate practice. Instead, distance simulation focuses on observing or participating in a case and discussing why certain actions are to be performed.

Tips: The learning objectives and/or outcomes of improved cognitive and behavioral skills drive the decision regarding simulation modality. If using distance simulation techniques, the real-time roles and responsibilities of the staff in the room and the participants on video need to be clearly defined prior to starting, and the expectations of the simulation must be made clear to faculty and learners alike. Also, there must be an emphasis on suspension of disbelief. Furthermore, since the debrief is on video, the facilitator must work hard to foster active participation. Limitations to distance simulation include the need for video communication to function correctly during the simulation, the internet capacity has to be compatible with needs, and the educators have to be familiar with the technology for the simulation to run without issues [9].

Modality: Tabletop Simulations

Definition: Two definitions of a tabletop simulation or exercise (TTX) are presented in the Healthcare Simulation Dictionary. The first is an educational tool intended to provide students/learners an opportunity to apply knowledge through formal discussion of a described scenario [10]. The second definition states, in the context of tabletop exercise, involves key personnel discussing simulated scenarios in an informal setting. TTX can be used to assess plans, policies, and procedures [11]. TTX simulations actively engage learners in discussions or board games and are most often used for emergency preparedness or crisis response. TTX is one of the most cost-effective simulation methods to use in contrast to a full-scale simulation which is resource intensive and time-consuming. TTX for emergency preparedness helps to bring together different disciplines who ultimately work side by side during an emergency. The emergency can be internal to an organization, external with multiple organizations, or on a global scale. A TTX addresses the progress of emergency planning and identifies gaps that may exist in a plan and special training necessary for different responders and system-level actions.

Scope: The TTX can be used for senior-level pre-licensure and graduate nursing courses that focus on leadership, public and community health, capstone coursework, and interprofessional work. The topics that can be covered include public health responses, mass casualty incidents, natural disasters such as hurricanes, earthquakes, or forest fires where patients may need to be evacuated, or any incident where healthcare systems are over-saturated. Evans and Schwartz [12] explained that tabletop exercises provide senior-level baccalaureate nursing students with open-ended decision-making opportunities to manage realistic practice problems. The TTX can be implemented in classroom settings for formative learning.

Tips: A TTX is well-suited for interprofessional exercises. It is important to have all different disciplines involved with disaster planning exercises so that all perspectives are represented and involved with the implementation. Extensive planning is necessary for a TTX and different templates are needed for planning. A TTX offers additional opportunities, beyond clinical care, including patient flow and discussions on how to assist vulnerable populations during an emergency. Examples of table top simulations for undergraduate and graduate nursing students are presented in Table 2.7.

Table 2.7 Examples for use of tabletop simulations in undergraduate and graduate nursing

	Undergraduate students	Graduate students
Tabletop simulation		
	Pandemic or epidemic Natural disasters Mass casualty incident Evacuation plan during fire emergency Implementation of a staffing decision tree in a leadership course	Response to sexual assault encounter Food poisoning for large group Interprofessional Leadership

Modality: Hybrid

Definition: A hybrid simulation is any simulation activity that uses two or more modalities [13].

Scope: The pairing of a standardized patient with a task trainer is a common hybrid solution to meet the objectives of providing emotional support during a sensitive exam or procedure. This protects the safety of the SP while giving the learner a higher fidelity experience by bringing human touch into the scenario. The task trainer can be a wearable device or a non-wearable device in the room. The scope of hybrid simulation does not stop there. Any two modalities can be used as per the examples below.

Tips: There are limitless possibilities for the use of hybrid simulations when combining all modalities. Future possibilities for hybrid simulations is to use virtual and extended reality technologies with other modalities.

Examples of hybrid simulations for undergraduate and graduate nursing students are presented in Table 2.8.

Table 2.8 Examples for use of hybrid simulations in undergraduate and graduate nursing

	Undergraduate students	Graduate students
Hybrid		
	CPR renewals combining computer-based simulation with in-person motor performance using a CPR task trainer or manikin	A well-woman gyn exam using a standardized patient for communication and a pelvic task trainer or breast simulator
	Using an SP as a parent or guardian during a pediatric scenario using a pediatric manikin	End-of-life care with a manikin and simulated participant as a family member to discuss advanced directives
	SP with a wearable tracheostomy to practice suctioning	SP amputee wearing a bleeding limb or cut suit for trauma response

References

1. Nestel D, Tierney T. Role-play for medical students learning about communication: guidelines for maximizing benefits. BMC Med Educ. 2007;7:3. https://doi.org/10.1186/1472-6920-7-3n.
2. Lewis KL, Bohnert CA, Gammon WL, et al. The Association of Standardized Patient Educators (ASPE) Standards of Best Practice (SOBP). Adv Simul. 2017;2:10. https://doi.org/10.1186/s41077-017-0043-4.
3. Gliva-McConvey G, Shannon GM, Pitt J, Clark L. The human simulation continuum: integration and application. In: Gliva-McConvey G, Nicolas CF, Clark L, editors. Comprehensive healthcare simulation: implementing best practices in standardized patient methodology. Cham: Springer; 2020. p. 31–50.
4. Foronda C, Fernandez-Burgos M, Nadeau C, Kelley C, Henry M. Virtual simulation in nursing education: a systematic review spanning 1996 to 2018. Simul Healthc. 2020;15(1):46–54. https://doi.org/10.1097/SIH.0000000000000411.
5. Dubovi I. Online computer-based clinical simulations: the role of visualizations. Clin Simul Nurs. 2019;33:35–41. https://doi.org/10.1016/j.ecns.2019.04.009.
6. Wüller H, Behrens J, Garthaus M, Marquard S, Remmers H. A scoping review of augmented reality in nursing. BMC Nurs. 2019;18(1):19. https://doi.org/10.1186/s12912-019-0342-2.
7. Okrainec A, Okrainec A, Henao O, Henao O, Azzie G, Azzie G. Telesimulation: an effective method for teaching the fundamentals of laparoscopic surgery in resource-restricted countries. Surg Endosc. 2010;24(2):417–22. https://doi.org/10.1007/s00464-009-0572-6.
8. Lioce L. (Ed). Healthcare Simulation Dictionary Addendum. V2.0 ADDENDUM: terms related to simulation at a distance. 2020. SSH dictionary Distance Simulation Addendum. Retrieved from https://www.ssih.org/Portals/48/Distance%20Simulation%20Addendum.pdf.
9. Diaz M, Walsh B. Telesimulation-based education during COVID-19. Clin Teach. 2021;18:121–5.
10. Lehtola CJ. Developing and Using Table-Top Simulations as a Teaching Tool. The Journal of Extension. 2007;45(4):27. https://tigerprints.clemson.edu/joe/vol45/iss4/27.
11. California Hospital Association. Emergency Preparedness. What is the difference between a tabletop exercise, a drill, a functional exercise, and a full-scale exercise? 2017. https://www.calhospitalprepare.org/post/whatdifference-between-tabletop-exercise-drill-functional-exercise-and-full-scale-exercise.
12. Evans CA, Schwartz R. Using tabletop exercises as an innovative and practical teaching strategy in response to external disaster scenarios. Nurs Educ Perspect. 2019;40(1):62–4. https://doi.org/10.1097/01.NEP.0000000000000308.
13. Lioce L (Ed.), Lopreiato J (Founding Ed.), Downing D, Chang TP, Robertson JM, Anderson M, Diaz DA, Spain AE (Assoc. Eds.), and the Terminology and Concepts Working Group, Healthcare Simulation Dictionary–2nd ed. Rockville: Agency for Healthcare Research and Quality; 2020. AHRQ Publication No. 20-0019. https://doi.org/10.23970/simulationv2.

Essentials of Debriefing and Feedback

3

Leland Rockstraw

Introduction

The International Nursing Association for Clinical Simulation and Learning definition of debriefing suggests a reflective procedure occurring after a simulation-based experience (SBE) which is conducted by a trained facilitator who uses evidence-based debriefing models [1, 2]. Debriefing is one of the pillars of healthcare simulation, which promotes clinical reasoning. Debriefing is a powerful tool and a strong educational technique in healthcare simulation training. The use of debriefing in healthcare simulation demonstrates improved team performance, improved behavioral skills, and increase patient outcomes [3, 4]. While there are many methods of debriefing, it is important to understand and incorporate core strategies that will aid in the debriefing process. This chapter will introduce the concept of debriefing, explore the International Nursing Association for Clinical Simulation and Learning's (INACSL) Best Practice in debriefing [1, 2], share strategies to create both an emotional and physical environment conducive to debriefing, and introduce some models of debriefing. With a better understanding of debriefing strategies and methods, learners will gain confidence, and clinical reasoning skills, enhance team performance, and improve behavioral and clinical skills of the learner [5]. Dreifuerst [6] suggests that debriefing should be focused on the identification of participants' perceptions and attitudes, a linking of the simulation experience to a learning theory or competency building and refinement, and a place where feedback on the participant's involvement, behavior, and choices made during the scenario. The practice of debriefing should be practiced by persons knowledgeable and skilled in facilitation/debriefing, and it is the goal of this author to provide an organized approach to obtain this knowledge and skills.

L. Rockstraw (✉)
School of Nursing, University of Nevada, Las Vegas, NV, USA
e-mail: leland.rockstraw@unlv.edu

Definition of Terms

This chapter will define simulation terminology related to debriefing to promote understanding and shared values in simulation as defined by INACSL. These definitions will assist in common understanding regarding this chapter on debriefing.

- Clinical Reasoning: A process that involves both thinking (cognition) and reflective thinking (metacognition) to gather and comprehend data while recalling knowledge, skills (technical and non-technical), and attitudes about a situation as it unfolds. After analysis, information is put together into meaningful conclusions to determine alternative actions.
- Critical Thinking: A disciplined process that requires validation of data, including any assumptions that may influence thoughts and actions, and then careful reflection on the entire process while evaluating the effectiveness of what has been determined as the necessary action(s) to take. This process entails purposeful, goal-directed thinking and is based on scientific principles and methods (evidence) rather than assumptions or conjecture.
- Debriefing: A reflective process immediately following the SBE that is led by a trained facilitator using an evidence-based debriefing model. Participants' reflective thinking is encouraged, and feedback is provided regarding the participants' performance while various aspects of the completed simulation are discussed. Participants are encouraged to explore emotions and question, reflect, and provide feedback to one another. The purpose of debriefing is to move toward assimilation and accommodation to transfer learning to future situations.
- Feedback: Information is given or dialog between participants, facilitator, simulator, or peer with the intention of improving the understanding of concepts or aspects of performance.

J. M. Kutzin et al. (eds.), *Comprehensive Healthcare Simulation: Nursing*, Comprehensive Healthcare Simulation,
https://doi.org/10.1007/978-3-031-31090-4_3

- Fiction Contract: The implicit or explicit agreement among participants and facilitator(s) about how the participant is expected to interact with the simulated situation and how the facilitators will treat that interaction.
- Reflective Thinking: The engagement of self-monitoring that occurs during or after a simulation experience. Considered an essential component of experiential learning, it promotes the discovery of new knowledge with the intent of applying this knowledge to future situations. Reflective thinking is necessary for metacognitive skill acquisition and clinical judgment and has the potential to decrease the gap between theory and practice. Reflection requires creativity and conscious self-evaluation to deal with unique patient situations.
- Simulation-Based Experience: A broad array of structured activities that represent actual or potential situations in education, practice, and research. These activities allow participants to develop or enhance knowledge, skills, and/or attitudes and provide an opportunity to analyze and respond to realistic situations in a simulated environment [1, 2].

A Standard for Debriefing: INACSL Standards of Best Practice

The act of learning is supported by the matching of what the participant experienced and their deliberation on the experience [7]. Reflection can lead to improved behavior and clinical reasoning [8, 9]. The ability to guide the participant is important to promote the best plausible learning results. The incorporation of debriefing activities should support learning and improvement of competencies and behaviors, which will lead to safe patient outcomes [10, 11]. In 2011, a group of healthcare simulation educators completed what was to become international standards in conducting simulation scenarios to include the standard of best practices in debriefing [1, 2]. These standards operationalize measures to promote a planned debriefing experience and improve the future performances of participants.

The five criteria are:

- The debrief is facilitated by a person(s) competent in the process of debriefing.
- The debrief is conducted in an environment that is conducive to learning and supports confidentiality, trust, open communication, self-analysis, feedback, and reflection.
- The debrief is facilitated by a person(s) who can devote enough concentrated attention during the simulation to effectively debrief the simulation-based experience.
- The debrief is based on a theoretical framework for debriefing that is structured in a purposeful way.
- The debrief is congruent with the objectives and outcomes of the simulation-based experience.
  [1, 2]

The incorporation of these five criteria into the practice of debriefing will facilitate positive outcomes, which include participant obtainment of improved skills, behavior, and competence [11, 12]. Understanding and incorporating the five criteria and the required elements will only improve the obtainment of participant outcomes and debriefing experience for all involved.

Phases of Debriefing

After significant events, debriefing assists the learner in reacting, analyzing what happened, and promoting the obtainment of new knowledge, skills (competencies), and improved behavior. Debriefing after healthcare simulations supports Simulation-based education (SBE) and is considered a cornerstone of the learning experience and promotes critical thinking and clinical reasoning [5, 6]. Having a structure or technique to guide debriefing aids in the organized movement from the experience of the simulation event to the application of what can be learned. One technique of debriefing includes three phases of debriefing which include reaction or description phase, a second the phase where insight, understanding, and analysis are encouraged, and the third, where the goal of the application of lessons learned and summarization of the experience happens [5].

Phase 1—the reactions phase: in this phase, participants are encouraged to share their feelings of how they were made to feel by the simulation experience, to blow off steam, if you will. The debriefing facilitator should use open-ended questions to encourage participants' involvement, review the experience of the simulation experience based on their memory of the facts of the event, and share common feelings and experiences with peer participants.

Phase 2—the understanding or analysis phase: is where the facilitator guides the participant to review simulation objectives with performance (or failure to perform) actions to accomplish stated outcomes. In this phase, the facilitator should assist the participant in exploring assessments, decisions made, performance of care, and evaluation of actions. The technique should include open discussions and inquiries from the facilitator. Questions such as 'What happened? Why did it happen?' will promote understanding of the simulation experience.

Phase 3—the application of lessons learned phase: in phase three, the facilitator should summarize take-home messages of what went well and what can be improved. It is important to assist the participant in applying lessons learned to future clinical experiences, which will assist in the inclusion of best practices as well as identifying and preventing future decisions with poor outcomes. Participants should be encouraged to ask questions in this phase, which follows the GAS model espoused by the American Heart Association [13].

Conducive Learning Environments in Simulation: Emotional and Physical

Debriefing of participants' experiences, memories, and thought processes to reflect on the clinical scenario should occur immediately after, within minutes, or a few hours of the simulation event [5]. This timing allows for the assessment and exploration of urgent issues raised by the simulation experience. Facilitators of debriefing must spent time on providing an environment conducive to debriefing. This allows for a feeling of safety which in turn provides for interpersonal risk-taking in exploring the simulation experiences positive events as well as mistakes that may occur. Psychological safety is important for learners to feel safe to talk about clinical reasoning, performance, and uncertainty, especially in the presence of the hierarchy of healthcare training. Learners need to feel safe to explore, question, and receive feedback without being worried about being humiliated or shamed [14]. Environments that include elements for psychosocial safety, a common understanding of expectations, a review of the fiction contract, use of open-ended questions, and effective use of silence will assist in establishing psychological safety in the debriefing process.

Debriefing should be conducted in a private, comfortable environment. If possible, arrange seating in a circle fashion; with facilitators sitting among participants rather than at the head of the table [15]. The process of debriefing should not be hurried but rather allow time for reflection on questions and actions. The introduction of the debriefing should include the objectives, a statement about shared confidentiality, and the development of trust. Asking open-ended questions allows for open discussion between participants and the facilitator and allows participants to critically reflect on their thoughts and actions. Decker [15] also suggests the use of silence will promote reflection and allow time to think. Effective elements of debriefing to facilitate the process include common rules which should be incorporated into the facilitator's frameworks and techniques [5, 16]. Table 3.1 includes debriefing components and their defining characteristics. The inclusion of these elements will promote a safe and effective debriefing environment to support the method of debriefing chosen.

Table 3.1 Essential elements of debriefing and its characteristics

1. Ensuring psychosocial safety
• "Behave or perform without fear of negative consequences to self-image, social standing, or career trajectory"
• Essential to optimize learning outcomes by providing a supportive climate
• Should be conducted during the pre-simulation briefing and then during the debriefing
2. Having a debriefing stance or "basic assumption"
• Predefined basic assumption statement, "We believe that everyone participating in simulation is intelligent, capable, cares about doing their best, and wants to improve"
3. Establishing debriefing rules
• A basic set of rules for debriefing among participants
• Confidential discussion
• Encourage all learners to participate actively
4. Establishing a shared mental model
• Review the event details with input from the facilitator
5. Addressing key learning objectives
• Incorporate and analyze clear learning objectives during debriefing
6. Using open-ended questions
• Helps facilitate discussion and foster reflection
• Avoid close-ended or (yes/no) questions
7. Using silence
• A brief period of silence after a facilitator asks a question
• Promote an internal process within the debriefing learner's mind
• Allows learners to formulate their thoughts and analyze their mental frames

Abulebda et al. [5]

Debriefing Methods

There are a plethora of debriefing methods which assist the facilitator and learner to maximize the learning from the simulation scenario and conduct a debriefing. This section will introduce five common styles, which are: structured debriefing, Socratic questioning, advocacy-inquiry and debriefing with good judgment, plus-delta, and promoting excellence and reflective learning in simulation (PEARLS).

Structured Debriefing

Structured debriefing assists with providing guidance in the educational process, assists with the collection of information, and provides insight to the learner of their understanding [17]. Cantrell [18] used structured debriefing questioning which was developed from questions originally created by Ham and O'Rourke [19] which facilitates the participants' learning process. These questions are:

- What were the patient's goals for this episode of care?
- Were these goals met by your nursing behaviors?

- How did you prioritize the patient's needs?
- What would you do differently if actually caring for him or her and the family in an acute care setting? ([18]: e20).

Socratic Questioning

Socratic questioning is a learning-centered approach that assists the learner to develop their clinical reasoning skills by engaging in analytic discussion and will lead to learning and thinking independently [20]. Socratic questioning will assist the learner in exploring ideas, uncovering assumptions, and exploring complex concepts. Questions of synthesizing concepts are preferred versus simple yes or no questions; thinking can be promoted by using "what if" questions and modifying key aspects of the learning to encourage learners to think beyond the encounter they experienced [6]. The benefits of using Socratic questioning include increasing the motivation and participation of the learner, encouraging the student to ask questions and answer questions, and promoting interaction, dialogue, and debate between the facilitator and student [21].

Advocacy-Inquiry and Debriefing with Good Judgment

Advocacy-inquiry and debriefing with good judgment are debriefing methods that contains three components which, when used, assist the participant to reflect on assumptions and clinical practice [22]. This nonjudgmental approach inquires as an advocate for the patient using "I" statements followed by the request of the participant to describe their thought process. Advocacy-inquiry includes three components which are (1) the participants' understanding of their thought process and actions; (2) a curiosity from the facilitator to understand from a non-judgmental standpoint; and (3) an evaluative judgment question of advocacy-inquiry [22]. The framing of the question contains two parts, an observation followed by an inquiry; an example could be when watching a participant when determining a pulseless individual during CPR and failing to start compressions for 3 min; the advocacy inquiry could be stated as 'I noticed that when you determined the patient was pulseless, compressions were not started for 3 min; according to the American Heart Association, compressions should be started immediately when an individual is determined to be without a pulse; I am curious as to your decision making here.' The facilitator calling attention to the delayed implementation of compressions is considered the 'good judgment' of the facilitator's view [23].

Plus-Delta

The Plus-Delta method is considered a formative assessment process that provides feedback on the participant's actions and assists with the collection of ideas, future actions, or behaviors for future improvement [24]. The Plus-Delta method involves dividing action up into good behaviors vs. those actions and behaviors which need improvement. This method allows the learner to actively participate in the discussion and easily categorize their actions and behaviors [25]. This technique is borrowed from flight crew debriefing and generally involves creating three columns on a white/blackboard; the three columns which include (1) actions of participants, (2) plus, and (3) opportunities for improvement (delta). The actions of participants column will be filled with actions and behaviors of individuals and the team members involved in the simulation scenario. The plus column describes the effective or positive actions and characteristics which will want to be replicated in future similar experiences (simulated and real). The delta column should list opportunities for improvement of actions and behaviors for future scenarios. A few advantages of using the Plus/Delta are the ease of learning and mastery by the facilitator, and learners can quickly and comfortably master this technique of exploring their actions and behaviors [23].

PEARLS

Promoting Excellence and Reflective Learning in Simulation (PEARLS) is a blended approach to debriefing strategies [26]. PEARLS blends the obtainment of goals such as clinical reasoning, improving clinical skills, promoting teamwork, and interprofessional collaboration. This debriefing approach suggests the development of a script to assist educators in providing a sense of psychological safety while assisting the learner in organizing and analyzing their performance. The PEARLS framework divides debriefing into four phases of reaction, description, analysis, and summary [26]. This strategy of debriefing is easy to follow and assists both the novice and experienced debriefer.

Summary

The process of debriefing in supporting the learner's critical thinking and reflection and promotes improvement in actions and behaviors. The inclusion of 'best practices' of debriefing will facilitate improved learner outcomes and increase safe patient care. The importance of the facilitator following a structured technique to guide their debriefing will aid in the organized movement of learners from the simulation event to application of new knowledge and improved competencies. The psychosocial safety and arrangement of the physical environment will aid the learners to be open to discussion and feedback to explore and question their actions. There is a shared understanding that debriefing plays a critical role in the learner's experience, and continued development by simulation facilitators will require excellence in the debriefing process. It is the hope of this author that this chapter sparks the desire to learn and practice debriefing techniques to reach a higher level of excellence.

References

1. INACSL Standards Committee. INACSL standards of best practice: SimulationSM debriefing. Clin Simul Nurs. 2016;12(Suppl):S21–5. https://doi.org/10.1016/j.ecns.2016.09.008.
2. INACSL Standards Committee. INACSL standards of best practice: SimulationSM simulation glossary. Clin Simul Nurs. 2016;12(Suppl):S39–47. https://doi.org/10.1016/j.ecns.2016.09.012.
3. Kessler DO, Cheng A, Mullan PC. Debriefing in the emergency department after clinical events: a practical guide. Ann Emerg Med. 2015;65(6):690–8.
4. Sawyer T, Loren D, Halamek LP. Post-event debriefings during neonatal care: why are we not doing them, and how can we start? J Perinatol. 2016;36(6):415–9.
5. Abulebda K, Auerbach M, Limaiem F. Debriefing techniques utilized in medical simulation. StatPearls [Internet]. 2020. https://www.ncbi.nlm.nih.gov/books/NBK546660/.
6. Dreifuerst KT. The essentials of debriefing in simulated learning: a concept analysis. Nurs Educ Perspect. 2009;30(2):109–14.
7. Cheng A, Eppich W, Grant V, Sherbino J, Zendejas B, Cook DA. Debriefing for technology-enhanced simulation: a systematic review and meta-analysis. Med Educ. 2014;48(7):657–66.
8. Ahmed M, Sevdalis N, Paige J, Paragi-Gururaja R, Nestel D, Arora S. Identifying best practice guidelines for debriefing in surgery: a tri-continental study. Am J Surg. 2012;203(4):523–9.
9. Rudolph JW, Simon R, Rivard P, Dufresne RL, Raemer DB. Debriefing with good judgment: combining rigorous feedback with genuine inquiry. Anesthesiol Clin. 2007;25(2):361–76.
10. Kolbe M, Grande B, Spahn DR. Briefing and debriefing during simulation-based training and beyond content, structure, attitude, and setting. Best Pract Res Clin Anaesthesiol. 2015;29(1):87–96.
11. Rudolph JW, Raemer DB, Simon R. Establishing a safe container for learning in simulation: the role of the pre-simulation briefing. Simul Healthc. 2014;9(6):339–49.
12. Der Sahakian G, Alinier G, Savoldelli G, Oriot D, Jaffrelot M, Lecomte F. Setting conditions for productive debriefing. Simul Gaming. 2015;46(2):197–208.
13. Salik I, Paige JT. Debriefing the interprofessional team in medical simulation. [Updated 2022 Apr 21]. In: StatPearls [Internet]. Treasure Island: StatPearls Publishing; 2022. https://www.ncbi.nlm.nih.gov/books/NBK554526/.
14. Madireddy S, Rufa EP. Maintaining confidentiality and psychological safety in medical simulation. [Updated 2021 May 9]. In: StatPearls [Internet]. Treasure Island: StatPearls Publishing; 2021. https://www.ncbi.nlm.nih.gov/books/NBK559259/.
15. Decker S. Integrating guided reflection into simulated learning experiences. In: Jeffries PR, editor. Simulation in nursing: from conceptualization to evaluation. New York: National League for Nursing; 2007. p. 73–85.
16. Gardner R. Introduction to debriefing. Semin Perinatol. 2013;37(3):166–74.
17. Wittmann-Price RA, Rockstraw LJ, Kirk T. Debriefing. In: Wilson L, Wittmann-Price RA, editors. Review manual for the certified healthcare simulation educator (CHS) exam. Springer Publishing Company. 2015. pp. 193–208.
18. Cantrell MA. The importance of debriefing in clinical simulation. Clin Simul Nurs. 2008;4:e19–23.
19. Ham K, O'Rourke E. Clinical strategies. Clinical preparation for beginning nursing students: an experiential learning activity. Nurse Educ. 2004;29(4):139–41.
20. Makhene A. The use of the Socratic inquiry to facilitate critical thinking in nursing education. Health SA. 2019;24:1224.
21. Ralph E. Oral-questioning skills of novice teachers. Any questions? J Instr Psychol. 1999;26(4):286–96.
22. Rudolph JW, Simon R, Dufresne RL, Raemer DB. There's no such thing as "nonjudgmental" debriefing: a theory and method for debriefing with good judgment. Simul Healthc. 2006;1(1):49–55.
23. Littlewood KE, Szylad D. Debriefing. In: Palaganas JC, Maxworthy JC, Epps CA, Mancini ME, editors. Defining excellence in simulation programs. Philadelphia: Wolters Kluwer; 2015. p. 558–72.
24. Bajaj K, Meguerdichian M, Thoma B, Huang S, Eppich W, Cheng A. The PEARLS healthcare debriefing tool. Acad Med. 2018;93(2):336.
25. Sawyer TL, Deering S. Adaptation of the US Army's after-action review for simulation debriefing in healthcare. Simul Healthc. 2013;8(6):388–97.
26. Eppich W, Cheng A. Promoting Excellence and Reflective Learning in Simulation (PEARLS). Simul Healthc. 2015;10(2):106–15. https://doi.org/10.1097/SIH.0000000000000072.

Part II

Undergraduate Nursing Education

4 Simulation Modalities for Undergraduate Nursing Education

Natalya Pasklinsky and Beth Latimer

Background

Clinical simulation is a dynamic and adaptable teaching and learning strategy that has and continues to transform healthcare education. Simulation, as defined by the Society for Simulation in Healthcare in its latest *Healthcare Simulation Dictionary* (1), is "a technique that creates a situation or environment to allow persons to experience a representation of a real event for the purposes of practice, learning, evaluation, testing, or to gain an understanding of systems or human actions" (p. 44).

Simulation in undergraduate nursing is a learner-centered pedagogy that helps students build clinical skills, demonstrate the application of clinical knowledge, develop critical thinking and decision-making skills, and practice team-based care to provide quality, safe patient care (2–4). Simulation can be designed to provide difficult-to-obtain clinical experiences for pre-licensure nurses (e.g., birth, blood transfusion reaction, rapidly deteriorating patient or anaphylaxis), as well as allow educators to advance student skill mastery and complex care management experience for patients with chronic and acute health conditions in a variety of settings. The range and breadth of simulation modalities allow for an expansive use of simulation teaching and learning throughout undergraduate nursing education. Effective use of simulation modalities allows students to actively learn and make mistakes in controlled environments with no harm to patients and give pre-licensure students opportunities to collaborate, debrief and reflect on their actions in meaningful ways that impact learning and future practice (4, 5).

Professional organizations, accrediting bodies, and the research literature support the integrated use of simulation in undergraduate nursing education to accelerate student knowledge acquisition, promote critical thinking and support the transfer of theory into practice (4, 6, 7). Clinical simulation holds an essential place in undergraduate nursing education and continues to be expanded into program curricula through the use of enhanced technologies, innovations, and immersive learning opportunities (5, 6). Students and nurse educators increasingly benefit from expanding modalities and the controlled, creative, contextual experiences and psychologically safe learning environments that effective simulation affords (8, 9).

Simulation pedagogy has foundations in several well-known learning theoretical frameworks, most notably experiential learning, social cognitive learning, reflection, cognitive load theory, and adult learning theory (10–14). These theories can guide educators in the selection of simulation strategies and modalities to optimize student engagement, enhance learning and facilitate the transfer of new clinical knowledge to practice. Simulation can be used to create effective learning situations that meet rapidly changing needs and help students lean into lifelong learning, develop and maintain clinical competence, and expand confidence and connectedness in safely caring for patients, families, and communities.

Simulation Modalities

The International Nursing Association of Clinical Simulation and Learning (INACSL) Standards Committee (15) definition of simulation highlights that " simulation can incorporate one or more modalities to promote, improve, or validate a participant's performance" (p. S44). Through the use of a range of simulation modalities, students are given reliable, experiential opportunities to achieve mastery learning where students can safely practice and make errors without causing harm to actual patients. Pairing modalities purposefully to the learning objective, level of the learner, available resources, and desired fidelity is a priority to successfully achieve learning outcomes. In the field of healthcare simula-

N. Pasklinsky (✉) · B. Latimer
New York University, Rory Meyers College of Nursing, New York, NY, USA
e-mail: veksln01@nyu.edu; beth.latimer@nyu.edu

J. M. Kutzin et al. (eds.), *Comprehensive Healthcare Simulation: Nursing*, Comprehensive Healthcare Simulation, https://doi.org/10.1007/978-3-031-31090-4_4

tion, a modality is defined as "a selected type or types of simulation equipment, concept, or technique that constitutes a method of simulation use" (1).

Simulation modalities for undergraduate nursing education can range from:

- **Task trainers** to develop psychomotor skills such as IV administration, injections, wound care practice, and Foley catheter insertion.
- **Standardized patients** to develop therapeutic communication skills or personal interaction skills while conducting health interviews, performing assessments, and planning care.
- **Hybrid** is a mix of task trainers and standardized patients to integrate skills and for skill mastery and communication competencies.
- **Computer-Based Virtual Simulation** is the use of a digital learning environment (computer, phone, tablet) for partially immersive screen-based learning experiences to improve learning outcomes.
- **Virtual Reality (VR)** is a technology that provides fully immersive virtual experiences through the use of a headset for psychomotor and cognitive learning.
- **Human Patient Simulator** fosters effective team performance, prioritization of care, situational awareness, and clinical decision-making for complex care of patients and entry to practice.

Simulation modalities will vary depending on the learning objectives, level of the learner, available resources, and expertise of the faculty or adjunct staff. Each modality needs to be carefully chosen to match the learning outcomes to the student experience. As simulation education is complex and multi-faceted, educators and faculty must be knowledgeable of each modality and well-prepared and equipped to facilitate simulation and ensure students are receiving the highest quality education (16, 17).

Task Trainers

Task trainers or skills simulators are commonly used in undergraduate nursing education and are useful for teaching psychomotor skills such as intravenous insertion and fluid administration, medication administration, tracheostomy care, nasogastric tube placement care, and urinary catheter insertion. Task trainers can be utilized for skill mastery acquisition (1, 15). For example, a foot can be staged with a pressure ulcer, and students measure, clean, assess, and practice dressing changes on this task trainer. Task trainers can be used to practice medication injections which include finding the correct landmark prior to administration of the injection.

Task trainers vary in complexity and provide opportunities for deliberate practice. For example, an intravenous arm task trainer allows students to practice in a safe and effective way with the ability to make mistakes, repeat the procedure numerous times, receive feedback from facilitators, and develop the skills necessary to reach proficiency. Task trainers can be utilized alone or in combination with a manikin or standardized patient to increase the fidelity of the simulated scenario. Task trainers wear and tear just like any other type of equipment and will need to be replaced over time. It is important to explore how many practices each task trainer can accommodate prior to needing replacement while keeping in mind how large or small the student body is.

Simulated Patients

The terms simulated patient, standardized patient, and simulated participant (SP) are often used interchangeably and refer to a person trained to portray a patient or other human role player in realistic and repeatable ways for healthcare education, evaluation, and research (1, 18). SPs can participate in undergraduate nursing high-stakes assessments in which SP responses to the learner are standardized though more recently, SPs have been included in more formative teaching scenarios. SPs are invaluable in undergraduate nursing education because they provide live, real-time interaction and feedback to students as to how they feel from a patient perspective in the delivery of nursing care students are providing. For example, in a medication administration simulation focused on safety and error prevention, students can receive a handoff SBAR report via an iPad, phone, or face-to-face, then proceed to an encounter with an SP. The SP portrays the patient in a medication administration encounter where the student's objectives are to perform a focused assessment, perform all the medication rights and checks prior to medication administration, and then proceed with the administration.

It is important to partner with SPs when the simulation modality to consider is focused on addressing specific learning outcomes that focus on the development of communication skills such as implementing behavioral health interventions, e.g., having difficult conversations in healthcare (breaking bad news), health interviewing and patient teaching (18, 19). Another example of integrating SPs into simulation curriculums is the adoption of SPs in Telehealth undergraduate nursing simulations where the SP plays the role of the patient in the community or psychiatric settings. SPs can serve as an asset in not only the scenario fidelity but provide invaluable feedback to participants students from the "patient" perspective. In the undergraduate psychiatric simulation, SPs can play various patient roles, from anxiety, depression, and bipolar disorder to schizophrenia, which allows for the simulation facilitator to observe, take notes, and provide detailed feedback on student participation and performance during the debrief. The SPs are trained on scenario responses, scenario progression, and student objectives to ensure consistency for all simulation experiences.

Another example of SP implementation in undergraduate nursing education is in the area of physical assessment. SPs receive training to portray one of several patient roles, e.g., a patient with appendicitis, COPD, or any other ailment or disease process, and students perform a head-to-toe exam with a history focused on their presenting illness. A designated rubric can be utilized for student competency assessment. Partnering with SPs improves student experience, critical thinking, and assessment skills (20).

Hybrid Simulation

Hybrid simulation, or the use of two or more simulation modalities in the same simulation activity to enhance fidelity, can involve, most commonly, the addition of a static task trainer to a dynamic SP (1). For example, the SP may wear a tracheostomy suction wearable, which keeps the SP safe yet allows for skill development and mastery over time with the contextual practice for the student. Or where an SP wears an intravenous arm sleeve that mimics the IV that a student would use to administer medication. This approach maintains SP safety while enhancing realism.

Another example of a hybrid modality is the use of an ostomy appliance partial task trainer worn by an SP to integrate the learning of the technical skills associated with ostomy management whilst demonstrating sensitive communication skills and effective patient education for complex self-care needs (1, 18). In a birthing scenario, an SP can wear a specialized suit to simulate labor or delivery while utilizing a human infant simulator to practice newborn care immediately post-delivery. SPs can be utilized to portray the roles of family members in diverse simulation scenarios. For example, if attempting to recreate an unconscious patient, the use of a human patient simulator portrays the patient while the SP is at the bedside as the family member. By merging these modalities, educators can create an engaging, realistic, and heightened approach to meet the requisite learning objectives.

Computer Screen-Based-Virtual Simulation

Virtual simulation is an area of rapid growth in the field of simulation and is increasingly accessible for undergraduate nursing education. The expanded use of new virtual technologies in clinical teaching, greatly accelerated by the need for online learning solutions in the midst of the coronavirus pandemic, creates a mounting interest in virtual modalities science, the use of "virtual" terminology, and virtual modalities used in the clinical simulation (21–23). Simulation education nurse researchers now suggest levels of immersion as a current distinguishing characteristic in virtual modalities, with Foronda proposing the definition of virtual simulation as: "the use of partial immersion through a digital learning environment (e.g., computer, tablet, phone, screen, etc.) to foster a perceived lived experience for an intended outcome (e.g., learning, entertainment, etc.)" (8). This differentiates it from the fully immersive experience of virtual reality (VR) simulation, which will be discussed in the next section (21, 24).

Research supports the use of virtual simulation in nursing education as a viable learning modality to enhance clinical judgment, critical thinking, self-confidence, and learner satisfaction and improve undergraduate nursing student knowledge, skills, and performance (24–26). Virtual computer screen-based simulation is frequently available to learners through a subscription to specialized software applications. This allows students to participate in a virtual environment through a screen-based device (PC, laptop, phone, or iPad) and interact with avatars and game-based platforms with branching choice scenarios to assess and intervene based on the patient's presentation (27–29). The benefit of computer-based simulation allows for participants to join from any location without restrictions to time and space. Learners log in from their own devices to participate in a virtual interactive simulation, allowing for student convenience.

In the virtual simulation environment, learners have encounters with life-like virtual patients or avatars to practice communication, assessment, documentation, and patient care skills (28, 29). Computer-based virtual simulation provides a safe setting to practice nursing skills. For instance, virtual simulation products often offer individualized analytics and feedback for learners on strengths and areas to improve. In addition, virtual simulation offers opportunities to repeat simulation experiences in order to improve clinical skills, clinical reasoning, and decision-making through repeated practice. Virtual simulation is a learning modality with the potential to be accessible, cost-effective, and can be used for remote simulation learning.

The rapid uptake of virtual simulation during the times of remote instruction highlights the expanding roles and learning needs of simulation educators for remote simulation facilitation and debriefing. To address this, Cheng et al. (30) point simulation educators toward the Community of Inquiry framework, highlighting the impact of social, teaching, and cognitive presence to support meaningful, collaborative learning in new remote simulation environments. Ongoing training, engagement, and development for simulation educators are essential for the use of virtual simulation modalities in undergraduate nursing education.

The creation and development of innovative virtual simulation scenarios can enhance critical thinking and decision-making through the use of interactive components that allow for and support student engagement throughout the simulation and debrief. For example, undergraduate students participating in Maternity clinical simulation at NYU Meyers College of Nursing in the USA have an opportunity to engage in active learning and reflection through virtual simulation workshops. Additionally, a virtual simulation on reproductive justice and healthcare develops students' awareness of the social determinants of health and inequality which prepares them for a facilitated video case review and debriefing about reproductive justice and nursing practice. This is achieved by using a variety of active learning approaches, such as game-based learning and immersive audio-visual elements. Students prioritize postpartum care while evaluating the effects of unconscious bias on potential maternal health outcomes. The most important "lessons learned" are to pair the appropriate virtual activity with the learner's level of expertise and ensure that appropriate pre-simulation preparation has been completed by the participants.

Virtual Reality (VR)

Virtual Reality (VR) is a digital technology that immerses the user's senses (vision, hearing, and motion) in a 3D virtual world. It requires a head-mounted display (e.g., VR headsets/goggles) and may also be enhanced by haptic devices, visual tracking, motion sensors, or speech recognition (22, 31). Augmented Reality (AR) is a digital technology that superimposes an image into the real world with which the user can interact. AR generally requires a smartphone or tablet (22, 31). Mixed Reality (MR) is sometimes referred to as Hybrid Reality. It is an immersive version of AR, where the virtual elements are not only overlaid onto the real world (AR) but are anchored within it, allowing the user to interact with it as if it were within reality (31).

In the VR environment with a headset or goggles, learners can manage patients in an immersive 3D environment. Aspects of care can include nursing assessment, nursing diagnosis, prioritization and implementation of care, interaction with a multidisciplinary team, and evaluation of care. Directive feedback on actions can be provided immediately or as close as possible after each encounter and while the student is fully immersed in the scenario (22). Similar to virtual simulation, the benefits of VR as a modality are that it can be replicated and can offer immediate, individualized feedback, including performance analytics, metrics, or scores. Virtual reality is a modality that requires little space, provides consistent fidelity, and provides opportunities for self-directed, repeated practice for skills mastery. The high level of immersion allows students to be fully engaged in the virtual environment and successfully achieve learning outcomes. It has also been found to increase student satisfaction and performance (32, 33).

It is necessary to work closely with virtual simulation vendors who specialize in VR in order to find the best products for learners customized to the available virtual simulations. VR can be utilized on-site and remotely if users possess a headset or goggles, although the "immersive" nature of the 3D VR environment is lost when the scenario is transferred to a screen-based platform. An important consideration is when VR is used asynchronously because although students receive real-time feedback, it is important to debrief on the learning experience to ensure all learning objectives are met, and students engage in active learning. The benefit of VR is that it can be used independently by students with unlimited scenario attempts to improve patient outcomes.

Human Patient Simulators

Human patient simulators are life-like, anatomically correct, computer-driven manikins with physiologic responses that mimic a real patient. These human patient simulators are controlled by instructors to create a structured learning environment in a clinically realistic setting where learning occurs (34). Human patient simulators can mimic diverse parameters of human anatomical physiology, for example, changes in cardiovascular, pulmonary, metabolic, and neurological systems. These simulators have the ability to respond to nursing or pharmacological interventions in real time (35). Additionally, human patient simulators are equipped with technology that can be displayed on bedside monitors to depict respiratory, cardiac, and hemodynamic instability. Eye blinking, tears, pulses, programmable voice responses, and intravenous line insertion are additional capabilities of high-fidelity manikins.

Human patient simulators are excellent when used to recreate or mimic an acute care environment. They allow students to assess the "patient" and, based on those findings, allow students to perform a range of nursing interventions. In a branching simulation scenario using a human patient simulator, students have the opportunity to make real-time decisions that impact patients' responses and outcomes within the scenario and increase student confidence (27, 34). Development of a simulation for patient management with a chest tube with the manikin developing respiratory distress due to kinked chest tubing is a great way for students to learn how to assess breath sounds and troubleshoot the tubing to ensure proper drainage. Once the tubing is fixed, the patient immediately improves.

Another example of high-fidelity manikin use is creating a simulation scenario with head trauma, using moulage to mimic an injury. Students can practice not only 'head-to-toe assessments but can place a Foley catheter and IV line and administer medications. By incorporating the physical findings with the patient's vital signs displayed on the bedside monitor, students can come to understand the whole patient presentation.

Birthing human patient simulators are high-fidelity manikins that are capable of simulating normal or abnormal delivery. This allows students to visualize contractions and vital signs on the patient's bedside monitor. Additionally, birthing simulators possess the ability to hemorrhage, therefore allowing students to learn about appropriate interventions in critical scenarios. A few examples of birthing scenarios can include normal vaginal delivery, complicated delivery caused by shoulder dystocia, and hemorrhage complications post-delivery. When the manikin hemorrhages, students can assess the color, consistency, and amount of blood loss to determine the severity of the situation and what is required for immediate intervention.

Pediatric and infant simulators have the capability to display the clinical presentation of a seizure, and their lips can become cyanotic to illustrate hypoxemia. Pediatric and infant simulators are considered essential resources because children often do not play the role of an SP. There are a range of scenarios where the use of pediatric human simulators is applicable. Students can practice basic skills, such as measuring the head circumference, or more complex skills, such as nasogastric tube feeding or providing care in a pediatric code.

Overall, human patient simulators provide life-like experiences for students where learning is optimized in a controlled, safe learning environment. It is immersive in nature and is where students can be given an opportunity to make real-time decisions to manage complex care (33–36).

Modalities and Simulation Fidelity

Modalities support the simulation educator in successfully setting the stage to mimic the reality of the physical clinical healthcare environment. Fidelity is another important consideration and determines how authentic the simulated environment is and how believable the clinical scenario is in relation to the environment. The higher the fidelity, the more realistic and believable the environment is for students (1). Simulation fidelity plays an integral role in immersing the learner into a particular clinical state or environment where the learner truly believes and reacts in meaningful ways to safely care for the patient. When a modality is chosen for a simulation experience in undergraduate nursing, testing the functionality of the modality and additional equipment is paramount for ensuring fidelity.

Low-fidelity simulation in undergraduate nursing can be used to develop student's knowledge and practical skills through the use of static models, two-dimensional displays, or partial manikins or task trainers for the practice of clinical skills such as IV insertion, urinary catheterization, or basic life support (1, 15). Low-fidelity manikins can be utilized for students to practice a basic 'head to toe' assessment, basic skills such as turning and repositioning a patient in bed, or basic wound care skills.

Medium fidelity simulation includes full-body manikins that can be controlled by an external, handheld device. They have more realism than low-fidelity simulators and can mimic cardiac, respiratory, and abdominal sounds. In undergraduate nursing, Medium fidelity simulation can include the use of manikins or task trainers that offer breath sounds, heart sounds, bowel sounds, or simulated blood but lack the authenticity of a realistic environment.

High-fidelity manikin-based simulation involves the use of sophisticated life-like situations where learners become fully immersed in a clinical scenario (1, 15). SPs provide the highest level of fidelity as they are 'live' and provide real-time, scenario-specific, and student-specific feedback in a constructive manner. To maximize the learning outcomes for students, it is important to train all SPs for each simulation experience and notify them of the expectations of both their roles and student roles and the time limit for feedback and debriefing. When SPs stray from the script or decide to throw students a "curveball," it is not beneficial to the scenario or learning outcome because, ultimately and unexpectedly, the outcome of the scenario may change. Conducting "just in time" training to answer questions, clarify any mood points, and role play, if necessary, is a good strategy to employ.

Moulage plays an important role in simulation fidelity because it helps create the realistic element of physical ailments, smells, and other features in a simulated environment, therefore, maximizing and increasing the level of simulation fidelity. Techniques used to simulate injury, disease, aging, and other physical characteristics specific to a scenario can be applied to a mannikin or an SP with their consent. Moulage supports the sensory perceptions of participants and supports the fidelity of the simulation scenario through the use of makeup, attachable artifacts (e.g., penetrating objects), and smells (37). Ready-to-use moulage molds are available for sale; however, mastering the art of moulage without causing damage to the simulator or task trainer is an art in itself and takes time, practice, and patience to perfect.

Operations and Modalities

Simulation operations are complex and intricate and have many moving pieces to consider when planning for a simulation-based experience. Modalities require financial resources and space considerations. These factors can be barriers if appropriate space and resource allocation are not established when budgeting for simulation expenses in a fiscal year. When operationalizing a clinical simulation scenario, it is important to match the appropriate learning modality available to the scenario objectives and to provide learners with the ability to meet these outcomes. To ensure student success in any simulation-based education activity, preparation is essential. This includes a student pre-brief assignment to prepare them for the simulation content, simulation room orientation, including the availability of supplies and functionality of the equipment in the simulation room, and environmental safety precautions to establish a safe environment (8, 38, 39).

Training of the faculty, facilitators, and educators is crucial to the operation of the simulation and the success of students. Orienting simulation educators to the simulated clinical environments allows for "hands-on" training and deliberate practice. It also helps to improve their skills when working with a variety of manikins, task trainers, standardized patients, and virtual reality platforms. As simulation modalities and their application in a simulated learning environment evolve, experienced educators are needed to best integrate these technologies and modalities into the simulated learning environment. Testing simulation equipment (manikins, task trainers) for functionality and conducting professional development for educators is crucial to ensure students are engaged, and there are no distractions. A team approach for planning, developing, and executing simulation scenarios, including 'dry runs' of newly developed and first-time simulations, are pivotal to addressing issues that may arise. Simulation operations staff also require training to accurately portray the environment to the expected fidelity of the clinical situation.

Conclusion

This chapter provides a broad overview of simulation modalities in undergraduate nursing programs. Simulation education in undergraduate nursing curricula continues to expand, with nursing educators striving to create innovative and high-quality simulated learning experiences for students. Undergraduate nursing education is now afforded a plethora of simulation modalities aimed at replicating the 'real world' clinical environment and the achievement of learning outcomes under dynamic conditions, emerging new technologies, and an evolving educational landscape. The array of simulation modalities provides rich opportunities for nurse educators to leverage the power of simulation to meet program outcomes and advance transformative learning for student readiness for entry into clinical practice.

References

1. Lioce L, Lopreiato J, Downing D, Chang TP., Robertson JM, Anderson M, Diaz DA, Spain AE. Healthcare simulation dictionary, 2nd ed. Rockville. 2020. https://doi.org/10.23970/simulationv2.
2. Cant RP, Cooper SJ. The value of simulation-based learning in pre-licensure nurse education: a state-of-the-art review and meta-analysis. Nurse Educ Pract. 2017;27:45–62. https://doi.org/10.1016/j.nepr.2017.08.012.
3. Cantrell MA, Franklin A, Leighton K, Carlson A. The evidence in simulation-based learning experiences in nursing education and practice: an umbrella review. Clin Simul Nurs. 2017;13(12):634–67. https://doi.org/10.1016/j.ecns.2017.08.004.
4. Hayden JK, Smiley RA, Alexander M, Kardong-Edgren S, Jeffries PR. The NCSBN national simulation study: a longitudinal, randomized controlled study replacing clinical hours with simulation in prelicensure nursing education. J Nurs Regul. 2014;5(2):S1–S64.
5. Aebersold M. Simulation-based learning: no longer a novelty in undergraduate education. Online J Issues Nurs. 2018;23(2):1.
6. Cant RP, Cooper SJ. Use of simulation-based learning in undergraduate nurse education: an umbrella systematic review. Nurse Educ Today. 2017;49:63–71. https://doi.org/10.1016/j.nedt.2016.11.015.
7. Institute of Medicine. The future of nursing: leading change, advancing health. Washington: The National Academies Press; 2011.
8. INACSL Standards Committee. INACSL standards of best practice: SimulationSMSimulation design. Clin Simul Nurs. 2016;12(S):S5–S12. https://doi.org/10.1016/j.ecns.2016.09.005.
9. Rudolph JW, Raemer DB, Simon R. Establishing a safe container for learning in simulation: the role of the simulation briefing. Simul Healthc. 2014;9(6):339–49.
10. Kolb DA. Experiential learning: experience as the source of learning and development. Englewood Cliffs: Prentice Hall; 1984.
11. Bandura A. Social cognitive theory: an agentic perspective. Annu Rev Psychol. 2001;52:1–26. https://doi.org/10.1146/annurev.psych.52.1.1.
12. Schon DA. Educating the reflective practitioner: toward a new design for teaching and learning in the professions. Hoboken: Wiley; 1987.
13. Sweller J. Cognitive load during problem-solving: effects on learning. Cogn Sci. 1988;12(2):257–85.
14. Knowles MS. Andragogy in action: applying modern principles of adult learning. San Francisco: Jossey-Bass; 1984.
15. INACSL Standards Committee. INACSL standards of best practice: SimulationSM simulation glossary. Clin Simul Nurs. 2016;12(S):S39–47. https://doi.org/10.1016/j.ecns.2016.09.012.
16. Hallmark BF. Faculty development in simulation education. Nurs Clin North Am. 2015;50(2):389–97. https://doi.org/10.1016/j.cnur.2015.03.002.
17. INACSL Standards Committee. INACSL standards of best practice: SimulationSM facilitation clinical simulation in nursing. 12:S16–S20.
18. Lewis KL, Bohnert CA, Gammon WL, et al. The Association of Standardized Patient Educators (ASPE) Standards of Best Practice (SOBP). Adv Simul. 2017;2:10. https://doi.org/10.1186/s41077-017-0043-4.
19. Rutherford-Hemming T, Alfes CM, Breymier TL. A systematic review of the use of standardized patients as a simulation modality in nursing education. Nurs Educ Perspect. 2019;40(2):84–90.
20. Slater LZ, Bryant KD, Ng V. Nursing student perceptions of standardized patient use in health assessment. Clin Simul Nurs. 2016;12(9):368–76. https://doi.org/10.1016/j.ecns.2016.04.007.
21. Foronda CL. What is virtual simulation? Clin Simul Nurs. 2021;52:8.

22. Cant R, Cooper S, Sussex R, Bogossian F. What's in a name? Clarifying the nomenclature of virtual simulation. Clin Simul Nurs. 2019;27:26–30. http://search.ebscohost.com/login.aspx?direct=true&db=edsbl&AN=vdc.100074516786.0x000001&site=eds-live.
23. Kardong-Edgren S, Farra SL, Alinier G, Young HM. A call to unify definitions of virtual reality. Clin Simul Nurs. 2019;31:28–34.
24. Foronda CL, Fernandez-Burgos M, Nadeau C, Kelley CN, Henry MN. Virtual simulation in nursing education: a systematic review spanning 1996 to 2018. Simul Healthc. 2020;15(1):46–54. https://doi.org/10.1097/SIH.0000000000000411.
25. Fogg N, Kubin L, Wilson CE, Trinka M. Using virtual simulation to develop clinical judgment in undergraduate nursing students. Clin Simul Nurs. 2020;48:55–8.
26. Foronda CL, Hudson KW, Budhathoki C. Use of virtual simulation to impact nursing students' cognitive and affective knowledge of evidence-based practice. Worldviews Evid Based Nurs. 2017;14(2):168–70. https://doi.org/10.1111/wvn.12207.
27. Pasklinsky N, Graham-Perel A, Villacarlos-Philip P, Slaka-Vella M, Tilley CP. Real-time decision-making in chronic illness branching simulation. Mhealth. 2021;7:14. https://doi.org/10.21037/mhealth-19-215.
28. Verkuyl M, Lapum JL, St-Amant O, Hughes M, Romaniuk D. Curricular uptake of virtual gaming simulation in nursing education. Nurse Educ Pract. 2021;50:102967. https://doi.org/10.1016/j.nepr.2021.102967.
29. Gentry SV, Gauthier A, L'Estrade Ehrstrom B, Wortley D, Lilienthal A, Tudor Car L, Dauwels-Okutsu S, Nikolaou CK, Zary N, Campbell J, Car J. Serious gaming and gamification education in health professions: systematic review. J Med Internet Res. 2019;21(3):e12994. https://doi.org/10.2196/12994.
30. Cheng A, Kolbe M, Grant V, et al. A practical guide to virtual debriefings: communities of inquiry perspective. Adv Simul. 2020;5:18. https://doi.org/10.1186/s41077-020-00141-1.
31. Moro C, Štromberga Z, Raikos A, Stirling A. The effectiveness of virtual and augmented reality in health sciences and medical anatomy. Anat Sci Educ. 2017;10(6):549–59. https://doi.org/10.1002/ase.1696.
32. Foronda CL, Alfes CM, Dev P, Kleinheksel AJ, Nelson DA Jr, O'Donnell JM, Samosky JT. Virtually nursing: emerging technologies in nursing education. Nurse Educ. 2017;42(1):14–7. https://doi.org/10.1097/NNE.0000000000000295.
33. Kardong-Edgren S, Breitkreuz K, Werb M, Foreman S, Ellertson A. Evaluating the usability of a second-generation virtual reality game for refreshing sterile urinary catheterization skills. Nurse Educ. 2019;44(3):137–41. https://doi.org/10.1097/NNE.0000000000000570.
34. Doolen J, Marian B, Atz T, Horsley TL, Rourke J, McAfee K, Cross CL. High-fidelity simulation in undergraduate nursing education: a review of simulation reviews. Clin Simul Nurs. 2016;12(7):290–302. https://doi.org/10.1016/j.ecns.2016.01.009.
35. Hanshaw SL, Dickerson SS. High fidelity simulation evaluation studies in nursing education: a review of the literature. Nurse Educ Pract. 2020;46:102818. https://doi.org/10.1016/j.nepr.2020.102818.
36. Labrague LJ, McEnroe-Petitte DM, Bowling AM, Nwafor CE, Tsaras K. High-fidelity simulation and nursing students' anxiety and self-confidence: a systematic review. Nurs Forum. 2019;54(3):358–68. https://doi.org/10.1111/nuf.12337.
37. Smith-Stoner M. Using moulage to enhance educational instruction. Nurse Educ. 2011;36(1):21–4. https://doi.org/10.1097/NNE.0b013e3182001e98.
38. The INACSL Standards Committee. INACSL standards of best practice: SimulationSM: operations. Clin Simul Nurs. 2017;13(12):681–7. https://doi.org/10.1016/j.ecns.2017.10.005.
39. Rutherford-Hemming T, Lioce L, Breymier T. Guidelines and essential elements for prebriefing. Simul Healthc. 2019;14(6):409–14. https://doi.org/10.1097/SIH.0000000000000403.

Writing Clinical Simulations for Undergraduate Nursing Education

5

Stephen Guinea and Patrea Andersen

A Structured Design Framework

Critical and pragmatic considerations are essential at every step of the simulation design process. Taking time to conceptualize a simulation and outline the key considerations for planning a simulation activity before using templates enables simulation educators to focus on the educational experience without being constrained or distracted by a simulation template. This ensures the greatest return on investment in relation to time, effort, and financial resourcing and enhances the longevity of simulation activities and programs.

The structured design process presented in this chapter incorporates key principles and best practice guidelines for simulation, educational design, and curriculum design. The process comprises a framework of nine focused design elements for consideration. These are:

1. *The need:* Considerations that result in a clear statement of purpose that justifies the need for the simulation activity and the theoretical perspective of learning that aligns the simulation activity with the broader curriculum.
2. *Participant group:* Understanding who the simulation experience is being designed for and their characteristics is important to inform the selection of simulation modality and the level of facilitation employed.
3. *Purpose and learning outcomes*: Clarifying the purpose or objective of the scenario informs the development of learning outcomes. The purpose describes what the simulation designers wish to achieve and the learning outcomes state the desired behavior or attributes students should be able to demonstrate by the end of the simulation.
4. *Simulation scenario*: When choosing a scenario, consideration should be given to the desired behavior expected of students to achieve the learning outcomes and potential practice-based situations that will allow students to demonstrate the desired behavior.
5. *Simulation modality and rationale:* An important consideration is selecting the modality based on the best fit for the specific simulation activity and which will provide the best opportunity for students to achieve the desired learning outcomes.
6. *Resources and preparation:* The environmental and human resources required for the simulation learning event must be identified.
7. *Pre-simulation brief:* Developing information and the orientation session before the scenario is necessary to adequately prepare students for the simulation experience. The participant group, learning outcomes, and antecedent knowledge and skills are key elements.
8. *Debrief*: This involves selecting a model or framework of debriefing that aligns with the purpose, theoretical perspective, objectives, and learning outcomes of the simulation.
9. *Evaluation/assessment:* This includes the designed strategies and measures that demonstrate the achievement of the purpose, objectives and learning outcomes and, thus, the value of the simulation learning experience.

The purpose of this chapter is to provide a framework in the form of a structured concept map. Once this process is complete, the simulation activity can be applied to any given simulation template. In addition, essential considerations are explored, providing the reader with the foundations of simulation design for undergraduate nursing education. While the context of this chapter is simulation design for undergraduate nursing education, the principles presented could translate to different contexts, disciplines, and learner levels.

S. Guinea (✉)
Australian Catholic University, Melbourne, VIC, Australia
e-mail: Stephen.Guinea@acu.edu.au

P. Andersen
University of the Sunshine Coast, Sippy Downs, Australia

J. M. Kutzin et al. (eds.), *Comprehensive Healthcare Simulation: Nursing*, Comprehensive Healthcare Simulation,
https://doi.org/10.1007/978-3-031-31090-4_5

What Is the Need?

Understanding the need is possibly the most important consideration when designing any educational activity, whether for teaching, learning, or assessment. Without understanding the need, a designed experience may be misdirected and fail to align with the intended purpose, learning outcomes, and evaluation and assessment. In the context of simulation, this impacts the outcomes of the curriculum and can also be expensive. A structured approach to exploring the need for simulation can ensure that all simulation learning events specifically addresses identified needs.

A needs assessment [1] should inform simulation activities, for it is a needs assessment that provides the evidence required for the justification of any educational activity [2]. A helpful way to consider a needs assessment is as a scoping activity, with the purpose being to think through the overall purpose of the simulation activity and the broader context within which the simulation will be situated. A good place to start is with the targeted participants and the learning context. In the context of this chapter, the target participants are undergraduate nursing students. Considerations may include:

- Who are the students, and what is known about them?
- What is the anticipated level of understanding, skill, and experience of the students in relation to practice and in relation to simulation?
- What is the anticipated outcome or the desired observable change in behavior students are expected to demonstrate after the simulation experience?
- What are the actual and potential constraints to effective learning? For example, time available for the learning experience, physical resources, human resources, including educators, and scheduling.
- What possible ways can the education or training experience be provided (didactic, practical skills, game, simulation)? What are the pros and cons of each? Why is simulation the best option?
- What is the timeline for development and implementation?

Undertaking a needs assessment as the first step in simulation design provides an opportunity to consider strategic drivers of education from the perspectives of accrediting bodies (standards, guidelines, legislation), organizational needs (strategic plans, missions, reports of near misses, patient safety incidents and sentinel events, curricula), and learners (performance gaps in relation to current and future skills or competency). Additionally, contemporary healthcare imperatives such as patient safety can be used to justify the purpose of specific simulation education and training programs [3].

Learning activities are designed, broadly speaking, for one of three purposes: teaching, learning, and assessment. These form the basis of the design process. It is equally important to align the purpose of the simulation activity with an appropriate theoretical perspective of learning, for example, behaviorism, cognitivism, constructivism, and social constructivism [1, 3]. Doing so enhances the quality of the simulation activity and advances simulation as a robust educational experience. Examples where theoretical perspectives have been used to inform simulation design, are provided in Chap. 4.

The outcome of this first step is a clear statement that justifies the planned simulation activity. The statement should make a clear connection between the need (e.g., curriculum, mission, legislation) and the intended learning as an outcome of the simulation experience. Once this statement is constructed, planning for the simulation can continue in more depth.

Participant Group

Understanding student characteristics for the designed simulation activity is an equally important early step in the simulation design process. Student group characteristics include discipline-specific considerations and simulation-specific considerations [4]. Discipline-specific considerations relate to curriculum, the knowledge, skills, and prior experiences students will bring to the simulation. These, in turn, will inform the types of situations to be simulated that the students can relate to [1]. Simulation-specific considerations relate to the number and type of previous simulation activities students have experienced. Importantly, do students understand how learning occurs through simulation, the pre-simulation brief, participating in the simulation scenario and in different simulation modes, and what is expected during the debrief. Understanding these characteristics is important to inform the selection of simulation modality and the level of facilitation employed [5, 6].

Purpose, Learning Outcomes

The needs assessment will provide the overall purpose of the simulation activity. The purpose is considered educator focussed in that its intent is to be aligned with the overall curriculum (course). For example, what is the desired level of cognitive effort [7, 8] of students when participating in the simulation? Is it envisaged that students participate in the simulation as individuals or in small groups? Does the simulation require students to engage in critical thinking and clinical reasoning? If the purpose of the designed simulation is to provide opportunities for students to use these higher-order skills, careful consideration should be given to the difficulty and complexity of the scenario and the expected standard of performance. For example, the difficulty of a scenario can be designed using cues and the cuing [9] provided to students during the simulation scenario. Examples are whether assessment findings are provided to students or whether students need to obtain the assessment findings themselves, whether the facilitator is embedded in the scenario to provide guiding cues to keep the scenario on track, or whether the scenario requires students to make all decisions themselves. These factors will all affect the difficulty of the simulation as experienced by students. The complexity of a scenario can also be planned. For example, the number of tasks or challenges presented to students or the complexity of the clinical presentation.

Cognitive effort should be aligned with the overarching pedagogical philosophy of a program (such as inquiry-based learning), the level of the student in the program of study, the simulation learning outcomes, and the structure and process of the debrief. Careful consideration is needed to determine the learning outcomes of the simulation, the experience level of the student group, and the expectations of performance. If the students are novice learners, then it may be advisable to design the scenario with the facilitator's presence to provide support.

In contrast to the purpose or objectives, learning outcomes should be student-focused and a statement of what students are expected to demonstrate as a result of the learning experience. In the design of any educational activity, the educator deliberately designs the learning experiences, including tasks with which students are able to participate, methods of assessment, and feedback processes, so that it aligns with planned learning outcomes [10, 11]. Put another way, learning outcomes inform all aspects of simulation design.

In the context of undergraduate and pre-registration nursing education, the scenario design must align with the overall curriculum learning outcomes and professional competencies. This requires mapping the simulation event to course learning outcomes and course content to ensure the simulation experience is integrated and adds value to the curriculum and professional requirements for practice. In relation to simulation design, learning outcomes inform the entire simulation learning event, including the debrief.

Learning outcomes provide the essential point of reference for quality education design. These outcomes should guide all aspects of simulation design, implementation, and evaluation [1]. Providing clear learning outcomes also provides transparency between teaching, learning, and assessment. To construct appropriate learning outcome statements, the seminal educationalist Robert Mager proposed that each statement should include the following:

a verb indicating the expected performance to be observed,

a statement of the conditions under which the performance is to take place, and

the criteria or the quality of the performance deemed acceptable [12]. See Box 5.1.

Box 5.1 Example of a Learning Outcome for a Simulation Experience

At the end of this simulation experience, students will be able to:

- Demonstrate (verb) basic life support in a simulation environment (conditions) in accordance with the Australian Resuscitation Council basic life support guidelines (criteria).

In addition, key principles for constructing learning outcome statements are to keep them specific, measurable, achievable, realistic, and timely (SMART) [13].

There will usually be two to three learning outcomes for a simulation. Learning outcomes provide the point of reference for the entire simulation, connecting the pre-simulation brief, the simulation scenario, the post-simulation debrief, and the assessment of learning. The more learning outcomes, the more complex a simulation tends to be. Quite often, up to three well-constructed learning outcomes will suffice for a simulation comprising a 5-min pre-simulation brief, a 15-min scenario, and a 30-min debrief.

Simulation Scenario

Choosing a simulation scenario involves considering the desired behavior expected of students to achieve the learning outcomes and potential practice-based situations that will provide students with the opportunity to demonstrate the desired behavior.

Elements for consideration when selecting and designing a simulation scenario include professional practice factors, physical requirements, environmental factors, psychological factors, and time.

Professional practice factors include replicating essential characteristics of real clinical situations and professional interactions in the simulation. For example, who are the people and the artifacts of practice required for the situation to be replicated? How many students would normally be present in a real practice-based situation? Will student roles in the scenario be that of a student or as a qualified professional? What are the implications for students' understanding of the scope of practice? Related considerations include the number of students in a class, the desired number of students who will interact directly in the simulation scenarios, and whether observational roles are appropriate.

Physical elements include considering the physical activities students will be expected to undertake during the scenario. What equipment is required to perform the physical activity? What space is required? Is what is proposed feasible? What is the risk to safety?

Environmental considerations include ensuring classes in nearby areas where a simulation will be taking place. One example is sound. If more than one simulation or class is being conducted within the same area, there is the possibility that sound will unintentionally carry from one room to another. This can result in disruption, breaches of privacy, and, depending on the simulation scenario, distress from classes overhearing the sounds arising from a simulation.

Psychological considerations relate to how students may respond emotionally to a simulation experience. It is not possible to know the impact simulation may have on students. Some simulated situations can be so real for students that they trigger strong emotional responses. Students may worry about their performance and become stressed. While debriefing is designed to ensure that events are managed appropriately and people are supported so that there is a successful outcome, there are times when additional support is required, such as when simulations are purposefully designed to evoke strong emotional responses such as anxiety, frustration, and sometimes fear. It is essential to plan for how student distress will be managed should this arise. Psychological considerations can include the likelihood that the topic of the simulation or the replicated situation may closely reflect negative experiences students have had either in practice or their private lives. Questions to ask include is it possible that the simulation may evoke a response? How will adverse responses be managed on the day? What supports are available for students should this be an issue during or after the simulation?

The environmental, physical, and psychological safety of the proposed simulation experience can be determined by completing a risk assessment.

Time

One of the greatest challenges when designing simulations is that of time. In the undergraduate context, time is a crucial consideration, particularly when matching scenarios to real-world expectations. Suppose the unfolding situation takes longer than the allocated scenario time. How can the scenario be presented to students that are sufficiently realistic and maintains coherence with the trajectory of a simulated situation to students?

If group numbers are small, it may be possible for participants as individuals or in pairs to complete the simulation one after the other in the allotted time. Using a group simulation design may be helpful when large groups of people are involved. This incorporates observational simulation. In this model, participants rotate through scenarios. For example, if there are 12 participants in a group, working in groups of three students could rotate through four simulations. At any given time, three would undertake the simulation, and nine would be observing. At the end of the simulations, all students will have actively participated in a simulation, will have observed all simulations, and participated in all debrief sessions. Tasks may be given to observers to enhance their involvement in the simulation. Their contributions can be included in the debrief.

A balance needs to be managed between the designer of the simulation replicating a real situation and ensuring opportunities for learning are provided. Whilst it can be tempting to authentically replicate an actual real-life situation, the simulation must not overwhelm the students and always remain focused on student learning. Consideration should also be given to the amount of experience students have had. It is reasonable for students to take longer to perform procedures than experienced clinicians. However, one of the objectives of simulation is to prepare graduates that are work ready and can meet the demands of the practice environment. This means students need to learn how to perform procedures promptly. Simulation provides excellent opportunities to learn these skills in a safe environment. The key is to maintain a balance between providing sufficient time to ensure success and maintaining realism.

Simulation Modality and Rationale

Many simulation users may prefer a particular modality of simulation. However, it is important to remember that there is no single best mode. The selection of simulation modality should be based on the best fit for each simulation activity. Importantly, sustainability is a critical consideration for simulation design, and pragmatic considerations are required to ensure longevity for the designed simulation experience.

A simulated practice-based situation can be delivered using a range of simulation modalities. Chapters 1 and 4 list and summarise common and emerging simulation modes used in pre-registration nursing education. When selecting a simulation modality, it is worth considering the following:

- Possible simulation modalities: What are the possible ways this situation can be simulated?
- Capability and capacity: What access is there to equipment, technology, technical support, staff experienced in modes of simulation, and staff availability to deliver the simulation?
- Realism/fidelity: What is the desired level of realism to be replicated? How real do the scenario, environment, and

roles need to be to enable participants to suspend disbelief and engage with the scenario?

In addition to simulation modality, how a simulation is structured also relates to the sustainability of a simulation design.

One of the common approaches to simulation structure is (1) Pre-simulation activity, ensuring students have been provided with the antecedent knowledge and skills required to fully participate in the simulation scenario; (2) Pre-simulation brief; (3) Simulation scenario; and (4) Post-simulation debrief. An alternative approach can be to omit the pre-simulation activity and the pre-simulation brief and expose students directly to the scenario. This approach is often used in professional practice situations where experienced health professionals are assumed to have achieved and maintained a certain level of competence (e.g., annual credentialing for CPR). If this approach is used, debriefing is vital to ensure learning occurs from the mistakes made. Invariably, individuals will feel unhappy with their performance. Hence, the debrief session needs to be allocated extended time and will need to be skilfully facilitated. For this approach to be successful and affirming, it is recommended that participants can have another attempt at the scenario, demonstrate what has been learned, and improve their perception of themself. This takes time. Whilst this 'baptism by fire' approach may be selected to provide a more authentic replication of a real situation, it can also be very stressful for novice learners and is not recommended for undergraduate students.

Pause and reflect is a simulation structure that can be particularly useful for inexperienced student cohorts or for very complex scenarios. Pause and reflect comprises two forms of debriefing. The first is during the simulation, where the instructor calls for 'time out' often when the student's performance is deviating significantly from that which is desired or when a teachable moment is reached. The pause enables the facilitator to engage students in a brief period of reflection, consideration of the presenting situation, and discussion of possible options to follow. Whilst there is no general rule, a pause should be brief, lasting no more than 1–2 min, and pauses should be limited to 2–3 per 15-min scenario. The longer the duration of a pause, the more likely the pause will result in a teaching session. The greater the number of pauses in a scenario, the greater the likelihood that students will have trouble suspending disbelief and disengage from the scenario. When using the pause and pause and discuss structure, the formal post-simulation debrief provides students with an opportunity to reflect on the whole scenario.

Tag Team Patient Safety Simulation provides another way that simulation can be structured. This approach draws on the theoretical underpinnings of Forum Theatre [14]. Tag Team stands for:

T = Theatrical. Embracing the dramatic contribution of acting to learning

A = Applied. Reflecting the functional and pragmatic realism of theatre

G = Guided. The 'Director' facilitates the learning experience

T = Tactical. Strategically designed to achieve pre-defined learning outcomes

E = Engaged. Immerses the learner in authentic learning experiences

A = Active. Interactive learning opportunities through the provision of dynamic simulation experiences

M = Meaningful. Memorable learning experiences [15]

This unique approach to simulation provides an opportunity for students to 'rehearse' a range of interpersonal, cognitive, and metacognitive skills in preparation for safe clinical practice. The scenario (play) incorporates a semi-structured script based on the Australian National Safety and Quality Health Service Standards [16]. The plot of the script is guided by a facilitator who assumes the role of the director. An actor (simulated participant, student, or masked educator [17]) assumes the role of a patient (the protagonist). The narrator introduces the patient and provides the prologue. Students (cast) respond to the pre-determined needs of the patient, drawing on their knowledge and skills and improvising to dramatize the essence of the scenario. The 'play' addresses key learning outcomes and generally comprises two or more acts. In the first act, the scenario is played out without interruption. Intermission provides the opportunity for the audience to reflect on the scene that unfolded and its outcomes. Socratic dialogue by the Director guides the discussion and facilitates the identification of key practice issues. Act Two follows, providing an opportunity for students to try out what they have learned from Act One and Intermission. During each act, students can 'Tag' players and replace them to try out alternative interventions. Complex plays with lots of players require careful consideration. Managing the level of interactivity can be problematic if the play is too complex. This simulation method can be used with very large student groups and utilizes observational simulation [18, 19].

Resources Required and Preparation

Resources include considering the environmental and human resources required to make the simulation work. The simulation modality chosen for the simulation will influence the type of technology, equipment, and human resources needed. For example, if high-technology manikin simulation is the modality chosen, it is important to consider the availability of the manikin. Who will be available to operate the manikin each time the simulation runs is an essential consideration. If dedicated technical staff are available and familiar with the technology, the simulation may run well 'on the fly.' If staff are less familiar with the technology, or if the person operating the simulator is also the class facilitator, it may be appropriate to run a pre-built scenario.

The type and amount of equipment to incorporate in the simulation depends on the desired realism level. Ensuring that the equipment provided to students in the simulation is current with what is used in everyday practice is important. In addition, the equipment provided to students in the simulation should be the same as those that students have practiced with in class unless the purpose of the simulation is to provide students with a more challenging experience. Many media- to high-technology manikins can provide the user with feedback in the form of pulses, respiration rate and breath sounds, blood pressure, heart rate, and heart sounds. Products such as Laerdal's Patient Monitor Software® and iSimulate REALITi® can simulate patient monitors using a manikin or simulated participant. When considering the use of such technology, it is worth considering the learning outcomes for simulation and the desired skills students will apply in this situation. For example, perform vital signs manually, or is it suitable for students to use a monitor?

It is worthwhile to consider the possible ways in which students may respond to the unfolding scenario. As it is impossible to predict every way students approach the situation, it is important to ensure that a range of equipment is available. Students' suspension of disbelief will 'drop out' if they go for a piece of equipment that is unavailable to them. Also, consider the props that might be needed to enhance realism.

Resource considerations are not just for technology-based simulations. In the example of using a role-play, what are the environmental requirements for this simulation activity? How much equipment and what are the props required to enable students to buy into the simulation and suspend disbelief? Which roles are required to authentically portray the desired interaction? Who will play these roles, and what form will the preparation for these roles take?

Preparation is an essential consideration but one that is easily overlooked. Preparation takes the form of environment, staff, and students.

Considerations for the preparation of the environment can be as simple as how much time is required to prepare the environment for the simulation. Is the physical space vacant to allow preparation? If the simulation is being run multiple times, are other simulations or activities using the same space, and how will this impact setup and pack-down? Are faculty staff available to do this work?

If moulage is being used, some important considerations include the time required to apply the moulage. How robust does the moulage need to be; is it for a visual cue, or will students be applying dressings that may damage the appearance?

It is always a good idea to have a 'backup plan'. In undergraduate education, classes cannot be canceled and are often difficult to be rescheduled. Like other classes, the simulation must run according to the timetable. Consider how you might manage a situation where a facilitator or simulated participant is unwell and unable to attend.

All staff involved in facilitating a simulation must be prepared for their role. Building in staff preparation is part of the design process. It is most useful to plan and conduct a special preparation session where teaching and technical staff are orientated to the environment in which the simulation will take place and, ideally, participate in a dry run of the simulation. Staff preparation should include the following:

- Course learning outcomes and content specific to the simulations.
- Learning outcomes for the simulation.
- Simulation modality and management.
- Roles and responsibilities of facilitators and support available.
- Review of the scenario.
- Preparation of simulated participants (if used).
- Preparation of students/participants.
- Simulation rules—Safety, Confidentiality, Consent, Filming, Security (if applicable).
- Expected demonstrated actions and reactions of students during the simulation and expected standard of performance.
- Debriefing model.
- Assessment (if applicable).

If using a simulated participant (also known as a simulated patient) methodology [20], scheduling a preparation session for the simulated patients/actors is essential. Such a preparation session should include:

- Venue dates/reporting times and time commitment.
- A summary of the course and content.
- Learning outcomes for simulation.
- What to bring (clothing, food, drink).
- Issues related to Safety, Confidentiality, Consent, Filming, and Security.
- The briefing document for the role will include key information relating to the role, including guidelines and boundaries within which the simulated participant can improvise. This allows simulated patients to be more responsive to students and provide a more authentic learning experience. Briefing for the role also includes mechanisms to manage situations during a scenario with potential harm to a student or the simulated participant.
- Orientation to the environment and equipment to be used.
- Opportunities to rehearse and receive feedback from facilitators.

- Whether the simulated participant will be involved in debriefing and what this will involve, such as providing students with feedback.
- Debriefing and support for the simulated participant.
- How the simulated participant's experience of this entire simulation process will be evaluated.

When engaging actors as simulated participants, it is important to understand the conditions of employment according to employment legislation and awards. Engaging members of the community as volunteers requires considerations for public safety, including public liability insurance, as well as understanding legislative requirements for the use of community members as volunteers. In addition, legal requirements exist when working with vulnerable populations such as children and aged populations, including issues such as gaining consent [21].

The focus of student preparation is to ensure the students have the required knowledge, skills, and attributes to participate in the simulation. How integrated the simulation is with the curriculum relates to how well the simulation scenario draws on the course content students have been exposed to, the simulation experiences they have participated in, and their experiences of professional practice during practicum. Student preparation may include pre-reading, videos, or skills stations. If the simulation activity includes students in a role, critical considerations include providing students with the resources to prepare for the role and giving students sufficient time to prepare.

In addition, the pre-simulation brief is the dedicated time in the simulation process that focuses on preparing students for the simulation.

Pre-simulation Brief

Pre-simulation briefing, or pre-briefing, is essential to the simulation process. The pre-simulation brief is essentially an orientation session conducted before the start of the simulation, where information about the simulation experience is provided to students, including the learning outcomes, the scenario, and the expectations of students [22, 23]. Some describe the value of the pre-simulation brief as creating a safe learning environment by establishing a mutual understanding of expectations, reducing students' insecurity of making mistakes, lessening the propensity for defensive behaviors, and setting the entire tone of the simulation learning environment [23, 24]. One way to structure a pre-simulation brief is using the funnel metaphor, starting broadly and narrowing the focus for students at the end. For example:

- Establish a Safe Learning Environment.
  - Permission to make mistakes, fiction contract, confidentiality, consent for filming if relevant, security of data collected, and supports available during and after the simulation experience if students experience distress related to the simulation.
- Outline of the simulation experience:
  - Course learning outcomes and knowledge and skills specific to the simulation
  - Simulation learning outcomes
  - Simulation modality being used
  - Phases of the simulation, such as pre-simulation brief, scenario, debrief, and duration of each. Any breaks?
  - Description of the debriefing model being used and the expectations of student participation in the debrief.
  - Expected standard of performance, criteria, and methods of evaluation.
- Focussed introduction to the scenario:
  - Statement of the scenario.
  - Statement of roles to be portrayed and preparation for roles.
  - Orientation to scenario time.
  - Orientation of students to the simulation environment and equipment used. Ensure students actively search for and manipulate equipment essential to the scenario. For example, if obtaining blood pressure from a manikin is essential to the scenario, ensure students obtain the blood pressure during orientation. This will significantly reduce anxiety during the scenario.
- Provide an opportunity for students to ask questions and seek clarification.

Providing sufficient time for students to prepare for roles is an important consideration that can be easily overlooked. Some roles require little preparation, for example, when a student nurse is portraying a student nurse role. However, it may be appropriate to provide students with a week or more to prepare for more complex roles or simulations. One approach to enhancing the authenticity of complex roles portrayed by students is to co-construct the roles with the relevant students over the weeks leading up to the simulation.

Another consideration relating to roles is that of observers. For many nursing schools, pragmatic constraints require simulations involving large class sizes whereby few students participate in the scenario, and many more observe. Some researchers report that observers typically learn less than learners with a 'hands-on' experience and are often less satisfied with the simulation experience [25, 26]. Evidence suggests that creating a role for students observing a simulation, providing role clarity, using tools that provide a focus for observers, and including observers' perspectives during the post-simulation debrief can increase the achievement of learning outcomes and satisfaction with the simulation experience [27, 28].

Debrief

Like all other simulation elements, the post-simulation debrief requires consideration as a designed element of simulation [29]. There are many models or frameworks of debriefing. Many follow a structured three-phase pattern of reactions, analysis/discussion, and summary [30]; a structure that has been suggested enhances learning [31]. It is, however, important to align a debriefing model with the purpose, theoretical perspective, objectives, and learning outcomes of the simulation.

For example, reflection and reflective learning are arguably the most important aspects and outcomes of the post-simulation debrief [32–34]. The engagement of participants in interactive critical reflection during the post-simulation debrief has been recognized as key to improved learning [35]. However, reflection is a skill that requires development, and reflective learning can be taxing. For student nurses enrolled in the early years of their program, a debriefing model such as Plus-Delta or Gather, Analyse, Summarise (GAS) [36] may be appropriate to introduce students to reflective learning. Debriefing models that require a more advanced level of reflective learning and foster the development of higher-order thinking include Debriefing for Meaningful Learning [37] or Debriefing with Good Judgement [38].

Regardless of the model, a critical consideration when designing the debriefing phase of a simulation is the level of competence of faculty with the debriefing model. This is for the simple reason that the student experience of post-simulation debriefs can largely depend on the facilitator's confidence and capability. Therefore, effective planning, education, and training are critical to ensure that educators understand the structure and timing of the simulation overall and the debrief specifically.

Finally, despite consensus about the essential role of debriefing in simulation-based learning, time restrictions too often compromise the length and quality of debriefing. Due consideration must be given when selecting a debriefing model in relation to the time required to facilitate the debrief for a specific simulation. Factors that will impact the time required include the number of learning outcomes to be addressed, the debriefing model selected, the complexity of the scenario, the number of students who will be involved in the debrief (direct participants, observers), and the involvement of simulated participants.

Evaluation/Assessment

Evaluation and assessment are essential considerations for any learning activity in nursing education. The resource intensiveness of simulation-based learning requires careful consideration of what and how to evaluate and undertake these considerations as part of the design process. Both evaluation and assessment should be directly related to the objectives and learning outcomes developed as step 3 of this structured design framework. By aligning the purpose, learning outcomes, and evaluation measures, it should be possible to demonstrate the value of a simulation learning experience embedded within nursing curricula and forms the foundation for education practice based on continuous improvement [1].

A range of evaluation tools and research instruments have been developed to measure simulation outcomes and promote continuous improvement from the perspectives of the participant (student) and facilitator. Examples include the evaluation of participant satisfaction [39–43], achievement of learning outcomes [44, 45], and facilitator self-evaluation of performance [46].

While the primary purpose of a simulation is to facilitate learning, simulation can be used as means to construct events to formally assess performance. If an assessment is the purpose, all the above design considerations should be addressed. However, in addition, students must be provided with the assessment criteria that clearly state what will be assessed and the expected standard. Careful consideration must be given if planning group assessments using simulation. Whilst possible, assessment criteria for group assessments must focus on teamwork and group dynamics rather than individual knowledge or technical skill.

Consideration should also be given to how the assessment will be moderated. One example is the use of video recordings. Important considerations for simulation learning environments with recording capability include which camera angles are best for capturing the activity in the scenario. For example, the assessment will not be valid if a student's back is to the camera at any time. Similarly, it is important to ensure any recording system is sensitive enough to capture communication during the scenario or not too sensitive that environmental noise drowns out communication.

Consideration is also required for the assessment of attributes such as critical thinking, clinical reasoning, and clinical judgment. If assessing critical thinking, clinical reasoning, and clinical judgment, it is important to consider strategies that enable students to demonstrate these attributes, such as 'Think Aloud' [47, 48], whereby students articulate what they think while they perform the various tasks. Importantly, measures are required to ensure the reliability and validity of the assessment process when using simulation and include designed scenarios and processes that facilitate a standardized experience for all students.

Conclusion

The design phase of simulation is critical to the quality, effectiveness, and sustainability of a simulation event or program. This chapter presented a framework that provides a structured and sequential process for simulation design. The framework provides a simple planner comprising nine focused design elements presented as a structured concept map. The description accompanying each design element provides many fundamental concepts, principles, and evidence of simulation practice.

There are many approaches to designing simulations. However, as one component of a coherent and integrated curriculum, simulation events must be designed as a constructively aligned educational learning experience embedded within curricula rather than an activity that is simply added on. In this chapter, the importance of understanding the priorities and the available resources of the organization and the target participant group for which a simulation is designed has been emphasized. This chapter has aimed to provide simulation designers with critical and pragmatic considerations deemed essential at every step of the simulation design process to ensure the greatest return on investment in relation to time, effort, and financial resourcing and enhancing longevity of simulation activities and programs. Whilst the process presented in this chapter may seem too onerous and unnecessary, educators may find that investing time in the design phase may well provide benefits in the longer term. The value of considered simulation design is explored further, with three examples provided, in Chap. 4.

References

1. INACSL Standards Committee, Watts PI, McDermott DS, Alinier G, Charnetski M, Nawathe PA. Healthcare Simulation Standards of Best PracticeTM Simulation Design. Clinical Simulation in Nursing. 2021;58:14–21. https://doi.org/10.1016/j.ecns.2021.08.009.
2. Sleezer CM, Russ-Eft D, Gupta K. A practical guide to needs assessment. 3rd ed. San Francisco: Wiley; 2014.
3. Levett-Jones T, Guinea S. The evolution of a mnemonic for quality simulation practices. Clin Simul Nurs. 2017;13(11):552–61. https://doi.org/10.1016/j.ecns.2017.07.004.
4. Chu EMY, Sheppard L, Guinea S, Imms C. Placement replacement: a conceptual framework for designing simulated clinical placement in occupational therapy. Nurs Health Sci. 2019;21(1):4–13. https://doi.org/10.1111/nhs.12551.
5. Fanning RM, Gaba D. The role of debriefing in simulation-based learning. Simul Healthc. 2007;2(2):115–25. https://doi.org/10.1097/SIH.0b013e3180315539.
6. Kelly M, Guinea S. Facilitating healthcare simulations. In: Nestel D, Kelly M, Jolly B, Watson M, editors. Healthcare simulation education: theory, evidence, and practice. Wiley Blackwell: Chichester; 2018. p. 143–51.
7. Reedy GB. Using cognitive load theory to inform simulation design and practice. Clin Simul Nurs. 2015;11(8):355–60. https://doi.org/10.1016/j.ecns.2015.05.004.
8. VanMerriënboer JJG, Sweller J. Cognitive load theory in health professional education: design principles and strategies. Med Educ. 2010;44(1):85–93. https://doi.org/10.1111/j.1365-2923.2009.03498.x.
9. Paige JB, Morin KH. Simulation fidelity and cueing: a systematic review of the literature. Clin Simul Nurs. 2013;9(11):e481–9. https://doi.org/10.1016/j.ecns.2013.01.001.
10. Biggs J, Tang C. Teaching for quality learning at university. 4th ed. Maidenhead: McGraw-Hill/Society for Research into Higher Education & Open University Press; 2011.
11. Andersen P, Guinea S, Reid-Searl K, Levett-Jones T. Designing Tag Team Patient Safety Simulation: an instructional design approach. Clin Simul Nurs. 2021;59:1–9. https://doi.org/10.1016/j.ecns.2021.05.001.
12. Mager R. Preparing instructional objectives. 2nd ed. Belmont: Fearon; 1975.
13. Bjerke MB, Renger R. Being smart about writing SMART objectives. Eval Program Plann. 2017;61:125–7. https://doi.org/10.1016/j.evalprogplan.2016.12.009.
14. Boal A. Games for actors and non-actors. London: Routledge; 2002.
15. Guinea S, Andersen P, Reid-Searl K, Levett-Jones T, Dwyer T, Heaton L, et al. Simulation-based learning for patient safety: the development of the Tag Team Patient Safety Simulation methodology for nursing education. Collegian. 2019;26:392–8. https://doi.org/10.1016/j.colegn.2018.09.008.
16. Australian Commission on Safety and Quality in Health Care. National safety and quality health service standards. 2nd ed. 2017. https://www.safetyandquality.gov.au/our-work/assessment-to-the-nsqhs-standards/nsqhs-standards-second-edition/.
17. McAllister M, Reid-Seral K, Davis S. Who is that masked educator? Deconstructing the teaching and learning processes of an innovative humanistic simulation technique. Nurse Educ Today. 2013;33(12):1453–8. https://doi.org/10.1016/j.nedt.2013.06.015.
18. Dwyer TA, Levett-Jones T, Flenady T, Reid-Searl K, Andersen P, Guinea S, Heaton L, Applegarth J, Goodwin BC. Responding to the unexpected: tag team patient safety simulation. Clin Simul Nurs. 2019;36:8–17. https://doi.org/10.1016/j.ecns.2019.06.007.
19. Levett-Jones T, Andersen P, Reid-Searl K, Guinea S, McAllister M, Lapkin S, Niddrie M. Tag team simulation: an innovative approach for promoting active engagement of participants and observers during group simulations. Nurse Educ Pract. 2015;15(5):345–52. https://doi.org/10.1016/j.nepr.2015.03.01416.
20. Nestel D, Bearman M, editors. Simulated patient methodology: theory, evidence, and practice. Chichester: Wiley; 2015.
21. Budd N, Andersen P, Harrison P, Prowae N. Engaging child actors as simulated patients in nursing and midwifery higher education. Simul Healthc. 2020;15(3):199–204. https://doi.org/10.1097/sih.0000000000000452.
22. Lopreiato JO (Ed), Downing D, Gammon W, Lioce L, Sittner B, Slot V, Spain AE (Associate Eds), and the Terminology & Concepts Working Group. Healthcare simulation dictionary, 2nd ed. Rockville: Agency for Healthcare Research and Quality; 2020. https://doi.org/10.23970/simulationv2.
23. Rutherford-Hemming T, Lioce L, Breymier T. Guidelines and essential elements for prebriefing. Simul Healthc. 2019;14(6):409–14. https://doi.org/10.1097/SIH.0000000000000403.
24. Rudolph JW, Raemer DB, Simon R. Establishing a safe container for learning in simulation: the role of simulation briefing. Simul Healthc. 2014;9(6):339–49. https://doi.org/10.1097/SIH.0000000000000047.
25. Hober C, Bonnel W. Student perceptions of the observer role in high-fidelity simulation. Clin Simul Nurs. 2014;10(10):507–14. https://doi.org/10.1016/j.ecns.2014.07.008.

26. Kettlewell K, Southcott C, Stevens E, McCrone T. Engaging the disengaged (NFER research program: from education to employment). Slough: NFER; 2012. https://www.nfer.ac.uk/publications/ETDE01/ETDE01.pdf.
27. Norman J. Differences in learning outcomes in simulation: the observer role. Nurse Educ Pract. 2018;28:242–2477. https://doi.org/10.1016/j.nepr.2017.10.025.
28. O'Regan S, Molloy E, Watterson L, Nestel D. Observer roles that optimize learning in healthcare simulation education: a systematic review. Adv Simul. 2016;1:4. https://doi.org/10.1186/s41077-015-0004-8.
29. INACSL Standards Committee, Decker S, Alinier G, Crawford SB, Gordon RM, Wilson C. Healthcare Simulation Standards of Best PracticeTM The Debriefing Process. Clinical Simulation in Nursing. 2021;58:27–32. https://doi.org/10.1016/j.ecns.2021.08.011.
30. Mariani B, Cantrell MA, Meakim C, Prieto P, Dreifuerst KT. Structured debriefing and students' clinical judgment abilities in simulation. Clin Simul Nurs. 2013;9(5):e147–55. https://doi.org/10.1016/j.ecns.2011.11.009.
31. Sawyer T, Eppich W, Brett-Fleegler M, Grant V, Cheng A. More than one way to debrief: a critical review of healthcare simulation debriefing methods. Simul Healthc. 2016;11(3):209–17. https://doi.org/10.1097/SIH.0000000000000148.
32. Dreifuerst KT. The essentials of debriefing in simulation learning: a concept analysis. Nurs Educ Perspect. 2009;30(2):109–14.
33. Kelly MA, Barragan E, Husebø SE, Orr F. Simulation in nursing education: international perspectives and contemporary scope of practice. J Nurs Scholarsh. 2016;48(3):312–21. https://doi.org/10.1111/jnu.12208.
34. Tutticci N, Coyer F, Lewis PA, Ryan M. Student facilitation of simulation debrief: measuring reflective thinking and self-efficacy. Teach Learn Nurs. 2017;12(2):128–35. https://doi.org/10.1016/j.teln.2016.11.005.
35. Husebø SE, O'Regan S, Nestel D. Reflective practice and its role in simulation. Clin Simul Nurs. 2015;11(8):368–75. https://doi.org/10.1016/j.ecns.2015.04.005.
36. Phrampus P, O'Donnell J. Debriefing using a structured and supported approach. In: Levine A, DeMaria S, Schwartz A, Sim A, editors. The comprehensive textbook of healthcare simulation. 1st ed. New York: Springer; 2013. p. 73–84.
37. Dreifuerst KT. Using debriefing for meaningful learning to foster the development of clinical reasoning in simulation. J Nurs Educ. 2012;51(6):326–33. https://doi.org/10.3928/01484834-20120409-02.
38. Rudolph JW, Simon R, Dufresne RL, Raemer DB. There's no such thing as "nonjudgmental" debriefing: a theory and method for debriefing with good judgment. Simul Healthc. 2006;1(1):49–55. https://doi.org/10.1097/01266021-200600110-00006.
39. Arora S, Ahmed M, Paige J, Nestel D, Runnacles J, Hull L, Sevdalis N. Objective structured assessment of debriefing. Bringing science to the art of debriefing in surgery. Ann Surg. 2012;256(6):982–8. https://doi.org/10.1097/SLA.0b013e3182610c91.
40. Leighton K, Ravert P, Mudra V, Macintosh C. Update the simulation effectiveness tool: item modifications and re-evaluation of psychometric properties. Nurs Educ Perspect. 2015;36(5):317–23. https://doi.org/10.5480/15-1671.
41. Levett-Jones T, Lapkin S, Hoffman K, Arthur C, Roche J. Examining the impact of high and medium fidelity simulation experiences on nursing students' knowledge acquisition. Nurse Educ Pract. 2011;11(6):380–3. https://doi.org/10.1016/j.nepr.2011.03.014.
42. Levett-Jones T, McCoy M, Lapkin S, Noble D, Hoffman J, Dempsey J, Roche J. The development and psychometric testing of the satisfaction with simulation experience scale. Nurse Educ Today. 2011;31(7):705–10. https://doi.org/10.1016/j.nedt.2011.01.004.
43. Simon R, Raemer DB, Rudolph JW. Debriefing assessment for simulation in healthcare (DASH): student version. 2010. https://harvardmedsim.org/debriefing-assesment-simulation-healthcare.php.
44. Adamson KA, Kardong-Edgren S, Willhaus J. An updated review of published simulation evaluation instruments. Clin Simul Nurs. 2013;9(9):e393–400. https://doi.org/10.1016/j.ecns.2012.09.004.
45. Kardong-Edgren S, Adamson KA, Fitzgerald C. A review of currently published evaluation instruments for human patient simulation. Clin Simul Nurs. 2010;6(1):e25–35. https://doi.org/10.1016/j.ecns.2009.08.004.
46. Simon R, Raemer DB, Rudolph JW. Debriefing assessment for simulation in healthcare (DASH): instructor version. 2012. https://harvardmedsim.org/debriefing-assesment-simulation-healthcare.php.
47. Burbach BE, Barnason S, Thompson SA. Using "thinking aloud" to capture clinical reasoning during patient simulation. Int J Nurs Educ Scholarsh. 2015;12(1):1–7. https://doi.org/10.1515/ijnes-2014-0044.
48. Verkuyl M, Hughes M, Fyfe MC. Using think aloud in health assessment: a mixed-methods study. J Nurs Educ. 2018;57(11):684–6. https://doi.org/10.3928/01484834-20181022-10.

Simulation in Pre-nursing Pipeline Programs

6

Kati Maxkenzie and Joilah James

Background

A pipeline program provides opportunities for youth and young adults to gain early exposure to different aspects of healthcare careers [1]. Through participation in a pipeline program, young adults can receive information and have experiences that can help them make informed decisions about their future careers. It is especially critical for youth from underrepresented backgrounds to have access to healthcare courses since, historically, students from these diverse backgrounds have been poorly represented [2]. Barriers to students entering healthcare careers are often due to their racial and ethnic background, low socio-economic status, limited educational attainment, and other aspects that make them more vulnerable to health disparities [3]. The recruitment and retention of students into healthcare positions through a pipeline program are critical to mitigate these barriers.

Amongst students in the United States pursuing science-related careers, reports have shown a need for more preparation [2, 4]. Over several decades, United States high schools have attempted to address these deficits by creating health pathways that students can select and apply for. A major concern with schools running these pathway programs is that they cannot readily address the practical application of health-related content. Health pathway programs at high schools often do not have a health professional teaching the material or being available to speak directly with students regularly. These programs also need more resources to provide students with hands-on experiences to gain practical knowledge and skills. The creation of health pathways in nursing education helps bridge the gap between health and science-related content covered in schools and students' preparedness for a future career in the health professions.

Providing a health pipeline program within nursing education offers a strategic plan to diversify the healthcare field through the implementation of experiential learning and skills-based training, thus taking some of the burdens from an already impacted school curriculum [1]. Pipeline programs provide professional development specific to the healthcare industry that results in students gaining both the hard and soft skills necessary to become worthwhile applicants for competitive programs in nursing. It also gives students face-to-face opportunities with health professionals. Experiential learning methods used in pipeline programs can include mentorship, job shadowing, and hands-on experiences, among others [5].

Pre-nursing students' ability to easily access career exploration opportunities such as job shadowing or volunteering in clinical settings can be limited [6]. This is due to many factors, such as their background and health clearance, regulatory requirements, patient privacy, and age requirements. Simulation-based education provides pre nursing students a platform to access realistic clinical environments, interact with clinicians, and have exposure to a range of service-based lines. It also can provide students with exposure to the different types of nursing opportunities as many simulation programs have simulated environments, including home health, clinic, emergency, inpatient, surgical, rehabilitation, and long-term care settings. Furthermore, unlike job shadowing, it allows students to immerse themselves in the nurses' role and perform some of the roles and responsibilities. Thessin, Scully-Russ, and Lieberman highlight the importance of this real-world context in helping students narrow their choices as to what to pursue in their post-secondary education [7].

Structure of a Pre-nursing Pipeline Program

Pre-nursing pipeline programs operate independently but may be linked to a high school, university, or healthcare institution. Although many programs work independently of

K. Maxkenzie (✉) · J. James
Alameda Health System, Alameda, CA, USA
e-mail: kmaxkenzie@alamedahealthsystem.org; jjames@alamedahealthsystem.org

J. M. Kutzin et al. (eds.), *Comprehensive Healthcare Simulation: Nursing*, Comprehensive Healthcare Simulation,
https://doi.org/10.1007/978-3-031-31090-4_6

schools, in some instances, there may be a collaborative effort between schools and pipeline programs as a recruitment method. Pipeline programs serve students from varying education levels, such as middle school, high school, work programs, college, and beyond. Through various learning modalities, students learn about careers they may not have otherwise been exposed to. Health pipeline programs provide a pathway for underrepresented youth to learn more about and gain skills necessary to pursue a career in the healthcare field. It gives them a snapshot of health careers to help them to make an informed decision about their desired career pathway. It also helps them to become viable candidates in competitive programs, teaching them the skills necessary to succeed in these careers.

Health pipeline programs provide various options depending on whether the program exists within the internal structure of a healthcare organization, university, or high school. It is often dependent on the staff size, the goals of the organization, and whether there is direct accessibility to a hospital.

Types of Pipeline Programs

Internal Programs are programs are housed at a healthcare institution and/or college or university and have direct access to clinicians and the breadth of healthcare professionals, both clinical and non-clinical.

Partnership Programs operate independently from the hospital setting.

Program Format

Programs are generally designed for a range of students and usually involve four main types of structures:

- light-touch techniques
- internship
- externship or job shadowing
- volunteering

Having a selection of different learning opportunities allows students to customize their learning depending on their preferences. It also gives students more flexibility based on their level of commitment and can meet the needs of a broad range of youth depending on their education path (Table 6.1).

It is also important to customize cohorts of students based on the desired goals and learning objectives. For instance, for internships, some cohorts may have a short experience with specific themes. Other cohorts may have a longer, more intensive experience where they can take a 'deep dive' into a general area of healthcare (Table 6.2).

Table 6.1 Types of pipeline programs examples

Exposure type	Length	Target audience
Light-touch experience	One to three touch points where students gain general information about healthcare careers through guest speakers, skills sessions, simulation experiences, or informational sessions	For students who are unable to commit a lot of time to the experience, it offers great flexibility in scheduling and is an option for schools and organizations who are looking to provide a short experience for a large group
Internship	It lasts a few weeks to a few months, sometimes longer. Give students a beginner's look at the diversity of careers within healthcare. In some cases, students can get class credit. These can be conducted in-school hours as linked learning or as after-school/summer programs. Internships, because they are longer, have more opportunities for guest speakers, didactic learning, skills and simulation experiences, informational sessions, and job shadowing	This option works for students who can make a long time commitment and seek a deeper learning experience
Externship/ Job shadowing	Approximately one day to eight weeks in length	Experiential opportunity for students needing to meet job shadowing requirements to apply to a post-secondary healthcare program. Also optimal for teachers and other non-healthcare professionals who work in a teaching capacity to gain exposure to healthcare
Volunteer	Short-term to long term	All-encompassing but often has an age requirement in hospital settings

Table 6.2 Type of internships

Types of internships	
Short-term	Short-term cohorts cover a broad range of topics at the surface level, such as: learning about what healthcare encompasses, taking vitals, bedside care, the different fields of healthcare, etc.
Themed	Covers a specific topic or area, such as life-saving techniques, preventative services, airway disorders, etc.
Intensive	Intensive cohorts allow for a deeper dive into various topics (or a specific one), with students understanding essential concepts and how to implement said concepts. For instance, covering social determinants of health, understanding body systems and how they work cohesively, etc.

Preparing for Simulations in Pipeline Programs

When developing simulations for pipeline programs, it is important to ask the following questions to ensure the goals of the simulation can be achieved:

1. What are the goals and learning objectives?
2. What simulation staff and nurse staff are needed to facilitate the simulation?
3. Who are your support staff?
4. What training and resources are required?

Coordinating Simulation Experiences

There are three prominent staff roles for coordinating simulation experiences for pipeline program students

- The ***pipeline program coordinator*** must have in mind the desired learning outcomes for the students and provide the expertise needed to design the curriculum and bridge the gap between the content and functionality of the simulation scenario.
- The ***simulation operation specialist*** who work in conjunction with the education team to implement and deliver the simulation. They may use a variety of technologies such as computers, audio-visual equipment, and networking technologies. Based on the goals of the simulation, the simulation operation specialist help to determines the simulation modality, setting, and functions.
- The ***clinical facilitator/s*** is needed to observe students to ensure they are taking the necessary steps in facilitating the simulated patient case, debrief the scenarios, and provide feedback.

Support Staff

Other clinicians can also be recruited from your home institution or outside of your institution to observe and support students during the simulations. It is important that the clinician is both an expert in the area of nursing that is being covered and is familiar with the specific scenario and goals to ensure the achievement of learning objectives. When recruiting clinicians, it is important to keep in mind the budget. Are you able to pay clinicians for their time, or are you looking for them to volunteer their time?

For many clinicians that have not had experience guiding students through a simulation, the following tips may be helpful:

- Create opportunities for students to think out loud and think through the scenario without jumping in immediately to provide answers.
- Have a guiding clinician in the simulation to assist the students. Remind them to keep their hands in their pockets. Try to direct students on how to do an action if there is a knowledge gap; avoid doing it for them.
- Ask foundational prompting questions and give options (e.g., what is normal here and what is not normal). Give time for them to formulate a response.
- Direct a question to an individual or ask someone you haven't heard from yet.

Simulation Curriculum Development

Curriculum design for pre-nursing pipeline programs shares many similarities with nursing simulation programs. Thomas et al.'s Six-Step Approach to Curriculum Development provides a useful framework. These include:

1. problem identification/general need assessment
2. targeted needs assessment
3. goals and objectives
4. educational strategies
5. implementation
6. evaluation and feedback [8].

When designing a curriculum for pre-nursing pipeline programs, the development process needs to be viewed through a different lens. While the curriculum is still cemented in healthcare situations, the expectations and objectives of the scenarios need to be applied to the pre-nursing student. Healthcare awareness, role delineation, and different workflows are unique considerations.

Some parallels can be drawn between Benner's Novice to Expert nursing competency model and the stage and age of the pre-nursing learner (Table 6.3) [9].

Younger students (pre-high school) often have little to no knowledge of healthcare roles, concepts, and terminologies. High-school-aged students often have limited knowledge of healthcare roles, concepts, and terminologies but

Table 6.3 Comparison between the pre-nursing and nursing learner

Level/ Type	Novice	Advanced beginner	Competent
Nursing	"Since novices have no experience with the situation they face, they must use these context-free rules to guide their task performance"	"This person has coped with enough real situations to note (or to have them pointed out by a mentor) the recurrent meaningful situational components"	"Competency, typified by the nurse who has been on the job 2–3 years, develops when the nurse begins to see his or her actions in terms of long-range goals or plans"
Pre-nursing	Pre-high school to early high school	Mid to late high school	Late to post-high school

are more motivated to explore their career options. Post-high school students will have a wider range of knowledge levels but will likely be extremely motivated to pursue their options.

Differences in the learner groups will help guide the curriculum design's needs assessment. For example, a grade 6 career exploration event for students interested in healthcare careers might focus on basic concepts such as what is the role of a nurse, what are some basic tasks of a nurse (vitals, auscultation, etc.), and how to become a nurse. Whereas a grade 11 career exploration event for high school students in a health pathway might elaborate on what is the role of a nurse and how it differs from a doctor, some basic tasks of a nurse and how to perform that tasks in relation to a doctor's order, and how to become a nurse including alternative pathways. Challenges for designing curriculum can arise when pre-nursing pipeline programs include learners of multiple age groups and educational backgrounds (e.g., different schools) and different levels of experience (e.g., previous internship programs). The curriculum must meet the needs of the most novice learner while providing enough stimulation for the most competent learner.

The biggest difference in designing curriculum for those exploring healthcare careers and those practicing healthcare is around the principles of Adult Learning Theory [10]. Younger students will respond better to a pedagogical rather than an andragogical approach. This will change the structure of the curriculum, especially in the educational strategies, implementation phases, and evaluation and feedback stages.

When delivering curriculum for younger learners, it is important to take the time to:

- Establish and enforce clear expectations and consequences for classroom behavior and engagement.
- Provide clear step-by-step instructions (with no more than 1–2 instructions at a time).
- Keep it short. Break the curriculum into short sections (under 20 min) to retain their attention.
- Provide the information in a clear written format (such as on an electronic presentation or whiteboard).
- Repeat everything multiple times using multiple formats (written, verbal, etc.).
- Don't underestimate your learners. They are smarter than you think but might need more time or encouragement to solicit the answer from them.

When creating a curriculum for pre-nursing pipeline programs, all these factors must be considered. While the curriculum design uses similar elements of designing a curriculum for a pre-licensure nursing student, it is also important to acknowledge the differences in order to design a successful curriculum.

Simulation Design and Operations

When implementing simulation-based education for pre-nursing pipeline programs, there are several factors to consider when deciding on simulation design and operations (Table 6.4):

Table 6.4 Matrix of simulation design features

Timing of program	Duration	Frequency	Type of learner	Learner level	Size of cohort	Resources	Recruitment of learner	Recruitment of faculty
In-school	Once	Single	Pre-high school	Novice	Small group/s	Space	School District	Volunteers/Paid
After-school	Recurring	Weekly/ Bi-weekly	High School and Continuing Ed	Advanced beginner	Large group/s	Facilitators	Workforce development programs	Organization staff
Summer		Monthly	College/University	Competent		Scheduling	Universities	Community partners
		Semester	Post-college/ University			Curriculum	Own organization	
		Yearly	Fellowship/ Externships			Costs		
			Volunteer programs			Equipment		

Creating Scenario-Based Simulations for Pre-nursing

It is important not to underestimate the capabilities of pre-nursing students when creating a scenario but to match their experience and knowledge base. A study of high school health pathway students participating in health internships reported that only 22% "often" had their experience linked back to their schoolwork [11]. The pre-nursing pipeline program coordinator must work with the school to determine objectives best suited to the pre-nursing student's curriculum. This can become more difficult in multi-age, multi-site cohorts as their knowledge and experience vary significantly.

Creating scenarios can be time-consuming [12], and creating scenarios for pre-nursing students is no different. When developing scenarios for pre-nursing students, a new scenario can be created, or a pre-written scenario can be adapted. If creating a new scenario, using a template ensures that all the appropriate information is included. An alternative to creating a new scenario would be simplifying or adapting an existing one. When choosing the scenario to adapt, selecting from a scenario designed for first or second year nursing students will be the most suitable one to align with novice pre-nursing students. For the more advanced beginner or competent pre-nursing students, a scenario for third or fourth year nursing students might be considered especially if it is for a longer pipeline program with reoccurring experiences.

Novice Pre-nursing Students

Novice pre-nursing students may include pre-high school and early high school-aged students, newcomer students (recent immigrants new to the dominant language), and older high school or non-clinical post-secondary students with no previous health experience. Initial scenarios for this group should focus on building the student's understanding and confidence in how to interact in a simulated clinical environment. Topics could include:

- Foundational patient and team communication skills
- Taking a patient history
- Assessing a patient's vitalsigns (HR, BP, RR, and Temperature)
- Providing a single intervention (such as CPR or giving oxygen) based on a single abnormal vital sign.

Where a typical scenario for a nursing student or a practicing nurse may contain three to five stages with many expected learner actions and take 15–20 min to complete, the pre-nursing student may take 15 min to complete the expected learner actions of the first stage of the same scenario. Start small with one to two concepts to orientate the students on how to interact with the simulated clinical environment, including other team members.

To help students be successful, strong structures should be put towards underlying pathophysiology and expected interventions. This can be provided through embedded participants and/or the clinician providing information such as types of medications, tests, or possible diagnoses.

Experienced Pre-nursing Students

Experienced pre-nursing students may include advanced beginners or competent pre-nursing students that are more senior high school or post-secondary students who have some health experience. Possible health experiences could be work-study programs, volunteer experience, previous internships, or health-specific curricula. These students may have a basic understanding of vital signs, exposure to the clinical environment, and different health conditions. Initial scenarios for these learners can focus more on the different roles and scope of practice of the healthcare team. Topics could include:

- Foundational patient and team communication skills
- Taking a patient history from a challenging patient
- Assessing a patient's vitals
- Providing multiple interventions (such as giving oxygen and antibiotics) based on multiple abnormal vital signs
- Building differential diagnoses
- Ordering and/or interpreting tests (such as imaging and labs) to narrow differential diagnoses
- Recognize decompensating patients

These pre-nursing students may get through two states and expected learner actions of a typical nursing student scenario in the same amount of time. Experienced pre-nursing students will be able to think critically through more options than novice pre-nursing students. The clinician can help guide the students by providing multiple options to choose from for interventions or next steps.

For pre-nursing scenarios, consider using unfolding scenarios to help students build on their knowledge and skills. Pre-nursing students respond enthusiastically to hands-on interventions such as starting IVs, delivering babies, airway management, and performing CPR. Incorporating a skills session into the curriculum before participating in a scenario can elevate the pre-nursing student's experience. Finally, aligning the topics with the school curriculum and/or the school community helps students relate to the subject matter.

Whether creating a new scenario or adapting a pre-written one, it is important to add instruction for the clinician to help guide them through the scenario. This mentoring role of the clinician requires a balance between allowing students space and time to think and providing the framework to bridge any knowledge gaps.

Debriefing Pre-nursing Students

Debriefing with a framework is the best practice [13]. The same principles of debriefing are utilized with pre-nursing students. However, the lens will be different. When debriefing with pre-nursing students, it is important to consider their age, knowledge level, and experience. For pre-nursing students, due to their lower levels of healthcare concepts, it is likely that less time will be spent on the pathophysiology of the patient and more time on the roles of the healthcare professionals.

Debriefing that focuses on the roles and responsibilities of healthcare professionals may be new to the debriefer. Open-ended questions that help pre-nursing students better understand the opportunities and workflow of a nurse will help achieve the career exploration objectives of the scenario. These questions may include:

- How did the doctor's role vary from the nurse's?
- What type of personality traits do you think would best be suited to an emergency room/critical care/home health/etc. clinician?
- What are some of the tasks the nurse performed during the scenario?

During the analysis phase of debriefing, it is critical to spend time linking the scenario's events back to the student's school curriculum. For example, if students have been learning about the circulatory system, during a debrief of a Cardiac Arrest scenario, the discussion should link back to how compressions move the blood through the heart's four chambers and into the vascular system. If available, the school teacher, intimate with the school curriculum, can assist during the debrief. However, if this approach is taken, the school teacher is likely not an expert in debriefing and may start to move into lecture mode.

Challenges of Debrief Pre-nursing Students

For the lead debriefer, there are a few additional factors to consider with the pre-nursing population which can hinder learning:

- The new learning environment may affect trust between students and debriefer;
- The fear of being judged, especially for students of color;
- For mixed cohorts, lack of peer-trusted relationships;
- Lack of familiar structure; and
- Adversity factors (stable access to sleep, food, etc.) [14]

These elements can result in students' disengagement or classroom behavior management issues. There are strategies debriefers can use to help mitigate some of these factors and minimize challenges.

- The debriefer can utilize basic classroom behavior management techniques familiar to the students, such as 'one, two, three, eyes on me' or clapping in a pattern to gain the student's attention.
- Provide snacks for students to access before or during the session.
- Teambuilding or icebreaker exercises to build relationships.
- Utilizing debriefers representing the student population (first-generation, person of color, etc.).
- Reinforcing that simulation is a space for failure and giving extra time and space for students to formulate their answers.

Like all debriefings, the debriefer must reflect on their experiences to continue to improve. Soliciting feedback from the school teachers, the pre-nursing students, and fellow simulationists will allow for richer, more engaging debriefs in the future.

Summary

The introduction of pre-nursing pipeline programs has given greater exposure to healthcare careers for a demographic of students who usually have little to no access. A large part of the curriculum for many pipeline programs includes simulation, as it is a valuable learning tool that provides a hands-on experience so that students can make informed decisions about their pursuit of a healthcare career. Using simulation in pre-nurse training helps to bridge the gap between knowledge and skills, reinforces learning, and gives students a competitive advantage to enter nursing degrees.

When using simulation to educate pre-nursing pipeline students, it is important to take into consideration the learner group, the development of relevant scenarios to meet the desired learning outcomes, and the logistics of the simulated scenario. Through simulation, pre-nursing pipeline students can focus on the hard and soft skills necessary to make them capable and successful nurses.

Case Examples

One Touch

A local high school science teacher approaches your Simulation Coordinator and inquires about bringing students for a tour next month. It is the busiest time of year for the small Simulation Program, and the Simulation Coordinator is unsure how to proceed. The Simulation Coordinator should begin by gathering more information from the teacher about the type of student population, objectives of the tour, the knowledge level, and basic logistics (number of students, ideal times/dates, length of visit). This information can be gathered with a tour request form and/or an initial planning meeting.

During the meeting, the teacher explains that there are two Grade 11 biology classes with 40 students total. The school is a 20-min walk from the Simulation Program. The students have been learning about physiology, and the objective of the tour would be to give students a hands-on introduction to healthcare careers that utilize physiology. Their friend, who is a nurse, mentioned that your Simulation Program would be a great place to take the students for some hands-on learning. They are flexible to either bring the students one class at a time and come twice or bring both classes at the same time. If the classes were to come separately, it would need to be two consecutive weeks. The tour must be on Wednesday afternoons from 12:40 to 3:20 p.m. on the following month's second, third, or fourth Wednesday. There would be two teachers and two parent chaperones will be available.

After obtaining this information, the Simulation Coordinator must consider the physical and human resources required to support the request and the school's objectives. As this is the busiest time of the year, there is only availability on one of the Wednesdays of the following month. The Simulation Coordinator will then need to determine if the Program can support 40 students at one time, allowing for hands-on experiences for the student. The Simulation Program has one larger and one small debriefing room, two simulation rooms with a high-technology birthing manikin and an adult, and a skills lab with five low-technology manikins. The total capacity of all rooms is 30 people. It is determined that the two classes can be split into two 50-min tours to accommodate all 40 students. The Simulation Coordinator has one faculty available who is willing to volunteer and a Simulation Operations Specialist. The following agenda is agreed upon to maximize the hands-on experience for the students:

Class 1		Class 2	
12:40–1:00	Class 1 walks to Simulation Program with one teacher and one chaperon	1:40–2:00	Class 2 walks to Simulation Program with one teacher and one chaperon
1:00–1:10	Welcome students and What is simulation? – Large debriefing room – Volunteer faculty	2:00–2:10	Welcome students and What is simulation? – Large debriefing room – Volunteer faculty
1:10–1:30	Group 1A—CPR – Skills lab – Volunteer faculty Group 1B—intro to manikin – Sim room 1 – Simulation operations specialist	2:10–2:30	Group 2A—CPR – Skills lab – Volunteer faculty Group 2B—intro to manikin – Sim room 1 – Simulation operations specialist
1:30–1:35	Groups switch	2:30–2:35	Groups switch
1:35–1:55	Group 1B—CPR – Skills lab – Volunteer faculty Group 1A—intro to manikin – Sim room 1 – Simulation operations specialist	2:35–2:55	Group 2B—CPR – Skills lab – Volunteer faculty Group 2A—intro to manikin – Sim room 1 – Simulation operations specialist
1:55–2:00	Wrap up	2:55–3:00	Wrap up
2:00–2:20	Class 1 walks to school with one teacher and one chaperon	3:00–3:20	Class 2 walks to school with one teacher and one chaperon

References

1. Katz JR, Barbosa-Leiker C, Benavides-Vaello S. Measuring the success owf a pipeline program to increase nursing workforce diversity. J Prof Nurs. 2016;32(1):6–14.
2. Melillo K, Dowling J, Abdallah L, Findeisen M, Knight M. Bring diversity to nursing: recruitment, retention and graduation of nursing students. J Cult Divers. 2013;20(2):100–4.
3. Jackson CS, Gracia JN. Addressing health and healthcare disparities: the role of a diverse workforce and the social determinants of health. Public Health Rep. 2014;129 Suppl 2(Suppl 2):57–61.
4. Hayes S. Preparation matters most in STEM. Issue brief. ACT, Inc. 2017.
5. Brooks Carthon JM, Nguyen TH, Chittams J, Park E, Guevara J. Measuring success: results from a national survey of recruitment and retention initiatives in the nursing workforce. Nurs Outlook. 2014;62(4):259–67.
6. Muncan B, Majumder N, Tudose N. From high school to hospital: how early exposure to healthcare affects adolescent career ideas. Int J Med Educ. 2016;7:370–1.
7. Thessin RA, Scully-Russ E, Lieberman DS. Critical success factors in a high school healthcare education program. J Career Tech Educ. 2018;32(1):51–72.
8. Thomas P, Kern D, Hughes M, Chen B. Curriculum development for medical education: a six-step approach. Baltimore: John Hopkins University Press; 2015.
9. Benner P. From novice to expert, excellence and power in clinical nursing practice, vol. 84. Menlo Park: Addison-Wesley Publishing Company; 1984. p. 1479.
10. Knowles M. Andragogy in action: applying modern principles of adult education. San Francisco: Jossey-Bass; 1984.
11. Warner M, Park CJ, Chen W, Benge C, Fikes A, McMurchy M. Evaluation of the Oakland Health Pathways Project: final report. Menlo Park: SRI Education. 2020. https://www.sri.com/publication/evaluation-of-the-oakland-health-pathways-project-final-report/.
12. Waxman KT. The development of evidence-based clinical simulation scenarios: guidelines for nurse educators. J Nurs Educ. 2010;49(1):29–35.
13. INACSL Standards Committee. Healthcare Simulation Standards of Best PracticeTM. Clinical Simulation in Nursing. 2021.
14. Darling-Hammond L, Cook-Harvey CM. Educating the whole child: improving school climate to support student success. Palo Alto: Learning Policy Institute; 2018.

Nursing Fundamentals Simulation

7

Mary Moran, Stephen Guinea, and Patrea Andersen

Nursing Fundamentals

Nursing fundamentals comprise the essential tenets of any pre-registration nursing curriculum. While a range of models describing nursing fundamentals exist, all represent a mechanism by which to understand the foundational theory and practice of nursing. These perspectives, in turn, often form the basis and structure of pre-registration nursing programs. An example by Kitson et al. [1] presents the fundamentals of nursing as 14 aspects of care (Table 7.1).

Key to teaching and learning nursing fundamentals is the development of knowledge, understanding, and applying knowledge and understanding in theoretical and practical contexts. Accordingly, courses focusing on the fundamentals of nursing care often emphasize developing psychomotor skills, communication strategies, and critical thinking [2] as interrelated dimensions of nursing practice. For example, when considering how to teach any of the nursing fundamentals presented by Kitson et al. [1], learning outcomes and the design of lessons would likely require students to apply theoretical knowledge and engage in interpersonal communication, critical thinking, and psychomotor skills to develop the desired knowledge, skills and attributes effectively.

Simulation is an ideal educational method for teaching nursing fundamentals as simulation promotes active learning, enhances self-confidence, and reduces anxiety [2]. Through simulation, many students encounter early experiences of nursing practice and, indeed, engage in their first experiences of applying theoretical concepts to practice-based situations. It is, therefore, essential that users of simulation have an understanding of the fundamentals of simulation pedagogy and practice.

Table 7.1 Nursing fundamentals [1]

1. Safety, prevention, and medication administration	8. Rest and sleep
2. Communication and education	9. Comfort (including pain management)
3. Respiration	10. Dignity
4. Eating and drinking	11. Privacy
5. Elimination	12. Respecting choice
6. Personal cleansing and dressing	13. Mobility
7. Temperature control	14. Expressing sexuality

Fundamentals of Simulation

Healthcare simulation has evolved significantly over the past 30 years, with pre-registration nursing education at the forefront of this evolution. Today, simulation is understood to be a valid and essential educational method utilized in many pre-registration nursing programs worldwide, supported by a strong and evolving evidence base. As an educational method, fundamental principles and concepts underpin simulation practice. A critical theme from the evidence is that understanding the fundamental principles and concepts of simulation practice is essential to ensure simulation activities and experiences are of high quality, are educationally sound, remain contemporary, and are sustainable.

There are many definitions of simulation. One that conveys the value, as well as the educational principles that underpin simulation in nursing, is provided by Bland, Topping, and Wood [3], who define nursing simulation as "a dynamic process involving the creation of a hypothetical opportunity that incorporates an authentic representation of reality, facilitates active student engagement and integrates

M. Moran (✉)
Columbia University School of Nursing, New York, NY, USA
e-mail: mbm4@cumc.columbia.edu

S. Guinea
Faculty of Health Sciences, Australian Catholic University, Sydney, NSW, Australia
e-mail: Stephen.guinea@acu.edu.au

P. Andersen
Waikato Institute of Technology, Te Kuratini o Waikato New Zealand, Hamilton, New Zealand
e-mail: patrea.andersen@wintec.ac.nz

J. M. Kutzin et al. (eds.), *Comprehensive Healthcare Simulation: Nursing*, Comprehensive Healthcare Simulation,
https://doi.org/10.1007/978-3-031-31090-4_7

the complexities of practical and theoretical learning with opportunity for repetition, feedback, evaluation, and reflection" ([3]: 668). Implicit in this definition is the understanding that simulation is a created activity, a learning experience in which authenticity, complexity, and reflective learning can be specifically designed for.

Simulation in pre-registration nursing education can take many forms. A summary of modalities commonly used in nursing education is presented in Table 7.2.

Whilst many simulation users may prefer a particular modality of simulation, there is no single best mode. The selection of simulation modality should be based on the best fit for a simulation activity, factoring in considerations such as the desired level of realism or fidelity, access to required equipment or technology, staff experience with modes of simulation, and staffing numbers required to deliver the simulation.

Regardless of the mode, simulation-based learning experiences typically take the form of three phases: (1) the pre-simulation brief, (2) the simulation scenario, and (3) the post-simulation debrief.

The purpose of the pre-simulation brief is to prepare learners for the simulation experience. The pre-simulation brief comprises two components. The first component comprises resources, materials, or activities required to ensure learners have the knowledge and skill to engage in the simulation scenario. Learners should be made aware of the learning outcomes for the upcoming simulation and be provided with materials and resources such as readings, videos, quizzes, or online games as preparation. The second component is the face-to-face information and orientation session conducted immediately before the simulation scenario. This often comprises a review of the learning outcomes, orientation to the simulation environment, preparation of roles, and an introduction to the scenario. The overall purpose of the pre-simulation brief is to create a safe learning environment, helping prepare participants for a constructive learning experience.

The second phase of a simulation experience, the simulation scenario, is a purposefully designed activity that provides participants with a simulated, authentic recreation of an actual situation, through which participants should be able to achieve the intended learning outcomes. The scenario provides the context for the simulation experience and can vary in duration and complexity.

The third phase of the simulation experience is the post-simulation debrief. The debrief immediately follows the simulation scenario. It is a process comprising feedback and reflection facilitated by an experienced facilitator. Feedback is provided regarding the participants' performance, and par-

Table 7.2 Common modalities of simulation

Mode/modality of simulation	Definition
Augmented reality	A technology that overlays digital computer-generated information on objects or places in the real world to enhance the user experience [4]
Haptics	Computer-based devices that provide tactile feedback to the user. In healthcare simulation, haptics can be used to simulate touching and palpating an organ or body part and the cutting, tearing, or traction of a tissue. Often used in combination with virtual or augmented reality, the purpose of haptics is to provide tactile feedback to inform participant decision-making [4, 5]
Hybrid simulation	The use of two or more simulation modalities aims to provide a more realistic experience. For example, using a part-task trainer (e.g., intravenous cannulation arm) is realistically attached to a simulated participant [4]
Insitu simulation	A simulation-based experience is conducted in the actual practice setting where the participants typically work. In-situ simulation aims to achieve a very high level of environmental and cognitive fidelity [4, 5]
Manikin-based simulation	Also referred to as human patient simulation. A simulation that utilizes full-scale human simulators or manikins. Manikins may be classified as no, medium or high technology, or low, medium, or high-fidelity [4]
Mixed reality	A category of simulation that encompasses the hybrid combination of virtual reality environments and reality, e.g., real environment, simulated participants, and manikin simulator [6]
Mixed simulation	The use of a variety of different simulation modalities in the same scenario [4]
Role-play	A technique used in education where topics are explored, using social interaction, from the perspectives of different roles. In role-play, learners are provided with specific roles and are projected into a fictitious situation where they adopt their role's values, attitudes, status, behaviors, and motivations. The purpose of role play is to enable learners to understand the experience of others through the exploration of ideas, perceptions, attitudes, and possibilities in social yet hypothetical situations [7]
Simulated participants (simulated patients, standardized patients)	Professional or amateur people trained to portray a patient or other individual in a scripted simulation scenario for the purposes of instruction, practice, or assessment [4, 5]
Task trainer / part-task trainer	Simulators are designed for teaching and learning specific parts of a skill. For example, the insertion of a peripheral intravenous cannula [4]
Virtual reality	Simulations that use a variety of immersive, highly visual, 3D characteristics to replicate real-life situations and/or health care procedures [4]. Virtual reality may include serious games

ticipants' reflective thinking is encouraged whilst discussing the various aspects of the simulation. Participants are encouraged to explore emotions and question, reflect, and provide feedback to one another. The purpose of debriefing is to provide a safe learning environment where the educator, through facilitation, assists learners to integrate theory and practice, assimilate and accommodate what has been learned from the simulation experience [5], extend the application of what has been learned to future situations, and to identify learning needs.

Domains of Learning

The appeal of simulation in pre-registration nursing education is in the various applications for which it can be used. Examples include skills training (priming an intravenous line), rehearsal of protocol-driven clinical scenarios (basic life support), or the development of complex cognitive skills (clinical reasoning). Indeed, simulation-based learning activities can be purposefully designed to develop specific learner knowledge, skills, and attributes, also known as *domains of learning*.

When designing any learning activity, it is necessary to consider the three domains of learning; cognitive (knowledge-based), affective (emotion-based), and psychomotor (action-based). The three domains of learning were first developed by Bloom and colleagues [8] (the cognitive domain—1956), Krathwohl, Bloom, and Masia [9] (the affective domain—1964), and Harrow [10] (the psychomotor domain—1972). Each domain has a taxonomy associated with it that specifies the principles of that domain and is presented as a classification structured from simple to more complex.

When designing simulation-based learning activities, it is not uncommon to focus on one domain of learning. For example, in higher education, the cognitive domain, revised in 2001 [11], is frequently used to structure learning outcomes. In the clinical education setting, when the assessment of clinical competence is required, the psychomotor domain may significantly inform simulation activity design. However, as simulation-based learning enables a recreated yet authentic representation of reality, simulation provides an opportunity to construct more holistic learning experiences by using all three domains of learning in the design. This approach helps create more well-rounded learning experiences, meets several learning styles, and assists recall and retention. In this chapter, the use of the three domains of learning will be demonstrated as the context for the teaching of nursing fundamentals.

Simulation Fundamentals: The Psychomotor Domain

The psychomotor domain of learning, also referred to as kinaesthetic learning, includes the use of motor skills and the ability to coordinate them. The psychomotor domain comprises a taxonomy of seven categories: (1) perception, (2) set, (3) guided response, (4) mechanism, (5) complex overt response, (6) adaptation, and (7) origination [10]. Psychomotor skill development is a central characteristic of nursing fundamentals. The curriculum design of nursing fundamentals courses often aligns theoretical and practical components, for example, the tutorial (theory) and skills laboratory (practice). This alignment assists students in acquiring knowledge through didactic instruction, complemented by the application of knowledge in a skills laboratory. The aim of this approach is for students to develop competency in performing skills over time.

Simulation has an essential role in teaching and learning fundamental psychomotor skills, as it enables students to apply knowledge and provide an experience from which they can draw on when refining their practice. A range of simulation modalities may be used in nursing education to develop fundamental knowledge, skills, and attributes. The selection of modality is based on the desired experience of learning using simulation, the experience of the educator with modalities of simulation, and the resources available. Simulation used for teaching and learning individual skills in nursing fundamentals courses may include role play, the use of part-task trainers, and increasingly virtual, augmented, and mixed reality. Regardless of the simulation modality, sound education models of instruction provide value for the design of psychomotor skill teaching. One example of an education model is Peyton's four-step approach to teaching a skill [12]. Developed for medical education, Peyton's approach provides four clearly defined steps to frame teaching psychomotor skills. They are:

Step 1 Demonstration: The educator demonstrates the skill in real-time and without commentary. This provides learners with an understanding of the performance of the skill at a proficient standard, the standard expected of a registered practitioner.

Step 2 Deconstruction: The educator demonstrates the skill while describing each procedural step in detail. For more complex skills, the skill may be divided into small subsections or chunks. This provides learners with an understanding of the rationale for the steps demonstrated.

Step 3 Comprehension: The learner describes every step of the skill. The educator demonstrates the skill according to the instruction from the learner. The description and demonstration do not occur simultaneously.

Step 4 Performance: The learner demonstrates the skill independently. This step may involve the learner describing each step of the skill whilst demonstrating the skill.

One example of teaching a psychomotor skill using an education model such as Peyton's four-step approach is the performance of blood glucose measurement.

The accurate measurement of a blood glucose level via finger stick constitutes a fundamental element of nursing care as it contributes to the promotion of safe care. Teaching the measurement of blood glucose is often one of the foundations of pre-registration nursing education, as it is this parameter that can guide further patient assessments and patient care. Simulation has a significant role to play in the teaching of blood glucose measurement in pre-registration nursing programs, providing an invaluable link between theory and practice.

The theory of blood glucose measurement is often taught, by requiring student to learn the name, function, assembly, and care of the equipment required via a didactic manner of instruction. It is common for students to rote-learn normal blood glucose ranges and memorize terms such as hyperglycemia and hypoglycemia and the associated signs and symptoms. Teaching psychomotor skills such as blood glucose measurement can often take the form of teacher demonstrations or instructional videos. These approaches to teaching may be teacher-focused and can lack student participation and engagement. There is a risk that when class sizes are large, learning activities such as blood glucose measurement can become disorganized and impede learning. The structure of Peyton's four-step approach provides a suitable framework for the teaching and learning of measuring a blood glucose level.

Step 1 Demonstration: The educator assembles the equipment required for measuring a blood glucose level and completes the procedure.

Step 2 Deconstruction: The educator demonstrates the skill of measuring a blood glucose level while describing essential components in detail. Through this step, the educator engages students in making connections between the theoretical content of blood glucose measurement and the skill. For example, the rationale for not touching the sensor pad is pricking the side of the finger rather than the fingertip.

Step 3 Comprehension: The learner describes every step of measuring a blood glucose level. The educator demonstrates the skill according to the instruction provided by the learner. The description and demonstration do not occur simultaneously.

Step 4 Performance: The learner demonstrates measuring a blood glucose level independently. The learner may describe each step whilst demonstrating the skill.

This structured approach to teaching a psychomotor skill can be applied to small or large groups of students. If being utilized for larger groups, the structure of Peyton's four-step approach [12] provides a means for the educator to monitor student progress and ensures students keep up. Importantly, by using Peyton's approach [12], student feedback is assured, with deliberate practice and instant feedback essential for clinical skill development [13].

Variation: Using a Simulator

Within nursing programs over the years, it has been accepted practice for students to be introduced to blood glucose measurement using pipetted glucose fluids of various concentrations, or to perform finger sticks either on themselves or undertake a role play, performing the skill on each other. The first of these practices does not allow for students to experience in any way the authentic activity of blood glucose measurement. In contrast, role play has the benefit of enabling students to practice locating anatomical landmarks, manipulating equipment, and trying out techniques required for blood glucose measurement under the supervision of an educator. Using role play, students can give and receive feedback from each other, which helps refine their technical skills and develop critical thinking. However, significant disadvantages of students learning blood glucose measurement on each other through role-play are fear and anxiety, the need for consent (and associated feelings of coercion), infection control, dissatisfaction, and potential disengagement with the learning experience.

Simulation using part-task trainers presents a suitable alternative to students gaining experience by administering a finger stick on themselves or others (Fig. 7.1). For example, a low-cost, high-fidelity simulator developed by Andersen, O'Brien, and Cox [14] has been shown to provide an effective tool in the development of core psychomotor skills that require sequencing and practice, in this case, blood glucose measurement. The approach presented by these authors maintains the learning characteristic of experiential learning, such as role-play, whilst overcoming risks to students and their learning.

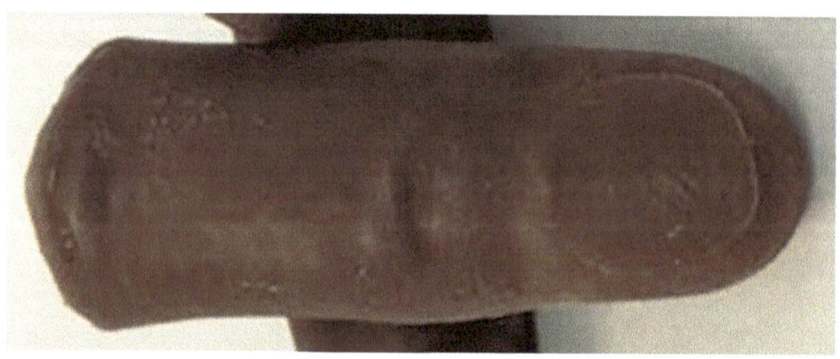

Fig. 7.1 Finger part-task trainer

Variation: Teaching Remotely

The COVID-19 pandemic of 2020 required education providers and educators to rapidly and significantly adapt to remote teaching. For many simulation users, this was the first time simulations were run via an online video communications technology such as ZOOM®. For the authors, teaching blood glucose measurement using remote learning was considered initially as requiring a significant change to the delivery of the simulation. However, Peyton's four-step approach [12] proved highly successful, requiring little modification to the structure of the skills session. The session plan is provided below.

Pre-simulation Brief

Each class in the course is comprised of 12 students. The class is welcomed by the facilitator. Students are asked to ensure their name is correct on their ZOOM® tile, their cameras turned on, and their microphones muted apart from when speaking. The pre-simulation brief commences with a statement of the learning outcomes and a question-and-answer session relating to the relevant course readings. Importantly, as students (and educators) have not participated in a skill session taught remotely, the structure of the session is explained. Of the 12 students participating in the session, one fulfills the role of the observer. This student uses a skills checklist for blood glucose finger stick to observe the performance of students during the session and use this information to provide feedback.

Simulation Scenario

In this example, when the focus is teaching a psychomotor skill, the scenario is straightforward. The technique of obtaining a finger stick is performed according to an evidence-based procedure or checklist. The technique is delivered using Peyton's four-step approach [12] as described.

Debrief

The debrief comprises two foci. One is the technique of obtaining blood glucose reading via a finger stick. The second is the experience of learning a technical skill remotely. Best practice recommends that the debrief commences with a description phase where the objectives of the simulation are revisited, and the purpose of the debriefing is stated [15]. It is anticipated that students will have some feelings about their experience of learning a skill remotely. The second phase of the debrief, the reaction/defuse phase [15], allows students to explore their responses to the simulation experience. During this phase, the debrief includes questions relating to their experience of learning a skill via remote learning. The reaction/defuse phase is followed by an analysis/discovery phase [15]. During this phase, students are asked questions directly relating to their experiences. The learning outcomes provide the focus of the debrief. The debrief concludes with a summary/application phase [15], where key learnings are captured in relation to the learning outcomes, and students are asked about the most significant learning for them to inform their future practice.

Simulation Plan: Obtaining Blood Glucose Via Remote Learning

Pre-simulation Readings

Hinkle JL and Cheever KH. Chapter 51: Assessment and management of patients with diabetes. In: Brunner & Suddarth's textbook of medical-surgical nursing. 14th ed. Philadelphia: Wolters Kluwer. 2018.

Taylor LP. Chapter X: Obtaining a capillary blood sample for glucose testing skills checklist. In: Taylor's clinical nursing skills: a nursing process approach, 5th ed. Philadelphia: Wolters Kluwer. 2018.

Learning Outcomes

Upon completion of this simulation, students will be able to:

(a) Identify the equipment required for performing a blood glucose finger stick.
(b) State the steps in sequence, and explain the rationale underpinning each step of performing a blood glucose finger stick to the facilitator.
(c) State three patient safety measures before and after measuring a blood glucose level via finger stick.

Equipment	
Part-task trainer (finger)	Simulated blood
Blood glucose monitor	Lancets
Cotton swabs	Reagent strips
Infections waste bin	Sharps container
Hand sanitizer	Non-sterile gloves
Eye protection	Sticking plaster / sterile dressing
Documentation— blood glucose record	

Setup

1. Arrange equipment on a clean flat surface following principles of best practice.
2. Position the camera so that the facilitator, the patient's hand/finger (simulator), and all equipment are in view.

Pre-simulation Brief

1. Welcome. Ask students to ensure their name displayed is correct, turn cameras on, and mute microphones unless speaking.
2. State learning outcomes for the simulation.
3. Q&A about course readings.
4. Explain to students the structure and sequence of the skills session. Describe Peyton's four-step approach to teaching a skill. Pause for questions at the end of each step.
5. Orientate students to the required equipment.
6. Instruct students to keep a copy of the skills sheet with them.
7. Explain that in place of a student demonstration each student will instruct the facilitator on performing the blood glucose finger stick procedure.
8. One student in the group is asked to observe the order in which students direct the steps to be performed and record this against the order on the checklist.
9. Ask students if they have questions before beginning.

Scenario

Step 1: The facilitator demonstrates the skill in real-time without description.

Step 2: The facilitator demonstrates the skill while describing the rationale for each step. At the end of the demonstration, the facilitator pauses for questions.

Step 3: One student at a time explains one step of the skill in sequence to the facilitator. The facilitator performs the procedure as instructed.

Step 4: Each student in the group is randomly assigned a step to direct the facilitator at the appropriate time. The student is required to explain the rationale for the step.

Checklist

Perform hand hygiene.

Apply non-sterile gloves.

Ask the patient to expose the finger of their choice.

Inspect the finger for any skin breakdown. Avoid fingers that have bruising, cracks, and rashes.

Wipe your finger with alcohol wipes and let dry.

Massage the finger gently to improve blood flow.

Turn on the glucometer. Insert the test strip into the glucometer.

Stick the skin with the lancet, expel, and wipe away the first drop of blood with gauze.

Squeeze the finger gently and allow blood to drop on the test strip.

Wait for and record the results.

Wipe the patient's finger and ensure bleeding has ceased.

Return the patient to a comfortable position.

Dispose of used items.

Wipe the glucometer & return it to its resting place.

Remove gloves & perform hand hygiene.

Report the results to the primary nurse immediately.

Debrief

The facilitator uses the following statements/ questions as prompts to facilitate the debrief.

1. Describe in one sentence your experience of learning a skill via remote.
2. The learning outcomes for today's simulation session were:
(a) Identify the equipment required for performing a blood glucose finger stick.
(b) State the steps in sequence, and explain the rationale underpinning each step of performing a blood glucose finger stick to the facilitator.
(c) State three patient safety measures before and after measuring a blood glucose level via finger stick.

Ask the observer/recorder how the learning outcomes were met.

What did you identify as three areas for improvement?

3. Ask each student at a time what has been the most important thing you have learned today. How will this inform your future clinical practice?

Nursing Simulation Fundamentals: The Cognitive Domain

The cognitive domain aims to develop students' thinking skills and knowledge. The cognitive domain comprises a taxonomy of six categories: remembering, understanding, applying, analyzing, evaluating, and creating [11]. Simulation-based learning provides an ideal medium for developing and assessing cognitive skills that may not be possible through more didactic learning and teaching methods. For example, the development of cognitive skills in the categories of apply, analyze, evaluate, and create. Using simulation, the development of cognitive skills can occur in all three phases of simulation. For example, revising course content during the pre-simulation brief can engage remembering and understanding. Participation in a simulation scenario engages students in application, analysis, evaluation, and potential creation. A well-structured and facilitated debrief presents an opportunity to engage students in all six cognitive domain categories.

Unlike psychomotor skills, students may find approaches for learning in the cognitive domain more daunting. This is because many strategies for the development of cognitive skills require making thinking visible [16]. This can expose students' need for knowledge and understanding. One such approach to learning that engages the cognitive domain of learning and makes thinking visible is the 'Think Aloud' approach.

When using Think Aloud in a simulation scenario, students verbalize their observations, thinking, and rationale for their actions during the scenario [17, 18]. In doing so, the Think Aloud approach makes thinking visible to observers, thus, enabling others to engage in collaborative thinking, reasoning, and judgment, and can potentially assist facilitators in identifying gaps in knowledge, clarifying concepts, reinforcing techniques, and facilitating students' learning and self-efficacy [17]. An example of a simulation experience for fundamentals nursing programs designed for learning in the cognitive domain is manual handling, more specifically, transferring a person from bed to chair.

Transferring a person from bed to chair is a fundamental skill. Yet the practice is complex, requiring students to combine the skills of assessment, analysis, planning, implementation, and evaluation. As a simulation activity, transferring a person is a complex learning activity comprising cognitive, psychomotor, and affective domains. For novice nursing students, remembering the steps for a complicated practice, such as transferring a person from bed to chair, can be a significant challenge. However, designing a simulation experience that engages strategies that target the cognitive domain of learning can make such a complex practice more memorable by making the cognitive or thinking processes visible. In this section, the design choices and the rationale for these choices are explained to aid in understanding the design of simulation activities for the cognitive domain.

Planning

This simulation activity intends to engage learning in the cognitive domain. The objective of the activity is to provide students with an experience of performing the practice of transferring a person from bed to chair. Accordingly, the learning outcomes are behavior-based, requiring students to *apply* theoretical knowledge and understanding such as assessment of the person and the environment, *analyz*ing assessment data in determining the person's fall risk, *creat*ing a plan for transferring the person from the bed to chair, and *implement*ing the plan.

In the planning phase, a key consideration for this activity is the role of the person to be transferred and the intended learning experience of the student. For example, using a peer or the facilitator (faculty) as the person to be transferred may provide a realistic experience for the student and enable feedback on student performance from the person being transferred. Disadvantages of this approach are that the student may not feel the dependent weight of a person during transfer, and there is a risk of injury to both the student performing the transfer and the person being transferred. In this simulation, the desired outcome is to provide the student with an experience of feeling the dependent weight of a person during transfer with minimal risk of injury. Hence, the use of a manikin is justified.

A second decision relates to the type of manikin. For this simulation, a no-technology manikin will suffice. Of importance is that the manikin has articulating limbs to accurately replicate human biomechanics during the transfer. For example, Laerdal Ultimate Hurt®.

A third and important consideration is of the environment being replicated, a home, an extended care setting, or a hospital. Determining the environment leads to considerations including the type of clothing for the manikin, floor surface, the type of bed and furnishings such as chairs, the availability and type of manual handling aides, and the type of clothing students are expected to wear, for example, a uniform. These considerations contribute to the visual replication of a real situation, as well as replicating factors such as sources of risk such as slippery surfaces, and physical constraints resulting from clothing.

Pre-simulation Activity

Prior to attending the simulation activity, students are introduced to the theory of manual handling and transferring a patient from bed to chair. This includes the theory of body mechanics, patient assessment, and safety and risk associated with this practice for both nurse and patient. Specific risk assessment tools, such as the Morse falls risk chart, are introduced, and their purpose and application are explained. A video of the procedure for transferring a patient from bed to chair and a skills checklist of the same skill are provided to students. This affords students the opportunity to view the practice in real time and reinforce the procedure by using the skills checklist.

Pre-simulation Brief

The pre-simulation brief commences with the facilitator welcoming the students by the facilitator and a statement of the learning outcomes. The learning outcomes for a simulation activity are designed to engage the cognitive domain of learning and focus on observable behaviors not achievable through other forms of formative or summative assessment. For example:

At the conclusion of the simulation, students will be able to

1. Implement relevant patient and environmental assessments before commencing the patient transfer.
2. Apply assessment findings in the planning, implementation, and evaluation of patient transfer from bed to chair, including preparing the environment, the patient, and self before, during, and after the skill.
3. Demonstrate the skill of transferring a patient from bed to chair to minimize risk to patient, nurse, and equipment while maximizing patient ability and patient safety.
4. Utilize the Think Aloud technique throughout the activity to explain thinking and decision-making.

Importantly, students are introduced to the Think Aloud approach, how it works, and the way it assists with the development of critical thinking, reasoning, and judgment. This is followed by a question and answer session relating to the relevant theory, pre-simulation course readings, the video, and the checklist. Socratic dialogue is used during the pre-simulation brief to assess the student's level of preparedness. This phase is concluded with an introduction to the scenario and an orientation to the simulation environment. This includes an introduction to the patient (manikin), Bailey Smythe. Students are informed that they are to ask their questions directly to the patient and that the patient will respond. The facilitator provides the voice of the patient. Finally, an explanation of roles and a call for volunteer participants occurs.

Simulation Scenario

During the simulation, students work in pairs to transfer a patient from bed to chair. Using the Think Aloud approach, students undertake a form of cognitive apprenticeship [16], talking through each step of the procedure prior to implementation. At the same time, the Think Aloud approach enables the facilitator to assess students' level of knowledge, observe students' techniques, and level of confidence with the skill. Importantly, it allows the facilitator to intervene in the event that an unsafe move is about to occur before this practice is implemented. In pairs, one student takes the lead, with the second on hand to assist when required. In this simulation, assistance may be helping with the transfer or providing advice on the next step. The remainder of the class takes on observer roles, following the demonstration with the skill checklist. Once Bailey is seated, a short debrief is conducted. After this, the next pair of students practice transferring the patient from bed to chair.

Debriefing

The debrief commences with the reactions phase and the question, "How did that feel?". Students often admit feeling "awkward and self-conscious initially." However, they may also report that these feelings soon subside once they focus on the task and think through each step. Using Think Aloud enables students to feel as if the situation is real, like they are practicing in the presence of an actual patient. Performing the skill in pairs boosts confidence when participating in the simulation, as well as when providing feedback during the debrief. Importantly the Think Aloud approach reported by students helps them remember the steps in a logical manner.

Each debrief is structured around the learning outcomes, first asking the students who performed the transfer what went well in relation to (1) assessing the patient and the environment, (2) planning for the transfer, and (3) performing the transfer of the patient from bed to chair. Observers are then asked what was observed to have been done well. The students who performed the transfer were then asked what could be improved, followed by the observers.

The simulation plan for this simulation activity is provided in Appendix 1.

Transferring a patient from bed to chair is a fundamental nursing skill yet one that few nursing skills textbooks address. Using the Think Aloud approach for complex practices and procedures which require multiple steps can prove useful to enhance meaningful learning in the cognitive domain. Think Aloud is a helpful teaching tool and a powerful student-learning strategy. It is a valuable strategy to prompt communication and knowledge sharing between students and model critical thinking and clinical reasoning. The simulation approach described has shown that Think Aloud is an effective strategy in providing a safe learning environment, encouraging peer engagement, providing structure, decreasing anxiety, creating realism, and improving student confidence.

Nursing Simulation Fundamentals: The Affective Domain

The affective domain of learning aims to engage and develop the learner's feelings, emotions, and attitudes. The affective domain comprises a taxonomy of five categories. These are (1) receiving phenomena, (2) responding to phenomena, (3) valuing, (4) organization, and (5) characterisation [9]. Receiving phenomena, or information relating to a situation, creates an awareness of feelings and emotions as well as the ability to utilize selected attention, for example, engaging in active listening with clients. Responding to phenomena is at the very heart of active learning and may be represented as active participation in a class or active listening to a client or patient in the practice setting. Valuing is significant to nursing education and for nursing professionals as it represents the ability of an individual to recognize the worth or value of phenomena and to express it. An individual's ability to prioritize one value over another and develop one's own value system is termed organization. The final category, characterization, relates to the ability of an individual to internalize values and allow them to form the basis of their behavior. In this third case study, resilience provides the context for simulation as a fundamental element of nursing to engage the affective domain of learning. This is because individuals' capacity to demonstrate resilience can be understood in terms of how they receive, respond, value, organize and characterize phenomena.

Resilience is a term commonly used to describe the ability to turn adversity into opportunities and to learn from demanding situations [19]. Whilst resilience may not be immediately recognized for inclusion as a 'nursing fundamental,' it provides an important contribution to nursing students' readiness to care. In this way, resilience has a place as a fundamental of pre-registration nursing education. However, this may be for nursing education to support nursing students to develop resilience. One such strategy using simulation is the Tag Team Patient Safety Simulation method [20].

Tag Team Patient Safety Simulation

Tag Team Patient Safety Simulation (TTPSS) [20] is a highly interactive simulation approach that promotes the active engagement of participants, including observers. Based on the tenets of Forum Theatre [21], TTPSS is designed to empower students to become agents of social change, specifically, to become advocates of patient safety. TTPSS is presented as a theatrical 'play' comprising five phases: (1) Setup and Briefing, (2) Act One (scenario), (3) Intermission (mini-debrief), (4) Act Two (repeat scenario), and (5) Debriefing [20]. Specific roles required for a TTPSS are Director, the Protagonist, Audience, and Cast. The Director is the facilitator who conveys the patient's story, promotes student learning, captures teachable moments, and facilitates the debrief. The protagonist (often a patient) is the central character in the play and has an authentic social and medical history that is relevant to the focus of the simulation scenario. The Audience members (students who are not members of the cast) are active observers who adopt the role of theatre critics and provide feedback to the cast during the intermission and debriefing. The cast are students who actively engage in the play by exchanging roles by tagging in and out of the unfolding scenario [20].

Tagging can be initiated by either the Director or cast members and is characterized by calling the word 'TAG' and the touch of hands or a tap on the shoulder. When tagged, the new cast member takes over where the previous cast member left off. Tagging supports students by managing performance anxiety during situations where students may feel overwhelmed or uncomfortable. Students can either 'tag out' or support another learner by 'tagging in' and offering an alternative solution. Tagging is not reflective of the level of performance; instead, it is a strategy that allows learners to rehearse different ways of responding to everyday practice-based situations and to work as a team to facilitate their learning. More information about the TTPSS methodology is available at Guinea et al. [20]

TTPSS aims to develop resilience in participants by placing students in everyday challenging situations whereby patient safety is threatened. The degree of the challenge created during the simulation is controlled by the director using antagonist cards, which instruct the protagonist to demonstrate a particular behavior, verbalize a specific statement, or adopt a particular attitude that may present students with a challenge. An example of the TTPSS used in this chapter is medication administration. In this simulation, the threat to patient safety is the buddy nurse leaving the student to administer medication unsupervised. The challenge resulting from antagonist cards aims to develop resilience in student nurses akin to the "Pushing Through" model of resilience [22] by first, 'stepping into' the adversity; second, 'staying the course', or being aware they must continue pursuing their goals; and third, 'acknowledging' that they have learned from their adversity and felt ready to meet another challenge [23]. Within this model, it is possible to draw parallels between resilience and the learning categories in the affective domain: receiving, responding, valuing, organizing, and characterization [9]. In TTPSS, students are encouraged to accept responsibility for their actions and to respond to the challenging situations resulting from Antagonist Cards. This approach allows students to persist by working through challenging situations and employing critical thinking, problem-solving, and teamwork. Collectively the outcomes of TTPSS assist students in building confidence and develop competence in managing challenging situations.

Setup[1]

This simulation scenario situates the nursing student in an acute care environment, caring for a post-operative orthopedic patient who is experiencing pain. The nursing student is working alongside a Registered Nurse and provides the opportunity for students to engage with clinical handover, pain assessment, neurovascular assessment, safe administration of medications, evaluating effectiveness of analgesic medications, recognition of adverse drug reactions, and responding to medication errors.

The setup for this simulation requires one simulated patient, who may be a student, to fulfill the role of the patient and the patient's family member. One of the principles of TTPSS is that these simulations can be conducted in any learning environment [20]. Hence only essential props are required with the following examples provided [24].

Environment: patient chair, footstool, chair for patient's family member, hand sanitizer, equipment for vital signs monitoring,

Patient: hospital gown, identification band, leg brace/bandages for the affected leg.

Documentation: Falls risk assessment tool, pressure injury risk assessment tool, medication administration chart, vital signs, neurovascular observations, and progress notes. Documentation complete with entries accurate to the date and time of the scenario.

Medications: medications as per medication chart, medicine cups, pharmacology reference, telephone.

[1]Scenario available online at https://www.cqu.edu.au/about-us/structure/schools/nm/simulation/ttpss

Pre-simulation Brief

The pre-simulation brief for the TTPSS scenario involves the statement of learning outcomes:

At the completion of this simulation, students will be able to:

1. Perform a patient assessment relevant to cues and the patient history.
2. Administer and monitor the therapeutic use of medications and respond appropriately to medication errors and adverse drug reactions.
3. Collaborate and communicate effectively with other members of the healthcare team.

As empowering students to be advocates for patient safety is a signature goal of TTPSS, the significance of this simulation as it relates to patient safety is discussed with students. The TTPSS approach is presented, including the rules of TTPSS, roles, and structure of this simulation method. Key characteristics of tagging, cue cards, and antagonist cards are also presented so that everyone understands how this specific simulation methodology works. The pre-simulation brief concludes with allocating roles and distributing briefing cards to the simulated patient and family member, briefing cards to participants in the student role (the cast), and briefing cards and cue cards to participants in the observer role (the audience). All participants are provided with 5 min to prepare for their role. Participants in the student role are provided with an orientation to the simulation environment. Finally, participants are reminded to use the Think Aloud approach and clear voice to explain the thinking behind their actions.

Simulation Scenario

Act 1 begins with the Director providing a clinical handover, following which the cast members participate in the unfolding scenario and tag in and out, working collectively to address the needs of the patient and their family members. When tagging occurs, the new cast member continues the role and influences the direction of the play through their actions and reactions to the unfolding situation. The director may use the antagonist cards to increase the complexity of the situation by presenting a challenge for the student to navigate. Responding to an antagonist card requires students to engage in critical thinking and to respond to a situation that may undermine patient safety. For example, in this simulation where the focus is on medication safety, one of the antagonist cards reads, 'As the registered nurse, you tell the student to leave the medication at the bedside so that the patient can take it with their next meal.' During the simulation, the audience members critically observe the performance with a focus on the information provided on their cue card. For example, in this simulation, one of the cue cards reads, 'Observe and provide feedback about the student nurses' adherence to scope of practice and any actions taken to seek supervision for medication administration.'

At the conclusion of Act 1, the director calls for Intermission. Intermission is a mini-debrief whereby the director uses Socratic questioning to facilitate reflection on action and for students to identify ways to improve their interaction in the scenario. The structure of the Intermission takes the form of the director asking audience members to provide their observations of Act 1 with specific reference to their cue cards. The focus is on making suggestions for improvement to be implemented in Act 2. The director then asks cast members to respond to the suggestions and to outline their plan to improve their practice in Act 2. If antagonist cards are utilized, the responses to these are explored in the context of developing resilience: recognizing the challenging situation confronting them and stepping into the adversity; staying the course by being aware they must continue pursuing the goal of providing care for the person within their scope of practice; and finally, acknowledging that they have learned from the adversity and feel ready to meet another challenge. The intermission should be no longer than 20 min.

Act 2 immediately follows intermission. This is a repeat of Act 1 with the key difference that the performance of cast members should have improved based on the feedback provided during the intermission. The aim of Act 2 is to provide students with the opportunity to demonstrate learning and build confidence and competence.

Debriefing

A structured Debrief follows Act 2. The director uses Pendleton's Rules of Feedback [25] to facilitate an in-depth exploration of what unfolded during the play with a specific focus on the perspectives of the patient and the actions and reactions of the cast members. The Patient Safety Competency Framework for Nursing Students [26] and the Australian National Safety and Quality Health Service Standards informs the discussion [27]. If the discussion does not cover all learning outcomes, the Director may use 'What if …' questions. For example: 'What if the patient refuses medication, but the Registered Nurse says you must force the patient to take it or hide it in their meal?'. Once again, a key focus of questioning during the debrief is developing resilience, helping students recognize challenging situations, manage these as opportunities for learning, and accept responsibility for their actions.

As mentioned earlier, resilience may not be immediately recognized for inclusion as a 'nursing fundamental.' However, using the case study of TTPSS, the need to develop resilience in pre-registration nursing students is evident. Simulations informed by the affective domain of learning can provide early years student nurses with simulation experiences that provide sufficient challenge to develop resilience:

- engaging heightened feelings and emotions (receiving)
- requiring students to manage heightened emotions while managing the challenging situation at hand (responding),
- reflecting on one's own perspectives and values as well as those of others (valuing),
- working out how to best prioritize and express these different perspectives and values in a given situation (organization), and
- through reflection, consider how these experiences inform the attributes of one's self as a nurse (characterize) [9].

The purposeful approach TTPSS to the use of tagging and replaying the simulation scenario contributes to the development of student nurses' readiness to care. Tagging provides student nurses with the opportunity to try different approaches to a situation, as well as to observe how different students interpret and respond to the same situation. Exploring these affective dimensions of learning during the intermission and the debrief provides invaluable insights with the aim of developing greater understanding of differing perceptions and perspectives, the role these play in challenging situations, and the role resilience plays in managing these situations as a registered nurse. TTPSS demonstrates that these learning experiences can occur as a direct participant in the simulation scenarios (cast) or vicariously as an observer (audience).

Conclusion

Simulation has an essential role in developing student nurses' knowledge, skills, and attributes through designed learning experiences. Within this chapter, three examples have been provided to illustrate the role simulation can play in the teaching and learning of nursing fundamentals. The choice to structure this chapter according to the three domains of learning—psychomotor, cognitive, and affective—has made it possible to demonstrate how the purposeful, focussed application of a learning domain can effectively guide the design of simulation activity for teaching, learning, or assessment. In addition, drawing on a particular theoretical perspective of learning for each example has provided insights into how learning theory can inform simulation design and assist simulation designers in developing educationally sound simulation experiences.

Equipped with an understanding of simulation practice's fundamental principles and concepts, educators can find that well-designed simulation activities readily translate to different simulation modalities. Educators may lament the time it takes to plan, develop, and document simulation activities. However, theory-informed practices provide structure, guidance, and strategies that aid in translating simulation scenarios to the suitable modality, practice context, and learning environment—including remote learning. In brief, the principles of simulation practice fundamentally do not change.

A note from the authors…
This chapter has been written at a time characterized by unprecedented social change requiring rapid and significant adaptation and innovation to the delivery of nursing education. The global COVID-19 pandemic has influenced this chapter insofar as considering the situations some early years student nurses have been confronted with that they would not have been previously exposed to. For example, lockdowns, being isolated from family and friends, online learning, and in the clinical field, wearing of PPE for extended periods, caring for critically ill patients, and witnessing death and dying on a scale not seen for several generations. These experiences have sparked critical conversations amongst the authors about ways to help students develop skills for practice, rehearsing processes for not only learning but surviving situations that are unfamiliar, stressful, and uncertain. The following vignette is a reflection of nursing education in 2020 from Mary Moran, RN.

Fundamentals Re-imagined During the COVID-19 by Mary Moran

Traditionally, students in the accelerated Master's Direct Entry Nursing Program at the Columbia University School of Nursing, New York, begin their clinical immersion at the end of their didactic classes in March of each year. The COVID-19 pandemic of 2020 made that an impossibility, as all clinical rotations were suspended. However, the School of Nursing and partner hospitals where the students did their course clinical rotations developed an innovative program offering the students the option of working as Patient Care Technicians (PCTs). By mid-March 2020, as the number of patients with COVID-19 soared, hospital nurses needed help. Approximately 50–90% students were enrolled in the PCT. Reviewing the job description and scope of practice for PCTs afforded the simulation educators needed information for program development.

The next step was to determine the framework to use. It was agreed to adopt the NLN Jeffries Simulation Theory [28]. The learning outcomes for the activities were based on the PCT's scope of practice. These included: post-mortem care (not previously covered), blood glucose monitoring (not an activity student nurses perform in hospitals), care of patients with COVID-19 on step-down units, applying leads for cardiac rhythm monitoring, and recording a 12-lead ECG. The content of the program was taught via remote videoconferencing (ZOOM®) and repeated several times to provide each learner to participate. The facilitator/educator worked in the simulation lab, where the manikin and equipment were close captured for greater fidelity. Students kept their cameras on and were unmuted so that they could ask questions during the demonstration. Thus, facilitating continued discussion between learners and facilitator. A block of 2 hours was allocated for each presentation.

The pre-brief allowed for questions and clarification. For the skills presentations, the Peyton four-step approach [12] was used: demonstration, deconstruction, comprehension, and performance, each followed by a question and answer session. The debriefing segment provided the students the opportunity to discuss how the experience made them feel. One or two students were asked to describe the activity and outcomes. The analysis portion included students discussing what went well. In summary, the students discussed how the session contributed to their learning and what they can take to their practice.

Prior to the presentation, students were sent the objectives of the session, the checklist from the skills test, and readings related to the topic, most of which required them to review their didactic notes. They were alerted that they would be called upon to instruct the facilitator how to perform the skill. The overarching objective was that each exercise simulated an in-person presentation as closely as possible. To achieve this, the number of participants per session was limited to 12. The materials used were made available on canvas. During the learner instruction sessions, they were charged with correcting errors made by the facilitator and explaining the possible outcome of such an error.

What Were the Challenges for Students?

There were a number of challenges experienced by students during this time. One of the biggest challenges was the paucity of PPE. At the beginning of their coursework in 2019, PPE training included proper disposal of gloves, masks, and gowns after each use. That all changed in the midst of the pandemic. Staff were using the same masks for days at a time; gowns were re-worn many times.

The lack of family members visiting the patients was especially challenging for all staff, patients dying alone as members said goodbye through FaceTime® on the phone with the nurse holding close to the dying patient or finding a deceased patient when entering a room.

What Were the Benefits of Providing Remote Videoconferencing During the Pandemic?

Students' responses ranged from feeling connected with faculty at a very "scary" time, knowing there was an option to continue learning, being able to ask questions without fear of pushback, seeing each other on (ZOOM®), a sense of belonging, support and empathy in the midst of a very trying time for hospital personnel.

How Was Learning Evaluated?

Having students involved in teaching the facilitator exposes their level of knowledge and emotional engagement in the activity. Assessing the psychomotor component of learning proves more challenging. However, some insight can be gained when for example, the facilitator receives corrective guidance from students, for example, applying a blood pressure cuff incorrectly or handling a syringe when giving an injection.

References

1. Kitson A, Conroy T, Wengstrom Y, Profetto-McGrath J, Robertson-Malt S. Defining the fundamentals of care. Int J Nurs Pract. 2010;16:423–34.
2. Stroup C. Simulation usage in nursing fundamentals: integrative literature review. Clin Simul Nurs. 2014;10(3):e155–64. https://doi.org/10.1016/j.ecns.2013.10.004.
3. Bland AJ, Topping A, Wood B. A concept analysis of simulation as a learning strategy in the education of undergraduate nursing students. Nurse Educ Today. 2011;31(7):664–70. https://doi.org/10.1016/j.nedt.2010.10.013.
4. Lioce L (Ed.), Lopreiato J (Founding Ed.), Downing D, Chang TP, Robertson JM, Anderson M, Diaz DA, Spain AE (Assoc. Eds.) and the Terminology and Concepts Working Group. Healthcare simulation dictionary. 2nd ed. Rockville: Agency for Healthcare Research and Quality; 2020. https://doi.org/10.23970/simulationv2.
5. INACSL Standards Committee, Molloy MA, Holt J, Charnetski M, Rossler K. Healthcare simulation standards of best practice: simulation glossary. Clin Simul Nurs. 2021;58:57–65. https://doi.org/10.1016/j.ecns.2021.08.017.
6. Hsieh MC, Lee JJ. Preliminary study of VR and AR applications in medical and healthcare education. J Nurs Health Stud. 2017;3(1):1–5. https://doi.org/10.21767/2574-2825.100030.
7. Arveklev SH, Wigert H, Berg B, Lepp M. The use and application of drama in nursing education: an integrative review of the literature. Nurse Educ Today. 2015;35:e12–7. https://doi.org/10.1016/j.nedt.2015.02.025.
8. Bloom BS, Krathwohl DR. Taxonomy of educational objectives: the classification of educational goals by a committee of college and university examiners. In: Handbook I: cognitive domain. New York: Longmans, Green; 1956.
9. Krathwohl DR, Bloom BS, Masia BB. Taxonomy of educational objectives: the classification of educational goals. In: Handbook II: affective domain. New York: David McKay; 1964.
10. Harrow AJ. A taxonomy of the psychomotor domain. New York: David McKay; 1972.
11. Krathwohl DR, Anderson LW, Bloom BS. A taxonomy for learning, teaching, and assessing: a revision of Bloom's taxonomy of educational objectives. New York: Longman; 2001.
12. Walker M, Peyton JWR. Teaching in the theatre. In: Peyton JWR, editor. Teaching and learning in medical practice. Rickmansworth: Manticore Publishers Europe; 1998. p. 171–80.
13. Kiernan LC. Evaluating competence and confidence using simulation technology. Nursing. 2018;48(10):45–52. https://doi.org/10.1097/01.NURSE.0000545022.36908.f3.
14. Andersen P, O'Brien S, Cox K. Developing low-cost, high-fidelity resources for blood glucose measurement and cord blood sampling. Clin Simul Nurs. 2016;12(11):504–10. https://doi.org/10.1016/j.ecns.2016.07.005.
15. INACSL Standards Committee, Decker S, Alinier G, Crawford SB, Gordon RM, Wilson C. Healthcare simulation standards of best practice: the debriefing process. Clin Simul Nurs. 2021;58:27–32. https://doi.org/10.1016/j.ecns.2021.08.011.
16. Collins A, Seely Brown J, Holum A. Cognitive apprenticeship: making thinking visible. Am Educ. 1991. https://www.aft.org/ae/winter1991/collins_brown_holum.
17. Burbach BE, Barnason S, Thompson SA. Using "thinking aloud" to capture clinical reasoning during patient simulation. Int J Nurs Educ Scholarsh. 2015;12(1):1–7. https://doi.org/10.1515/ijnes-2014-0044.
18. Verkuyl M, Hughes M, Fyfe MC. Using think aloud in health assessment: a mixed-methods study. J Nurs Educ. 2018;57(11):684–6. https://doi.org/10.3928/01484834-20181022-10.
19. Amsrud KE, Severinsson E. Development of resilience in nursing students: a systematic qualitative review and thematic synthesis. Nurse Educ Pract. 2019;41:102621. https://doi.org/10.1016/j.nepr.2019.102621.
20. Guinea S, Andersen P, Reid-Searl K, Levett-Jones T, Dwyer T, Heaton L, et al. Simulation-based learning for patient safety: the development of the tag team patient safety simulation methodology for nursing education. Collegian. 2019;26:392–8. https://doi.org/10.1016/j.colegn.2018.09.008.
21. Boal A. Games for actors and non-actors. London: Routledge; 2002.
22. Reyes AT, Andrusyszyn MA, Iwasiw C, Forchuk C, Babenko-Mould Y. Nursing students' understanding and enactment of resilience: a grounded theory study. J Adv Nurs. 2015;71(11):2622–33. https://doi.org/10.1111/jan.12730.
23. Lanz JJ. Evidence-based resilience intervention for nursing students: a randomized controlled pilot trial. Int J Appl Posit Psychol. 2020;17:1–4. https://doi.org/10.1007/s41042-020-00034-8.
24. Reid-Searl K, Flenady T. Medication safety. Rockhampton: CQUniversity; 2017. https://www.cqu.edu.au/about-us/structure/schools/nm/simulation/ttpss.
25. Pendleton D, Schofield T, Tate P, Havelock P. The new consultation: developing doctor–patient communication. Oxford: Oxford University Press; 1984.
26. Levett-Jones T, Dwyer T, Reid-Searl K, Heaton L, Flenady T, Applegarth J, Guinea S, Andersen P. Patient safety competency framework (PSCF) for nursing students. Sydney; 2017. http://patientsafetyfornursingstudents.org/
27. Australian Commission on Safety and Quality in Health Care. National safety and quality health service standards. 2nd ed. https://www.safetyandquality.gov.au/our-work/assessment-to-the-nsqhs-standards/nsqhs-standards-second-edition/.
28. Jeffries P. The NLN Jeffries simulation theory. Philadelphia: Wolters Kluwer; 2015.

Medical-Surgical Nursing

8

Georgina Willetts

Introduction: Background

> It is the general conception of any field of inquiry that ultimately determines the kind of knowledge that field aims to develop as well as how that knowledge is to be organized, tested, and applied. Such an understanding involves critical attention to the question of what it means to know and what kinds of knowledge are held to be of most value in the discipline of nursing [1].

The overall objective of teaching with simulation in medical-surgical nursing is to provide authenticity of clinical practice while creating a safe space for the student to develop nursing knowledge, skills, and attributes. Authentic simulations provide a significant opportunity to introduce students to the fundamental concepts of professional practice. The learning outcomes across all simulations within an undergraduate nursing program are best when they focus on the following:

- Reaction—exposure to the professional environment
- Learning—learning to think like a nurse
- Behavior—modeling and appropriate nursing behavior
- Results—competence and capable nursing practice

The aim is to move to introduce holistic, immersive, and authentic learning experiences that develop students' ability to reflect on and in practice.

Our medical-surgical simulation teaching was scaffolded throughout our pre-registration course. It was loosely aligned to Benner's (1984) novice to expert continuum with the expectation that the student would only reach the advanced beginner level on completion of their nursing course due to their limited real experiences with patient care [2].

When students first commenced (as in Benner's novice phase), we implemented simulation strategies that help students predict patient situations and perform patient care skills while also providing structure and guidelines to meet their needs. By the end of their pre-registration course, students are expected to have enough simulated experience to identify and meaningfully respond to components of a clinical situation, particularly within the medical-surgical environment. The students are then ready to enter the graduate world with the strategies to undertake clinical practice safely and prepared to progress along the novice-to-expert continuum through real-life in-depth clinical experience.

Medical-Surgical Nursing

Even though nursing contexts of practice are everchanging, medical-surgical nursing remains the backbone of nursing and is a focal component of undergraduate nursing education. Many curriculum hours are devoted to simulation that prepares nurses for the medical-surgical environment. This, therefore, creates an opportunity to ensure the skills developed during these learning experiences address the key nursing practice concepts. If the concepts are taught appropriately, the practice should be translatable to the varying clinical contexts in which the nurse will find themselves.

Medical-Surgical Simulation

In our simulation spaces, we created clear and consistent processes. One of these processes was to ensure consistency in the simulation episodes that enable familiarity with the environment. The significance of the consistency of the process was to decrease cognitive load allowing the students to focus on the learnings within the simulation itself [3].

Simulation is about holistically preparing students for clinical practice, not just developing psychomotor skills. Several key elements should be considered in designing medical-surgical simulations as part of the curriculum design process. These elements are most appropriately introduced at the beginning of the nursing program, which are then

G. Willetts (✉)
Federation University Australia, Ballarat, VIC, Australia
e-mail: g.willetts@federation.edu.au

J. M. Kutzin et al. (eds.), *Comprehensive Healthcare Simulation: Nursing*, Comprehensive Healthcare Simulation,
https://doi.org/10.1007/978-3-031-31090-4_8

scaffolded across different stages of the course so that students can grasp simple to complex concepts using practical examples aligned to best practice approaches in nursing. Many of these elements are not limited to simulation and Clinical Learning Environments (CLE) teaching and learning but are undoubtedly core to simulation in medical-surgical education. Many of these elements have been borrowed from best practices in the areas of simulation, nursing, and pedagogy and include:

- Code of conduct
- Strengths-based [4]
- Becoming person-centered [5]
- The fundamentals of care [5]
- Clinical reasoning—thinking like a nurse [6]
- Patient assessment skills [7]
- Therapeutic and empathic communication [8]

These elements represent specific aspects scaffolded across the curriculum that underpin student learning. These elements were used to guide the development and implementation of the simulation cases, lesson plans, and debriefing methods to promote situated thinking. Having faculty with clinical expertise in nursing practice is critical to ensure the narrative of nursing practice is developed in real-time for the student learning experience. Having standard elements to situate their teaching is also fundamentally important for faculty so they can focus on their clinical expertise rather than the teaching modality.

Design Consistency of Simulation Using Evidenced-Based Specific Elements

Code of Conduct

A code of conduct was introduced on the first day of the student's simulation experience and was used in all clinical learning environments. It was expected that this would be adhered to whenever students entered the simulated space. This created an expectation similar to what would be encountered by the students in a real clinical environment. We further developed this expectation to include professional attire during simulation activities that replicate the clothing students wear in the hospital (in our case, a uniform inclusive of appropriate footwear). Arriving on time and entering the clinical learning environment (CLE) safely by adhering to hand hygiene practices and other requirements were adopted within the simulation setting.

These expectations commence immediately in the first year, with students' first medical-surgical simulation enabling and continuing throughout the course, thus developing students' ability to think like a nurse and encouraging appropriate development of their professional identity.

Strengths-Based Nursing

To move the nursing student along the learning trajectory during the medical-surgical curriculum, the underpinning conceptual element used was Strengths-Based Nursing, an approach developed by Gottlieb [4, 9, 10]. This approach changes the focus of clinical practice away from an illness deficit model to a strengths-based model with eight underlying principles that develop nursing practice by promoting empowerment, self-efficacy, and hope [9]. These are fundamental principles for contemporary nursing practice. All our teaching episodes were developed with these core values, and in any given simulation, there would always be a consideration for the patient's strengths and what they could do rather than the traditional focus only on their deficits.

Becoming Person-Centered

Becoming person-centered emphasizes the professional focus of nursing practice and the need to communicate, collaborate and authentically demonstrate empathy [11]. Person-centered approaches were central when developing lesson plans for both CLEs and simulations in medical-surgical scenarios [12]. Practically speaking, lesson plans were often co-created with those who have had lived experiences as consumers of care. Students are challenged to think about components of person-centredness including:

- Being in relation
- Being in a social world
- Being in place
- Being with self [12]

An example of this co-creation was an Indigenous Simulation [13] developed with Indigenous leaders and an interprofessional healthcare team. This simulation focused on developing therapeutic communication skills in the first year. The evaluations demonstrated the authenticity of the simulation had a profound effect on the students.

Fundamentals of Care

Following on from the elements of person-centredness are the fundamentals of the care framework. This framework developed by Kitson et al. [14] identifies three core elements: "(1) nurse–patient relationship, (2) integration of care needs, and (3) the context in which care is delivered" [15].

Fundamentals of care were incorporated into the medical-surgical simulations. The effectiveness of the simulation was very much determined by faculty promoting these elements throughout the simulation, with observation and reflection used to drive the debriefing after the simulation has occurred [16].

Clinical Reasoning: Thinking like a Nurse

The next progression from person-centredness and fundamentals of care was the clinical reasoning cycle. In our simulation sessions, we used the clinical reasoning cycle as a learning process to develop the nursing student's capability to think like a nurse [17]. This framework steps the nursing students through a structured process to develop their care plan and then evaluate it. This framework, again introduced at the beginning of the CLE and simulations within the medical-surgical component of the curriculum, was used as a structured approach throughout the nursing program. This must be revisited and embedded into every session to enable the nursing student to reason through planning nursing care. The clinical reasoning cycle allows the nursing student to systematically work through a patient care process to develop a care plan. This was only one part of simulated learning, particularly in the early phases of the medical-surgical curriculum [18].

Patient Assessment Skills

We taught patient assessment skills in the very first sessions of medical-surgical CLEs. It is at the initial stages that part-task training occurs. This was where we broke down psychomotor skills for skills attainment within our CLE environment, which helped prepare the nursing students for the more complex patient scenarios they would encounter in the simulation space. The focus was on the acute setting of the medical-surgical hospital situation, and we began with teaching the concept of collecting data/cues or information as the first step of the clinical reasoning cycle. The concept of objective and subjective data was introduced, then primary and secondary assessment was taught using the acronym of DRSABCDE (see Box 8.1) [19].

Box 8.1 The DRSABCDE Approach to Health Assessment

D: Danger—is the environment safe for you and your patient? e.g., are there spills on the floor? electrical cords? trip hazards? 'don' any protective equipment such as goggles and gloves

R: Response—is your patient able to respond to vocal stimuli?

S: Send for help—do you need extra assistance? If so, call for help

A: Airway—is the patient's airway patent? Is it clear and open? Are there any drooling or voice changes?

B: Breathing—is the patient breathing? Is the chest rising and falling? Is there work of breathing or use of accessory muscles?

C: Circulation—is the patient warm? what is their capillary refill?

D: Disability—does the patient have any neurological deficits?

E: Environment/Exposure—consider things such as privacy in the current environment, as well as exposure to the external environment. Are they cold? expose the patient and check all limbs, abdomen and back

The nursing student then practices primary assessment using the mnemonic FGH

F—Full set of vital signs

G—Give comfort measures

H—History and Head-to-Toe

Once this was taught and practiced in the CLE environment, we introduced the secondary assessment, which was broken into a systems-based approach. Initially, this teaching commenced with taking a history, and we continued to provide mnemonics so that the novice nursing student had clarity on the steps to take. Specifically for the medical-surgical cases, we encouraged the students to use the pneumonic SAMPLE (See Box 8.2) [7].

Box 8.2 Secondary Assessment

S—Signs/Symptoms: what brings them to the health care setting? What is their clinical complaint?

A—Allergies: do they have any allergies to medications or foods?

M—Medications: what medications are they currently taking, including prescription and over-the-counter medications?

P—Past Illnesses: what relevant past medical history or illnesses could be contributing to their current problem?

L—Last input and output: when did they last eat or drink? when did they last void (urinate) or have a bowel movement?

E—Events leading up to present illness/injury: what preceded this event occurring?

The CLEs focus on teaching a systems approach assessment where the skills of- inspection, palpation, percussion, and auscultation relevant to each body system were introduced. Once this part of task training had been mastered, the nursing students were then equipped to move on to more complex case scenarios in the simulation space.

Teaching Therapeutic and Empathic Communication

The last approach used when teaching medical-surgical simulations was a clear structure to communication. This was developed from Amanda Henderson's (2019) book on communication for healthcare practice and has three elements: understanding, participation, and respect, which all pivot around the concepts of person-centredness. See Fig. 8.1.

Again, these concepts were incorporated into lesson plans and interactions and questioning approaches with the nursing students as they undertook their simulations and debriefing exercises.

Scaffolding of communication again happened across the curriculum to firstly ensure that students 'understanding' was sufficient as they develop their communication skills, then increase their 'participation' with 'respect' being the final developmental stage so that communication becomes 'person-centered.' Communication skills are complex skills that need time to develop. The facilitation by faculty is particularly important to enable the students to adapt and refine their therapeutic communication to a range of medical-surgical nursing situations.

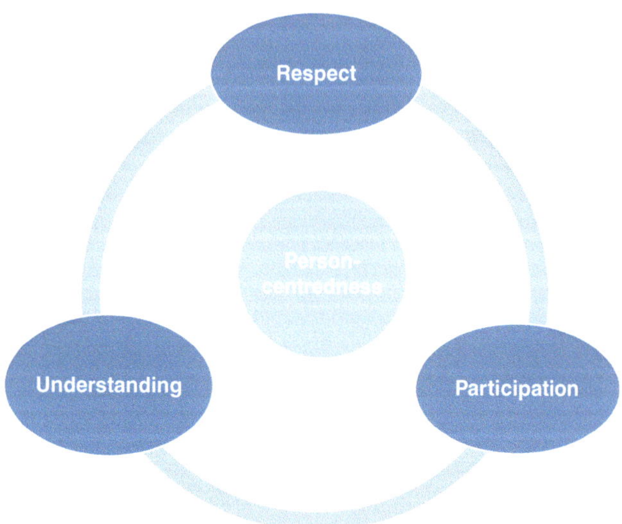

Fig. 8.1 Elements of communication [8, 20]

Best Practices, Challenges, and Solutions

This section discusses the best practices used to implement medical-surgical simulations successfully. Challenges encountered and possible solutions are also discussed in this section.

Best Practices

The overarching aim of the medical-surgical simulation is to practice skills and behaviors in a simulated learning environment in preparation for clinical practice. We discuss mastery further in this section; however, for simulation sessions to be successful, students need to undertake prior learning and practice to be able to navigate a simulation session successfully. As mentioned, the clinical learning environments (CLEs) where part-task training is taught are critical preparation before an actual simulation session. The best sequencing of this is for the student to **prepare** through the pre-learning, **explore and practice** in the CLEs and then **apply** this during the simulation episode. Nursing practice is made up of a range of complex skills, including psychomotor, clinical reasoning, and professional skills, inclusive of effective communication. We scaffolded this learning with more CLEs in the early stages of the course and fewer simulations. As the tasks were mastered, we increased complexity with more frequent simulation sessions and fewer CLE sessions. This was a staged approach in preparation for the complexities students will encounter in their clinical placements.

To utilize simulation for its intended purpose, it is important to scaffold the learning throughout the nursing degree. This approach starts with teaching technical skills early in the course using part-task trainers and skills-focused laboratory classes in the CLE episodes. These technical skills are then built upon in the simulation setting as students perform technical and other skills needed for professional practice.

Developing Professional Practice

Traditionally, in a simulation setting, students will focus on the tasks and skills they feel they need to master for practice. However, developing capability extends beyond procedural skills. As a rule, three categories of learning outcomes are to be achieved in a simulation session: professional skills, clinical reasoning, and psychomotor skills.

Professional Skills

Professional skills include learning a nurse's everyday behavior and expectations, such as communicating with the patients and their family/community, with each other, and within an interprofessional team. The development of professional skills is a crucial part of simulated learning. We set this up through several initial orientation processes before the students enter the CLE or simulation space. When we first orient the nursing student to the CLE and simulation space, our expectation was a professional presentation, and therefore, the nursing student would enter the CLE and simulations dressed as if they were ready for a real clinical practice environment. For our students, this meant wearing their student uniform, removing jewelry, and making sure their hair was tied back for safe clinical practice. They were expected to arrive early or on time for their simulation sessions as they would in a real clinical environment. A code of conduct, including hand hygiene, was adhered to on entering the space. At orientation to their first CLE, we undertook an exercise called 'above the line and below the line behaviors.' The students identifed appropriate behaviors that should occur in a nursing practice space. These were then recorded and displayed in the CLE and simulation rooms to remind the students and empower them to call out behaviors below the line and acknowledge when behaviors are above the bar. This encourages confidence and empowers the students to develop appropriate professional behaviors. This also keeps faculty in check who were also expected to demonstrate above-the-line behaviors.

Clinical Reasoning Skills

As mentioned in the "Medical-Surgical Simulation" section, developing the ability to clinically reason is fundamentally important for the nursing student, and promoting this in the simulation space should underpin all learning activities. It is through the ability to clinically reason that the nursing student will develop skills in critical thinking, empathy, reflection, self-determination, and resilience. All our simulation sessions had clinical reasoning components structured using the frameworks discussed in section "Medical-Surgical Simulation".

Psychomotor Skills

Psychomotor skills are particularly important to ensure safe patient care and encompass procedural skills such as taking vital signs. Initially, these were introduced in the part-task training sessions (within the CLEs) and expanded in scenarios involving more complex tasks, such as administering blood products. These skills translate into many areas of nursing and are the building blocks of nursing practice. Performing these skills takes significant manual dexterity and practice and will be discussed later in practice for mastery.

The optimal simulation session facilitates students practicing all three categories of professional skills, clinical reasoning, and psychomotor skills. For example, if the scenario is based on removing a drain tube:

- The professional skills are reinforced through the conduct and presentation, and communication skills demonstrated by the nursing student
- The clinical reasoning skills are demonstrated by the nursing student working through the cycle, making sure nursing care is evaluated and reflected upon
- The psychomotor skill is the technical performance of drain tube removal.

This episode of learning becomes an experiential opportunity requiring the nurse to consider the risks and safety of the patient. This is a complex and dynamic opportunity for the novice nursing student. The professional skills and clinical reasoning process are repeated similarly in other scenarios with differing skills. The overall learning process is aimed to embed all three elements (professional, clinical reasoning, and psychomotor) of skill mastery into the long-term memory of the nursing student. Overall, developing professional practice facilitates integrating theory, professional identity, and safe clinical practice.

Types of Simulation

Tag Team

The Tag Team Patient Safety Simulation (TTPSS) [21] is to enable meaningful engagement to large student groups when undertaking simulation sessions. There is a particular process, and the emphasis is on developing patient safety concepts and enabling large groups to remain engaged during the simulation even if they are not directly involved in the simulation activity. This form of simulation does not necessarily require high-fidelity manikins and can be flexible in location (e.g., simulation and tutorial spaces). The students can tag in and tag out of the simulation, and those observing are given questions with a specific focus while watching the simulation. These observations are then used in the debriefing session. In the medical-surgical space, we have used detailed cultural simulations and medical-surgical cases to foster empathy, cultural safety, and patient safety while developing skill capability. Many of the resources we used come from the work of Levett-Jones and her team at The University of Technology Sydney located at https://www.virtualempathymuseum.com.au/.

Interprofessional Education and Simulation

Interprofessional education (IPE) simulation is now important to most pre-registration nursing curriculums. IPE has become essential in developing teamwork and communication among healthcare students. We introduced the concepts of IPE early in the medical-surgical sessions, with at least one session being run in each medical-surgical clinical unit. IPE sessions are important to teach the differing roles and perspectives each profession brings to patient care. In these sessions, it is essential to 'unpack' how each profession has a different lens, and therefore, critical thinking and clinical reasoning can look quite different and sometimes quite similar depending on the profession. The lesson plan for an IPE simulation session is similar to a simulated ward plan with a strong emphasis on teamwork. Usually, the lesson setup takes a little longer, with an icebreaker to introduce the differing undergraduate health professional groups and to ensure students feel more comfortable working together. The focus is on all students practicing interprofessional communication and collaboration while caring for their allocated patients.

The Simulated Ward

The concept of the simulated ward is an important session of medical-surgical simulations. It is usually the last simulation of the semester aimed at bringing together all the learnings that have preceded throughout the semester. Generally, the aim is to culminate medical-surgical training before attending clinical placements. Using standardized patients is essential to the simulated ward and creates the most realistic experience for students. This experience aims to provide real patient cases so students can identify, plan and manage patient care. This can also be undertaken as an interprofessional session [22]. There is usually more than one patient in the session, increasing the complexity for the student.

Lesson Plan

The components of a lesson plan that we used for medical-surgical simulation were as follows:

Intended Learning Objectives (ILO)

- To apply skills learned during the semester
- To undertake care & planning for a variety of patients
- To appropriately document and handover relevant nursing care for a variety of patients

Part 1 Intro and a reminder of simulation rules: safety and confidentiality—what happens in simulation stays in simulation (10–15 min)

Part 2 Prebrief: set the scene and ensure the students know what they are expected to do so that they get the most out of the scenario (10 min)

Part 3 Scenario: students carry out care and assessments for the patient (1 h)

Use of assessments as discussed at the beginning of the chapter

Follow ISBAR format

Proposed Nursing care:

Part 4 Debrief: explore what happened in the scenario and make sure everyone goes away knowing exactly what has happened and why (20–30 min)

Have one student from each group handover their patient to the facilitator

Debrief on the experience of looking after a similar patient similar during clinical placement

Discussion of cases:

Probe with specific questions about cases regarding the care delivered

Any other questions about the cases

Challenges and Solutions

There are, of course, many challenges when undertaking simulation for medical-surgical nursing. These challenges are not necessarily unique to medical-surgical nursing, but as this is usually undertaken in the early years of the nursing curriculum, there are some specific areas to focus on. These include:

- Enabling enough time for practice to achieve mastery
- Ensuring the availability of appropriate resources
- Enabling debriefing and reflection
- Assessing the performance of the student in delivering safe clinical practice

Skills Mastery

It is not enough for the student to attend the CLEs and simulations and expect to master clinical skills. To obtain mastery, students need to practice outside the limited time of the face-to-face interactions scheduled in the timetable. The challenge is resourcing opportunities outside scheduled timetabled CLEs and simulations to provide the same informal feedback needed to promote clinical reasoning and skill attainment.

We tackled this challenge by constructing our CLEs to maximize the opportunity for deliberate practice to enable skill mastery. Deliberate practices are learning activities that are designed to optimize improvement, as identified by Gonzalez and Kardong-Edgren [23]. It is important for skill attainment. We also sanctioned practice times within the timetable to ensure the CLE spaces were accessible for deliberate practice. Increasingly this became challenging as the availability of the CLE space beyond formal teaching was continually reduced.

Availability of Resources

The challenge of resources relates to equipment, learning spaces, and human resources.

Equipment

The availability of simulation equipment, including manikins and consumables, impacts the ability to undertake effective and authentic simulation. Simulation is an artificial environment, and to create an authentic experience, expensive equipment is necessary to simulate the real healthcare world. This has often been addressed through government initiatives that have funded some organizations to establish their simulation infrastructure and equipment needs. An example of this was the work undertaken in Australia in the early twenty-first century committing $75.92 million for both capital and recurrent investments across sectors to "expand capacity for learning through simulation" [24]. This contributed significantly to mainstreaming this requirement at all healthcare workforce training levels [25]. However, the ongoing expense of purchasing and maintaining equipment remains challenging for many education providers. Equipment is not limited to the physical requirement of mannikins and consumables but also the requirement of appropriate technology to enable successful execution of simulation.

The Space

The availability of space can be complex in teaching medical-surgical simulations. It is possible for a successful simulation to be undertaken in a relatively small space, but as these simulations are core to nursing practice, there is a need to replicate the acute hospital ward/unit. This poses a significant challenge in ensuring enough hospital beds relative to the number of students and the adjunct equipment that support this space. As a rule, 3–4 students are assigned to a bed during part-task training. With full simulation scenarios, this can vary depending on the team makeup required for the scenario. Other logistical challenges include having a dedicated setup space, storage space for extra equipment and consumables, and a debriefing area that needs to be appropriately located relative to the simulation training rooms.

The People

The human resource requirements warrant consideration, including teachers, laboratory technicians, managers, and simulation specialist staff. Those teaching with simulation must be trained appropriately to be confident with the technology and know-how to facilitate simulation and conduct the debriefing process. We have found that our technicians, whose sole responsibility is the setup and organization of the simulation, are essential to the success of the simulation experience. They understand the setup of each CLE, the flow of the simulation, and the functionality of the technology and equipment. Having capable technicians means that faculty can focus their energies on teaching. The technicians also deal with equipment failures or other issues during the simulation.

Management is also integral to the success of simulation. From a budgetary perspective, it is important that there is buy-in from upper management to ensure that the resources required for simulation are a priority to graduate capable healthcare professionals.

Debriefing and Reflection

A debriefing occurs after or during the simulation and is paramount to student learning [26]. The medical-surgical rotation may be the first time students are introduced to debriefing and feedback. The challenge is to develop good feedback practices and the ability to reflect on and in practice. For the novice nursing student, the educator needs clear and consistent guidance to ensure feedback is student-centered and develops clinical reasoning abilities—'to think like a nurse.' We introduced specific approaches of debriefing, feedback, and reflection that were taught initially in the medical-surgical spaces in the early years and continued throughout the course. Consistency in these approaches decreased the student's cognitive load, knowing that they will always use the same approach in the CLE and simulation space enabling them to focus on the specific skill or scenario. Consistency across the whole years of training also mitigates challenges associated with debriefing and reflection.

Developing Assessment of Capabilities

The chapter on assessment in simulation covers the overall challenges of assessment in simulation. However, specific to the medical-surgical simulation teaching are the part-task assessments required for competency before initial entry into the clinical environment. The challenges we encountered centered on providing assurances of safe practice before entry into the real world of the hospital environment. Our approach was to identify the students struggling to pass a clinical assessment. We emphasized that mastery must be achieved to ensure safe practice once on clinical placement. We aimed to enable the student to undertake the skills assessment in an environment that did not exacerbate unnecessary anxiety. Our challenge was to enable a realistic assessment devoid of unnecessary anxiety and enable the demonstration of skill acquisition and mastery. This was achieved by providing the marking rubric well before the assessment was undertaken and providing time in the face-to-face CLEs to practice, with additional practice time made available on request by the student. Probably the most important aspect of decreasing the student's anxiety was to ensure that the educators undertook an inter-rater-reliability practice before the assessment to ensure consistency between markers.

Integrating into the Existing Curriculum: Pedagogy Underpinning Simulation for Medical-Surgical Learning in Nursing

The opportunities when teaching medical-surgical simulation in the design of a curriculum can progressively develop the students' levels of autonomy in knowledge, skills, and attitudes. It is, therefore, important to scaffold learning to enable this progression. The scaffolding of curriculum design enables increasing complexity in content skill and assessment, with the final year focussing on the management of complex medical-surgical patient care scenarios.

Kolb's Experiential Learning Theory [27] is one of the most relevant theoretical designs to match the desired outcome of the simulation. Experiential learning encourages active learning by doing. This active approach in the simulation space has shown that clinical learning acquisition is not restricted to clinical placements but complements and builds on placement experiences. The active learning approach can influence the instructional development of medical-surgical simulations.

It is also important to consider the cognitive load of the students when undertaking medical-surgical simulations introduced at the beginning of a nursing program. It is important to set the scene to enable student confidence within this learning space. The focus is on learning the content and skills, not the simulation process. Therefore, consistency of the process is important to ensure the intrinsic load is given to the essential learning and not the process. This, in turn, enables the students to perceive, think, and solve problems rather than rote learning, facilitating deep rather than surface learning. This approach draws on current understandings within cognitive learning theory [28].

Finally, we gave due consideration to the concept of self-determination. Nursing students require intrinsic motivation to develop a healthy professional identity.

Below is an example of our scaffolded curriculum across the 3 years, from less complex part-task training in the CLE space progressing to case-based simulations in the final third year. This is not an exhaustive list but rather an example of the way we built clinical practice from the simple to more complex over the years. The clinical reasoning cycle introduced in year one and then deconstructed for each area of practice. Moving novice students to the stages of evaluation and reflection takes time. Increasing the complexity of the scenarios in the simulations helps to develop these clinical reasoning skills. The importance of explicit scaffolding cannot be underestimated in the learning journey.

Year 1

CLEs only in the first half of year 1:

1. Introduction to the CLE	2. Vital signs: Respiratory rate; temperature; pulse
3. Vital signs: Blood pressure	4. CVS assessment
5. CNS assessment and pain assessment	6. Respiratory assessment
7. Neurological assessment	8. Renal assessment
9. Endocrine assessment	10. GIT assessment

The second half of first-year simulation is introduced every second week

CLE: Hand Washing, manual handling	Simulation
CLE: Medication administration	
CLE: Risk screening assessments	Simulation
CLE: Admission and discharge management	
CLE: Basic life support	Simulation: Case scenario (Post-op management)
CLE: Managing emergencies and codes	
CLE: Bed-making, showering, toilet	Simulation: Case scenario
CLE: BGL + Oxygen	
CLE: ISBAR and handover	Simulation: Case scenario
CLE: wound dressings	
Simulated Ward Aged Care: Communication, Safe Practice, and Foundations of Nursing Care	

Year 2

The CLEs increase in complexity, and the simulations continue to occur every second week

CLE	
IV meds, IVT, FBC, secondary lines	Simulation
CVADs, ECG	
Venepuncture, UWSD & ICC's	Simulation
Drain tube removal, BGL management (hypo/hyper)	
GCS, IDC, NGT & suction	Simulation
Wounds, sutures & staple removal, neurovascular observations	
Make up sessions and revision	Simulation
Simulated Ward	

Year 3

In year 3, there are only simulations, and these are more complex case scenarios whereby each week the nursing students are expected to undertake the teamwork activity.

Simulations
Shock
Heart failure
DKA & HHS
Acute kidney injury
Upper GI bleeding and anemia (incorporates blood transfusion
Stroke & Aneurysm
Deteriorating patient

Regulatory Bodies

Nursing curriculums are governed nationally by regulatory bodies regulating curriculum development and monitoring implementation. These vary internationally, but all have in common the need to ensure that nurses are safely and adequately prepared to undertake safe practice upon completion of their education. Simulation is now an accepted, important, and required inclusion within the nursing curriculum in most countries. There is much debate by regulatory bodies around best practices, and this includes minimum clinical placement hours required, the standards and scope of practice, and the potential for simulation to replace clinical placement hours [29]. What is now accepted and expected is that simulation is important and essential as a learning technique. This is particularly essential in the early training of medical-surgical skills to ensure safe practice in a context free space with debriefing opportunities. All regulatory bodies agree that simulation is an essential and necessary requirement across all levels of a nursing program [30–33]

Conclusion

Simulation in the medical-surgical undergraduate nursing curriculum is a fundamental learning strategy enabling safe, capable, and professional nurses to be developed. This chapter overviews our experience in developing a medical-surgical simulation curriculum scaffolded across an undergraduate nursing program. Important concepts to consider when designing simulations for a medical-surgical curriculum include strengths-based nursing, person-centredness, the principles of fundamentals of care, the use of the clinical reasoning cycle, patient assessment, and communication skills. Training for best and professional practice is imperative when designing and implementing medical-surgical simulations. Types of simulation that work well in this context are tag team simulation, interprofessional simulation, and a simulated ward.

Cases Example: Medical Surgical Nursing: The Simulated Ward

Authors: Associate Professor Loretta Garvey and modified by Professor Georgina Willetts

In each of the simulations the facilitator acts as a confederate. The confederate is an experienced registered nurse who supports the learners. This assistance can be as simple as locating equipment, or as complicated as supervising a student performing a procedure or rationalising their nursing interventions. The confederate is also a support person for the students when they require extra help. The confederate is considered a team member of the simulation scenario and can help to guide the scenario back to the intended learning outcomes.

This simulated is undertaken as an interprofessional simulation with Nursing students and occupational therapy students.

Lesson Plan

Part 1 Reminder of Simulation rules: Safety and confidentiality - what happens in simulation stays in simulation

Part 2 Prebrief: Set the scene and ensure the students know what they are expected to do so that they get the most out of the scenario

Part 3 Scenario: Students carry out care and assessments for the patient

Part 4 Debrief: Explore what happened in the scenario and make sure everyone goes away knowing exactly what has happened and why

Part 1: Reminder of Simulation Rules

Reiterate this is a learning environment. The aim of simulation is to contextualise the clinical skills practiced in the lab and to apply clinical reasoning to the scenario. Take this opportunity, in a safe environment, to apply diligent and deliberate practice of the skills that you learned from your instructor, literature, skills labs, and clinical time. You won't be perfect, and that is okay. They are not mistakes, they are learning opportunities and they will be discussed in detail in the debrief component of simulation so you can learn from them. Remind students of the confidentiality waiver they all signed and ensure they are familiar with simulation rules and that they are maintained throughout the scenario

Part 2: Prebrief

This part of simulation is to set the scene for the students so that they are aware of the situation. Provide a handover to the students using the information below. This will also be laminated and at the bedside for student referral.

- ISBAR is followed as the handover procedureIntroduction
- Situation
- Background
- Assessment
- Recommendation

Learning Objectives:

At this point, go through the learning objectives listed on the whiteboard. It's imperative that the learning objectives are made clear to the students so that they can focus on the appropriate tasks and get the most out of the experience.

Part 3: Scenario

Initiate the beginning of the scenario and request the students begin as students to care for the patient. Ensure they discuss their plan of treatment and allocate tasks before entering the room. Remind students they could ask a confederate for help if required, or to call a time out if they are stuck. This scenario is timed to run for approximately 15–20 min.

Cases:

Time: 7:40 h *Geriatric evaluation and management ward*

Identification:

John Smith DOB: 26/09/1943 Patient ID: 25685451

Situation:

John injured his right hip when he tripped over at the cricket club and required a surgical revision. He has been discharged to the Geriatric Evaluation and Management (GEM) unit to promote independence and mobility prior to discharge home. Overnight John fell whilst getting out of bed to go to the toilet. It was an unwitnessed fall so the doctor would like 2/24 neurological observations.

Background:

John is 75-years old and lives alone. John worked on building sites for many years as a carpenter and towards the end of his working life was a site manager. John has a 25-year history of osteoarthritis which now affects his right shoulder (cortisone injection 7 months ago to relieve pain), and both hips (Elective Left THR 7 years ago; Elective Right THR 9 years ago and Emergency RHR 4 months ago).

Assessments:

John is currently using a walking frame and only walking short distances. He is very fearful of falling again. Whilst in hospital, John is requiring assistance from the nursing staff with showering and dressing. John is also having some difficulty opening the packaging on his meal trays, and feels he is a bother to the nurses when he buzzes them to help him to open the packaging.

Recommendation:

John will require a review by an occupational therapist for an activities of daily living (ADL) assessment and discuss the potential for completing a home visit to assess his home setup.

Time: 7:40 h *Rehabilitation ward*

Identification:

Nancy Toh DOB: 06/08/1968 UR: 21598457

Situation:

Nancy has been admitted to the rehabilitation ward following discharge from the acute setting after having a serious fall at home.

Background

Nancy is 50 and lives with her partner and two children (16 and 19). Nancy was diagnosed with MS 5 years ago, which came as a shock to her family when the diagnosis was confirmed following MRI. Nancy was surprised but also relieved to have a diagnosis. Her symptoms included blurred vision and fatigue.

Assessments:

Nancy is no longer working and following an occupational therapy driver assessment is no longer driving. Nancy has had three falls in the last year. Nancy can walk short distances with a single point stick but needs a lot of encouragement. Nancy is complaining of some abdominal pain and states she has not opened her bowels for 4 days. She normally opens her bowels every day but since being in hospital has not been having her usual high fibre diet.

Recommendations:

Nancy will require an OT home visit to assist with promoting safety, independence, energy conservation and task simplification. The OT needs to meet Nancy on the ward to discuss this and to review her mobility equipment.

Time: 7:40 h *GEM ward*

Identification:

Mary Williams DOB: 15/03/1940 UR: 11549568

Situation:
Mary is a 78 year old lady who is admitted to the GEM ward following a UTI.

Background:
Mary has recently been diagnosed with dementia. She currently lives at home with her daughter Thelma. Things have been getting a little more difficult at home for Mary. Sometimes Mary refuses to get dressed in the mornings and does not always remember to have breakfast. Mary seems to need a lot more help planning what to do.

Assessment:
The handover from the night duty nursing staff reported that Mary was unsettled and attempting get out of bed and find the kitchen, as she thought she should make a start on preparing the roast for lunch after church. Mary's confusion is consistent with the nursing notes from last evening, which state Mary became upset and unable to understand why these people were in her house. Mary ambulates independently without any aids. The medical staff are wanting to assess Thelma's post void residual volume so nursing staff should perform bladder scans on the patient post urination.

Recommendation:
Mary had a UTI which has now resolved. The OT will conduct a cognitive screen as well as assess her ability with ADLs including dressing and putting on shoes. The OT will discuss home safety and the possible need for a home visit.

Time: 7:40 h *GEM ward*

Identification:

David Janckovic DOB: 04/07/1951 UR: 59874589

Situation:
David is a 67 year old gentleman. David had a fall one week ago and had surgery to fix his fractured left neck of femur. He has been admitted to the GEM ward to increase his mobility and assess his need for services prior to discharge home.

Background:
David has recently been diagnosed with Parkinson's Disease. He lives at home with his wife Zara but she has been struggling to look after him since his diagnosis. David is very anxious and is worried about going home and burdening Zara with his increased dependence.

Assessments:
David is ambulating with a gutter frame, but requires a lot of encouragement and support to do so. Upon showering David this morning, the nurse noticed David has a stage two pressure injury to his right heel which will require a wound assessment and dressing to be completed.

Recommendation:
The OT should assess David and discuss falls risk, an ADL assessment on the ward, a home visit prior to discharge and carer support options.

Time: 7:40 h *Rehabilitation ward*

Identification:

Khoa Nguyen DOB: 15/01/1956 UR: 95987415

Situation:
Khoa has been transferred to the Rehab ward today form the inpatient setting. He fell off his bicycle and fractured his right collarbone. He had surgery last week to repair the damage.

Background:
Khoa is a 62 year old divorced gentleman who lives at home alone. He has a very supportive family who all live close by. He is a recently retired accountant. He has a past history of GORD.

Assessment:
Khoa has just arrived at the ward and needs all of his admission paperwork attended to. Khoa has limited movement in his right arm and has been having difficulty using his hand for eating. His arm is also required to be in a sling and immobilised. Khoa walks independently with nil aids.

Recommendation:
The OT staff should assess Khoa's eating and provide him with assistive technology so that he is able to eat independently. The OT will also need discuss his ability to cook at home by himself with the possibility of training in one handed cooking techniques and a home visit.

References

1. Carper BA. Fundamental patterns of knowing in nursing. ProQuest Dissertations Publishing; 1975.
2. Benner P. From novice to expert. Menlo Park. 1984;84(1480):10–97.
3. Reedy GB. Using cognitive load theory to inform simulation design and practice. Clin Simul Nurs. 2015;11(8):355–60.
4. Gottlieb LN. Strengths-based nursing care health and healing for person and family. In: Ebooks C, editor. New York: Springer Publishing Company; 2012.
5. Crisp J, Douglas C, Reberio G, Waters D. Potter and Perry's fundamentals of nursing. 5th ed. Melbourne: Elsevier; 2019.
6. Levett-Jones TE. ProQuest. Clinical reasoning: learning to think like a nurse. 2nd ed. Melbourne: Pearson Australia; 2018.

7. Limmer D, O'Keefe M, Grant H, Harvey D, Murray B. Emergency care. 11th ed. Hoboken: Prentice Hall; 2008.
8. Henderson A. Communication for health care practice. Oxford: Oxford University Press ANZ; 2018.
9. Gottlieb LN, Gottlieb B. Strengths-based nursing: a process for implementing a philosophy into practice. J Fam Nurs. 2017;23(3):319–40.
10. Hubley P, Gottlieb LN, Durrant M. Influencing work culture: a strengths-based nursing leadership and management education program. Nurs Leadersh (Tor Ont). 2022;35(1):24–37.
11. Saunders A, Green R, Cross M. Making the most of person-centered education by integrating flipped and simulated teaching: an exploratory study. Nurse Educ Pract. 2017;27:71–7.
12. McCormack BE, McCance TE, Hwof K. ProQuest. Person-centered practice in nursing and health care: theory and practice. 2nd ed. West Sussex: Wiley Blackwell; 2017.
13. Garvey L, Mackelprang JL, Bhowmik J, Cassar N, Delbridge R, El-Ansary D, et al. Enhancing cultural capabilities amongst health professions students: a pilot study of Interprofessional tag team simulation. Clin Simul Nurs. 2022;62:83–91.
14. Kitson A, Conroy T, Kuluski K, Locock L, Lyons R. Reclaiming and redefining the fundamentals of care: nursing's response to meeting patients' basic human needs. Adelaide: School of Nursing,The University of Adelaide; 2013.
15. Feo R, Conroy T, Jangland E, Muntlin Athlin Å, Brovall M, Parr J, et al. Towards a standardized definition for fundamental care: a modified Delphi study. J Clin Nurs. 2018;27(11–12):2285–99.
16. Crisp J, Douglas C, Rebeiro G, Waters D. Potter & Perry's fundamentals of nursing ANZ edition. 6th ed. Elsevier Health Sciences. 2020.
17. Levett-Jones T. Clinical reasoning: learning to think like a nurse. 2nd ed. Frenchs Forest: Pearson Australia; 2019.
18. Levett-Jones T, Hoffman K, Dempsey J, Jeong SY-S, Noble D, Norton CA, et al. The 'five rights' of clinical reasoning: an educational model to enhance nursing students' ability to identify and manage clinically 'at risk' patients. Nurse Educ Today. 2010;30(6):515–20.
19. Brady A-M, McCabe C, McCann M. Fundamentals of medical-surgical nursing: a systems approach. Hoboken: Wiley; 2014.
20. Henderson A. Communication for health care practice. Brisbane: CQUniversity; 2019.
21. Dwyer TA, Levett-Jones T, Flenady T, Reid-Searl K, Andersen P, Guinea S, et al. Responding to the unexpected: tag team patient safety simulation. Clin Simul Nurs. 2019;36:8–17.
22. Kelly MA, Barragan E, Husebø SE, Orr F. Simulation in nursing education-international perspectives and contemporary scope of practice. J Nurs Scholarsh. 2016;48(3):312–21.
23. Gonzalez L, Kardong-Edgren S. Deliberate practice for mastery learning in nursing. Clin Simul Nurs. 2017;13(1):10–4.
24. Rudd C. Enhancing the uptake of learning through simulation in health. Sydney: Office for Learning and Teaching, DIICCSRTE; 2013.
25. Mason J. Review of Australian government health workforce programs. Brisbane: Commonwealth Department of Health and Ageing; 2013.
26. Nagle A, Foli KJ. Student-centered reflection in debriefing: a concept analysis. Clin Simul Nurs. 2020;39:33–40.
27. Kolb DA. Experiential learning: experience as the source of learning and development, 2nd ed. PH Professional Business; 2014.
28. Brown PC, Roediger HL, McDaniel MA. Make it stick: the science of successful learning. Cambridge: Harvard University Press; 2014.
29. Hayden JK, Smiley RA, Alexander M, Kardong-Edgren S, Jeffries PR. The NCSBN National Simulation Study: a longitudinal, randomized, controlled study replacing clinical hours with simulation in prelicensure nursing education. J Nurs Regul. 2014;5(2):S3–S40.
30. ANMAC. Registered nurse accreditation standards 2019. In: Australian Nursing and Midwifery Accreditation Council, editor. 2019.
31. CCNE. Standards for accreditation of baccalaureate and graduate nursing education programs. In: USA CoCNE, editor. 2018.
32. NCSBN. Simulation guidelines for prelicensure nursing education programs. In: USA NCoSBoN, editor. 2016.
33. NMC. Standards framework for nursing and midwifery education. In: UK NaMC, editor. 2018.

Maternity Nursing

9

Kellie Bryant and Julia Greenawalt

Background

The first use of simulation in recent history is attributed to aviation, creating a simulator called Link that was used to train pilots in a "life-like" environment [1]. The next evolution emerged in WWI, where training was needed for complex flight crews so that they could work together seamlessly. For 'bomber' type missions, these crews consisted of a pilot, co-pilot, navigator, and bombardier. Communication was vital for successful operations, and Cockpit Resource Management (CRM) was born [2]. With CRM, interpersonal skills were used to mitigate errors that might arise from power inequalities within the cockpit. In the early 1980s, this was expanded to include flight attendants and was changed to Crew Resource Management to foster safety for the ship and crew. The training was then expanded to include not only interpersonal risk mitigation but also human factors topics such as situational awareness, team building, and stress management. In the 1990s, James Reason expanded CRM to include factors that could impact safety and the hazards within a flight, such as fatigue, work overload, and stress on performance [3]. At this time, reporting shifted from a blame culture to a review of procedures and performance to fix the problem, and confidentiality was ensured for error investigation. This took a significant shift in philosophy to policy and was done to increase safety for the flying public.

Not only was simulation introduced into pilot training, but other areas of the military also embraced simulation. Examples include simulated war training for officers to shape future military leaders and training for cadets about strategy and operations that addressed not only winning but methods that fostered enhanced communication and safety of troops and self. For active-duty troops, simulation was integrated into professional development courses, such as Squadron Officer School courses, whereby all disciplines came together to train for the mission of the military.

While simulation was evolving in aviation and the military, medicine adapted it to the healthcare environment. Most notable was the work of Dr. David Gaba, a pioneer in anesthesia science, who adapted CRM to a curriculum for anesthetists. He used principles from the aviation field to improve the ability of anesthesiologists to manage crises [4]. The principles of CRM were also translated to other disciplines to foster team training, communication, and patient safety [5]. Within the obstetric field, simulation was adopted due to the rise of sentinel events in healthcare that were becoming a focal point for the public and accreditation agencies. During the early 2000s, the US Agency for Healthcare Research and Quality (AHRQ) offered grants to researchers to investigate how to mitigate errors in healthcare. Other agencies, including obstetrics, followed suit, targeting areas for investigation such as post partum hemorrhage, fires in the operating room, and shoulder dystocia. From there, nursing started adopting and expanding simulation, applying this to meet the learning needs of students.

One of the first areas in nursing to adopt simulation was maternal health. This stemmed from medicine, where sentinel events were used to guide practice and mitigate errors for many low-frequency but high-impact events such as postpartum hemorrhage, shoulder dystocia, and maternal cardiac arrests during childbirth. These events were targeted for simulation to increase healthcare providers' ability to plan and train for such events and to teach patient safety [6–10]. Nursing followed suit to target the use of simulation for scenarios that were difficult to teach and not commonly seen in practice for every nursing student. Simulation became a mechanism by which all students could be exposed to the same "dose" of difficult nursing situations. Example scenarios included magnesium toxicity for a preeclamptic patient on a continuous infusion of magnesium sulfate, the obstetri-

K. Bryant
Columbia University Medical Center, New York, NY, USA
e-mail: kdb2146@cumc.columbia.edu

J. Greenawalt (✉)
Indiana, Pennsylvania, USA

Nursing, Columbia University, New York, NY, USA
e-mail: kdb2146@cumc.columbia.edu

J. M. Kutzin et al. (eds.), *Comprehensive Healthcare Simulation: Nursing*, Comprehensive Healthcare Simulation,
https://doi.org/10.1007/978-3-031-31090-4_9

cal patient that experiences a seizure post-partum, or an obstetrical patient that experiences an unattended stillborn birth [11, 12].

A key growth area that emerged next was interprofessional simulation, where members from more than one profession participated in a simulation scenario. Such simulations in maternity nursing were developed to enhance communication and teamwork and to mitigate team errors. This was the premise by which Team STEPPS was created [13]. TeamSTEPPS was developed in 2002 by the Agency for Research and Quality to improve teamwork and foster communication in response to the To Err is Human report which showed that deaths were attributable to medical errors. A central tenet of this report was that an interprofessional learning approach should be used to transfer new knowledge and enhance communication and safety [14]. In undergraduate maternal health nursing, interprofessional simulation included nurse anesthesia and obstetric nurses training to work together on tasks, care management, and communication [15]. Often, obstetrics teams were combined with nurses in the NICU to mitigate errors or to foster communication between the two professions [16, 17]. As this area was being developed, many nursing schools were not affiliated with medical centers. Many universities partnered with local theatrical training centers or drama schools to address this issue and optimize communication training. With a long history of integrating standardized patients into medical education, this was a new pedagogy for nursing education. Theater students became integrated into mainstream education to optimize teaching and the learning of communication skills in real-time [18].

Maternity nursing simulation is an active learning strategy designed to foster maternity nursing skills and optimize patient care and safety outcomes. It is used to teach tasks and skills, demonstrate care management strategies, and portray sensitive clinical situations that are not easily reproducible for students. It also fosters teamwork and communication during high-incident care situations such as shoulder dystocia leading to a maternal cardiac arrest or a postpartum hemorrhage event.

Best Practice

The International Nursing Association of Clinical Simulation Learning (INACSL) has established Standards of Best Practice, which focus on eight key components of simulation, including simulation design, outcomes and objectives, facilitation, debriefing, participant evaluation, professional integrity, simulation enhanced interprofessional education, and operations [19]. These eight guiding standards should be utilized when creating simulation activities for undergraduate nursing students learning about maternal health.

The educational content for creating maternity simulation experiences should come from evidence-based resources. In the United States, organizations that set the standards for maternity care include the Association of Women's Health, Obstetric and Neonatal Nurses (AWHONN) and the American College of Obstetricians and Gynecologists (ACOG) and can provide the most up-to-date guidelines for care for maternal health. ACOG has gone a step further by creating a task force with a mission of establishing simulation as an essential component of education on women's health through collaboration, advocacy, research, and the development of simulations activities (ACOG, https://www.acog.org/education-and-events/simulations/about). The International Federation of Gynecology and Obstetricians, the World Health Organization, the Maternal Health Taskforce, and the Australian College of Midwives are additional organizations that provide guidelines for promoting safe practices in maternal health.

Sample Maternity Nursing Curriculum

There are many variables to consider when designing and implementing a maternity nursing curriculum. For many schools, the maternity rotation is considered an upper-level course offered at more senior levels of undergraduate education, although some programs introduce it in the earlier years, such as the sophomore year or first year of nursing, justifying this as an aberrancy of normal, not pathological. However, most universities include it in the later years of a course of study.

When maternity simulation was first introduced in undergraduate nursing, many faculties were originally resistant to standardized approaches to teaching and learning clinical skills. It has now become more accepted with greater access to shared scenarios. Other considerations for curriculum development include the number of students to be taught, the number of faculty skilled in teaching with simulation, the number of mannikins or space allocated for teaching, and how simulation can fit into the curriculum. For most nursing programs, resources are tight. Funding often goes towards purchasing mannikins and task trainers with very little funding allocated to faculty development, a major mistake when considering the sustainability of a program. The physical space needed to teach with simulation is also a major driver, including providing ample room to store simulation equipment and mannikins. Another consideration is ensuring students can be fully immersed in the replicated hospital environment. The space should include an area for prebriefing or preparatory work before commencing the simulation experience. This is often delivered to students through formal teaching or via online learning through a learning management system. Another new variable is how much simulation will "count" towards the overall educational process. Until recently, simulation was considered part of the clinical experience and was a 1:1 replacement for clinical experience. Newer research has demonstrated that some academic institutions offer a ratio of 1:2 or even 1:3 as a replacement for clinical practice [20].

The simulation teacher is often a self-taught individual, often with additional qualifications beyond the basic certification, with the premier schools providing formal training for simulation facilitators, such as the Certified Healthcare Simulation Educator (CHSE) course in the US or Graduate Certificates in Clinical Simulation in Australia. Many schools of nursing lack technicians who support those who operate healthcare simulation technology.

The drivers for implementing simulation in maternity nursing often depend on the willingness of management and administration to adopt simulation in nursing schools and the level of financial support that can be provided. The field of obstetrics is traditionally seen as an early adopter of simulation due to the high incidence of adverse events. Still, there is wide variability in the way in which simulation has been incorporated into the nursing curriculum. A factor impacting finances in higher education is the length of the course. Most university maternity nursing courses are offered for 15 weeks, but some programs pair obstetrics with pediatrics limiting its duration to only 7.5 weeks. Some have even experimented with a 5-week course delivery, although that is not currently mainstream in the undergraduate context. In some countries, maternity nursing is not included in undergraduate nursing and is a separate Midwifery pre-registration qualification. As a result, the amount of simulation that is offered is limited. Some schools allow 6–8 h of simulation per course; others allow 12–18 h. Likewise, simulation is either offered early in a course or toward the end so that students can apply all concepts and consolidate their learning. For most nursing programs, simulation is offered only in a formative environment. While some nursing schools have experimented with high-stakes maternal health learning or used simulation as Objective Structured Clinical Examinations (OSCEs), there has been much resistance to its implementation. In addition, the strain of the pandemic of 2019–2020 imposed further restrictions. While it did create more work for simulation faculty, due to many clinical sites prohibiting students, the use of simulation during the pandemic increased. Instead of just an "exposure dose" for students, up to 25–30% of clinical time was replaced with simulation. The benefits of this were the standardization and repeated exposure of simulated learning and teaching for all students.

A contemporary maternity nursing curriculum at the junior/senior level often includes a full or half semester of learning (about 75–90 h for clinical placement and one to two full days of simulation). Students may be exposed to approximately 6–9 simulations during this time. This would include pre-briefing, review, scenario participation, and debriefing for each scenario. Common scenarios can be seen in Table 9.1.

Table 9.1 Suggested syllabus for a Maternity Nursing Curriculum

Patient safety • Overdose, missed medication dose • Preeclamptic overdose of magnesium sulfate • Restraining a pregnant patient • Assisting with epidural • Immediate postoperative abdominal hysterectomy • Opioid intoxication • Hemorrhage • Normal childbirth with symptomatic Covid-19	*Patient-centered care* • Occiput posterior delivery • Term premature rupture of membranes • Normal maternal history and labor • Umbilical cord prolapse • Instruction with breast feeding • Mild and Severe Preeclampsia • Preparation for c-section due to umbilical cord prolapse • Providing discharge instructions to a new mother/father
Teamwork and collaboration	
• Post-partum hemorrhage • Retained placenta • Precipitous breech delivery • Shoulder dystocia • Instrument delivery • Premature labor at 30 weeks gestation • Rupture of membranes-meconium stained fluid • Maternal obesity • Chronic obstructive pulmonary disease-spontaneous pneumothorax	• Unattended delivery • Assisting with external version • Chorioamnionitis • Prolonged stage 1 • Partial placenta Previa • Group B strep positive • Fetal distress due to maternal hypotension • Fetal distress due to uterine Tachysystole • Delivery with risk of shoulder dystocia
Quality improvement • Fire in the operating room	
Informatics • Documenting suspected child neglect or battered woman while in hospital • Documenting an NST/CST and/or biophysical profile in the electronic health record	

Integrating Maternity Simulation into Existing Education

In the past, simulation was integrated into the nursing curriculum disjointedly, lacking a theoretical framework or integrative pedagogy [21]. Simulation has traditionally been used to complement the theoretical and clinical components of nursing education. However, simulation can also be used as a make-up for missed clinical opportunities, clinical skill attainment, competency testing, and to provide opportunities for remedial learning [21]. Although there is very little available in the literature regarding a standardized process for integrating simulation into the curriculum, some common best practices exist. One way to accelerate the implementation process is to create a team of simulation champions that will assist in developing and supporting the simulation curriculum. These champions are knowledgeable about simulation-based education and help promote simulation's importance within the organization. Another source of support and guidance is from university-based committees that oversee the curriculum. These curriculum committees can offer guidance and provide approval for implementing simulation programs. Buy-in from the leadership team is imperative in creating a successful simulation program. A leadership team that understands the value of simulation will be more likely to provide financial support, staffing, release time for simulation educators, and other necessary resources needed for a successful simulation program [22].

One of the most challenging steps to curriculum integration is developing the implementation plan. There are many steps to implementing a successful simulation activity. The first step is to conduct a needs assessment to identify learning priorities, gaps in education, patient safety goals, systems analysis, and feedback from stakeholders [23]. Simulation activities should be designed to meet course and program outcomes. Implementing simulation activities into the curriculum starts with establishing clear, measurable, attainable, and appropriate objectives/outcomes for the level of the learner. The learner should be able to complete the simulation in the allocated time frame. Thinking of the end goal for the learner can help develop the specific learning outcomes for the simulation activity.

Choosing the most appropriate scenarios should be well thought out and based on a need assessment. Normal vaginal delivery is an example of a scenario that all students in maternity need to know; however, it is a high-frequency/low-acuity scenario. Another frame of thought is to select scenarios that do not occur at high frequency but are important due to a high risk for mortality/morbidity, such as a cord prolapse scenario. The structure of the simulation should be purposeful and designed with an appropriate level of fidelity to meet the learning objectives [23]. For example, a scenario focused on providing intrapartum nursing care to a laboring woman may require a birthing simulator or standardized patient with a birthing task trainer. To assist with the implementation of simulation activities, a simulation template should be used to ensure consistency and key elements are included in the simulation design [24]. Before implementation of any scenarios, a dry run should be conducted of the simulation to confirm the validity of the scenario and identify any revisions.

The structure of the simulation session should define the details of the pre-brief, simulation, and debrief sections. Learners should be provided with simulation assignments and preparation materials before the session. The brief includes a review of the learning outcomes, simulation format, assigned roles, guidelines for establishing a safe learning space, evaluation, and orientation to the simulation environment. The simulation activity should be facilitated by someone who has received formal training in simulation pedagogy. Each simulation should follow with a debriefing or feedback component. A framework for providing feedback should promote reflection and improve future performance. It is also important to have an established evaluation process for the learner to evaluate their simulation experience [19].

Once a simulation program is implemented, it is important to collect utilization data, learner evaluations, and any other measurable learner outcomes that will provide data to support sustaining or expanding a simulation program. Simulation success stories should be shared through social media, newsletters, and other media outlets to garner additional support and sustain leadership buy-in [22].

Challenges and Solutions

Implementing a maternity simulation curriculum does come with obstacles and challenges. Some of the biggest challenges are the number of resources needed to run an effective simulation program. Time, money, supplies, equipment, and faculty development training are some of the resources needed to run an effective simulation program. Maternity simulation can also require a high-fidelity birthing manikin and unique maternity supplies that are an added expense for a university and may not seem a priority compared to other courses. Scenario design templates should list supplies, equipment, medications, documentation, and standard participants/simulation staff needed to run the session. Having a relationship with a nearby hospital can help with obtaining necessary supplies and equipment, including donations of expired supplies. Any supplies (such as birthing kits) should be reused as much as possible to conserve supplies.

A unique obstacle associated with maternity simulation is that many nursing curriculums have less time allocated to the maternity course than medical-surgical courses. In addition, some universities may not have a maternity clinical rotation due to the lack of clinical placements. Maternity simulation can be a great method for meeting course outcomes.

The lack of trained simulation facilitators is another major obstacle many universities face. Becoming an effective simulation facilitator requires formal training in best practices in simulation education. Training requires money, travel, and time. Many simulation facilitators were trained by human patient simulator vendors who are not experts in simulation-based education. It is essential that educators are skilled in debriefing techniques to best achieve student outcomes [24]. Due to the growing use of simulation, there are many more opportunities for simulation-based education, such as attending conferences, formal educational degree offerings in simulation, online training modules, and companies that will provide onsite educational sessions. A great free resource for simulation facilitators is the 7-week Clinical Simulation Massive open online course George Washington University offers at https://nursing.gwu.edu/clinical-simulation-mooc.

The lack of additional simulation staff, such as simulation operators, is a challenge for many simulation programs. Although facilitators are a key component of a simulation program, additional staff may be needed to assist with operating manikins, providing technical support, performing preventative maintenance, and preparing rooms for simulation sessions. One cost-saving measure to assist with staffing issues is using student volunteers, teaching assistants, and/or work-study students to help with some day-to-day simulation operations.

Interface with Regulatory Bodies

Nursing accrediting bodies have become increasingly supportive of simulation and its integral role in nursing education. The 1999 Institute of Medicine to Err is Human report and the 2010 National Council of State Board of Nursing (BON) Simulation study was monumental in providing research and evidence that simulation-based education is an effective teaching/learning strategy [25]. The American Association of Colleges of Nursing (AACN) and the Commission on Collegiate Nursing Education (CCNE) encourage the use of simulation in conjunction with direct patient care [26].

State Boards of Nursing in the USA regulate required clinical hours for licensure, including determining how many clinical hours can be completed using simulation [27]. More than half of the boards of nursing have specific regulations regarding simulation hours; however, the regulation varies widely among states. The covid-19 pandemic has resulted in some BON allowing wider use of simulation to meet clinical hour requirements [28]. However, due to the lack of research on learning during clinical training, the inconsistency in standards for using simulation for clinical hours will continue to exist [27].

Conclusion

The use of simulation in maternity nursing can increase leaners' knowledge and skills, reduce errors, and promote patient safety. Use of well-designed maternity simulations for healthcare providers has been proven to improve patient outcomes for mother and child. Maternity is a unique specialty and requires specific equipment, mannikins, and content expertise to implement an effective simulation. Standards of best practice in simulation include developing well-defined learning outcomes, designing a scenario that meets the needs of the learners, and allowing ample time for debriefing by trained facilitators.

References

1. Jeon C. The virtual flier: the link trainer, flight simulation, and pilot identity. Technol Cult. 2015;56:28–53.
2. Povenmire HK. Cockpit resource management: a selected annotated bibliography. Dayton: University of Dayton Research Institute; 1989.
3. Reason J. Human error. New York: Cambridge University Press; 1990.
4. Gaba DM, DeAnda A. The response of anesthesia trainees to simulated critical incidents. Anesth Analg. 1989;68(4):444–51.
5. Aebersold M. The history of simulation and its impact on the future. AACN Adv Crit Care. 2016;27(1):56–61.
6. Deering SH, Weeks L, Benedetti T. Evaluation of force applied during deliveries complicated by shoulder dystocia using simulation. Am J Obstet Gynecol. 2011;204(3):234.e1–5.
7. Ramseyer AM, Lutgendorf MA. Implementation of low-cost obstetric hemorrhage simulation training models for resident education. Mil Med. 2019;184(11–12):e637–41.
8. Turkelson C, Keiser M, Sculli G, Capoccia D. Checklist design and implementation: critical considerations to improve patient safety for low-frequency, high-risk patient events. BMJ Simul Technol Enhanc Learn. 2020;6(3):148–57.
9. Egenberg S, Karlsen B, Massay D, Kimaro H, Bru LE. "No patient should die of PPH just for the lack of training!" Experiences from multi-professional simulation training on postpartum hemorrhage in northern Tanzania: a qualitative study. BMC Med Educ. 2017;17(1):1–12.
10. Argani CH, Eichelberger M, Deering S, Satin AJ. The case for simulation as part of a comprehensive patient safety program. Am J Obstet Gynecol. 2012;206(6):451–5.
11. Garber A, Rao PM, Rajakumar C, Dumitrascu GA, Rousseau G, Posner GD. Postpartum magnesium sulfate overdose: a multidisciplinary and interprofessional simulation scenario. Cureus. 2018;10(4):e2446.
12. O'Gorman N, Penna L. Maternal collapse. Obstet Gynaecol Reprod Med. 2015;25(5):115–22.
13. Sheppard F, Williams M, Klein VR. TeamSTEPPS and patient safety in healthcare. J Healthc Risk Manag. 2013;32(3):5–10.
14. Baker DP, Amodeo AM, Krokos KJ, Slonim A, Herrera H. Assessing teamwork attitudes in healthcare: development of the TeamSTEPPS teamwork attitudes questionnaire. Qual Saf Healthc. 2010;19(6):e49.
15. Egbase E, Ferns J, Kandasarmy G, Murray F, Hall-Jackson M. O23 'A TOAST to team work': the impact of team obstetrics and anesthetics simulation training on attitudes to effective teamwork. BMJ Specialist Journals; 2018.
16. Brolinson M, Tondo-Steele K, Chan M, Gable B. Multidisciplinary in situ simulation to improve emergency obstetric care. BMJ Simul Technol Enhanc Learn. 2020;6(3):190–1.
17. Reed D, Hermelin R, Kennedy CS, Sharma J. Interdisciplinary onsite team-based simulation training in the neonatal intensive care unit: a pilot report. J Perinatol. 2017;37(4):461–4.
18. Le Lous M, Simon O, Lassel L, Lavoue V, Jannin P. Hybrid simulation for obstetrics training: a systematic review. Eur J Obstet Gynecol Reprod Biol. 2020;246:23–8.
19. INACSL Standards Committee. INACSL standards of best practice: Simulation©: simulation. Clin Simul Nurs. 2016;12:S5–S50.

20. Zyniewicz T. Simulation as a replacement for traditional clinical in pre-licensure nursing education: outcomes of different ratios of replacement time for traditional clinical with simulation. 2019.
21. MacKinnon K, Marcellus L, Rivers J, Gordon C, Ryan M, Butcher D. Student and educator experiences of maternal-child simulation-based learning: a systematic review of qualitative evidence protocol. JBI Database System Rev Implement Rep. 2015;13(1):14–26.
22. Lazzara EH, Benishek LE, Dietz AS, Salas E, Adriansen DJ. Eight critical factors in creating and implementing a successful simulation program. Jt Comm J Qual Patient Saf. 2014;40(1):21–9.
23. INACSL Standards Committee. INACSL standards of best practice: simulation SM simulation design. Clin Simul Nurs. 2016;12:s5–s12.
24. Jeffries PR, Dreifuerst KT, Kardong-Edgren S, Hayden J. Faculty development when initiating simulation programs: lessons learned from the national simulation study. J Nurs Regul. 2015;5(4):17–23.
25. Durham CF, Alden KR. Enhancing patient safety in nursing education through patient simulation. In: Patient safety and quality: an evidence-based handbook for nurses. 2008.
26. American Association of Colleges of Nursing. AACN statement on the use of simulation in nursing education. AACN. 2017. https://www.aacnnursing.org/News-Information/News/View/ArticleId/20713/Statement-Simulation.
27. Bradley CS, Johnson BK, Dreifuerst KT, White P, Conde SK, Meakim CH, et al. Regulation of simulation use in United States prelicensure nursing programs. Clin Simul Nurs. 2019;33:17–25.
28. American Association of Colleges of Nursing. AACN response to COVID-19 frequently asked questions. AACN; n.d. https://www.aacnnursing.org/News-Information/COVID-19/Frequently-Asked-Questions.

Psychiatric Mental Health Nursing

10

Louise Alexander

Background

Mental health nursing education (MHNE) has been slow to embrace simulation as an educational strategy and even slower to embed it into modern undergraduate curricula. The uptake of simulation in MHN is in contrast to other healthcare professions that are founded in the studies of human behavior, such as psychology and psychiatry, where simulation is used frequently and progressively. Allied health education, such as occupational therapy, paramedicine, and physiotherapy, likewise have embraced simulation. Only more recently has the use of simulation in MHNE garnered more traction.

One of the major challenges facing education in the MHN field is the translation of theory to practice. For many students, the first time they encounter someone with a severe mental illness is as a student on clinical placement. Understanding the diagnostic criteria and symptoms of schizophrenia, for example, is very different from the nuance of engaging with someone who actually has the condition. Learning about symptoms and seeing and reacting to them are two very different things. Not only does this pose significant risks to consumers in the mental healthcare system, but students report high anxiety levels about their MHN placement, and this, in turn, has significant impacts on the recruitment of graduates into an already underappreciated specialty [1]. We know that when students have a positive experience of placement, they are more likely to choose mental health nursing as a career [2], and the educational leadup to their placement is imperative in learning and applying skills and alleviating anxiety. Simulation with Standardize Patients (SPs) is a best-practice educational modality that can give students an opportunity to practice their interviewing and assessment skills and demonstrate these skills under examination conditions, where they are then deemed 'safe' to go on clinical placement.

L. Alexander (✉)
Mental Health Nursing, Deakin University, Burwood, Australia
e-mail: louise.alexander@deakin.edu.au

A broad range of simulation modalities is currently used in MHNE across various mental health contexts. The most common is role play, followed by simulation with SPs. Manikin-based simulation and, more recently, novel virtual simulation are also reported. It is likely that as technology progresses, virtual simulation may become more prominent, provided it can be delivered cost-effectively.

Best Practice

The success of an MHN simulation program hinges on the rigor of the simulation scenario design and the SP's ability to accurately portray the mental health condition. The simulation designer must always return to the learning outcomes of the scenario and ask, 'Is this the best way to teach this skill'? The following section will explore current best-practice in mental health simulation education.

Consumer Involvement

There has been increasing movement from mental health consumer groups, and clinicians, to ensure that an accurate voice of mental illness is heard through all the symptoms, assumptions, and terminology common to MHN. The consumer's voice has often been missing in MHNE, and processes that seek to use consumer input have become the norm rather than the exception. MHNE is somewhat of a dichotomy, caught between a medical model and a consumer-led recovery-oriented model of care. This can result in challenges in education design and delivery, particularly when trying to honor the recovery model whilst still teaching what is a highly medicalized subject. Simulation educational developers need to ensure they honor both models when developing the MHN curriculum so that it is articulated in a meaningful way for students who are novices to both concepts.

J. M. Kutzin et al. (eds.), *Comprehensive Healthcare Simulation: Nursing*, Comprehensive Healthcare Simulation,
https://doi.org/10.1007/978-3-031-31090-4_10

Best practice, therefore, is to have input from a consumer or someone with a lived experience of mental illness [3–5]. When consumers are included in the curriculum development process, students report how it helps them develop empathy and perspective, an appreciation of the admission and treatment process, and a knowledge of how mental health services could be enhanced [3]. At the very least, mental health consumers should be included in the peer-review process of a nursing simulation to ensure it accurately depicts the lived experience of a person with a mental health issue. The consumer will often have valuable contributions about their experiences of the mental healthcare system, their treatments, and their interactions with mental health nurses. It is now considered common practice to be consumer-inclusive in most aspects of mental health research, and now progressively education [4].

Standarized Patients should be carefully selected. Mental illness is a highly emotive topic, and many people can relate to mental health issues personally. While an SP with a lived experience could give a very accurate account of a condition, care must be taken so they do not put themselves at risk. The SP should be given frequent breaks and an opportunity to debrief with someone after they have finished. Obviously, scenarios featuring depression can be emotionally taxing, but alternatively, mania and schizophrenia can be physically exhausting, too [6].

Script Development

The development of a detailed script is also very important. This is because the mental health interview can be unpredictable and can often deviate from what is expected; therefore, providing as much detail as possible is necessary. This ensures SPs can understand, for example, their character's family history of mental illness so they can answer health assessment questions appropriately, or in the event the SP is given full discretionary power in how they portray their role, they can adapt their behavior to fit the student's responses. Where SPs are required for assessments, however, the SP should not have discretionary power as this results in an interaction that is not standardized. In this instance, an even more detailed script and pre-brief are necessary. An example scenario is included in this text to highlight the required level of detail.

SPs need to be given ample preparation time in order to prepare for characterization, and it is important that the mental health nursing faculty be available to field any questions in the lead-up to the simulation via email or phone.

Debriefing

Debriefing is covered in its own chapter in this text; however, as it comprises a significant part of an MH simulation, it is worth discussing specific considerations here. Debriefing is a learner-centric process to facilitate self-reflection and seek to inform future practice. It is a critical process following a MHN simulation scenario. There are several different models of debriefing that work well in the undergraduate nursing context. Some are more complicated than others. The length of the debrief will also depend on the complexity of the MHN scenario and the degree of emotional involvement by the student, but most mental health simulations warrant a lengthy debrief. Simulations involving complex emotional states that address highly emotive subjects require a more thorough debrief to ensure the psychological safety of participants. Debrief has been identified as one of the most significant phases of a simulation or role play as it is often where much of the learning occurs, and contemporary simulation practices suggest that this process also involves participant reflection [7, 8]. The debriefing process should be conducted by a mental health facilitator well versed in the process, who observed the simulation, which promotes an environment free from judgment, is professionally respectful, and encourages confidentiality and confidence. Regardless of the method of debriefing, it is the role of the facilitator to ensure that the group re-visits the learning outcomes in light of "performance gaps" [8] in a sensitive manner.

In the context of undergraduate MHNE, a number of debriefing approaches are advocated.

Gather, Analyse, Summarize Method (GAS)

The GAS debriefing method is a good option for novice and expert mental health nursing facilitators because it has a simple, guided format. The inclusion of guiding or pointed questions is also helpful for a facilitator who is new to debriefing. It involves three steps:

1. **Gather**—involves active listening to participants' experiences (usually, the team leader begins).
2. **Analyse**—involves the facilitation of reflection and exploration of the participant's actions. During this process, the facilitator may draw on their observations of the simulation and clarify any errors they noted. This needs to be done sensitively.
3. **Summarise**—Review learning outcomes and briefly recap comments. What would participants change next time?

"+/Δ" Plus—Delta Method

The **Plus–Delta** is a simplistic method of debriefing. This approach provides rapid feedback and clearly outlines where there is room for improvement in skills. This method is effective in scenarios where time for extensive debriefing may be an issue [9], or the mental health scenario is not overly complicated. The facilitator will need a whiteboard with two columns. The plus (+) or positives noted during the simulation are on one side. On the other side is the Delta (Δ), where change is documented. Scripting has also been demonstrated to be beneficial in knowledge retention, making it a good option for student nurses. This style is useful for visual learners, but care needs to be taken when describing delta actions as understandingly some students may be very sensitive about their simulation 'performance.' While this method is useful for novice debriefers, it may lack the necessary depth required to debrief a complex mental health simulation and, therefore, should be used with caution.

Advocacy/Inquiry

The benefit of this model is the provision of necessary feedback, delivered in a manner that reduces defensiveness in participants but is best suited to a facilitator experienced in this method. This may be a good fit for mental health simulation because, by nature and training, mental health educators are potentially more attuned to managing interpersonal communication where feedback is necessary. The facilitator uses both advocacy (by making a statement or observation) and inquiry (by asking a question).

The facilitator guides the discussion with statements such as:

- I noticed when the patient told you they felt hopeless, you changed the topic. Can you help me understand your reasoning for doing this?
- I observed the patient muttering to himself while you were distracted, taking notes. Why do you think that was the case? [9]

Like any teaching modality, the debrief session (regardless of which method is used) can encounter challenges. The facilitator should attempt to tune into students who are being self-critical of their performance and ensure that they provide constructive and useful feedback. Issues with the debrief are often related to participants' reluctance to contribute, antagonistic or unprofessional attacks from other participants, or a facilitator who applies blame in the process of trying to inform others. Debriefing is a skill that does not come naturally to every educator. It is important to ensure the mental health facilitator is prepared for this task and has the confidence to use different approaches for MHN debriefing situations.

Sample Curriculum

In an ideal world where money is no obstacle, an undergraduate MHN program would have multiple opportunities for learning through a range of activities that include simulation and would culminate with an assessment such as an objective structured clinical examination (OSCE). The program could encompass major mental health conditions such as schizophrenia, major depression, bipolar disorder, and borderline personality disorder. Foundational learning prior to the simulation is imperative because this provides the student with the necessary theoretical underpinnings to support the demonstration of the required skills.

You may first need to undertake an analysis of the literature to demonstrate how MHNE is strengthened when simulation is embedded into the curriculum. While it is unlikely you will find an abundance of supporting literature because in mental health this is sparse, there is emerging evidence to suggest that simulation in MHN complements existing pedagogical approaches [10–12]. The benefits are varied, yet overwhelmingly positive, and include reducing pre-clinical placement anxiety, decreasing stigma, attracting graduates for future work in MHN, and closing the theory-to-practice gap [5, 11].

Learning Outcomes

This leads to how one would go about developing a mental health nursing curriculum with embedded simulation. It is imperative that any role-play activity or simulation has a place in the curriculum and is aligned with learning outcomes or objectives. The curriculum within an undergraduate degree or course is generally thought of as the entirety of learning practices offered to students so that they may accomplish general skills and knowledge in diverse areas of learning [13]. This may consist of materials, books, lessons, and experiences. Learning outcomes or objectives are often a set of capabilities reflective of the long-term learning in a unit or subject. To successfully complete the unit, the student must pass the learning outcomes, often through means of assessment such as an examination or written assignment [13].

While most tertiary institutes will differ, commonly a *unit* of study might be devoted to learning mental health nursing and will have around 5-7 learning outcomes. This obviously differs from *simulation*-specific learning outcomes (which should stem from the *unit* ones). Some examples of MHN *unit* learning outcomes may include:

- demonstrate an understanding of mental states that are not neurotypical, underpinned by a sound comprehension of wellness and illness models of care;
- apply ethical and legal frameworks within a recovery-focused model in care planning for individuals experiencing a mental health issue;
- demonstrate an understanding of psychotropic medications and non-pharmacological therapeutic interventions for consumers living with mental health issues;
- describe the impacts of mental illness on consumers in the biopsychosocial context;
- demonstrate the skills necessary to engage safely and therapeutically with someone experiencing a mental health issue.

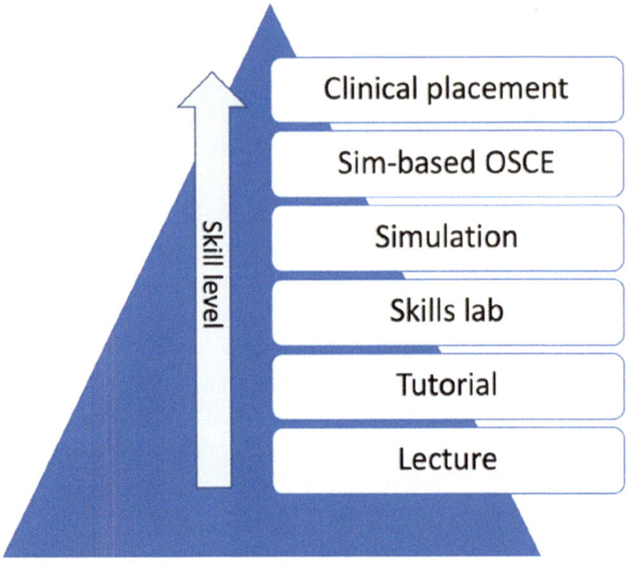

Fig. 10.1 Scaffolding knowledge and skill mastery in simulation-embedded curricula

Scaffolding

Simulation, like all other learning, is most effective when learning has been scaffolded. Scaffolding is a term coined from Vygotsky's zone of proximal development and refers to the support learners need to reduce the difference between what they can do *independently* and with *assistance* [14]. The notion of scaffolding implies that assistance is a temporary aid and that concepts are built upon to develop independence. The ability of facilitators to scaffold learning in MHN curricula is supported by using a variety of teaching and learning strategies such as didactic lectures, case-based scenarios, role play, skills laboratories, consumer-led sessions, and simulation. A suggested way to scaffold learning is demonstrated in Fig. 10.1. As a learner's skill level and mastery increases, so does the curriculum's complexity.

In Fig. 10.1, you can see that learning begins with lectures and tutorials, and this progresses to skills laboratories. A skilled laboratory might include practicing skills with each other, for example, through role-play. Role play or simulation should scaffold both *forward* and *backward* to the unit's objectives and the activity's learning outcomes. *Backward* scaffolding refers to the culmination of learning up to 'this point.' It implies that those skills and knowledge already learned are useful or necessary for the development of future skills to be embarked upon. Scaffolding *forward* implies that the skills to be addressed in the role-play or simulation will be necessary at a later date, for example, during an OSCE or clinical placement.

Roleplay

Role play is a teaching methodology beneficial in the development and training of communication skills, engagement, ethical considerations, empathy, and caring, which are all pivotal in a nursing degree [15]. Role play allows the participant to immerse themselves in the environment the simulation is replicating and is useful in the development and augmentation of existing and new skills [16] in addition to practicing communication skills [17]. Due to the immersive nature of role-play, participants are required to become active contributors, which is associated with the development of critical thinking skills [16].

Participants will generally be given a character or role to play (e.g., a patient) and will interact with another student also playing a role (e.g., a healthcare worker) with the aim of achieving a task or skill. This is known as peer-based role-playing. At the discretion of the educator, the character/s development will vary from minimal characterization with a requirement to 'ad-lib'; to a well-developed character with more information (e.g., anticipated responses, social information, degree of cooperativeness, etc.). Ideally, when the characterizations are developed by the facilitator, they should consider offering more than one option so that students have a choice in which mental health experience they want to portray. This will prevent a student from having to portray a condition that is too close to their own experiences, which may result in distress. Care should also be taken when asking participants to 'ad-lib,' as they may be more inclined to fall back to what they know personally and provide too much 'real life' input. It is important to understand that the greater the resemblance to 'real life' a teaching modality is, the more skills are absorbed faster and more efficiently [16], but we need to make sure this is distanced from people's real, personal experiences. This is a dichotomy from traditional, didactic methods of teaching.

While role-playing is an acceptable form of simulation, it is not without potential issues, and facilitators need to ensure that students are comfortable playing the role, that they depict it accurately (without stereotypes and prejudice), and that they take it seriously. These are not trivial or even easily overcome issues. Using 'role play cards' with character information and using a range of theatre or drama-inspired approaches can be useful. If your university has an Arts Faculty that has a drama school, you may find their expertise helpful. Facilitators working in the arts are skilled and experienced at using engaging techniques to make learning fun and interesting. Input from the arts has been effectively used in some simulation programs where simulation with SPs is not possible (or to compliment the teaching), and drama-inspired role play can be used instead [18]. These concepts are easy to teach for both facilitators and students, and instructions and resources are readily available. The following concepts offer novel ways of embedding engaging and unique role-play activities into teaching, and a simple internet search provides instruction on how to apply these techniques in an undergraduate program:

- Teacher-in-role
- Hot seating
- Tap and talk
- Freeze frame
- Flash back/flash forward

Immersive Simulation

Once students have mastered the theory and practiced skills with each other, they can then practice and/or observe with simulation, which can then be later assessed in an OSCE. Once all of these processes are complete, they are ready to go on clinical placement. The following is an example of how simulation in a theoretical mental health unit which encompasses the entire MHN component of a nursing degree, may be threaded. For many curricula, this will look like a theoretical mental health unit (skills and theory *learned*) and a practical mental health unit (skills and theory *implemented* or *practiced*). In short, all mental health skills are taught in these units, and students will have an accompanying clinical placement. While the nursing curriculum is moving towards more immersive and integrated mental health content that is embedded across multiple units of a nursing degree, for clarity, it is easier to demonstrate how this would occur in a discrete mental health unit.

Table 10.1 provides an example curriculum and reveals how learning is scaffolded over a 10-week period. A range of common mental health conditions are theoretically described and then brought to life with SPs in simulation. Students are then assessed in an OSCE based on one of the presentations already observed in the simulation. This table reveals the role of scaffolding in bringing all the concepts of MHN together in a meaningful way for students. The continuity of cases through tutorials, skill labs, and simulation are also beneficial to student learning. Figure 10.2 demonstrates how the simulation for week three from Table 10.1 might be scaffolded.

Figure 10.2 shows how the continuity in case studies helps consolidate these concepts for student learning. Using a variety of role-playing techniques in the skills laboratories gives students the confidence for the simulation. As men-

Table 10.1 Frameworke for inter professional education

Week	Lecture	Tutorial	Skills lab	Simulation
1	Introduction to MHN	Stigma & perceptions of people with mental illness	Empathy workshop	Virtual simulation: hearing voices
2	Mental State Examination (MSE) & risk assessment	MSE: Applying & making sense of terminology	Role play: MSE question development & practice role play	
3	Schizophrenia and schizophrenia spectrum	Case study: Bill 24 yo male with schizophrenia	Focus MSE: perceptual disturbance & thought	Bill MSE: perception, thought content & insight
4	Major depression	Case study: Alice 44 yo female with depression	Focus MSE: mood, affect & therapeutic silence	Alice MSE: mood, affect and speech
5	Bipolar I & II	Case study: Mohammed 69 yo male with mania	Focus MSE: mania & hypomania	Mohamed: de-escalation and medication refusal during a manic episode
6	Anxiety-based disorders	Case study: Shanice 19 yo female with OCD	Focus: managing panic	
7	Child & adolescent MH	Case study: DeShawn 8 yo male with autism	Focus MSE: interviewing the young person	
8	Substance-use disorders	Case study: Emily 31 yo female in alcohol withdrawal		
9	Personality disorders	Case study: Sofia 22 yo female with borderline personality disorder	MSE focus thought, self-harm & suicide	Sofia MSE: suicide & self-harm risk assessment
10	Neurocognitive disorders	Case study: Bert 77 yo male with Alzheimer's		
OSCE with any of the four simulated case studies				
Clinical placement				

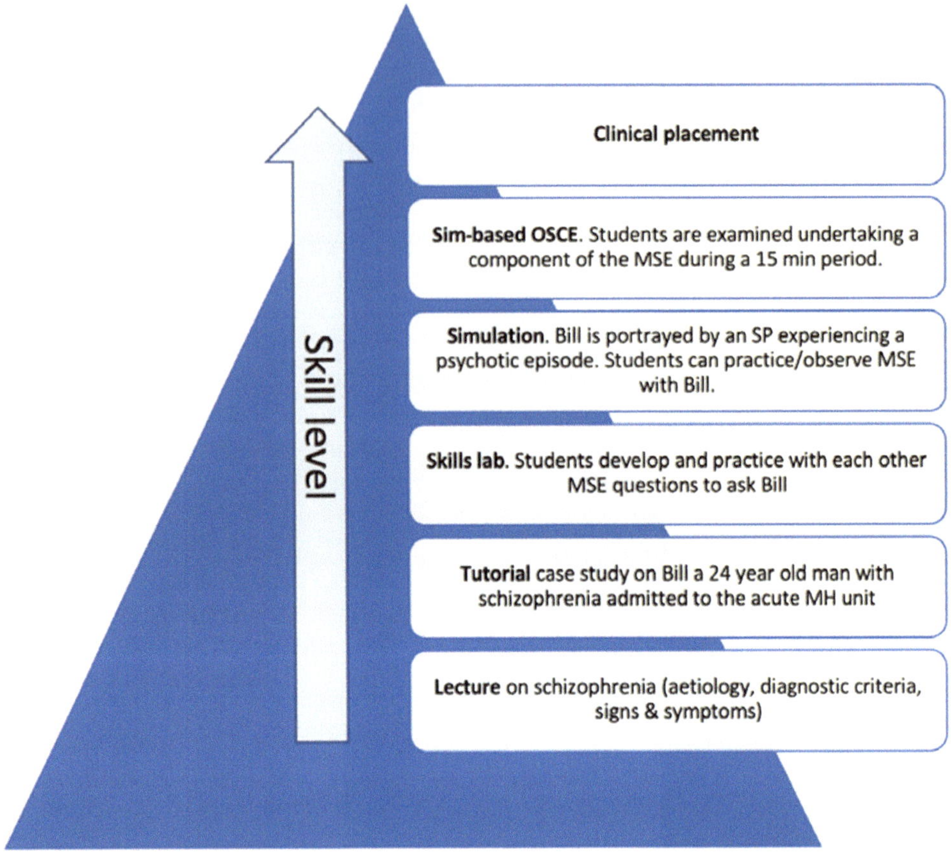

Fig. 10.2 Scaffolding knowledge and skill mastery in simulation-embedded curricula with example

tioned, this simulation can be adapted to a variety of contexts and does not have to include an SP.

Virtual Simulation

Virtual simulation is a technology replicating three-dimensional environments creating a realistic experience for participants [19], and in MHN is novel with very limited empirical research to support it. The required equipment and ever-changing nature of technology may be cost-prohibitive for many institutions, but it is still worthwhile keeping abreast of this type of simulation as it lends itself to scenarios where empathizing with the consumer experience is indicated. Virtual simulation, in particular, has been reported to support and facilitate the transition from classroom to clinical practice in the mental health context [20], and there is evidence to suggest its potential in MHN skill development.

Evaluation

The evaluation of simulation is an important part of curriculum development and ensuring quality simulations. High-fidelity simulations that involve lengthy planning and development often benefit from a peer review and, where possible, a practice 'run through' to ensure learning outcomes are met and to identify any hurdles to overcome. Student participants will often have valuable experiences and perspectives on improving future simulations, and they should be allowed to contribute to their improvement. This can be done through online surveys after the unit of study or a link to the survey at the conclusion of the simulation.

It is important to note that because most universities operate under a customer service model (where the student is the customer), positive evaluations of simulations may result in an increased budget for simulations. This is why collecting and collating these evaluations is important because you may be able to use this data later when demonstrating the benefits to students. Consider also evaluating clinical partners experiences of students on placement. They are in the ideal position to provide evidence of improvement in clinical skills when simulation has been added to the curriculum (particularly where there is a change).

Integrating into Existing Curriculum

The simulation options mentioned earlier are feasible possibilities that can be integrated into an existing curriculum. The simulation scenario would need to be adapted to the existing unit learning outcomes, although most universities will have provisions for making a curriculum change. This can be a lengthy process. It may be preferable to adapt the simulation to what is existing, and then when it is time for a curriculum review, embed simulation based on the outcomes from the review.

Mental health simulation can be 'switched' for any existing skills education currently used in your program. You are only limited by your unit learning outcomes; many of these are generic enough that you can be creative in applying them to a teaching method.

Challenges & Solutions

There are undoubtedly many challenges in implementing simulation in MHNE. However, the educational benefits far outweigh any perceived limitations. While there is a dearth of literature on mental health simulation, what evidence there is strongly supports its inclusion in nursing curricula [5, 11, 21, 22].

Cost

One of the biggest challenges for MHN simulation will be to 'sell it' to the appropriate faculty leads. This is because simulation with SPs is often considered cost prohibitive. MHN is often a minority specialty in academia and may not have a 'loud enough voice' in a general nursing-focused department. MHNE, without simulation, generally has no additional overheads in education. There are usually no consumables such as syringes, IV fluids, manikins, or simulated ward spaces. This means that for many departments, MHNE overheads are simply the facilitators' cost.

So how can you overcome this when pitching the idea of adding simulation to an existing program? Well, there are a few options. Firstly, it is not necessary to run multiple simulations in MHNE in order to have successful outcomes. Simulation in mental health does not need to be at an expensive 1:1 ratio with an SP, provided student observers are given an education-designed task. Observer roles provide very positive learning experiences [23]. Research regarding vicarious learning in simulation strongly suggests its worthy place in education and is considered even more effective than active participation in simulation [24]. For example, one SP could be interviewed by a tutor/lecturer in order to obtain an MSE in front of an entire cohort of students in a large lecture theatre. The observing students can then be divided into groups, where they take notes and construct a nursing entry note for a particular component of the MSE. For example, some students need to focus on general appearance and mood, others' perception and thought, and so on. The cost here is negligible. Indeed, just one simulation can successfully achieve multiple learning outcomes. If your SP agrees to allow the simulation to be recorded (usually for an increased fee), you can utilize this for years to come.

This leads us to video recording, which is a low-cost simulation option. There are many scenario possibilities when you consider recording content for later use, and these include:

- de-escalation techniques (e.g., facilitator deescalates SP);
- 1:1 MSE interview (e.g., between SP and facilitator);
- hearing voices exercise (e.g., recording of 'voices' for use on headphones);
- medication administration (e.g., between facilitator and SP);
- 'good' versus 'great' interaction (e.g., between facilitator and SP);
- legal frameworks (e.g., SP requesting explanation of legal rights in involuntary/compulsory admission to hospital);
- demonstration of symptomatology (e.g., SP demonstrating referential delusions);
- family meeting (e.g., discussion between a few SPs and the facilitator).

Ensuring that your general nursing colleagues only use SPs for simulations when necessary can help ensure any SP budget is used for the most appropriate scenarios. This would arguably be communication simulations such as those seen in mental health. A manikin is arguably a cost-effective way of teaching vital signs but is not an appropriate modality for a mental health simulation 5. While SPs would ideally be used for all scenarios where interaction is required, this is not usually financially feasible. Therefore, facilitators need to ensure that any SP budget is spent on the most suitable, often high-stakes scenarios.

One other option to consider, which has been successfully implemented at the Australian Catholic University in Melbourne, Australia, is to consider putting one week's worth of course content online and using the money saved from this (e.g., sessional academic wages, overheads, etc.) to finance a simulation with SPs. This would mean your students would not be on campus that week. This is particularly beneficial in universities where a large contingency of face-to-face teaching is undertaken by costly sessional or contract staff. Alternatively, you may wish to replace a written assessment that requires correction with an online exam (which is automatically corrected through a learning management system) and use the funds allocated to marking for your SP budget. There are certainly novel ways of delivering a curriculum to free up finances that could be spent on simulation.

As mentioned previously, consider the use of the Arts Faculty in your university with drama students acting as SPs who either volunteer their services or are paid a small fee. This could be a mutually beneficial option.

Choosing Wisely

When you do have an approved budget and have the opportunity to decide on the best use of simulation, the key is choosing the most appropriate scenario to fit the learning outcomes of the unit of study. Generally speaking, regardless of what part of the world you practice in, acute mental health care will have a high frequency of consumers with:

- schizophrenia
- mania
- depression
- borderline personality disorder
- drug-induced psychosis
- medication non-adherence
- suicide and deliberate self-harm
- a need for an assessment

In an ideal world, it would be beneficial if every MHN student could have exposure to more obscure conditions because we know that this is often where serious adverse events occur. There is unfamiliarity in knowing how to manage the situation. This is not practical. However, more common mental health scenarios are likely to be the focus. Once you have identified the right condition to present, you must decide which skills you want the student to learn and practice. Again, these should align with the unit's learning outcomes. Any of the following are well supported by simulation with SPs:

- de-escalation;
- mental state examination (MSE);
- risk assessment;
- medication administration;
- psychoeducation;
- admission

Once you have determined the skill and scenario, you can decide how to run the simulation. As mentioned, if your program is on a tight budget, you can run a very successful simulation with an SP for an entire group of students (rather than individually).

Student Preparation

Students in an MHN simulation may become anxious about the behaviors they are likely to experience from the scenario, performing in front of their peers or having their skills critically deconstructed in front of others. One of the best ways to avoid disengagement is to ensure students are fully prepared for the simulation. At a basic level, the student should have met the learning objectives from a theoretical perspective. Preparatory content would be delivered using lecture material and pre-reading.

Some students find the process of role-play and simulation anxiety-provoking, and this is seen as one of the disadvantages of this learning modality [16]. It is, therefore, important to promote a safe learning environment for students, with expectations of behavior clearly outlined. For units that involve prolonged periods of role-play or simulation across a semester, it may be worthwhile developing a confidentiality disclaimer for students to sign. This will ensure that what occurs in the learning environment stays there, thus making apprehensive learners more comfortable. Starting in small groups is also helpful to build confidence which can be extended to demonstrations in larger groups.

A pre-brief is an important part of any simulation. Orientation to the simulated learning environment is important (context), in addition to time in 'active' roles. Reiteration of learning outcomes and expectations is also necessary. Informing students about the opportunity for a 'time out' or a ‘pause’ should be a requirement for any simulation activity that is highly emotive or requires complex skill application. If this is the case, participants must be briefed about this process.

Student Disengagement

Fortunately, disengagement is not a common occurrence in mental health simulation. Students tend to be anxious about their clinical placement and therefore take all opportunities to practice skills they will later be assessed on (e.g., MSE). Despite this, disengagement is an unfortunate by-product of education, regardless of the specialty. It is important to be clear and explicit about learning expectations, what the role-playing or simulation requirements are, and how these relate to the successful completion of the unit. Where role-play scaffolds into simulation with SPs and then further scaffolded into an OSCE, students tend to take it more seriously. The stakes are higher.

Ensuring that vicarious participants or observers have a role while observing is also important. Not only does this involve them in the simulation, but it ensures they are aware of the expectations of their participation.

Emotionally Charged Topics

Mental health conditions are often highly relatable, and students may have their own mental health issues, which are triggered or exacerbated during a simulation. This is not a plausible justification for changing the way mental health nursing is taught, but care must be taken to provide visible and available support systems. Being open at the commencement of the course about appropriate channels of support for students who experience distress is important to reinforce. Before a MHN simulation, make it clear that anyone who finds the content upsetting can leave at any time. Set ground rules for respecting each other so that students feel safe and seek a confidentiality contract to ensure students respect the experience and its potential effects. The facilitator should be present and vigilant during role plays and simulations to ensure participants are focused, professional, and feel psychologically safe.

SP Training

SP training can be a lengthy and costly process, particularly if the SP does not have the skills to portray the behaviors and symptoms commonly seen. Preparation can include the use of YouTube clips and a detailed script. There are educational resource videos freely available on YouTube to help SPs develop an understanding of mental health conditions, nuance, and interview behaviors. For example, a detailed script and link to an educational video between an actor and a psychiatrist can be helpful in demonstrating the level of elevation needed for mania. It can also give the SP an example of what to expect and even how to dress for the occasion. There are also vintage YouTube resources (from the 1960s) that use real patients and psychiatrists to demonstrate accurate mental states.

It is important to note that you may wish your SP to present as disheveled or unkempt for the simulation or alternatively have a few changes of clothes. Understanding your SP's comfort level with clothing and behavior is also important. Your scenario, for example, may include a woman with mania who is provocative and suggestive. It would not be appropriate to require this of the SP on the simulation day without any prior warning.

This leads us to props on hand for mental health simulations, including eccentric accessories, such as bibles and newspapers. A notebook with comments on a particular character's delusional system can be useful for a simulation. For example, if the SP character has mania and believes he/she can cure cancer by adding up and subtracting numbers from supermarket catalogs, then have some brochures as props. The SP could also write these numbers down and use a calculator to add them up and subtract them. This can add another layer of authenticity to the SP's character and provide a distraction that is common to the real clinical environment.

Having a bank of SPs who are highly suited to portraying mental health scenarios is advantageous. You will find that some SPs are very good at depicting one mental health condition, but perhaps not others. It is important to ensure the depiction is realistic and believable, not a caricature. Noting the suitability of each SP in a database is useful. This may also save you time when looking for the right SP to characterize the right condition.

Simulation in OSCEs

When the simulation is used in high-stakes assessment conditions such as an OSCE, it is imperative that scenarios and roles are standardized when more than one SP will be portraying the same role. This will ensure that students are exposed to the same level of portrayal. To mitigate this, a specific and detailed script and a rigorous moderation process is needed to ensure consistency between SPs when presenting the same case, and inter-rater reliability for assessors. A structured briefing is required for all SPs where expectations of the role and how to react to certain situations can be discussed. Engaging in a few practice encounters together is also beneficial and helps the SP demonstrate their interpretation of the role to you.

Predicting what a student will say is impossible, but preparing SPs for typical responses (either very good or very poor, and anything in between) is required. SPs need to know what their triggers are. For example, the SP playing the role of someone who is depressed needs to know how to react to the student who lacks empathy or does not respond to their suicidality in a way that is clinically plausible and therapeutic. One way of addressing this is with the use of a decision-making tree. The following is an example to show how the more empathetic and engaging the student is, the more responsive and engaging the SP becomes:

SP Alan: I just don't know how I can go on anymore. I am a burden to my family. They are better off without me. I have nothing to live for … I am better off dead.

Student: What I'm hearing is you feel like everything is just too much for you at the moment, Alan. Like you are in a really dark place.

SP Alan: Yeah. I've never felt this bad in my life before … I've never wished myself dead before.

Student: It sounds like you have thought about your death a lot Alan. Could you tell me more about this?

SP Alan goes on to describe, in detail, his plan to die by suicide, and the student undertakes a thorough risk assessment.

The following example demonstrates how this same statement can go down a different path, depending on how the student responds to the SP Alan.

SP Alan: I just don't know how I can go on anymore. I am a burden to my family. They are better off without me. I have nothing to live for … I am better off dead.

Student: Oh ok … Right, um, Alan, do you drink alcohol?

SP Alan: What?
Student: Do you drink alcohol?
SP Alan: (sighs) … No

The interview continues, and SP Alan provides monosyllabic responses to questions.

Here the second student is not reading cues from SP Alan, which obviously impacts rapport and engagement. Discussing with the SP team before they commence should involve standardized ways to react to common situations like this. These reactions should all be informed by the aims or learning outcomes of the simulation, and they should try an adopt consistency between reactions.

Standardized participant's must be briefed about the learning outcomes to standardize their responses as much as possible. Ensuring that SPs know how to respond to positive and undesirable interactions is integral for students to develop the necessary skills to provide safe and effective therapeutic interactions when on placement.

Underpinning all this is the debrief. Regardless of the debriefing technique, facilitators should consider including the SP in this process. SPs can make a valuable contribution to student learning when incorporated into the debrief, and students may be more inclined to take their feedback on board because they, too, experienced the simulated session. Consider how you want the SP to give feedback. Caution should be taken if asking the SP to remain in the role as students may be reluctant to speak freely if they believe they are still speaking to the 'patient' rather than the actor who portrayed the patient.

Sample Cases

The following is an example taken from the Bachelor of Nursing at the Australian Catholic University. It presents Alice from week four of the exemplar curriculum. This scenario differs from many standardized templates as it has more emphasis on the characterization, which is required for the SP. This simulation can be done in small tutorial groups or larger groups. It is important to consider that very large groups may impact student participation. The SP would need to be sent the section titled 'characterization' at least one week prior to the simulation to ensure she is prepared for the role.

ACU Mental Health Simulated Patient Scenario

Acknowledgement: Bachelor of Nursing, Australian Catholic University, Melbourne Australia

Author: Dr Louise Alexander

Simulation Overview

Curriculum	
Unit Code	Mental Health Nursing Theory
Semester	Semester 1
Complexity	High
Roles	
Active Participant Roles (list each role)	Undertake MSE
Observer Roles (list each role and number in each role)	Observe, take notes for later comment
Facilitator Roles (list each role)	Guide, observe, lead pre/de brief
Technical Assistance Required (specify)	N/A
Time Allocation	120 min
Pre-simulation brief (including orientation to the simulation environment)	15 min
Scenario	60 min
Debrief	>30 min
Quality Assurance	
Has this simulation plan been peer-reviewed?	Yes
Has this simulation been reviewed by a lived-experience consumer?	Yes
Has this simulation been piloted prior to implementation?	No
How will the student experience be evaluated?	Student unit feedback
How will the staff experience be evaluated?	Debrief

Description of the Simulation

The aim of this simulation is to provide students an opportunity to observe and/or engage in a therapeutic interaction with a mental health consumer by undertaking an MSE. Simulated participants provide the most authentic learning experience for students in the mental health context as role playing and mannequin-based simulation often fail to provide correct diagnostic presentation and appropriate affect. Students participating in this activity will have undertaken 10 weeks of theoretical and practical mental health content.

Curriculum Alignment

Please indicate the horizontal and/or vertical alignment of knowledge and skills required to participate in this simulation (e.g., students will be required to expand on their understanding of taking a patient history in first year, to providing a verbal hand-over to the multidisciplinary team).

Past course content: HLSC111

Current course content: NRSG210 & NRSG262

Future course content: NRSG370

Unit-level learning outcome

By the end of this unit, learners should be able to:

1. *Assess and document a person's mental health status within the context of a holistic health assessment.*

Simulation-level Learning Outcomes

By the end of this session, learners should be able to:

1. *Recognise and respond to a mental state that deviates from a neurotypical presentation.*
2. *Practise and/or observe therapeutic communication skills and rapport development.*

By the end of this session, learners should be able to:

Perform a mental state assessment in a realistic, clinical presentation and under realistic conditions

Pre-simulation Activities

Attend lecture on major depressive disorder
Attend lecture on mental state examination and risk assessment
Rapport development

Set-up & Preparation

Simulated Participant

Please provide a brief profile of the Simulated Participant.

NOTE: Simulated Participants require a detailed characterisation four weeks prior to the scheduled date of simulation. If the simulation requires any diagnostic procedure, exposure or close contact (e.g., BP, chest auscultation), this must be identified and negotiated prior to confirmation of the Simulated Participant.

Item	Response	Equipment Required
Role of SP (e.g., client, patient, relative of patient)	Consumer Alice Russel	Tissues, chairs, table
Gender	Female	
Age Range	31–45 years	e.g., 12/08/1974 DOB
Clothing and appearance (e.g., dishevelled)	Dishevelled, unkempt, messy, poor attention to grooming	
Description of the presenting problem	MDD (post-partum onset)	
Onset and setting of the problem (frequency, factors precipitating/exacerbating)	? peripartum MDD progressing into post-partum period	
Person's perceptions of the problem	Some insight present but feels beyond saving Guilt +	
Past medical history (general health, medications, past illness/hospitalisation, family history)	IVF pregnancy P/H: DSH, but denies prior MH history	
Psychosocial history (living arrangements, relationships, employment, education, drug & alcohol use, hobbies)	See below	
Medical Record Details (name, DOB, allergies)	To align with approx. age of SP	
Moulage		
Simulated blood (if yes, indicate volume and location)		
Bruising		
Wounds		
Dressings		
Other		
Consent		
Will you be filming? If YES access the [INSERT NAME OF FORM]	No	
Please complete the Simulated Patient Case Template		

Characterisation

Name: Alice Russel

Background: You are a successful lawyer and a partner in a law firm. You love this job; it has been your identity for years. Being a mother is not what you thought it was going to be. This is a much-wanted IVF baby (have been trying to conceive for 11 years with your husband Tom). You have good leave entitlements, can take as much time off as needed. Tom is an engineer and took 4 weeks off after baby Andrew was born. Tom has been becoming increasingly concerned about your mental health. The house is in disarray when he comes home from work, Andrew is often in his bassinet crying, and you look like you haven't showered all day. You have poor family supports. Situation escalated when Tom came home early today, and you were in the bathroom with a "heap of pills". You hadn't taken any yet but were about to. You had written a suicide note. You are devastated this plan was thawed… "I can't even get that right". Tom called an ambulance, and you were brought into ED, assessed by psych triage and are now being admitted to the ward.

Appearance: Dishevelled, unkempt and messy. You are suffering from depression, but also managing the day-to-day issues of having a newborn baby. Psychomotor retardation. Poor eye contact.

Social: Majority of your friends are career-minded people or have older children and you feel very much isolated by this baby. You are estranged from your father, and your mother (with whom you were very close to) died 2 years ago. You have a brother, but he lives overseas. You are as close as you can be given the distance, e.g., Skyping often etc. Tom's parents live interstate and has a good relationship with them. You went to the local mother's group once "I can't connect with them …They're all very young and were thrilled to stop working. They're nice people but I cannot relate to them."

Mental State Examination

Speech

- latency of responses (not profoundly so)
- difficult to engage
- monotonous
- no spontaneous speech

Mood

- Anhedonia (inability to experience pleasure)
- Distressed
- 'Depressed'
- Rates mood 1/10—this is consistent/congruent to affect
- Ongoing lethargy and fatigue
- Feeling 'down' for about 2 months now … "I just need sleep really, I'll be fine if I get a good night's sleep".
- ***Appetite***—Poor, can't remember what you had for dinner last night. "Tom thrusts food in front of me when he comes home from work …"
- You have lost your appetite
- You weigh less than your pre-pregnancy weight by about 4 kg.
- ***Sexual relationships***—Has not been intimate with Tom since about 21 weeks pregnant, "We did it once then, but I was so terrified of something going wrong with the pregnancy we didn't do it again and now it's the last thing I can think about".
- This lack of intimacy has extended to no longer kissing, hugging etc.
- Tom is being "sweet" about this at the moment.
- Prior to this you had an active sexual relationship with Tom
- ***Sleep***—"I just can't get enough". Sleep became difficult in the later stages of pregnancy but you're not sleeping well when Andrew is asleep. "I just lie there with my eyes closed, but I can't sleep. I'm exhausted".
- "I just want to go to sleep and never wake up again, I'm so tired".

Affect

- Flat
- Congruent to mood

Thought Content

- Self-deprecating
- Focus on failures and how you miss working as a lawyer "motherhood is not what I thought it was … why am I being punished?"
- Ruminating about what a 'bad mother' you are
- Thoughts re. death—distressed that suicide plan didn't work
- Worthlessness
- Hopelessness
- Guilt +++
- "Better off dead"
- Guilty about not spending time with Tom and Andrew. "Tom is such a great dad … he deserves a better wife and Andrew deserves a better mother"
- No evidence of delusions
- Remains risk of suicide—feels beyond help
- Risk of homicide (stated only if asked by students and causing ++ distress) "Sometimes I think Andrew would be better off dead too …and then I think what kind of a monster thinks like that?! But then I grew up with a shitty dad and look where I am now …."
- Significant risk of suicide
- Plan was well-established

- Had means
- Had written a detailed 'apology' note
- Had enough meds to succeed in dying
- *Current:* Planned attempted OD as above today intercepted by partner
- *Past:* denies
- DSH: Past History of self-harm (cutting) when teenager…" everyone was doing it. Things were difficult at home. I saw a psychologist for a little while and it helped".
- *Eth:* Increase in alcohol consumption ("I never drank at all when trying to get pregnant or when I was pregnant, but now I'm drinking almost every night")
- *OD:* Cannabis "a few times as a teenager"
- *Interpersonal Violence:* Denies
- *Homicide:* as above.

Perception:
- Denies perceptual disturbance & no evidence of same

Cognition:
- Admits to having issues with concentration and memory
- Cannot remember what you ate last night
- Sometimes you forget to feed Andrew but then think the screaming may be hunger and not wind and you feel 'terrible' when you feed him and he's starving.

Insight:
- You understand you are depressed but cannot see a way out of this now. "Nothing will fix me, I'm too broken"
- Will accept help but believes "I'm well and truly beyond anything you can do for me"

Judgement:
- Poor. Leaving baby unattended, issues with missing feeds, ? homicidal ideation.

Environment

Describe the environment to be simulated and the desired set-up.

Item	Response	Equipment Required
This simulation can be run in a classroom, lecture theatre or skills laboratory.		Requires table, chairs & whiteboard

Equipment

Please indicate below what type of equipment (including amount) you will be using.

Item	Response	Equipment Required
Documentation[a]		
Monitors / Monitoring		
Props		
Consumables		

[a]It is the responsibility of the Facilitator-in-Charge to prepare and provide completed documentation for the simulation

Information for Learners

Detail information that will be provided to learners at the commencement of the simulation.

Pre-Simulation Brief:

Orientate students to simulated environment (private/confidential area of a hospital)
Remind students of simulation rules

By the end of this session, learners should be able to:

Perform a mental state assessment in a realistic, clinical presentation and under realistic conditions

Learning Outcomes

1. Recognise and respond to a mental state that deviates from a neurotypical presentation.
2. Practise and/or observe therapeutic communication skills and rapport development.

Handover (to commence scenario)

Alice Russel is a 44-year-old woman brought into the MH unit by her husband via ED after an OD suicide attempt. Alice is 15 weeks post-partum. Alice needs an admission MSE after a review in ED with psych triage.

Information for Facilitators

Detail information that will be used to guide the facilitation of the simulation.

Background & Briefing Information:
This simulation will be set up in a manner where the SP is at the front of the room and the students are seated in a semi-circle around her. The week prior to the simulation, students will be asked to volunteer to be active participants in this simulation.
Students will take turns in asking questions to the SP in front of the class. They can pause at any stage, to ask the facilitator for assistance, or other members in the class. When they want to finish, or when the facilitator decides to move to another student, the simulation will be paused. Students will 'pick up' where the previous student left off to ensure continuity and avoid repetition. At the conclusion, the facilitator will lead a debrief which includes the SP (who is out of character).
Learners will be expected to:
Active participants:
- Interview SP asking appropriate MSE questions
- Engage therapeutically and demonstrate their understanding of the MSE by asking relevant questions

Observers:
- Note the positive interactions they observed
- Note the areas needed for improvement and consider how to structure this to give constructive peer feedback
- Write the observed interaction as a nursing file entry

Facilitator Roles:
Primary Facilitator
- Conduct the pre-brief with SP
- Orientate students to the simulated environment
- Provide input and assist students as needed
- Pause and discuss as needed
- Facilitate debrief including guiding SP to give feedback

Secondary Facilitator (can be run without, however if available, role as follows)
- Monitor students who are observing
- Assist the primary facilitator in debrief

How will students know the scenario has started?
- Facilitator will use the word "start" when commencing

How will students know the scenario has ended?
- Facilitator will use the word "pause" when stopping

Student Roles:
Hands-on student roles:
- Interview SP asking appropriate MSE questions
- Engage therapeutically and demonstrate their understanding of the MSE by asking relevant questions

Observer student roles:
- Note the positive interactions they observed
- Note the areas needed for improvement and consider how to structure this to give constructive peer feedback
- Write the observed interaction as a nursing file entry

Facilitator notes & observations

Facilitator notes & observations

Debrief

Please develop a debriefing framework for this simulation activity. Include:

- The setup for the debriefing environment
- The pre-simulation brief including the rules of simulation
- Identification of the debriefing model to be used
- Detailed description of the process the debriefing will undertake using the structure of
  - Reactions Phase
  - Analysis Phase
  - Summary Phase

  Include suggested timing for each phase and example questions

Quality Improvement

In this table, please indicate what aspects of the simulation went well and those that need improvement.

What went well?
What needs to be improved?
What did not work well?

Conclusion

Simulation in mental health nursing continues to grow albeit at a slower rate than more traditional areas of nursing practice largely due to the costs associated with incorporating SPs as a modality of learning. This chapter has identified a number of cost-effective and even cost-neutral ways of supporting a simulation program in mental health nursing undergraduate curricula. Simulation developers need to pay close attention to both unit and simulation learning outcomes and ensure that they are developing a fit-for-purpose scenario which meets these requirements.

The burden of mental illness is a global health priority with nurses comprising the largest mental health workforce. To effectively assist people with mental illness, we need a future workforce capable of supporting and helping people living with mental illness. Simulation can positively influence a student's experiences of learning about mental health illness, and perhaps even inspire them to make a career out of this important speciality.

References

1. Happell B, Platania-Phung C, Harris S, Bradshaw J. It's the anxiety: facilitators and inhibitors to nursing students' career interests in mental health nursing. Issues Ment Health Nurs. 2014;35(1):50–7.
2. Foster K, Giandinoto J, Furness T, Blanco A, Withers R, Alexander L. 'Anyone can have a mental illness': A qualitative inquiry of pre-registration nursing students' experience of traditional mental health clinical placement. Int J Ment Health Nurs. 2021;30(1):83–92.
3. Happell B, Byrne L, McAllister M, Lampshire D, Roper C, Gaskin C, et al. Consumer involvement in the tertiary-level education of mental health professionals: a systematic review. Int J Ment Health Nurs. 2014;23(1):3–16.
4. Happell B, Waks S, Bocking J, Horgan A, Manning F, Greaney S, et al. Int J Ment Health Nurs. 2019;28(4):950–9.
5. Alexander L, Coyte B, Evans A, Dickson J, Guinea S, Foster K. The educational value of mental health simulation in undergraduate Bachelor of Nursing education: An integrative review. Clinical Simulation in Nursing 2023;84:101459.
6. Gerzina AH, Poreli EJ. Mindfulness as a predictor of positive reappraisal and burnout in standardised patients. Teach Learn Med. 2012;24(4):309–14.
7. Jaye P, Thomas L, Reedy G. 'The diamond': a structure for simulation debrief. Clin Teach. 2015;12(3):171–5.
8. Decker S, Fey M, Sideras S, Caballero S, Rockstraw L, Boese T, et al. Standards of best practice: simulation standard IV: the debriefing process. Clin Simul Nurs. 2013;9(6):S26–9.

9. Cato ML. Debriefing and guided reflection, National League for Nursing. 2012. Available from http://sirc.nln.org
10. Alexander L, Dearsley A. Using standardised patients in an undergraduate mental health simulation: a pilot study. Int J Forensic Ment Health. 2013;42(2-3):149–64.
11. Alexander L, Sheen J, Rinehart N, Hay M, Boyd L. Mental health simulation with student nurses: a qualitative review. Clin Simul Nurs. 2018;14:8–14.
12. Kidd L, Morgan KI, Savery J. Development of a mental health nursing simulation: challenges and solutions. J Interact Online Learn. 2012;11(2):80–9.
13. Marsh CJ. Key concepts for understanding curriculum. 4th ed. Taylor & Frances; 2008.
14. Orey M. Emerging perspectives on learning, teaching and technology. Global text. https://textbookequity.org/Textbooks/Orey_Emergin_Perspectives_Learning.pdf
15. Riera JRM, Cibanal JL, Mora MJP. Using role playing in the integration of knowledge in the teaching-learning process in nursing: assessment of students. Texto Contexto Enfermagem. 2010;19(4):618–26.
16. Clapper TC. Role play and simulation: returning to teaching for understanding. Educ Digest. 2010;75(8):39–43.
17. Lane C, Rollnick S. The use of simulated patients and role-play in communication skills training: a review of the literature to August 2005. Patient Educ Couns. 2007;67(1-2):13–20.
18. Jacobs AC, van Jaarsveldt DE. 'The character rests heavily within me': drama students as standardised patients in mental health nursing education. J Psychiatr Ment Health Nurs. 2016;23(3-4):198–206.
19. Bracq MS, Michinov E, Jannin P. Virtual reality simulation in non-technical skills training for healthcare professionals: a systematic review. J Soc Med Sim. 2019;14(3):188–94.
20. Verkuyl M, Romaniuk D, Mastrilli P. Virtual simulation of a mental health assessment: a usability study. Nurse Educ Pract. 2018;31:83–7.
21. Hall K. Simulation-based learning in Australian undergraduate nursing curricula: a literature review. Clin Simul Nurs. 2017;13(8):380–9.
22. Witt MA, McGaughan K, Smalldone A. Standardized patient simulation experiences improves mental health assessment and communication. Clin Simul Nurs. 2018;23:16–20.
23. O'Regan S, Molloy E, Watterson L, Nestel D. Observer roles that optimise learning in healthcare simulation education: a systematic review. Adv Simul. 2016;1(4):1–10.
24. Stegmann K, Pilz SM, Fischer F. Vicarious learning during simulations: is it more effective than hands-on training? Med Educ. 2012;46(10):1001–8.
25. Phrampus PE, O'Donnell JM. Debriefing using a structured supported approach. In: Levine AI, DeMaria S, Schwartz AD, Sim AJ, editors. The comprehensive textbook of healthcare simulation, vol. 73. New York: Springer; 2013. p. 84.

11 Pediatric Nursing

Andree Gamble, Melissa Ciardulli, and Kiralee Ciampa

History & Development

Simulation in nursing has a long history. Historically, nursing students practiced on each other, including invasive skills such as nasogastric tube insertion and injection technique [1]. The literature identifies the use of manikins for practical training as early as 1911 with the inclusion of Mrs. Chase - an adult manikin [2, 3]. The inclusion of 'Baby Chase' approximately three years later appears to be the earliest pediatric manikin-based simulation. Both Mrs and Baby Chase were involved in nursing education for six decades until more specialized manikins arrived on the scene in the 1970s [4].

By the early 1990s, simulation with manikins of increasing technological capability became more ubiquitous in nursing education. However, the first high-fidelity pediatric simulator, a manikin representing a 5 to 7-year-old child, was not developed until 1999. Two high-fidelity infant manikins followed in 2005 that afforded learner's opportunity to monitor vital signs, conduct physical assessments, and allow for treatment interventions such as IV cannulation and intubation [5]. Since these early manikins, the range and technological capabilities have increased. Manikins can reflect a diverse age range of children, offer basic to advanced skills learning, enable the practice of invasive procedures, and offer a visual display of a suite of assessment findings. These have helped fill the void left in pediatric nursing education by reducing the opportunity for learner exposure to actual pediatric patients.

In addition to inclusive manikin simulation, historical and contemporary literature acknowledge simulated patients/participants (SPs). In the literature by Barrows [6], SPs were first recognized as trained lay people to act as patients in medical education. The first reports relating to the engagement of SPs in pediatrics involved SP mothers, introduced into the medical curriculum to help learners develop interviewing skills. Pediatric OSCEs were introduced in the 1980s to evaluate the clinical skills of medical residents, along with the inception of child and adolescent SPs in medical education [7].

Current State

Children are not little adults, yet many nursing students come to pediatric education thinking the only differences lie in physical development. Experiences in teaching students over the past five years have also revealed that students come to nursing education with much less exposure to children in their past personal or employment experiences. Undergraduate students often lack the necessary skills, such as developmentally appropriate communication, to successfully transition to clinical placement. Didactic teaching sessions, such as lectures or tutorials, cannot teach these skills; however, simulation provides a feasible alternative to meet the learner's needs.

Simulation as a technique for learning has rapidly evolved in pediatric education, with many undergraduate nursing programs now including it as a teaching strategy. Identifiable drivers for the use of simulation arise from both within and external to the education setting, such as a reduced number of available clinical placements, increased acuity of illness making patients less suitable for learning encounters, rapid resolution of symptoms, and high patient turnover. In addition, the focus on patient safety and family-centered care has both contributed to reducing access of learners to patients already seen as vulnerable [8].

Supplementary Information The online version contains supplementary material available at https://doi.org/10.1007/978-3-031-31090-4_11.

A. Gamble (✉)
Faculty of Medicine, Nursing & Health Science, Nursing & Midwifery, Monash University, Clayton, Australia
e-mail: andree.gamble1@monash.edu

M. Ciardulli
Monash University, Clayton, VIC, Australia
e-mail: aMelissa.Ciardulli@monash.edu

K. Ciampa
Holmesglen Institute, Melbourne, Australia

J. M. Kutzin et al. (eds.), *Comprehensive Healthcare Simulation: Nursing*, Comprehensive Healthcare Simulation,
https://doi.org/10.1007/978-3-031-31090-4_11

The realism of clinical practice can be emulated in simulation, providing a reasonably safe learning environment for undergraduate nursing students. Integrating the three domains of learning—cognitive, psychomotor, and affective into the simulation resembles what should happen in actual clinical encounters [9], allowing students to immerse themselves in an experiential learning situation. Simulation complements learning that occurs using more traditional methods such as lectures and, as a result, allows the linking of theory to practice without the risk of harm to actual patients [10].

In pediatrics, the utilization of simulation develops psychomotor skills such as vital sign monitoring and injection technique. In addition, simulated learning scenarios can provide students with the most realistic option outside of the clinical setting to practice communication, decision-making, teamwork, and leadership skills. As students in clinical practice, they may never have these opportunities, so preparing them through simulation can ensure they accrue these professional attributes before graduation.

There is a recognized dearth of pediatric clinical placements for undergraduate nursing students. Although many education programs allocate some time for a pediatric nursing curriculum, the number of available matching placements does not meet the requirements. Simulation can therefore provide students with exposure to pediatric patients they may never otherwise receive.

Simulation has several benefits in pediatric nursing education. It can expose students to common presentations they need to develop confidence and competence in managing while also offering exposure to rare conditions to stimulate learning [11]. Simulation is amenable to diverse students by adjusting the complexity within the scenario according to the student experience. In addition, the number of students who can be involved in the simulation and the ability to repeat the scenario multiple times is an added positive aspect [12].

Adequate preparation of students is the primary goal of pediatric undergraduate nursing education, ensuring students can consistently and safely care for children and adolescents with a multitude of healthcare needs in a manner that recognizes the role of children as part of a family unit. Although the gold standard in achieving this may be actual patients, this is not always possible or ethical. Simulation can assist in achieving this goal by exposing students to a variety of ages, clinical conditions, and care requirements. The inclusion of manikins, parent SPs, and child/adolescent SPs can assist students in developing the fundamental skills necessary for safe practice.

The focus of many simulation scenarios in pediatrics lies in emergency and crisis management. These are essential areas, but the reality of practice environments for undergraduate nursing students necessitates exposure to frequently encountered clinical situations that will enable them to provide safe care. Aspects of interactions such as developmentally appropriate assessment, communication, and preparing children for invasive procedures may be considered more mundane but crucial aspects of professional practice preparation.

Future Uses in Pediatric Nursing

There are limitless possibilities for pediatric simulation that could enhance the preparedness of nursing students to care for children. These relate to content, method, and technology (Table 11.1).

An example that may fulfill many aspects found in Table 11.1 is a scenario including multiple cases represented by manikins and SPs of differing ages. Although complex 'ward for a day' type simulation is in existence, there is scope to broaden these to include culturally diverse patients represented by either SPs or manikins with different skin tones. Child, adolescent, and parent SPs ably complement infant and child manikins. Patient conditions within the scenario can range from more common pediatric presentations such as asthma or gastroenteritis to less frequent illnesses that students may not gain exposure to during routine clinical placements.

The inclusion of virtual reality (VR) and augmented reality (AR) technology can also expose students to rare occurrences and those conditions that all students should know about yet often do not see because of a lack of clinical placement availability. VR and AR are increasing in their realism and can be very engaging for students. The cost of simulation-related technology can be prohibitive, so VR may be a good alternative for financially constrained settings. Sharing VR scenarios may also enable clinical placement providers to gain insight into the student's learning, so their level of knowledge and skills is evident to those supporting their clinical development.

Table 11.1 Matrix of pediatric simulation

Content	Method	Technology
Empathy Patient-centered care Patient safety Increasing scenario complexity as students progress through their learning Exposure to rare situations such as COVID-19 Establishing simulation in untapped markets such as family violence, mental health, LGBTQI, cultural diversity, and disability	Manikins of varying ages and skin tones Moulage Cross-functional simulation with both education provider and healthcare setting staff Increased engagement with allied health	Virtual reality Augmented reality

Best Practice

In healthcare today, human error can have devastating effects on unwell children. The controlled and safe learning environment of simulation can be an effective way to replicate real-life pediatric events [12], with the optimal outcome being the provision of high-quality care to pediatric patients once the graduating student enters the workforce. The overarching goal of simulation should therefore focus on patient safety and quality improvement, but equally important is that undergraduate students must experience innovative, evidence-based simulation conducted in a safe learning environment.

As simulation is a powerful and valuable educational modality, curriculum planners must ensure the design and implementation of simulation align with learning aims and objectives. A best practice approach is to follow published standards, such as those produced by the International Nursing Association for Clinical Simulation and Learning (INACSL) and the Association of Standardized Patient Educators (ASPE) [13, 14]. The field of pediatric simulation has experienced steady growth internationally, as evidenced by the establishment of societies and networks such as the International Pediatric Simulation Society (IPSS), a global community of pediatric healthcare providers focusing on multi-disciplinary simulation-based pediatric care through research and training.

The most successful development and execution of pediatric simulation incorporate the acquisition of knowledge, skills, and behaviors conducted in a risk-free environment [15]. The best practice encompasses curriculum, resources, student learning needs, faculty executives/educators' considerations, and instructional design. These form two key areas, teaching and learning considerations, and organizational considerations (Table 11.2).

Table 11.2 Best practice approaches for pediatric simulation

Teaching and learning considerations	Organizational considerations
Conform to international standards of best practice for simulation design, e.g., INACSL & ASPE	Invest in faculty- expert pediatric educators who can mentor less-experienced colleagues [13, 16]
Conduct a systematic learning needs assessment addressing potential curriculum gaps	Foster the professional development of simulation laboratory personnel and technicians on the essentials of pediatric simulation
Develop a pediatric syllabus that is reflective of learning needs, aims, and objectives	Ensure there is management commitment and engagement to pediatric simulation to enhance educator 'buy-in.'
Prepare high-quality simulation resources, e.g., scenarios, SP scripts using approved templates, and resources to supplement simulation	Provide specialized pediatric resources such as low or high-fidelity simulation manikins
Scaffold simulation is part of a varied approach to teaching methods, e.g., classroom lectures, tutorials, role-play, part-task skills training, distributed practice, and immersive simulation scenarios.	Ensure simulation scenarios do not exhaust or place unachievable demands on resources
Provide engaging teaching methods pitched at the appropriate level for the student	
Ensure pediatric scenarios reflect everyday clinical situations; where appropriate, offer complex, rare scenarios that may not otherwise be seen on clinical placement [16]	Collaborate and negotiate with simulation companies and innovative technologies such as VR/AR to produce realistic simulations
Conduct evaluations of simulation gathering data from all stakeholders (learners, facilitator(s), faculty, and support team)	
Consider faculty educational research of simulation to build on the body of evidence for simulation;	
Adopt and test new simulation technologies	
Allow for multisite educational facilities [13]	

Examples of Successful Programs

Two examples of best practice simulation programs that have been successfully implemented within undergraduate curricula include:

1. Pediatric CPR (RESUS4KIDS) which focuses on the use of mannikins
2. Pediatric End of Life Care based on students working with simulated participants.

Both programs demonstrate exemplary best practice curriculum and instructional design, use of high-quality resources, the importance of gaining buy-in from faculty executives and educators, and benefits to undergraduate nursing students.

Paediatric CPR

As a foundational clinical skill for undergraduate nursing students, basic life support (BLS) is a critical component of a pediatric curriculum. Simulation-based training is an effective modality to ensure that the students can respond to an infant or child experiencing cardiorespiratory arrest.

RESUS4KIDS is a standardized, evidence-based pediatric life support simulation course developed and governed by the Sydney Children's Hospitals Network in Australia (https://www.resus4kids.com.au/). One of the critical attributes of the course is its effective instructional design with well-defined learning objectives and the opportunity for repetitive practice and immediate feedback. Resources required to implement RESUS4KIDS are easily accessible, cost-effective, and designed to be delivered at undergraduate or postgraduate levels to medical, nursing, allied health, or paramedic participants to provide them with the mandatory skills required to manage the first ten minutes of a pediatric collapse.

The course comprises an e-learning module and a short practical session. The e-learning uses both interactive steps and video to guide participants through the stages of pediatric resuscitation. The concisely written course consists of two sections: firstly, teamwork and communication (30 min), and secondly, a scenario-based, pause-and-discuss format, hands-on practice (60 min). The course needs minimal equipment, including an infant mannikin such as the ALS baby (Laerdal), and uses a train-the-trainer and super-trainer model to allow it to be delivered Australia-wide [16]. Table 11.3 [16] outlines the RESUS4KIDS program, highlighting the various components, including the 60-minute pause-and-discuss scenario-based teaching.

Course evaluation indicates an improvement in human factors, knowledge retention, and the mechanics of resuscitation for components of the course. RESUS4KIDS has also received anecdotal feedback from participants who have used skills learned in the course to help real pediatric patients [16].

Preparing a future pediatric nurse to respond to the complex and sensitive needs of a child and their family in the terminal stages of care requires more than didactic content taught in a classroom. Classroom discussion of the impact, expectations, and emotions nursing students may experience when faced with a pediatric death is limited [17, 18].

End-of-life care (EOLC) is not routinely associated with high technology; however, simulations have the potential to improve EOLC nursing education and, subsequently, practice [19]. Pediatric EOLC situations can be stressful experiences, with a study suggesting that high-fidelity simulations about pediatric end-of-life care decrease students' anxiety levels [20].

In the USA and UK, there are several pioneering undergraduate pediatric programs that introduce nursing students to the concepts of EOLC, death, and unexpected death. Undergraduate pediatric EOLC simulations involving simulated participants can assist in developing students' non-technical skills, such as empathy, trust, patient/family education, and shared decision-making.

In Texas, USA, the Department of Nursing at Concordia University developed a pediatric EOLC simulation scenario involving simulated participants portraying the parents of the dying child. Students were aware that the baby in the simulation would not survive and that the primary objective was to support the baby's family. A chaplain from the local hospital and staff members from the local organ donation group also participated in the simulation, allowing students to practice interdisciplinary communication. Trained counselors were available to any participant experiencing emotions after the simulation. Results from this initiative showed that when simulated participants portray the parents in an EOL simulation, the fidelity of the simulation dramatically increases. Careful planning, training, and attention to psychological safety were vital to having simulated participants contribute consistently [21].

At the University Health Science Center, Texas, USA, a pediatric EOLC simulation focused on the death of an infant from a preventable communicable disease is embedded into their undergraduate curricula to improve student attitudes towards teamwork and communication and enhance their understanding of their role in providing care. The simulation involves simulated participants, family members, and healthcare providers. Medical, pharmacy, public health, and nursing students participate and are required to demonstrate a coordinated team approach to a complex case and interact appropriately with emotional parents [22].

The Department of Nursing and Midwifery at the University of West of England, UK, source simulated participants from the university's drama department with students playing the role of adolescents. Reflective of the subject aims and learning objectives, students engage with these young actors in the role of a person experiencing EOLC, replicating a rare and complex situation for pediatric student nurses who do not usually work in this specialist field. It allows students to utilize their generic communication skills and transfer these to an area of clinical practice they may not commonly experience [23].

Table 11.3 The Resus4Kids Program [16]

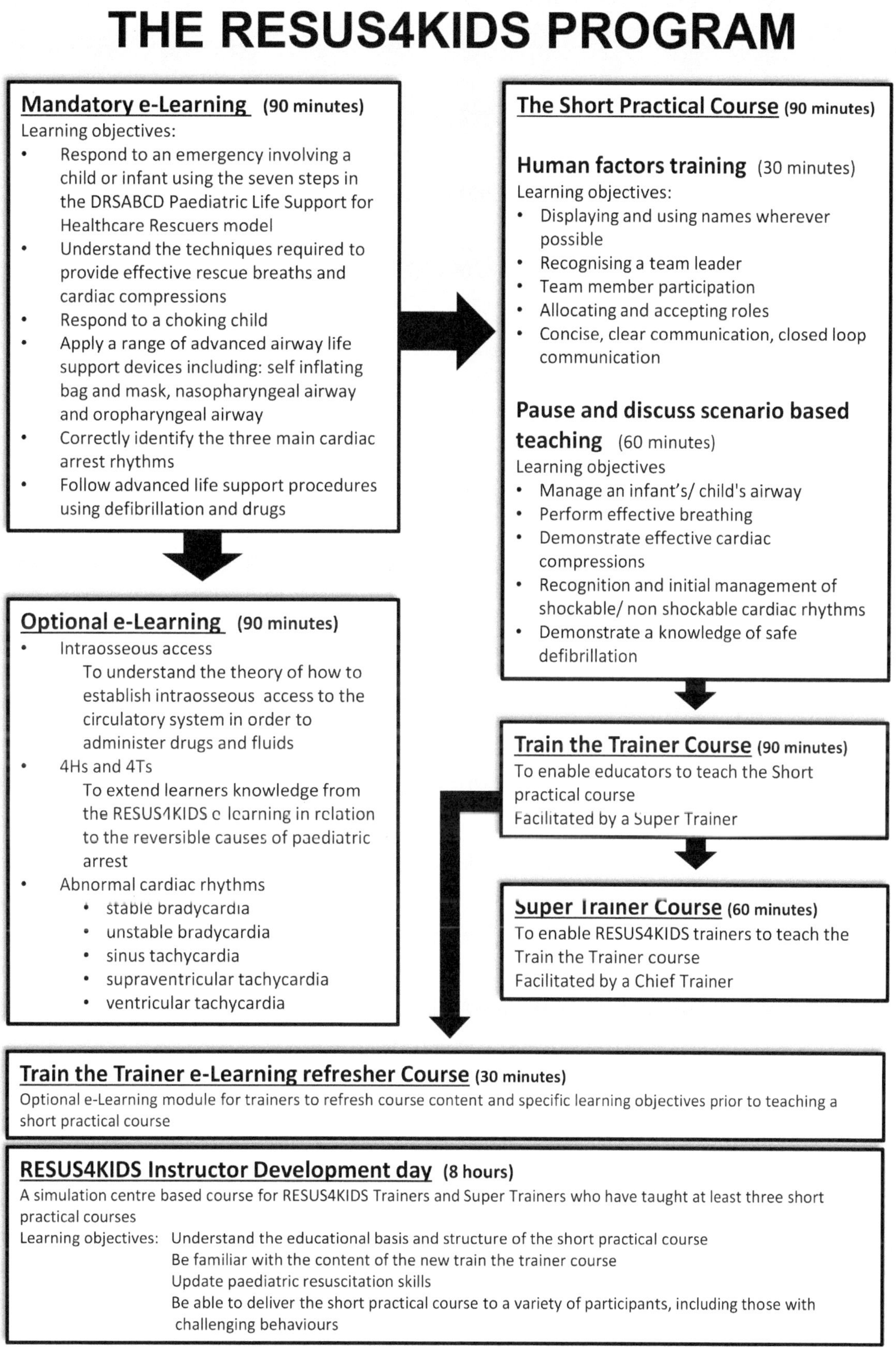

Sample Curriculum

Preparing undergraduate nursing students for pediatric practice can be grueling in an era of reducing clinical placements and financial constraints limiting equipment purchase. Particularly so for pediatrics, the age range of 0–18 years necessitates a suite of manikins and associated equipment that may well be out of reach. It is also more challenging for child SPs to adhere to child employment laws and consider their safety and well-being in a primarily adult learning space.

Holmesglen Institute in Melbourne, Australia, is a leading provider of nursing education. Students in the Bachelor of Nursing program at Holmesglen undertake a core specialty subject focused on caring for children and adolescents. In the first iteration of the BN (2009–2013), students had the opportunity to complete a pediatric elective in their final semester. Incorporated into this elective was a pediatric-specific simulation that is the focus of the following discussion.

Pediatric Elective

The critical learning goal of the pediatric elective is for students to develop a deeper understanding of the core principles of pediatric care. Undergraduate students enter clinical placement feeling more confident in their pediatric nursing skills and knowledge with this education. As this unit falls within their final semester, a significant focus of learning is on professionalism and ensuring adequate preparation for placement and their imminent graduate nurse practice.

The core learning outcomes focus on essential and crucial pediatric-specific areas: Child and adolescent development and the impact of this on interventions, communication with children and families, family-centered care, common presentations requiring hospitalization, care of the child postoperatively, and the emergency management of the child following non-accidental injury (NAI). The introduction of EOLC also occurs in this unit. Skills-based learning focuses on engaging with children in a developmentally appropriate manner that encourages cooperation, assessment and management of the unwell child, and medication administration. More generic learning outcomes focus on developing professional skills, including time management, prioritization, leadership, and teamwork.

Simulation is an adjunct to more traditional forms of teaching and learning. In this elective unit, simulation complements the academic and skills program to provide opportunities for students to experience a pediatric ward as realistic as possible, yet one without the potential for harm to actual patients.

Crucial aspects to the success of this curriculum include:

- Ensuring the content is aligned to the overall unit learning outcomes
- Scaffolding the content to ensure students have the required knowledge and skills to practice in a supervised capacity.
- Effective pre-briefing and preparation of students for their roles

The Integration of Pediatric Simulation

The pediatric elective unit incorporates three separate compulsory simulations that students attend. Each has a running time of approximately 3.5 h.

Simulation 1

Simulation1 involves three separate scenarios to maximize the number of active participants while also offering a suite of learning opportunities related to the theoretical and skills-based learning of the previous weeks. Scenarios 1 and 2 involve the use of manikins, and scenario 3 involves an SP. Scenarios 1 & 2 take place in an extensive simulation apartment to fit the multiple patients, while scenario 3 occurs in one room with the patient/parents in another room, with Skype technology reflecting the telehealth experience. In all scenarios, students are encouraged to take accountability for the patient group and seek help from 'senior staff' if they cannot find a solution amongst themselves. The 'patients' within each simulation are identified below (Table 11.4)

Simulation 2

This simulation involves providing EOLC to an infant girl whose parents, along with the medical team, have elected to cease active Leukemia treatment, with a small simulation suite resembling a single patient room. A total of 4 students are involved to ensure support is available during a potentially emotive and distressing scenario. SimNewB, reflecting the infants' minimal involvement, is utilized, focusing on communication with SPs playing the role of parents. Students are encouraged to 'create memories' with the parents and then provide after-death care to the infant, ensuring the support of the 'parents' at all times. A thorough pre-briefing and debriefing are crucial for this scenario, as the infant dies during the simulation.

Table 11.4 Patient details

Bed	Admission	Name	Age	Diagnosis	Care
SCENARIO 1 Duration: 45 min Students participants: $n = 6$					
Bed	Admission	Name	Age	Diagnosis	Care
1	13.8.14	Katie ALEXANDER	6M	Poor feeding, general irritability, decreased urine output & loose stools	Needs IV line commenced for IV AB's Regular Panadol Neuro assessment ?LP
2	13.8.14	Cooper MAXTON	3Y	Runny nose & cough 10/7 PHx Asthma with multiple admissions	20 minute Ventolin Regular respiratory assessment Needs NPA, ?O_2 Oral steroids
SCENARIO 2 **Duration: 45 min** **Students participants:** $n = 4$					
1	13.8.14	Felix DALLARD	10Y	Febrile Neutropenia 5/7 post-CHTHx. Pain at CVC site (red) & mouth	IV AB's GCSF for Neutropaenia NGT change required Encourage mouth care Weight
SCENARIO 3 **Duration: 30 min** **Students participants:** $n = 2$					
1	Telehealth Consultation	Andrew JOHNSON	16Y	Acopia following severe head injury – poor concentration, memory, academic performance & R) hemiparesis	Overall coping assessment of both Andrew and parent

Simulation 3

Although scenarios in the pediatric arena have improved, most still involve one or several students working with a single SP. Although that may be useful for teaching skills, it may not reflect clinical reality, where a nurse works simultaneously with multiple patients. The simulation curriculum in the elective unit culminates in a day-long complex scenario that aims to "Bring it all together" in a 'ward for a day' simulation.

Gamble's (2017) 'ward for a day' simulation, a realistic, complex, extended multi-patient environment, is designed to emulate an actual pediatric ward with several patients, diverse conditions, and multitudinous needs. Students perform multiple tasks to demonstrate various psychomotor, physical assessment, decision-making, prioritization, delegation, leadership, and teamwork skills. Other professional attributes integral to a successful transition to clinical placement are encouraged. Notably, the students must demonstrate competency in these core skills without compromising patient safety, all achievable in a more extended simulation experience.

Each group commences their 3.5 h shift at designated times during the day, with the first shift arriving at 0700. The simulated ward (in an existing nursing skills laboratory) includes nine patients. To ensure the ward adequately reflects a general pediatric environment, the patient group includes infants, children, and adolescents experiencing a diverse range of medical and surgical conditions.

Various medium and high-fidelity manikins reflect the desired clinical conditions, reproduce clinical assessment findings, and display appropriate responses to expected nursing interventions. For a deteriorating case scenario and invasive procedures, students work with a high-fidelity child manikin. A medium-fidelity manikin represents a child distressed by gastroenteritis but whose actual assessment data is not a critical element in the achievement of realism.

To further enhance realism and facilitate effective communication and engagement with adolescents, two SPs are employed to play two roles: a 17-year-old boy with unstable diabetes and a 16-year-old girl with osteomyelitis. Four adult SPs play the role of parents. The use of SPs provides learners with the unique opportunity to further develop skills in communicating with parents, particularly parents of a sick child, and enables them to recognize the importance of family-centered care (Table 11.5). Engagement with SPs who are casual employees of the Institute is a unique and defining characteristic of the nursing undergraduate program.

This best-practice scenario demonstrates that a complex extended multi-scenario ward simulation is a valuable adjunct to didactic lectures, clinical skills laboratories, and 'snapshot simulations' to facilitate learning and knowledge

Table 11.5 Simulated patient group

Patient age	Condition	Skills	Technology
6 months	Croup	Respiratory & hydration assessment IV care, O_2 administration, NPA	Infant manikin SP mother
4 years	Multi-trauma	IDC, NGT insertion IV fluids & Blood transfusion	Child manikin
7 years	Appendicitis	Theatre preparation IVC care & IV Antibiotics	Child manikin SP father
2 months	Open SB lesion – repaired 16.9	Neurological assessment Staple removal & simple dressing change	Infant manikin SP Grandmother
3 years	ALL: Febrile Neutropaenia	Central Venous Catheter care IVF, AB's, dressing change and bloods	Child manikin SP mother
10 months	Gastroenteritis	Infection control & Barrier Nursing Specimen collection NGT insertion & feeding	Infant manikin
17 years	Unstable T1 Diabetic	BGL & Insulin administration Neurological assessment	Adolescent SP
16 years	Osteomyelitis	Neurovascular observations Pain assessment & management	Adolescent SP
5 months	Scald burns to mid trunk	Pain assessment & management NG/Oral feeds Wound care	Infant manikin

retention for undergraduate nursing students enrolled in a pediatric elective subject and experienced the extraneous variables often present in the pediatric clinical environment.

Logistical Considerations

A consistent and logical approach to all simulation programs is required.

Pre-briefing

The definition of pre-briefing is "an information or orientation session held before the start of a simulation activity in which instructions or preliminary information is given to the participants. The purpose of pre-briefing is to set the stage for a scenario and assist participants in achieving scenario objectives" [24]. Pre-briefing involves preparing faculty, simulation technologists, and students for the simulation.

Faculty: Inclusion in the script development of all facilitators involved in running the scenarios is considered best practice. A 'simulation rehearsal' also occurs at least one week before the scheduled simulation date to ensure the scenario has no flaws, that all equipment is available, and identify any potential technical or scenario-specific concerns.

Students: Should receive a written document outlining the schedule, expectations of behavior and engagement, and a brief overview of the scenario. This latter inclusion serves to encourage students to ensure their knowledge and skills are at an appropriate level. In addition, the expectation is that both students and faculty attend a formal pre-briefing session where an overview of the simulation should occur (PowerPoint) and a discussion of expectations should occur. An attendance register is maintained as students cannot safely undertake simulation without attending the pre-brief. During the pre-brief, the designation of an active participant or observer role to the students occurs. In the absence of volunteers, the assignment of students by faculty who have considered prior participation occurs. It is essential in this elective unit that all students can actively participate, an achievable goal for a small student cohort.

SPs: The preparatory process for SPs is multi-faceted. A written script outlining their role and the opportunity to provide any feedback should occur. Immediately before the simulation, SPs run through their role with faculty, who then prepare any SP-specific equipment requirements, such as insertion of an IV cannula or a wound dressing. Should more than one SP be involved, an additional time allocation is given for all SPs to discuss their role and how they will work together.

Immersion & Expected Activity

Although students are not yet registered nurses, they participate as independently as possible. Responsibility to seek supervision or guidance rests with the student, an aspect identified during pre-brief. Actively participating students plan, provide, and hand over the care of their patient/s to a team leader. Students have a brief overview of each patient's care, planning, and prioritizing aspects of the student's responsibility. Student observers focus on specific aspects of the scenario, such as infection control, teamwork, or communication with children and families. It is an expectation that students will offer feedback specific to their area of focus during debriefing.

Conclusion of Simulation

With the students experiencing an immersion in the pediatric simulation scenario, calling an end to a scenario can be challenging. However, ensuring all participants have adequate opportunity to achieve the learning outcomes or end the scenario timely is essential. The conclusion of simulation scenarios occurs in one of three ways: (1) The shift is over, and students must complete their work and handover to the incoming staff, or (2) The shift is over, and students' handover care to the 'senior staff' (faculty) or (3) Cessation of the simulation by faculty staff either by microphone or by entering the simulation environment.

Debriefing and Feedback

A debriefing occurs immediately after the following simulation and is facilitated by all staff, the discussion led by the facilitator involved in the scenario. The Debriefing technique is very flexible and staff-dependent, but the Pendleton model of feedback is standard. All students are encouraged to participate and, importantly, take away learning points they believe they need improvement on before clinical placement. Electronic evaluation of the simulation by the students should occur while still in the simulation space, encouraging survey completion. Faculty debrief as one and discuss elements including how the simulation progressed, any student concerns, identification of learning needs, and ideas for improving future scenario iterations. SPs also offer feedback regarding elements such as faculty preparation to enable future improvements.

Integrating into Existing Education

The idea of caring for younger people can be daunting for many students without prior experience. Children are different and not just physically. Preparing students to interact, communicate, assess, and competently care for young people is challenging for many undergraduate nursing programs. A lack of focus on specialist areas of nursing in generalist undergraduate degrees, challenges securing equipment, unavailability of appropriately trained staff, and difficulty securing enough quality clinical placements to achieve learning outcomes are just some reasons for reducing or even omitting pediatric nursing undergraduate programs.

The learning of psychomotor skills in nursing laboratory settings is not without value, and it is these opportunities that can provide a scaffolded approach to learning. However, including a manikin, child SP, or an adult SP simulating a parental role does encourage students to take the care of their patients more seriously during simulation [25]. Simulation can provide a good starting point and a safer environment in which students can develop and practice their interpersonal and psychomotor skills without the risk of potentially impacting the care experience of children and their families, giving them time to build their confidence.

Simulation provides learners with the opportunity to develop critical thinking skills in a safe learning environment. However, for critical thinking skills to develop as intended, simulation should complement rather than replace alternative learning methods. A need to identify the value (or value add) of simulation to the current curriculum should always precede resource allocation to creating scenarios, purchasing equipment, planning, and facilitating simulation-based learning. Without solid structural foundations and experienced faculty, there is the risk that learners do not achieve the intended learning outcomes [26]. For implementing pediatric simulation into the curriculum to be successful, stakeholder buy-in is a crucial element.

The allocation of at least one or two key project coordinators will ensure the success of the simulation structure and timelines, ensuring that they have the required time and resources. Crucial stakeholders included are:

- Dean of Faculty
- Current learners/students
- Local health organizations who provide clinical placement and employment to students and graduates
- Faculty staff members are willing to help get the project up and running, involving them in the delivery of simulation to develop a sense of ownership, share ideas and expertise, and spread the workload. Explore the current readiness, experiences, and attitude towards simulation with immediate faculty members.

In deciding the quantity of simulation introduced within the course, determine the viability and necessity of including simulation according to content specialties or topics, for example, learning outcomes relating to pediatric nursing may only account for a small component, so the amount of simulation included should reflect this [27].

Draw upon key learning outcomes already within the curriculum and focus on a select few to further expand upon simulation. Assess and prioritize learning needs for students relevant to pediatric nursing. Determine whether it is more important for learners to explore common pediatric presentations or clinical situations rarely seen in clinical practice, providing an opportunity to replace learning outcomes on placement with simulation. An excellent opportunity exists here to consult with and connect with current and potential clinical facilities that provide clinical placements for the student cohort to determine what skills and knowledge they require and expect nursing students to attend clinical placement in their pediatric areas. This collaboration aims to determine how the simulation curriculum can assist students in readiness for clinical practice.

Successful strategies used previously to incorporate pediatric simulation into the existing undergraduate nursing curriculum include:

- Holmesglen Institute model of high-fidelity simulation involving child and family SPs (or manikins or both) on scheduled simulation days held throughout the semester, with simulation run on class-free days
- Low to mid-fidelity clinical nursing laboratories- weekly opportunities for students to apply theoretical knowledge in practice using demonstration, return demonstration, role-play, scenarios, manikins, with or without SPs.
- One-off bootcamp-style workshop providing short glimpses or exposures to different pediatric conditions that students are less likely to see in the clinical environment [28]
- Telehealth sims are delivered remotely using simulation video recordings or SPs.
- Interactive web-based simulation activities [29]
- Ward for a day [30]

If not already present within the curriculum, regular timetabled nursing laboratory classes can be a more manageable way to introduce simulation techniques rather than developing high-fidelity simulation programs in the initial stages. Simulated nursing laboratories complement the content being delivered elsewhere within the curriculum rather than further crowding the curriculum to promote students' best learning outcomes and experience [27]. Nursing laboratories use medium-fidelity simulation methods such as a child manikin with respiratory function, including breath sounds, chest movement, and pulse capability—students guided by clinical teachers to assess children who present with respiratory compromise or distress. Individual skill stations can enable small student groups to practice skills such as the application and use of adhesive pulse oximeter probes on children of different age groups, utilizing a medication resource to review asthma medication for children, and simulated medication administration using training inhalers and spacers according to the medication order provided.

Faculty members who are involved in more didactic areas of the course should also be involved so that they can evaluate student strengths and weaknesses holistically, identify students at risk, and work to implement strategies in other areas of the curriculum to further support learning [27]. Learning then continues after simulation through structured debriefing and reflection and then further during clinical practice if the opportunity arises. Students can draw upon their experiences in simulation and apply them to the care of children and families, increasing students' confidence in their abilities.

Once successful integration of pediatric simulation has been integrated into an undergraduate curriculum, there may be the need or the interest to further expand the complexity and build the level of fidelity.

To ensure expansion is effective, staff need to receive further education and training to design, plan, and deliver programs according to guidelines. It also needs to be a viable option for available resources, including workload, time, budget, professional development costs, and expertise.

As course cohort sizes grow, clinical placement opportunities for students generally remain consistent, thereby leaving a gap that leaves institutions with the challenge of providing alternative practical learning experiences while meeting curriculum and registration requirements. The research is mixed regarding the suitability of simulation to replace clinical practice requirements.

Challenges and Possible Solutions

Although there are many challenges/barriers to simulation in the undergraduate pediatric curriculum, there are many solutions to help address these. We have categorized the unique pediatric undergraduate nursing challenges/barriers as either educational or organizational for ease of understanding (Table 11.6).

Table 11.6 Challenges, Barriers, and Solutions

Educational Challenges and Barriers	Possible Solutions
Absence of pediatric curriculum in undergraduate courses	Advocate to regulatory authorities and senior management for the inclusion of pediatrics in undergraduate nursing
Diminished opportunity to consult, collaborate and share scenarios amongst existing and new pediatric undergraduate courses.	Establish an undergraduate pediatric nursing education community of practice to encourage sharing and collaboration
Lack of scaffolded learning opportunities for students to apply theory to practice	Introduce essential pediatric skills and knowledge in achievable blocks throughout the preceding weeks' content, providing ample opportunity to practice psychomotor skills and achieve learning objectives.
A focus on adverse or rare events rather than more common pediatric presentations students are likely to see during clinical placement.	Value each and construct a curriculum that can address both types of events through a variety of teaching methods. E.g., peer-reviewed online resources, skills demonstration videos, and simulations for high-risk scenarios.
Triggering of an emotionally charged response in students to an unwell child	Provide appropriate self-care education for nursing students. Prepare learners to identify and recognize their emotional responses. Conduct structured and thorough debriefing after the simulation
Undergraduate pediatric nursing SIM programs based on limited evidence to support learner outcomes	Encourage involvement of simulation facilitators in research that demonstrates evidence of improved patient and learner outcomes
Shortage of pediatric clinical placement hours and inability to use simulation as a replacement.	Consider a pilot research project aimed at measuring the impact of replacing clinical hours with simulation.
Financial outlay associated with the purchase of differing-sized manikins.	Consider sharing of resources to reduce organizational financial outlay. Sponsorship from pediatric medical companies Adopt the use of alternative simulation technologies such as VR/AR that does not require physical mannikins or equipment
Human resource and ethical concerns if child/adolescent simulated patients are involved	Identify and adhere to employment laws related to the engagement of young people. Ensure that ethical considerations are planned and addressed.
Ensuring availability and adequate training of staff in pediatric simulation methodologies	Offer training programs to staff in pediatric simulation methods. Build working partnerships with nursing education staff from pediatric hospitals/ units (especially those from clinical placement partners), providing them with simulation education, and supernumerary simulation days
Engagement of staff is suitably qualified to monitor the health and well-being of learners and any child-simulated patients.	Employ casual teachers who currently work in pediatric clinical practice, training them in the role of "confederate." Ensure availability of staff with pediatric / child health qualifications and working with children clearance.

Interface with Regulatory Bodies—How Simulation Can Help or Hinder Accreditation

The gold standard of learning in practice-based professions such as nursing has long been clinical exposure. Students undertake placements of variable duration in a diverse range of healthcare settings where the opportunity to plan, provide and evaluate the care of actual patients is on offer. However, the number of students requiring placement is increasing simultaneously, that access to quality clinical placements is reducing. The identification of simulation as a possible replacement for placement by the NBCSN study was published in 2014 [8]. Based in the USA, this study indicated that up to 50% substitution of placement with simulation has no detrimental impact on nursing students' preparedness for professional practice. Interestingly, to date, there has been no replication of this study in the Australian context, and there remains ambiguity amongst regulatory bodies as to whether substitution of placement with simulation is a viable option.

The Nursing and Midwifery Accreditation Council (ANMAC) is the accrediting authority for nursing and midwifery education programs in Australia, and in 2019 produced a set of standards underpinning nursing and midwifery practice [31]. Standard 3.5(d) identifies the need for learners to integrate the knowledge of care across the lifespan and different contexts of nursing practice. Standard 3.11 further suggests that undergraduate nursing education includes simulated learning experiences designed to prepare students for clinical placement. Accreditation also mandates that every nursing student complete a minimum of 800 clinical hours across their degree in a clinical setting. Given the relatively small proportion of pediatric healthcare settings compared to adult care settings, this can be challenging to achieve.

Lack of quality clinical placements, increasing patient acuity and decreasing length of stay, parents denying learner access to their child, and the global focus on patient safety have impacted education providers' ability to secure pediatric placements for their students. This challenges accreditation if the pediatric placement is a compulsory aspect of the education program. Should this dearth of quality pediatric placement persist, further research is required to find alternatives that better prepare learners for pediatric care using simulation.

Exemplary Cases—Adolescent mental health template (See Electronic Supplementary Material)

Conclusion

The value of simulation to undergraduate pediatric nursing students has yet to reach its full potential. This chapter has provided an overview to guide both novice and experienced simulation users in integrating or expanding the use of simulation into undergraduate pediatric nursing education. The most common outcome measures currently relate to student's perceptions of the learning experience. Conclusions are commonly focused on a demonstrable increase in student self-confidence and satisfaction with the learning. It is now necessary to build on these outcomes to demonstrate the impact of simulation learning on graduate performance in the pediatric clinical setting with long-term knowledge retention and the improvement of pediatric patient outcomes. Although there are both challenges and barriers to overcome, the solutions and best practice examples offered in this chapter can assist educators with how to design, deliver, and evaluate simulations in current and future pediatric undergraduate courses.

References:

1. Aebersold M. Simulation-based learning: no longer a novelty in undergraduate education. Online J Issues Nurs. 2018;23(2):1–3.
2. Nickerson M, Pollard M. Mrs. Chase and her descendants: a historical view of simulation. Creative Nurs. 2010;16(3):101–5.
3. Herrmann EK. Mrs. Chase: a noble and enduring figure. Am J Nurs. 1981;81(10):1836.
4. Anonymous. A brief history of nursing simulation: the evolution of health care manikins over the past 100 years; 2015. https://www.bc.edu/bc-web/schools/cson/csonnews/Abriefhistoryofnursingsimulation.html
5. Mai CL, Szyld D, Cooper JB. Simulation in pediatric anesthesia. In: Coté CJ, Lerman J, Anderson BJ, editors. A practice of anesthesia for infants and children. 6th ed. Elsevier; 2019. p. 1204–11. https://doi.org/10.1016/B978-0-323-42974-0.00053-7.
6. Barrows HS. Simulated (standardized) patients and other human simulations. Chapel Hill, NC: Health Sciences Consortium; 1987.
7. Joorabchi B. Objective structured clinical examination in a pediatric residency program. Am J Dis Child. 1991;145(7):750–4. https://doi.org/10.1001/archpedi.1991.02160070053021.
8. Hayden JK, Smiley RA, Alexander M, Kardong-Edgren S, Jeffries PR. The NCSBN national simulation study: a longitudinal, randomized, controlled study replacing clinical hours with simulation in prelicensure nursing education. J Nurs Regul. 2014;5(2):S3–40.
9. Penn BK. Mastering the teaching role: a guide for nurse educators. Philadelphia, PA: FA Davis; 2008.
10. MacKinnon K, Marcellus L, Rivers J, Gordon C, Ryan M, Butcher D. Student and educator experiences of maternal-child simulation-based learning: a systematic review of qualitative evidence. JBI Database Syst Rev Implement Rep. 2017;15(11):2666–706.
11. Wyllie E, Batley K. Skills for safe practice - a qualitative study to evaluate the use of simulation in safeguarding children teaching for pre-registration children's nurses. Nurse Educ Pract. 2019;34:85–9.
12. Clerihew L, Rowney D, Ker J. Simulation in pediatric training. Arch Dis Childhood Educ Pract. 2016;2016(101):8–14.
13. Bryant K, Aebersold ML, Jeffries PR, Kardong-Edgren S. Innovations in simulation: nursing leaders' exchange of best practices. Clin Simul Nurs. 2020;(41):33–40.
14. Lewis KL, Bohnert CA, Gammon WL, Hölzer H, Lyman L, Smith C, Thompson TM, Wallace A, Gliva-McConvey G. The association of standardized patient educators (ASPE) standards of best practice (SOBP). Adv Simul. 2017;2(1):1–8.
15. Lin Y, Cheng A. The role of simulation in teaching pediatric resuscitation: current perspectives. Adv Med Educ Pract. 2015;6:239.
16. O'Leary F, Allwood M, McGarvey K, Howse J, Fahy K. Standardising pediatric resuscitation training in New South Wales, Australia: RESUS 4 KIDS. J Pediatr Child Health. 2014;50(5):405–10.
17. Lindsay J. Introducing nursing students to pediatric end-of-life issues using simulation. Dimensions Crit Care Nurs. 2010;29(4):175–8.
18. Cole MA, Foito K. Pediatric end-of-life simulation: preparing the future nurse to care for the needs of the child and family. J Pediatr Nurs. 2019;44:e9–12.
19. Moreland SS, Lemieux ML, Myers A. End-of-life care and the use of simulation in a baccalaureate nursing program. Int J Nurs Educ Scholarship. 2012;9(1)
20. Megel ME, Black J, Clark L, Carstens P, Jenkins LD, Promes J, Snelling M, Zander KE, Bremer A, Goodman T. Effect of high-fidelity simulation on pediatric nursing students' anxiety. Clin Simul Nurs. 2012;8(9):e419–28.
21. Aldridge MD. Standardized patients portraying parents in pediatric end-of-life simulation. Clin Simul Nurs. 2017;13(7):338–42.
22. Stout-Aguilar J, Pittman A, Bentley R, Livingston J, Watzak B. The effects of interprofessional pediatric end-of-life simulation on communication and role understanding in health professions students. Nurs Educ Perspect. 2018;39(6):360–2.
23. Kenny G, Cargil J, Hamilton C, Sales R. Improving and validating children's nurses communication skills with standardized patients in end-of-life care. J Child Health Care. 2016 Jun;20(2):145–52.
24. Lioce L. (Ed.), Lopreiato J. (Founding Ed.), Downing D., Chang T.P., Robertson J.M., Anderson M., Diaz D.A., and Spain A.E. (Assoc. Eds.) and the Terminology and Concepts Working Group (2020). Healthcare simulation dictionary—2nd Ed. Rockville, MD: Agency for Healthcare Research and Quality; 2020. AHRQ Publication No. 20-0019. doi: 10.23970/simulationv2
25. Akselbo I, Killingberg H, Aune I. Simulation as a pedagogical learning method for critical pediatric nursing in Bachelor of Nursing programs: a qualitative study. Adv Simul. 2020;5(1):1–9.
26. Park MY, McMillan MA, Conway JF, Cleary SR, Murphy L, Griffiths SK. Practice-based simulation model: a curriculum innovation to enhance the critical thinking skills of nursing students. Aust J Adv Nurs. 2013;30(3):41.
27. Masters K. Journey toward integration of simulation in a baccalaureate nursing curriculum. J Nurs Educ. 2014;53(2):102–4.
28. Hogewood C, Smith T, Etheridge S, Britt S. Clinical Boot Camp: an innovative simulation experience to prepare nursing students for obstetric and pediatric clinics. Nursing education perspectives. 2015;36(6):410–1.
29. Cleveland LM, Carmona EV, Solis L, Taylor B. Baby boy Jones interactive case-based learning activity: a web-delivered teaching strategy. Nurse Educ. 2015;40(4):179–82.
30. Gamble AS. Simulation in the undergraduate pediatric nursing curriculum: evaluation of a complex 'ward for a day 'education program. Nurse Educ Pract. 2017;(23):40–7.
31. Registered Nurse Accreditation Standards; 2019. https://www.anmac.org.au/search/publication

12 Interprofessional Simulation

Marie Gilbert and Debra Kiegaldie

Background

The Interprofessional Education (IPE) movement, having begun in the early 1960s, acquired greater prominence in the late 1970s when the World Health Organisation (WHO), in the Declaration of Alma-Ata, sought "urgent action by all governments, development workers, and the world community to train and work socially and technically as healthcare teams" ([4], p.1). The evidence supporting the implementation of IPL stretches across more than four decades, with the drivers having emerged from multiple imperatives, including rapid workforce changes, the need for a coordinated approach to the complexity of patient care, and the rise of the quality movement [5, 6]. The underpinning premise in all the drivers for IPL is that if individuals learn together, they will work better together, thus improving care delivery.

Despite the same drivers and historical timeline, and the fact that simulation is largely focused on team training, there has been little reference to IPP in the simulation literature, and most systematic literature reviews have focused on either medicine *or* nursing. What is concerning about this is that it continues to perpetuate a discrete and separate approach which can result in outcomes that are likely to be considered different and distinct for each professional group. One possible explanation for this distinction is that the language and outcomes of IPL have not been easily transferred to the simulation context, where references to 'team training' is more common. There is frequent reference to 'the team' in simulation literature. Still, the professional membership of the team is often not explicit or the focus of attention, nor is there reference to the importance of profession-specific roles within the team and how these impact relationships and communication. In short, simulation focuses on team capabilities, and IPL focuses on interprofessional capabilities. Rosen et al. [7] highlight the importance of team performance measurement in simulation and how it is frequently overlooked. However, the authors do not elaborate on the interprofessional configuration of the team itself and how it should be measured. A study by Hobgood et al. [8] did not witness any changes post-intervention regardless of the education modality, but what was interesting in this research was that typical outcomes commonly measured in IPL interventions were not included, such as an awareness of professional identity, understanding, and appreciation of the roles of self and others and patient-centeredness skills.

Problems also exist in the IPL literature, where there are many examples of simulation as a teaching approach. Still, there is scant attention to best practice features for simulation [9]. What is clearly needed in this space is the recognition that IPL and simulation both attempt to achieve the same goals of teamwork, collaboration, patient-centredness (patient safety), effective communication, and an understanding of the roles of self and others. A future commitment to combine forces, share a common language, include capability and education frameworks, and examine outcomes across a broad front would further extend and enhance the evidence base for both. This chapter is a step forward in acknowledging IPL and simulation's significant role in undergraduate education.

Best Practices

Five vignettes are presented to describe best practices and for the reader to gain insight into successful interprofessional simulation approaches that have been used in undergraduate nursing. These international examples have been selected to reflect a variety of programs and activities and illustrate creative strategies for IPL simulation.

M. Gilbert
Eastern Health Clinical School, Monash University, Melbourne, VIC, Australia
e-mail: mgilbert@mail.fresnostate.edu

D. Kiegaldie (✉)
Eastern Health Clinical School, Monash University, Melbourne, VIC, Australia

Victorian Simulation Alliance, Melbourne, Australia
e-mail: debra.kiegaldie@monash.edu

J. M. Kutzin et al. (eds.), *Comprehensive Healthcare Simulation: Nursing*, Comprehensive Healthcare Simulation,
https://doi.org/10.1007/978-3-031-31090-4_12

Vignette No. 1:

Title and Location: Simulation-Based Interprofessional Education Learning Activities; Des Moines Area Community College Healthcare Simulation.

Creator: Melody Bethards, EdD, RN, Health and Public Services/Nursing Simulation Coordinator

Des Moines Area Community College (DMACC) Healthcare Simulation provides a variety of simulation-based IPE learning activities for nursing and other healthcare students. IPE experiences are developed using the INACSL Standards of Best Practice [10]: The IPEC Core Competencies for Interprofessional Collaborative Practice provide the foundational competencies for all IPE experiences [11].

Nursing and Paramedic IPE Simulation

DMACC nursing and paramedic students participate in a simulation that follows a patient from the home to the emergency room. The experience begins with all students sharing about their program and roles and responsibilities as healthcare team members. All students listen to the Emergency Medical Services (EMS) dispatch report and plan care for the patient based only on this report.

While paramedic students see the patient, nursing students prepare the emergency room and review routine orders and protocols. The paramedic students then call the report to the simulated Emergency Department (ED) prior to transport. Nursing students finalize their plan of care based on the paramedic report. Once the paramedic students arrive at the simulated ED, they give bedside reports and include any updates based on what occurred during transport. Paramedic students then watch the ED portion of the experience via live feed.

Debriefing focuses on teamwork, communication, and roles and responsibilities with students from each program providing feedback to the other. Nursing students report that the experiences help them better understand the role of EMS providers, and paramedic students report that they gain a greater understanding of how the information they gather during a patient call and the report they give can impact the patient's care.

Capstone Events

DMACC students from multiple programs and campuses participate in two large-scale (capstone) simulation-based events. The capstone events provide a unique opportunity for students to hone discipline-specific communication, collaboration, prioritization, and critical thinking skills.

The Fall capstone event is a simulation of a hospital that is experiencing a blackout during a massive winter storm. DMACC EMS, nursing, respiratory therapy, social services, and nursing assistant students work together to care for patients in a hospital functioning on only one small generator. The limited power creates challenges in patient care in a technology-driven healthcare system.

The Spring capstone event simulates a multiple-victim motor vehicle accident and receiving emergency room. DMACC criminal justice, fire science, medical laboratory technology, nursing, nursing assistant, paramedic, respiratory therapy, social services, and surgical technology students work together to treat the victims at the accident scene and transport them to the emergency room for further assessment and treatment. At the same time, students from the early childhood program participate in a mock lockdown of the child development center. More information about these capstone events can be found on the DMACC website: https://www.dmacc.edu/programs/health/simulation/Pages/capstone.aspx

Des Moines Area Interprofessional Education Collaborative (DMAIPEC) Activities

DMACC Healthcare Simulation provides simulation-based learning experiences as a partner in the Des Moines Area Interprofessional Education Collaborative (DMAIPEC). More information about DMAIPEC can be found on their website at https://www.grandview.edu/ipe-collaborative. DMACC Healthcare Simulation offers a live and virtual simulation-based learning experience designed for nursing students, second-year medical students, P3 pharmacy students, and social services students who have an advanced understanding of interprofessional collaboration and a strong foundation of knowledge and skills in their profession.

The live simulation experience focuses on critically ill patients' care. It is designed for final-semester nursing students, second-year medical students, and P3 pharmacy students. In this simulation, the team plans to care for a patient with a critical condition requiring multiple IV medications. Students determine the protocols that will be implemented and add any orders they desire. Simulation faculty and staff set up the scenario based on the team's decisions. The scenario is designed to help students understand the important role each profession plays in the care of critically ill patients.

Designed to meet IPE learning opportunities during COVID restrictions, the virtual simulation experience focuses on the impact all aspects of a healthcare system have on the care of pediatric patients. The simulation is designed for final-semester nursing students, second-year medical students, P3 pharmacy students, and social services students. In this simulation, the team explores the role of interprofessional teams and health systems in pediatric patient situations. Based on the positive responses to this virtual IPE learning experience, the plan is to continue over this experience regardless of COVID restrictions.

Vignette No. 2

Title and location: CovSim: Coventry University Simulation, Coventry, UK

Creator: Natasha Taylor, EdD, Associate Professor and Lead for Simulation

Coventry University, a large university in the United Kingdom, has developed and currently runs large-scale, cross-discipline simulation events several times a year. Although CovSim is not healthcare-specific, its learning outcomes, ethos, and implementation are focused on employability skills. These employability skills, or collaborative capabilities as called within the School of Nursing, Midwifery, and Health, are central to the outcomes of the event and allow learners to develop these skills together, regardless of discipline.

Fifty years of inquiry support interprofessional education (IPE) to prepare healthcare students for the workforce. This integration of care strongly correlates to improved health outcomes, higher staff satisfaction, and better acceptance of care. The effective transition from higher education to the work environment is fundamental to ensure care integration in the health workforce. To support this, there has been an emphasis on developing capabilities that develop these common employability skills, and a framework for these has been developed at Coventry University School of Nursing, Midwifery, and Health. These collaborative capabilities allow learners to develop these skills together, regardless of discipline. However, difficulty may occur in operationalizing effective and innovative pedagogical tools to engage learners and provide collaborative learning outcomes.

To prepare for this event, a new, relevant simulation story, consisting of separate but interlinked simulations, is written every year. The 'story' is chosen based on the learning outcomes for each station and what event could potentially precipitate the learning required. For organizational ease, all stations are 30 min long exactly; learners all experience the simulations in the same order, in a linear fashion. There is no assumption or requirement for pre-learned knowledge. For example, CovSim2018 was based on a fire at a music festival, CovSim2019 was a nerve agent release, and CovSim2020 was a "dirty bomb" explosion simulation. Each simulation station is facilitated by a subject expert who has general knowledge of the other simulations in the story and works together to provide a seamless transition from station to station to ensure learners feel that each station forms part of the whole linear story.

Feedback from learners and facilitators (and observers) has been overwhelmingly positive, with these events now being integrated into the interprofessional education curricula in all courses across the School. Each year's events also have a research theme to ensure effective evaluation and purposeful learning for all involved.

Examples of factors organizers thought were valuable during the planning of these interprofessional simulations:

- Scope out what 'spaces' or facilities you have available. There might be spaces outside your immediate area that willing to share, such as a mock courtroom, boardroom, etc.
- Plan dates for the year as soon as possible by getting together with the facilitators and put in at least one event every semester. Use any online timetabling to ensure spaces are free. This collating of dates can be the most challenging part of setting up these events.
- Once dates are set, send electronic calendar invitations to ensure facilitators (and helpers) cannot back out!
- Use electronic sign-up software (several free ones available) to create a booking event for groups of six to eight, starting 30 min after each other. Putting simple instructions, maps, etc., is useful to fend off the most asked questions.
- Identify someone to manage the day to ensure everyone is keeping to time, students and facilitators have everything they need, and can be available for emergencies. It is too difficult to facilitate a simulation and run the day.

Vignette No. 3

Title and Location: Escaping the Traditional in Interprofessional Escape Rooms, The University of Tennessee Health Science Center, College of Pharmacy, Memphis, Tennessee

Creator: Chasity M. Shelton, BS, PharmD, Assistant Dean for Student Success & Associate Professor, Department of Clinical Pharmacy & Translational Science,

Escape rooms are a creative method for encouraging individuals to work together to solve puzzles and complete the task of escaping the room. While commercially available for entertainment purposes, the same structure can be applied in the academic environment to a clinical scenario to promote recall and application of prior instructional material and strengthen problem-solving, teamwork, and communication skills to encourage interprofessional team development. With a multidisciplinary team of participants, the escape room structure presents an enjoyable and non-traditional method to encourage interprofessional collaboration and the development of Interprofessional Education Collaborative (IPEC) core competencies [11].

Faculty from an academic health science center's College of Pharmacy and an undergraduate college of Nursing at a public university met to discuss integrating an escape room into their interprofessional education (IPE) curriculum. This simulation approach was chosen as the specific learning outcomes for each learner group included: (1) effective employment of communication skills, (2) supporting a team approach in the care of a patient, (3) applying relationship-building values and the principle of team dynamics to develop a care plan, and (4) exhibiting behaviors and values that are consistent with the tenets of professionalism.

The purpose of the interprofessional escape room was to place learners in a simulated environment designed to be stressful to address the learner outcomes in a clear, concise, and considerate manner while maintaining mutual respect. Faculty identified the need for an activity that was case-based, appropriate for second-year students, would reinforce communication and teamwork, and required minimal set-up and clean-up. An advanced healthcare IPE escape room developed and vetted at another institution was identified to incorporate into the IPE curriculum for each college. The learner groups for this activity included undergraduate nursing students and second-year pharmacy students. This IPE activity focused predominantly on the IPEC competencies of interprofessional communication and teams/teamwork.

Faculty from pharmacy and nursing met to discuss the logistics and possible barriers/challenges to implementing the escape room and identify resources needed. The time allotted for the learning activity was 2 h for each learner group, which included the pre-brief (20 min), simulation escape room activity (60 min), and debrief (40 min). Due to the time needed to complete the activity and the large cohort of students, the decision was made to conduct the simulation a total of five times using four simulated inpatient hospital rooms to run simultaneously over 1.5 days. Faculty from each profession served as co-facilitators. Additional volunteers were recruited to assist in setting up the rooms, reassembling puzzles, and cleaning up each day. Pictures of the set-up were used to ensure accurate room recreation for all learner groups. The task of resetting the rooms was conducted while facilitators were debriefing the learner groups.

During the brief, four preassigned interprofessional teams of students were brought in at a time as one larger cohort. The session started with an web-based icebreaker activity and introduced the team to solving puzzles and working together within their team. Additionally, students were provided with an overview of the escape room activity and the rules. After the brief session, learner teams were brought to their simulated inpatient hospital room, and the patient hand-off was read aloud. The team was charged with developing a patient-specific discharge plan, hoping to leave within the hour. Learners were permitted to enter the room and given 60 min to complete the activity. Clues were permitted. Simulation puzzles consisted of an electronic medical record, lockboxes, sound recordings, black lights/pens, sound recordings, and video recordings of patient interactions. Unlike traditional escape rooms, participants were permitted the use of electronic devices. Learners were then brought together for a large group debrief at the conclusion.

In the large group debrief, learners were asked to identify moments of success and challenges encountered during the simulation. Many commented on the strength of their roles as contributing to the team's overall strength. Challenges that some teams identified were uncertainty as to what clues to start with, lack of familiarity with the puzzles/locks, and the inclination to work in silos versus working in a large group. A post-participation survey was used to assess learning outcomes. Survey findings identified that learning outcomes were met and student satisfaction with the activity was high. Most students reported that this activity improved their understanding of respectful communication with other healthcare professionals and increased their confidence in effectively collaborating with other team members.

This activity demonstrated that using gamification as an escape room is a feasible and effective method to meet objectives for interprofessional education competencies. The co-debriefing following each simulation provided an environment for advocacy and inquiry, which enhanced learning. Participants identified communication and the importance of collaboration as a team to be integral in providing the best care for a patient and that roles are equally important as each healthcare team member brings value from a different perspective.

Example of factors participants thought was valuable during the interprofessional simulations:

The value of other's perspectives when trying to solve a problem (Nursing student)

Communication, active listening, and asking questions when needed is very important (Pharmacy student)

Acknowledgment: Friedrich C, Teaford H, Taubenheim A, Sick B. 2018. *Advanced Escape Room Guidebook for Health Care Education.* Minneapolis, MN:1Health Interprofessional Education Program.

Vignette No. 4

Title and Location: Clinical Partnerships between Healthcare and Academic Institutes; California State University, Fresno, California

Creator: Marie Gilbert, DNP, RN, Director, Central California Center for Excellence in Nursing

Clinical partnerships have the potential to mitigate challenges faced by organizations and nursing programs attempting to implement interprofessional simulation. For organizations, the challenges of establishing their simulation program may include expensive and inexperienced healthcare simulation educators. The barriers to implementing interprofessional simulations may include limited access to multiple healthcare-related professional students and/or clinicians for nursing programs. A clinical partnership between a healthcare and academic institute allowed sharing human and financial resources. It allowed nursing students to work autonomously with clinicians, residents, and interns in simulation.

Faculty from an undergraduate nursing program at a local public university and a pediatric residency program at a local hospital met to discuss whether a partnership between the programs could provide interprofessional learning opportunities for students and residents. Faculty agreed that a learning experience including learners from these different groups would be valuable and decided to conduct an in situ interprofessional simulation pilot study that would include nursing students and pediatric residents at the clinical site.

Permission was obtained from senior leadership at the clinical site where the in situ simulations were being proposed. Before the initiation of the pilot study, Pharmacy at the clinical site identified that pharmacy residents onsite would benefit from the opportunity to participate in the in situ interprofessional simulations.

The learner groups for the pilot included undergraduate nursing students during their pediatric clinical placement at the clinical site, pediatric residents completing their residency at the clinical site, and pharmacy residents at the clinical site.

The simulations aimed to develop insight, shared knowledge, teamwork skills, and collaboration among nursing students, pharmacists, and physicians and assess the feasibility of an in situ program.

The simulation scenario was developed by clinical/faculty representatives from pharmacy, medicine, and nursing and included specific learning outcomes for each learner group and collaborative learning outcomes for all learners. The same representatives facilitated the pre-brief, interprofessional simulation, and debrief.

The pilot was conducted during one academic semester. Participants included nursing students, medical residents (pediatric & family practice), medical students, and pharmacy residents and students.

Findings from the pilot identified that learning outcomes were met and participant, student, and faculty satisfaction were high. The debriefing following each simulation provided a rich learning environment for all involved. Participants identified they worked well as a team, found the learning experience valuable, and reported a high readiness for interprofessional learning.

The pilot demonstrated it was feasible to include students from different programs and organizations in insitu interprofessional simulation.

The collaborative interprofessional simulations continued for three years. The purpose and goals of the simulations during that time were to develop and maintain the core competencies for interprofessional collaborative practice enhancing communication, collaboration, quality of care, patient outcomes, patient satisfaction, and staff/learner satisfaction for current and future practitioners.

The learner group expanded to include social work students from the same public university as the nursing students, medical students and pharmacy students from different academic programs completing rotations at the clinical site.

This clinical partnership between healthcare and academic institutes combined the expertise of both sites to develop and implement high-quality interprofessional simulations. The success of the interprofessional simulations somewhat contributed to them being discontinued. The positive feedback from all learner groups led faculty and organizational leaders to identify the value of interprofessional education (IPE) and the desire to expand learning experiences to include more students and clinicians.

This led to a formal inter-agency IPE collaborative being established. Opportunities for student involvement extended beyond nursing and social work students to include all programs within the College of Health and Human Services at the local University. All healthcare providers at the clinical site were also invited to attend the IPE workshops. Participant interest was too large to continue with simulations, so an alternate approach was adopted for the IPE.

The clinical partnership successfully combined the academic and clinical expertise of both sites to develop, implement and sustain for several semester effective interprofessional simulations.

Example of factors participants thought was valuable during the interprofessional simulations:

Working with the other professions. Get to experience everyone's roles, so I know what my role is (Nursing student)

Realistic roles/team members and everyone's importance, how to help each other become stronger in the roles (Pediatric resident)

Stress environment mimics chaos, and communication skills are needed (Pharmacy intern)

Learning in ACTION. Debriefing with experienced professionals and perspectives was beneficial and solidified challenge areas (Social Work Student)

Vignette No. 5

Title and Location: The Delirium Program, Monash University

Creator: Debra Kiegaldie, PhD, RN, Professor and Clinical Chair - Health Workforce & Simulation, Holmesglen Institute, Healthscope Hospitals, and Monash University.

For over 10 years, Monash University in Melbourne, Australia, has delivered an IPL learning experience for undergraduate nursing and medical students called The Delirium Program. More than 12,000 students have experienced this program which is focused on the collaborative management of delirium (a common, poorly recognized clinical problem). The program has evolved to become a full-day immersive experience integrating a delirium simulation scenario. In the simulation, students not only learn about delirium but also learn how to work collaboratively in the management of a simulated patient with delirium, where they could demonstrate patient-centered care, interprofessional communication, effective teamwork, and an understanding of the respective healthcare team members' roles. The program commences with an icebreaker; there is content delivery about delirium in the form of a professionally produced video where senior clinicians talk about the key features of delirium and the need for interprofessional practice.

A small group case study exercise culminates in the simulation scenario of a simulated patient portraying the role of delirium titled "Lorna is looking for her purse."

A large-scale randomized controlled trial of this initiative was conducted in 2008 [12, 13], with results indicating that the IPL approach increased students' knowledge of delirium ($p < 0.01$), increased students' ratings of how IPL influenced effective interprofessional collaborative practice ($p < 0.01$); improved nursing and medical students' knowledge and appreciation of each other's roles; developed attitudes of appreciation, trust, and respect amongst the two professions; and increased students' confidence and perceptions of their personal development in interprofessional collaborative competencies. Other important outcomes of the study showed:

- the importance of placing equal emphasis on the students learning about a clinical topic as well as learning about IPP;
- the value students place on an authentic blended learning approach such as simulation.
- A large-scale IPL is possible if logistical and organizational barriers are overcome, but it takes a lot of work [12].

Sample Curriculum Framework

Given the complexity of both IPL and simulation, Kiegaldie [12, 14] suggests a curriculum development framework that begins with the work of the WHO framework on IPL [2]. It encompasses four key steps (the 4Bs) and includes key questions to ask yourself when designing IPL.

Build on Existing Links

Before commencing, consider the current clinical context and the existing team environment. Questions to ask include:

- How many health professions could be involved?
- How are these members currently linked in terms of health care delivery?
- Is the learning program a small or large-scale initiative?
- What ability is there to grow the program into the future?

Build Opportunities in Clinical Settings

This focuses on embedding the experience into a relevant contextual setting. Questions to ask include:

- What is the clinical context and setting for the potential IPL program, course or activity? (Is it a classroom, acute, sub-acute context, or is it in a community, regional, rural, or remote setting)
- What clinical topic(s) should be considered and why? Remember learners often value the clinical topic just as much as the opportunity for IPL.

Benefits Demonstrated to All Stakeholders

Before planning the program, it is critically important to identify how the program aims to benefit each stakeholder group because, without their support, the educational initiative is unlikely to succeed. Stakeholders include learners; teachers, the faculty, the healthcare system, organization or health service; and, most importantly, patients. Describing the benefits to each stakeholder group is integral to success.

Based on Best Evidence Approaches

One evidence-based approach to designing educational experiences for students is the Biggs 3P model, which is very well suited to work-based learning situations [15]. It comprises three main components: Presage, Process, and Product.

Presage factors: These factors exist prior to learning and relate to the student and to the teaching context.

Process factors: The approach that learners use to process tasks. Biggs refers to this as either a deep or surface approach to learning [15]. In the context of this chapter, this process could be simulated.

Product factors: The product phase is related to qualitative differences in learning outcomes. In other words, deep approaches produce high-quality learning outcomes, while surface approaches produce lower-quality outcomes.

Freeth and Reeves adapted this model for IPL by presenting a range of choices open to the IPL designer in the Process area [16]. They emphasized teacher characteristics more and included interprofessional capabilities in the Product section. This model has been used extensively in the IPL field. It was further extended in 2015 to enhance the teaching and learning process by including an extra "P" for planning [12, 14]. This was to emphasize the requirements for careful preparation and planning of all IPL interventions. Presage and Planning go 'hand in hand.' Presage is used to identify the issues, and Planning is seen as the way to determine what is needed to address the Presage. Presage is the 'what', Planning is the 'how'. Figure 12.1 presents the iterative, multi-directional process of the 4B-4P model that requires equal attention on every component. Ignoring any could very well make the difference between failure and success.

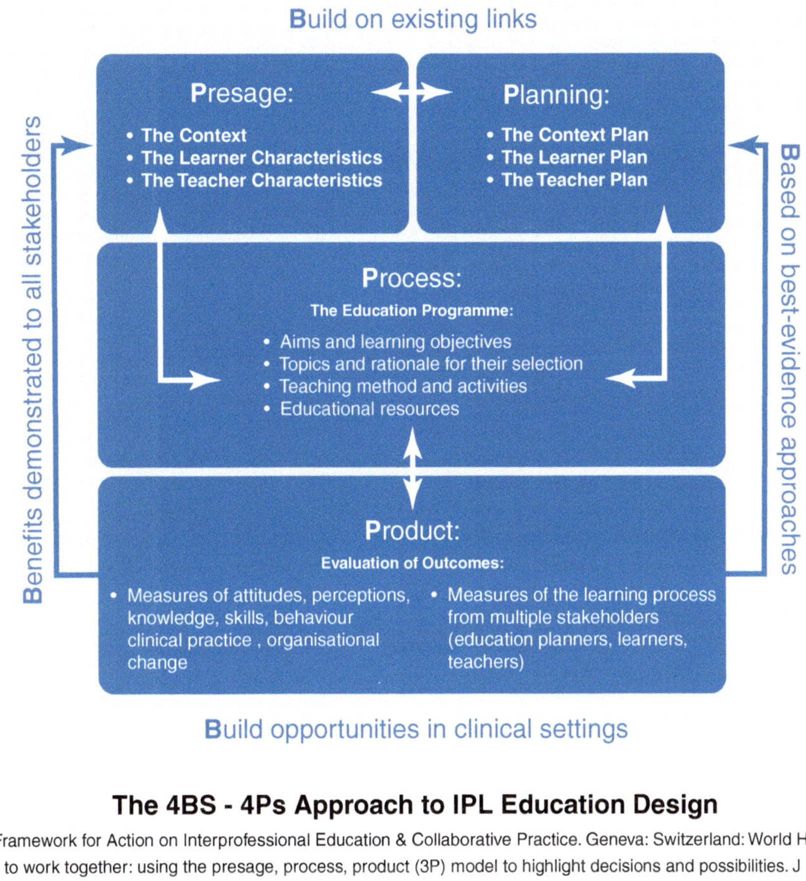

Fig. 12.1 The Kiegaldie 4B-4P model of IPL [12, 14, 16, 17]

An example curriculum framework using the 4Ps approach is provided in Table 12.1. This model was used for the pilot and first iteration of The Delirium Program. It provides a template that could be adapted to any IPL initiative in undergraduate nursing education. While the answers to key questions may not always be the same, each question warrants careful consideration. This will ensure that all features of the 4Ps are addressed, inclusive of the process of learning and how it could be evaluated from a learning and process perspective.

Table 12.1 The 4Ps educational design model for IPL using the Australian example of The Delirium Program

Items	Presage components (What are the issues?) Key questions to ask yourself	Planning components: (The Action Plan) What do you need to do?
THE CONTEXT		
Political climate	At the local level, in what way is the political climate right for introducing IPL?	The Australian Learning and Teaching Council funded a consultation to increase the capacity of the higher education sector to graduate health professionals who have acquired IPL and IPP capabilities. The political climate was ready for IPL
Regulatory framework	Are there any hindrances or considerations from accreditation or regulatory authorities?	The Australian Medical and Nursing Education Accreditation Bodies and Health Care regulators expect and mandate IPL and IPP as National Standards for Nursing and Midwifery and National Standards for Quality and Safety.
Funding	How much will it cost to deliver, and where will the funds come from?	A small 'seed' grant was provided by the University. This assisted in embedding the program as a routine curriculum initiative.
Management support	What is your current organizational structure? Have you got management support?	The medical and nursing Deans were made aware of and were fully supportive of the program, and the Heads of Schools became members of the advisory committee.
Relationship with stakeholders	Who are your stakeholders, and how will they be informed of the program (e.g., learners, health service, teachers, patients)?	Stakeholders included the program planners, faculty, teachers, and students. All stakeholders were fully informed of the project.
What is the learning environment?	Where will the learning take place? What challenges will the environment pose (clinic, community practice, hospital ward, simulated clinical environment)?	The program took place over 6 days, with approximately 40 students attending each day. The classroom components of the teaching were delivered in tutorial rooms. The simulations and debriefing were conducted in the clinical skills simulation laboratories of the School of Nursing, which mimicked a typical general ward setting. The duration of the teaching was 4 h and included light refreshments.
What resources do you have?	What resources will you need (technical, physical)	Trained simulated participants, DVD player, ppt presentations, and fully set up ward environment.
Competing interests	Are there any competing educational demands? Who will you manage this?	The timetabling was a challenge. For medical students, it needed to be delivered during an Aged Care Clinical Rotation, and for nursing students, it was a clinical placement day in their Mental Health Rotation.
THE LEARNERS		
Learner characteristics	How many learners will be involved?	Two hundred eleven medical and nursing students completed the pilot program ($n = 123$ nursing students; $n = 88$ medical students). The parity of numbers was considered important but was not always attainable.
	Where are they located?	Students were in metropolitan Melbourne.
	Are the demographics similar (age, gender, culture)?	Nursing: 6.6% of nursing students had a prior Diploma in Nursing, and more nursing students were over 25 years of age than medical students Medicine: 28.8% of medical students had a prior Bachelor of Medical Sciences. Most students were female, and significantly more females were studying nursing (consistent with the nursing workforce in Australia)
	Will this be compulsory or optional?	The pilot program was not compulsory, but from 2010 to current, the program was compulsory for all medical and nursing students.
	What are their prior knowledge, skills, attitudes, and conceptions of collaboration and learning?	Approximately 30% of medical and 16% of nursing students indicated prior opportunities to participate in IPL, with most occurring informally on clinical placements.
	Are there competing learning needs?	None Identified
	Are there social factors that might impact delivery?	Students may not have interacted with each other previously. An icebreaker and catering were therefore planned for social interaction purposes.
THE TEACHERS		

Table 12.1 (continued)

Items	Presage components (What are the issues?) Key questions to ask yourself	Planning components: (The Action Plan) What do you need to do?
Teacher characteristics	Who will be your teachers/facilitators? What is their prior experience with IPL? How will you select them? Will they need training? How will this be managed? Who will be your IPL local champions?	Each group of students had a medical and nursing facilitator, with eight being needed each day (4 medicine; 4 nursing). Sixteen facilitators were recruited for the program based on their enthusiasm for IPL and ability to lead small group learning and simulation. Being a role model for IPL was a priority for selection. Very few facilitators had prior experience with IPL The selection was voluntary and included faculty and senior clinicians from partnering health services The training was provided, and a comprehensive manual on IPL, IPP, and how to deliver each of the teaching and learning activities was provided A medicine and nursing team lead was designated the local 'champions.'

PROCESS

What is the overall direction of the simulation? What are the anticipated learning objectives?

Aim: For students to learn with, from, and about each other to recognize and respond to a patient who presents with delirium

Learning objectives:

1. Describe the prevalence, significance, and prevention strategies for delirium
2. Recognise the clinical features of delirium through joint patient assessment
3. Implement immediate strategies to ensure patient safety, including calling for help
4. Apply the confusion assessment method to diagnose delirium
5. Differentiate delirium from other possible diagnoses
6. Collaboratively identify risk factors and causes of delirium
7. Collaboratively manage a patient with delirium, including treating the underlying causes
8. Demonstrate effective teamworking and interprofessional communication
9. Demonstrate an understanding of own and other roles in the care of the cognitively impaired patient

Topics: What topics will you include in the teaching? What is the rationale for their selection?

- Delirium prevalence, significance and prevention
- Health assessment and diagnosis of delirium and the application of diagnostic tools
- Escalating care
- Patient safety measures for cognitive impairment
- Underlying causes of delirium and their collaborative management
- Collaborative management of delirious behaviors
- Interprofessional communication strategies

What **teaching approaches and activities** will you select? (Interprofessional case-based discussion, working in pairs in a community health center identifying roles, leading a grand round on collaborative management of a clinical problem, developing joint care plans, participating in immersive simulations, quality improvement projects, etc. Are the learning activities constructively aligned to the learning objectives? What will the learners and teachers be doing?

- Ice Breaker (30 min) (LO 9)
- Video (20 min): An Interprofessional Conversation about the collaborative management of Delirium (with a Senior Nurse and Medical Clinician (LOs 1-7)
- Small Group Case Study (60 min) (LOs 1-7)
- Simulation Scenario (60 min) (LOs 2-9)

What additional resources will you need? (Scenarios, case studies, simulated participants, facilitator training materials, videos, role plays, written learning activities)

Simulated participants, Facilitator Manual, Videos, Case study material and instructions for students, Supportive materials on delirium

PRODUCT (Evaluation of outcomes)

What theory-based **evaluation framework** will you use? (e.g., Kirkpatrick, Realist, other)

Kirkpatrick's hierarchy of outcomes modified for IPL (For more information, see Chapter on Assessment and Evaluation)

What aspects will you evaluate? (e.g., learner perceptions of their ability to work collaboratively in clinical practice; learner perceptions of their development in knowledge, skills, and attitudes; learners' perceptions of the learning experience (process), behavior outcomes, organizational outcomes, patient-related outcomes, and patient satisfaction.

What **instruments** will you use to measure outcomes?

Pre and Post Survey

- Student demographics,
- Readiness for Interprofessional Learning Scale
- Global IPL rating scale
- Likert scale and open-ended questions on student perceptions of the teaching and learning approaches

Barriers, Challenges, and Solutions for IP Simulation

While there are many reasons for developing IPL programs, significant limitations need to be overcome. Table 12.2 summarizes common barriers and challenges to interprofessional simulation based on current literature [18–23]. Best practices in simulation [10, 24–27], IPE frameworks/models [2, 28], and experiences cited in the literature [18, 20, 22, 29] guide the proposed solutions identified to mitigate these barriers and challenges.

Table 12.2 Barriers, challenges, and proposed solutions for IP simulation

Barriers and Challenges	Proposed Solutions
Characteristics of the Learner: Professional stereotype/bias toward other professions. Lack of understanding of own role and the roles of others. Learners lack experience with interprofessional education or simulations. Learner feeling uncomfortable being observed.	The development and implementation of a program or workshop to orientate learners to IPE and simulation. This would include orientation to roles and responsibilities of all professions included. Follow best practices in simulation and begin all simulation-based experiences with the briefing. Incorporate activities that help establish an environment of integrity, trust, and respect into the briefing. Require confidentiality of learners' performances and scenario content. Promote psychological safety throughout all phases of the simulation-based learning experience.
Characteristic of the facilitator: Lack of experience or education/training of the facilitator/s.	The requirement is that all facilitators complete initial education on using simulation through formal coursework/training. The requirement is that all facilitators pursue ongoing continuing education offerings and/or targeted work with an experienced mentor. The requirement is that all facilitators demonstrate competency in simulation pedagogy.
Characteristics of the Simulation: Lack of realism—including scenarios only aimed towards one discipline. Inadequate preparation/orientation/pre-brief. Debriefing is not multidisciplinary.	Develop mutual goals among the professions included in the IP simulation. Incorporate authentic, challenging, reality-based activities/scenarios. Scenarios should be developed and reviewed by the professionals involved in the simulation. Dry run (practice) the session with a group of interprofessional volunteer learners who reflect the composition of the target group. Activities should be based on learning objectives, participants' knowledge, skills, needs, and experiences. Provide team-based structured debriefing and feedback as appropriate for the goal of the simulation. Consider uniprofessional debriefings followed by interprofessional debriefing (or vice versa). Consider personal reflection on assumptions of other involved professions before debriefing. Scaffold the simulation activity to provide the learners with scenario-specific skills and knowledge, an understanding of the roles and responsibilities of other professional students in the scenario. Consider developing and implementing scenarios that promote interprofessional thinking, information and knowledge exchange, mutual understanding, mutual acceptance, respect for learners and professions within the scenario, and the reduction of hierarchies.

Table 12.2 (continued)

Barriers and Challenges	Proposed Solutions
Characteristics of the institute: Culture: Interprofessional formal or informal "Turf Wars" Logistical barriers: Scheduling—Coordinating schedules from more than one professional program Scheduling—Parity of student numbers Curriculum integration Cost	Promote an institute culture of IPE and support for IP simulation. This will include: A shared vision The development and implementation of a strategic plan that coordinates and aligns resources for IP simulation. Strong leadership and consistent engagement of deans and program directors. Supportive IPE and Simulation institutional policies. A willingness to update, renew and revise existing curricula. A champion/s who is/are responsible for coordinating IP simulation activities and identifies barriers to progress. Respect and appreciation of the benefits of IPE. The development and implementation of an interprofessional faculty steering committee supported by senior leadership that is not controlled by any one school or program. The development and implementation of a single academic calendar that identifies dedicated time for IPE and IP simulation. The development and implementation of a program or workshop to orientate learners to IPE and simulation. Identifying core graduation requirements that include interprofessional collaboration competencies adopted by all schools and programs. Incorporating interprofessional collaboration/education competencies that are indicated in program accreditation standards. Identifying and adopting a funding model that meets the needs of the IP simulation program and institutional structure (Centralized, Blended, Decentralized, and/or a combination of these 3 funding models). The maintenance and management of financial resources to support the stability, sustainability, and growth of the IP simulation program.

Conclusion

Interprofessional simulation is complex to design and deliver, yet it is a highly valuable teaching and learning strategy. In the context of undergraduate nursing education, it can develop students' interprofessional capabilities and prepare them for their future practice as effective healthcare team members. This chapter has provided an overview and practical examples of using IPL simulation in nursing, including their mutual historical beginnings. Using an educational framework such as the 4B-4P model of IPL education design can assist course planners in overcoming the many reported challenges of IPL simulation implementation. Educating our students to have a shared understanding of interprofessional learning and practice can ensure that the best collaborative care is delivered to meet the needs of patients and their families.

References

1. CAIPE. Defining IPE: Centre for the Advancement of Interprofessional Education; 2002 http://caipe.org.uk/resources/defining-ipe/.
2. WHO. Framework for action on interprofessional education & collaborative practice. Geneva, Switzerland: World Health Organization; 2010.
3. L-TIPP. Interprofessional health education in Australia: the way forward. In: University of Sydney and the University of Technology S, editor; 2009.
4. WHO, editor. Declaration of Alma-Ata. International Conference on Primary Health Care. USSR: World Health Organisation; 1978.
5. Braithwaite J, Travaglia J. In: Health A, editor. Inter-professional learning and clinical education: an overview of the literature. Canberra: Braithwaite and Associates and the ACT Health Department; 2005.
6. Reeves S. Why we need interprofessional education to improve the delivery of safe and effective care. Interface. 2016;20(56)
7. Rosen M, Salas E, Wilson K, King H, Salisbury M, Augenstein J, et al. Measuring team performance in simulation-based training: adopting best practices for healthcare. Simul Healthcare [Internet]. 2008;3:33–41.
8. Hobgood C, Sherwood G, Frush K, Hollar D, Maynard L, Foster B, et al. Teamwork training with nursing and medical students: does the method matter? Results of an interinstitutional, interdisciplinary collaboration. Qual Saf Health Care [Internet]. 2010;19(25):1–6.
9. McGaghie W, Issenberg S, Petrusa E, Scalese R. A critical review of simulation-based medical education research: 2003-2009. Medical Education [Internet]. 2010;44:50–63.
10. INACSL standards of best practice: SimulationSM simulation-enhanced interprofessional education (Sim-IPE). Clin Simul Nurs. 2016;12:S34–S8.
11. Brashers V, Haizlip J, Owen JA. The ASPIRE Model: Grounding the IPEC core competencies for interprofessional collaborative practice within a foundational framework. J Interprofess Care. 2020;34(1):128–32.
12. Kiegaldie D. Learning about delirium in a simulated clinical environment: an interprofessional learning intervention for final year medical and nursing students. Melbourne: Monash University; 2015.

13. Kiegaldie D, editor. Learning about delirium in a simulated clinical environment: an interprofessional learning intervention for final year medical and nursing students. Barcelona: Association of Medical Education in Europe (AMEE); 2016.
14. Kiegaldie D. Learning and teaching in clinical settings: expert commentary from an interprofessional perspective. Clin Educ Health Profess. 2021:1–21.
15. Biggs J. Approaches to the enhancement of tertiary teaching. Higher Educ Res Dev [Internet]. 1989;8(1):7–25. https://doi.org/10.1080/0729436890080102.
16. Freeth D, Reeves S. Learning to work together: using the presage, process, product (3P) model to highlight decisions and possibilities. J Interprof Care. 2004;18(1):43–56.
17. Lewallen LP. Practical strategies for nursing education program evaluation. J Profess Nurs. 2015;31(2):133–40.
18. Connolly F, De Brún A, McAuliffe E. A narrative synthesis of learners' experiences of barriers and facilitators related to effective interprofessional simulation. J Interprof Care. 2022;36(2):222–33.
19. Granheim BM, Shaw JM, Mansah M. The use of interprofessional learning and simulation in undergraduate nursing programs to address interprofessional communication and collaboration: an integrative review of the literature. Nurse Educ Today. 2018;62:118–27.
20. Homeyer S, Hoffmann W, Hingst P, Oppermann RF, Dreier-Wolfgramm A. Effects of interprofessional education for medical and nursing students: enablers, barriers and expectations for optimizing future interprofessional collaboration—a qualitative study. BMC Nurs. 2018;17:13.
21. Lee CA, Pais K, Kelling S, Anderson OS. A scoping review to understand simulation used in interprofessional education. J Interprofess Educ Pract. 2018;13(1):15–23.
22. Palaganas JC, Brunette V, Winslow B. Prelicensure simulation-enhanced interprofessional education: a critical review of the research literature. Simul Healthc. 2016;11(6):404–18.
23. Southall TM, Macdonald S. Fostering undergraduate medicine, nursing, and pharmacy students' readiness for interprofessional learning using high fidelity simulation. Cureus. 2021;13(1)
24. INACSL Standards of Best Practice. SimulationSM simulation design. Clin Simul Nurs. 2016;12:S5–S12.
25. INACSL Standards of Best Practice. SimulationSM professional integrity. Clin Simul Nurs. 2016;12:S30–S3.
26. INACSL Standards of Best Practice. SimulationSM facilitation. Clin Simul Nurs. 2016;12:S16–20.
27. INACSL Standards of Best Practice. SimulationSM operations. Clin Simul Nurs. 2017;13(12):681–7.
28. Carney PA, Bearden DT, Osborne ML, Driessnack M, Stilp CC, Gedney Baggs J, et al. Economic models for sustainable interprofessional education. J Interprof Care. 2018;32(6):745–51.
29. Mladenovic J, Tilden VP. Strategies for overcoming barriers to IPE at a health sciences university. J Interprofess Educ Pract. 2017;8:10–3.

International Innovations in Simulation: Case Studies from Four Countries

13

Michelle A. Kelly, Diane Dennis, Sissel Eikeland Husebø, Yun Kang, and Gary Francis

Case Study 1: Australia

AuthorsPle: Michelle Kelly, Diane Dennis

Title: Promoting Empathy in pre-licensure health Professionals through Simulation and Interprofessional Education in the Context of Patients with Obesity.

Location: Faculty of Health Sciences, Curtin University; Sir Charles Gairdner Hospital, Perth, Western Australia. Directions Disability Services, Perth, Western Australia.

Acknowledgments: Siana Critchett[a], Tracey McKernan[a], Sharon Keesing[a], Alison Kelly[c]

Funding: This work was supported by a Curtin University seed grant (2018)

M. A. Kelly (✉)
Curtin School of Nursing, Curtin University, Kent St Perth, Perth, Western Australia, Australia

Clinical and Health Sciences, University of South Australia, North Terrace, Adelaide, Australia
e-mail: Michelle.Kelly@unisa.edu.au

D. Dennis
Curtin School of Allied Health, Curtin University, Kent St Perth, Perth, Western Australia, Australia

Intensive Care Unit, Sir Charles Gairdner Hospital, Western Australia, Perth, Australia

S. E. Husebø
University of Stavanger, Stavanger, Norway

Y. Kang
School of Nursing, Teagu Science University, Daegu, Republic of Korea

G. Francis
School of Health and Social Care, London South Bank University, London, UK

AECC University College, Parkwood Road, Bournemouth, Dorset, UK
e-mail: GFrancis@aecc.ac.uk

Background

Simulation learning activities are particularly useful for teaching ethically challenging topics, rare events, high-stakes situations, or where the patient's well-being is compromised [1]. One ethically challenging topic is caring for a patient with obesity, particularly considering the social stigma associated with larger people. Obesity is one of the most prevalent public health issues in economically developed countries, with about 13% of the world's adult population (11% of men and 15% of women) reported as obese in 2016, and the worldwide prevalence tripling between 1975 and 2016 [2].

A recent survey of inpatients demonstrated an increased prevalence of extremely obese patients in an Australian hospitalized cohort compared to the general Australian population [3]. One example of legislation to address discrimination, the Western Australian Equal Opportunities Act, protects individuals from discrimination, including those with physical impairment, such as obesity, which limits the capacity to complete activities [4]. As such, health services globally must ensure the availability of appropriate facilities and equipment to accommodate consumers who are obese. This extends to the training and understanding by professionals working in all healthcare fields of this group of patients' specific physical and psychosocial needs.

Although health professionals play an important role in the management of patients who are obese, evidence suggests that they may, in themselves, hold strong negative attitudes about this group of patients. These judgments may impact the quality of the care provided [5–7]. In 2003, Schwartz et al. established that a high level of bias existed among healthcare professionals, whereby the stereotypes of obese individuals being lazy, stupid, and worthless were endorsed [8]. This bias extends to students-in-training for a range of obesity-related occupations within the health sector, including doctors, nurses, dietitians, psychologists, and

J. M. Kutzin et al. (eds.), *Comprehensive Healthcare Simulation: Nursing*, Comprehensive Healthcare Simulation,
https://doi.org/10.1007/978-3-031-31090-4_13

nutritionists, and may involve derogatory and cynical humor being directed at patients with obesity [9, 10].

What Was the Need?

Across the healthcare spectrum, university curricula for pre-licensure health professionals contain variable content around managing a patient with obesity. In addition, a recent meta-analysis of 17 studies concluded that there is a lack of research to reduce bias in health professionals around the stigma of weight [11]. Interprofessional education (IPE) and training are vital in relation to this aspect of healthcare, with the literature suggesting that even the words used during interactions with obese patients are important [5]. Given the incidence of obesity as a global health issue, we recognized the need to incorporate an IPE simulation to address the gap in this area of practice for healthcare professional students. This activity needed to align with and complement existing curricula, be a sustainable, repeatable educational activity that met the needs of interprofessional scopes of practice, and be delivered innovatively.

What Did We Do?

The project aimed to use a common case study to deliver and evaluate an IPE simulation-based learning activity related to specific care requirements for patients with obesity. Areas of interest were pre-licensure students' level of empathy in relation to the obese patients' social and functional health patterns and understanding of others' professional contributions to patient care. Pre-licensure students from four health professions (nursing, physiotherapy, occupational therapy, and radiation science) were the target group for this 12-month funded project. The choice of professions was based on convenience and the willingness of the faculty to extend and combine facets of existing simulation scenarios relating to interactions with, or care of, patients with obesity.

A layered approach to learning was used to develop the IPE simulation:

- a master case was created, merging information from four case studies;
- two audio-visual resources were created featuring an actor (the case patient) in an obesity suit;
- student surveys explored levels of empathy and readiness for IPE learning at various time points; and
- a voluntary, interactive IPE simulation activity was offered to all students, which featured the live 'patient.'

Creation of a Master Case: Justin Davies

The project team workshopped and merged existing case material into one master case study. Each faculty member incorporated relevant factors from their own scenarios into one master case study to maintain their profession-specific learning outcomes related to the care and management of a patient with obesity. The opening clinical context was kept fluid—either an emergency presentation to the hospital or inpatient case management within the first few days of hospital admission. The background and context of the patient were modified to ensure the credibility of care and treatment requirements to suit the learning needs of all four student groups.

Justin Davies became our master case study patient. In brief, *Justin* was a 55-year-old man, father to two children, recently divorced, and who lived alone. He was employed as a supermarket manager and enjoyed golf and computer games. Additional detail was provided to ensure adequate social and health contexts for all students, including his weight at 160 kg (nearly 353 pounds) and 175 cm tall (5 foot 9 inches). With a detailed backstory, two of the lead project team members briefed and worked with the actor to feature *Justin*, who then related his personal stories by adopting an interview approach (Fig. 13.1).

Creation of Audio-visual Resources

Health issues that *Justin* revealed in the simulated pre-hospital audio-visual (A.V.) clip (https://youtu.be/quGpKFbVrf4) included his diagnosis of diabetes, having to take time off work, social isolation, eating 'fast food' and not being able to exercise much, and a wound on his foot that was slow to heal. The latter was the reason for hospital admission. In the second simulated A.V. clip, just before being discharged home (https://youtu.be/a0ldPs0Wopw), *Justin* revealed the unexpected diagnosis of bowel cancer, which arose from other hospital test results. With limited mobility due to his foot wound, follow-up clinic visits, and preparation for bowel cancer treatment, *Justin* shared multiple concerns about coping independently after being discharged from the hospital.

Discipline-specific Simulations of the Master Case

The obesity simulation was introduced two years ago to 1st-year 1st-semester nursing students (undertaking a 3½ year Bachelor of Science (Nursing) degree). The same type of obesity suit was used in clinical laboratories, with a student volunteering to wear the suit to 'become the patient' in a hospital bed. The clinical focus was working and communicating with the patient about moving around and positioning in bed and specific skin care needs. The simulation aimed to prepare students for their first clinical experience, to enhance

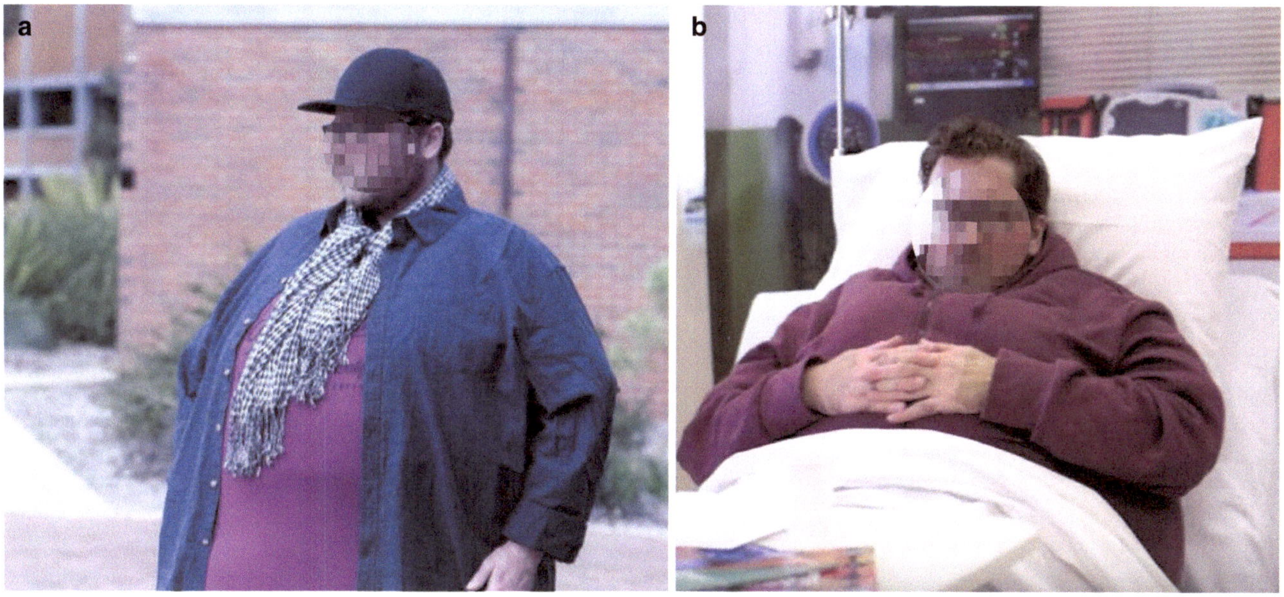

Fig. 13.1 (**a**) *Justin Davies* pre-hospital; (**b**) in hospital. Images reproduced with permission: Sources: Curtin University and The Experience Lab.

their understanding of obesity on patients' physical and psychological states, and the restrictions in undertaking activities of daily living.

For physiotherapy, the obesity simulation has also been incorporated into curricula for several years, targeting students in the 2nd year of a Bachelor's degree or in the 1st year of a graduate entry master (GEM) program. For these students, the focus was on patient mobility, positioning in bed, and ways to transfer the patient from bed to chair (and vice versa). Communication also featured within the context of difficult conversations related to strategies for weight loss and adopting a healthy lifestyle.

In Radiation Therapy (R.T.), treating patients with obesity with radiation therapy requires consideration of several aspects of practice. Maneuvering the patient onto a high, narrow, hard bed requires skill and tact, and ensuring that the position is reproducible over the course of several weeks is essential, with careful thought given to the placement of the positioning tattoos. First-year Bachelor's degree R.T. students were asked to start thinking about these aspects, with particular emphasis on safe manual handling, the communication skills required to deliver what could be very personal instructions to the patient, and professional communication within the team.

For Occupational Therapy (O.T.), an obesity simulation was incorporated into the curricula for the 2nd year Bachelor's program. Classroom activities were designed to provide students with information and practical activities to simulate the difficulties experienced (grooming, dressing, toileting, and showering) by people with bariatric needs. Opportunities were provided for students to modify these self-care activities to complete them independently, as well as the provision of assistive technology.

Delivery of the IPE Simulation

The IPE simulation was a culmination and coming together of all four student groups at a time point in the scenario where *Justin* was about to be discharged from the hospital. The activity was, in essence, *forum–theatre* involving the project team, students, and *Justin*, portrayed by the actor, who joined the session at a pre-determined time to field questions and provide feedback. A particular focus of the event was to portray the I.P. nature and person-centered approach to patient discharge planning.

Specific learning outcomes and objectives were set:

- To provide an opportunity for students to work collaboratively with students from other disciplines
- To increase understanding of how to deliver person-centered care
- To facilitate increased insight into some of the challenges for people with obesity
- To provide information about resources that may assist when working with larger people with co-morbidities

Format for the IPE simulation: students to work in small groups; expectations of students to be honest; to share ideas and opinions in a respectful way with the whole group; to ask for assistance if needed. The A.V. clip of *Justin* in the hospital was shown to all students to set the scene.

Case Conference

Each faculty member summarized what they had done with *Justin* thus far—the discipline-specific simulations. The aim was to role model each profession's discourse and offer insight into care responsibilities. *Justin* arrived and was seated alongside the faculty at the front of the stage. The last faculty member asked *Justin* if he had any questions, and he responded by addressing both students and faculty:

> "Over the last few weeks, you have addressed various aspects of my care and well-being. I do appreciate your support and expertise in helping me. I have a few questions that I would like to ask you all (addressing the students). I understand that some of the questions might be difficult for you to answer, but I only ask for honesty and respect. I notice that you have all been sorted into interprofessional healthcare teams, which is a great start. I encourage you all to work together to answer the questions."

In groups, students addressed one of *Justin's* comments and questions below:

> "While I have been in hospital, I have noticed how many different people work together in a healthcare team."

Question 1: What are some ways you communicate and work together to ensure you know what is happening with my care?

> "I am concerned about my outpatient appointments, especially my radiation therapy appointments. Sitting for long periods is painful; I have a lot to coordinate, and I can't walk very far."

Question 2: Can you suggest anything to help me address my concerns about outpatient care?"

"I hear people talking about me behind my back or to my face, and I am called the 'bariatric patient,' 'the morbidly obese man,'.... or worse. This makes me feel angry, embarrassed, and reluctant to ask for help. Sometimes I almost feel like health professionals are implying that it is my fault that I am unwell."

Question 3: What can you do to make me feel valued and listened to?

> "I am being discharged in a few days, and it seems like no one is listening to me what I say. I am worried about how I will manage at home alone."

Question 4: What can you do to help me manage better at home?

Each of the four I.P. groups had 10 minutes to consider and discuss one of the questions and then present their collective response to others in the room. A joint collegial discussion was facilitated by faculty for each question in turn, including ad-lib contributions from *Justin* himself. Faculty also addressed any other uncertainties or differences of opinion within groups.

Session Review by Staff

- Staff re-iterated what had been overheard in their group
- Re-visited learning objectives
- Useful resources were listed on the PowerPoint presentation (see resources at the end of the chapter)
- *Justin* concluded with a monologue (below), then left the lecture theatre

Justin's Closing Statement

> "Thank you all for coming today and for your honesty and respect. It has been very helpful for me to hear about your thoughts and perspectives, just as I hope it has been helpful for you to hear about things from my perspective. It is important to me that health professionals treat me as a person first before treating any of my illnesses. I don't want to be treated as an 'obese person'; I just want to be treated as a person. You may have even learned more about yourselves as future health practitioners by participating in these activities.
> When you work together as an interprofessional team, life is so much easier for me. I understand things more easily; I don't have to decide which profession's advice I want to follow, my care becomes more coordinated, and my quality of life starts to improve. When you all work together, I start to feel like the healthcare system cares about me and my well-being instead of just being another cog in the big health system machine.
> I really hope that the activities you have participated in today and throughout the semester have increased your understanding of interprofessional care and encouraged you to lead with empathy. You, as our future health professionals, have so much opportunity to transform the lives of others and communities. Thank you".

What Was the Impact?

From 'meeting' *Justin* within each profession's laboratory classes and working through individual learning objectives, the added pre-hospital A.V. clip of *Justin brought the case study to life*. The second A.V. clip was purposely used during the I.P. simulation as an introduction to the 'live patient' and consolidated the case study presentation by *Justin* relaying his concerns about going home. These layering and connecting learning strategies saw students develop a therapeutic alliance with *Justin*. They understood the level of empathy for the patient; developed a context of interprofessional practice and the contribution of each profession to the overall patient journey. The added psychosocial contexts within *Justin's* case study, in particular overhearing others talk about him in the doctor's waiting room, taught students to be more aware of the person's experience and the impact of their experiences on them.

Students were engaged, and the insights they developed went beyond the patient context to the I.P. dimension. Some examples of student feedback:

I particularly liked [when] *we talked about obesity and did the simulation on treating bariatric patients.*

I didn't know the difference between an O.T. and a Physio; now I do.

Students also recognized the value and relevance of the non-compulsory I.P. learning component:

[the] *Obesity sim was great—I would suggest making the adjunct obesity workshop compulsory.*

The IPE simulation surfaced assumptions and biases about people with obesity but extended to other patients with perceived disabilities. Indeed, the concept of 'disability' was raised and discussed. The scenario triggered the emotional aspects of learning in the context of the case study. Through small groups and facilitated discussions, students became more attuned to the role, responsibility, and contributions each discipline offered to health consumers. The focus on patient discharge and being more attuned to promotion of patient self-care highlighted to students the often forgotten patient issues related to mobility and independence.

What Lessons Were Learned?

We learned that prelicensure healthcare training could model interprofessional collaboration. In this project, a group of motivated facilitators from different professions created a bespoke activity that served both the discrete learning outcomes of each craft group as well as the collective outcomes serving the delivery of interprofessional patient-centered care. This was achieved by adapting a master case for each profession's educational needs and massaging these composite narratives into one patient journey that culminated in a discussion around their discharge from inpatient hospital care. In this discharge planning space, synergies were identified between groups, and common and overlapping goals were evident.

We overcame scheduling issues by successfully vertically integrating the simulation activity. This was achieved through the sequestration of common free time at a University level, as well as the commitment of all groups to making it work.

We also learned that having students from each craft group with variable levels of training within their specialties—that is, they were at different levels within their course—did not impede the learning process. In fact, it provided a richness that contributed to the interprofessional learning whereby students either felt confident to speak up or were satisfied to learn from their clinically more experienced interprofessional peers. That said, the guidance provided by the faculty ensured oversight such that each professional group was represented in interprofessional discussions.

Key Points

- The literature suggests health professionals lack empathy for people with obesity.
- Empathy may be enhanced through experiential simulation-based activities
- Interprofessional activities may enhance pre-licensure healthcare provider empathy

Case Study 2: United Kingdom

Author: Gary Francis
Title: Introducing a new simulation for first-year Bachelor of Science (Hons) and Postgraduate Diploma Pre-Registration Nursing students
Location: London South Bank University, Institute of Health & Social Care, United Kingdom.

Background

In the United Kingdom (U.K.), registered nursing education and training programs are only run at approved educational institutions. Courses usually take a minimum of three years, e.g., the Bachelor of Science (BSc) (Hons), although condensed entry routes are available which take into account previous learning and life experience, e.g., the two-year Postgraduate Diploma (PgDip) [12]. Learning through simulation is fundamental to pre-registration nursing education and training in the U.K. The Nursing and Midwifery Council (NMC) define simulation as 'an artificial representation of a real-world practice scenario that supports student development through experiential learning with the opportunity for repetition, feedback, evaluation and reflection. Effective simulation facilitates safety by enhancing knowledge, behaviors, and skills [12].

The 2018 Nursing and Midwifery Council 'Future Nurse: Standards of Proficiency for Registered Nurses' removed the 300 hour cap on simulation activities, allowing more hours to be used provided program outcomes were met, and these hours could count towards the required clinical practice hours [12]. The European Parliament and Council Directive 2005/36/EC states: Clinical training is that part of nurse training in which trainee nurses learn, as part of a team and in 'direct contact with a healthy or sick individual in hospital and/or community' [12]. This stipulation makes a clear distinction in how simulation can be used in terms of augmenting the 2300 h of "theory" or attributed towards the 2300 h of "practice" time (NMC, 2018). Francis [13] suggests this is an opportunity to re-think delivery in how simulation can support theory and practice. As the pressure on placement capacity in the U.K. grows, the simulation may need to form a new and expanding role in providing robust simulated placement experiences for the development of pre-registration nursing student's clinical skills [13].

What Was the Need?

SBE has previously taken place in the second year of the (BSc and PgDip) and the third year of the (BSc) programs as part of theory modules. Included were a variety of manikin scenarios, including medical/surgical and critical care presentations such as hypovolemia, sepsis, respiratory failure, and emergency situations featuring increasing complexity and challenge. The initiative reported here was to bring forward and introduce SBE into year one of the programs, to combine and consolidate standard skills with a simulation scenario to prepare students for their first practice experience. These were new SBE hours added to the curriculum. McNamara [14] identified the importance of preparing first-year students for clinical practice. Doolen et al. [15] also discussed preparing students early within their program through the use of simulation. Familiarising students with SBE about what to expect is an important step in gaining buy-in, and for learners to become comfortable and engaged, so they appreciate SBE as a valued approach to applying clinical learning [16].

To ensure we situated the simulation to include 'real people' and for it to count towards 'practice' hours, we looked to develop a scenario inclusive of a simulated participant. Simulated participants (SPs) are people who are trained, and coached to act as real people presenting with realistic patient presentations [17, 18]. By engaging service users, students from the drama school, students from other fields of healthcare professions, or fellow academics to role-play the different parts, we were able to cost-effectively replicate a real-to-life scenario.

We also aimed to focus the SBE on teaching fundamental skills for nursing practice. Blows [19] highlights, as a fundamental part of safe nursing practice, the importance of understanding, competently measuring, and interpreting vital signs as an indication of the patient's physiological state. The NMC [12] clearly states that this is a fundamental skill that needs to be acquired. Francis and O'Brien [20] suggest that for novice learners becoming familiar with these skills can be challenging, both in terms of perfecting the physical skill and also knowing how and when to deploy these in clinical practice. A scoping review by Kunst et al. [21] indicated that nursing is not only about theory and acquiring psychomotor skills but how theory and skills are applied in a practice context in a supported and developmental way. They suggest that structured simulations play a critical part in supporting learners in this regard.

What Did We Do?

Francis and O'Brien [20] suggest a range of approaches to teaching clinical skills and simulated activity incorporating: virtual, blended, and face-to-face activities. However, in line with our current university approach, students were prepared using a Hybrid Learning Model (HLM). Our cohort consisted of some complete novices and other students with more healthcare experience from paid work. Marshall [22] describes the HLM as engaging students in a combination of ways, including remote synchronous delivery as well as asynchronous activity, and can also incorporate face-to-face delivery. Preparatory theory lectures were synchronously delivered via the university's virtual learning environment (VLE), thus creating consistent delivery for all. Bovill et al. [23] acknowledge the benefits of such delivery. Forums were used for students to communicate with each other and for the skills teaching team to engage in supporting students in their self-assessment and formative assessment tasks. Prior to attending the clinical skill sessions, students attended virtual workshops focused on good communication with patients and clients. To practice the psychomotor skills, students rotated around face-to-face skills stations, which included: basic patient assessment—*look, listen, smell, feel.* Temperature, pulse, blood pressure, respiratory rate, pulse oximetry, an alert, verbal, pain, and unresponsive (AVPU) score, using the National Early Warning Scoring Version 2 (NEWS-2) chart (RCP, 2017) and creating a handover using Situation, Background, Assessment and Recommendation (SBAR) [24]. Students were then invited back in groups of five to run through a patient simulation. Preparation included watching an online video introducing the concept of simulation, what to expect, and participant psychological safety within the simulation. Students were also able to access a video pre-brief online, which included the scenario, the wider context, and behavior expectations for the simulation.

To help students begin to systematically and critically examine all aspects of their thinking and actions, the *Clinical Reasoning Cycle* was introduced [25]. This model provided a framework through which the SBE activity could be structured and explored, as well as acting as a tool to help students clinically reason in their ongoing practice. Hunter and Arthur [26] advocate the use of such models, from novice to experienced learners, as the level at which concepts are explored can be made incrementally more complex.

Clinical Reasoning as a Framework

The simulation was divided into three parts using the *Clinical Reasoning Cycle* as a structure. Each part was timed and represented 60 min of activity:

Box 13.1 Outline of Year 1 Simulation ActivitiesS

Part 1	**Students meet the patient (15 min)**, consider the patient's situation, collect cues, process information, and identify problems or issues.
Part 2	Students discuss a proposed care plan with the clinical supervisor (15 min), *establish goals, take action, and evaluate outcomes (possible).*
Part 3	Students debrief with a facilitator (30 min), *reflect on the process and new learning*

Our S.P. scenario was gender-dependent on who could portray the patient's role. The S.P. was always briefed before the day and then briefed again on the day. The scenario was set in the simulated ward with the patient in bed, wearing a gown an I.D. band, and a nasal cannula. To illustrate, one scenario featured a 55-year-old patient who had just been admitted to the medical ward with shortness of breath and breathing difficulties.

For part 1, students in groups of five were asked by their clinical supervisor to welcome the patient to the ward, undertake a basic assessment, and take a set of baseline vital signs. Students needed to demonstrate a professional approach towards the patient and each other, during which they were required to perform an initial assessment of the patient, using appropriate questioning and explanations. As a group, they had fifteen minutes to decide how to approach and allocate tasks. They were to demonstrate the correct technique for taking manual vital signs, after which they were given a set of case-specific pre-determined vital signs to record on the NEWS-2 chart. Next, they were to correctly calculate the NEWS-2 score and prepare an SBAR communication tool handover to their clinical supervisor. Once they had done so, they moved to part 2 to discuss the findings with their clinical supervisor. Information the students had to convey included: vital signs, the NEWS-2 score, their impressions of the patient, and, depending on their questioning, the patient's back story and recent medical history. With the support of the clinical supervisor, the students were encouraged to interpret the vital sign measurements, the NEWS-2 score, and the circumstances and then propose a plan of care. In part 3, students debriefed their experiences with the facilitator. This space allowed students to reflect on their experience and their performance and to discuss the challenges and the perspectives of all included participants.

The S.P. (out of role) also provided feedback to the students about interactions. This provided valuable insight for all groups of students. The students then reflected on their learning and how to take that forward. The facilitator helped to scaffold further learning activities, which included revisiting either skill techniques, certain aspects of the theoretical underpinning, or looking more widely at the immediate and longer-term care of the patient.

What Was the Impact?

This was the first time the historically separate skills sessions were incorporated into a simulation to consolidate learning. Despite being nervous, students enjoyed applying the skills they had learned in the preceding weeks. They valued being asked to prepare for a scenario which could easily be something they would face on day one of their first placement. For some, the scenario felt strange in that they were talking to a 'pretend' patient, but for others, it was a good way to build confidence. Students highly valued the opportunity to practice a handover to a 'clinical supervisor' and experience the types of discussions that might be expected of them in the clinical setting. Students felt comfortable and generally well-prepared for the simulation. Several students mentioned they enjoyed working as a team in the scenario. However, some students with prior healthcare experience said that aspect was not as realistic.

In terms of learning, students recognized how the experience challenged their theory, optimized their skills practice, and, most importantly, prepared them for clinical practice. Students felt they gained an insight into what being a 'real' nurse would be like, especially when the S.P. shared their personal experiences with them. During the debrief, students talked about working as a team and the importance of identifying a leader. The academics reported high levels of student engagement. They felt it was a good way to bring the skills together. While the use of the virtual learning environment was challenging at times, the value was seen in ensuring the delivery of consistent theory to all students, with forum posts being an interesting way of capturing students' thoughts and assessing understanding. Academics also commented on a sense of team working among students and on good professional communication skills. Academics felt that while the time invested in preparing and delivering the SBE was significant, it was justified by the obvious benefits and engagement of the students.

What Were the Lessons Learned?

The benefit of introducing a new simulation for first-year nursing students was to integrate the teaching of psychomotor skills with communication and teamwork skills. The simulation experience also introduced the structured 'observer role' described by O'Regan et al. [27], which enhanced opportunities for student participation and self and peer critique. Working with S.P.s provided added benefit in enabling first-year student nurses to have an authentic interaction experience as their introduction to SBE. The clinical reasoning cycle provided a structured process for discussing and determining nursing care. Hunter and Arthur [26] comment that the C.R. cycle is a way of unpacking simple to complex concepts that allow students to discuss and reflect upon their actions in both simulation and in their forthcoming practice. Introducing clinical reasoning and critical thinking skills early in our course provided structure to student's thinking which assisted in the development of their problem-solving and decision-making abilities—an important aspect in the delivery of open-minded, safe, and holistic care [25]. This format has been used to expand and develop other fundamental skills training in an applied way. The HLM of delivery enabled us to standardize theory and ensured a consistent approach across the different student groups. It also provided a repository for the pre and post-simulation activities and engaged both students and staff in a new and different way.

Key Points

- Providing psychomotor skills within an applied context is important preparation for year one student nurses before their first clinical placement experience
- Working with S.P.s is a good way to introduce novice learners to simulation without overloading them
- Using a model such as the clinical reasoning cycle helps guide and promote a deeper level of student thinking

Case Study: Norway

Author: Sissel Eikeland Husebø

Title: Evaluation of a simulation-based course in clinical facilitation

Location: Faculty of Health Sciences, University of Stavanger and Department of Surgery, Stavanger University Hospital, Stavanger, Norway.

Background

The Bachelor of Nursing program in Norway is a 3-year program at universities or regional colleges and includes both theoretical and clinical learning components. The structure and content of nursing education is regulated by the Norwegian Ministry of Education [28]. Clinical placement studies in Norwegian Bachelor of Nursing programs account for fifty percent and comprise clinical studies in, for example, hospital surgical units and is emphasized as an important learning arena for nursing students. During clinical placements, clinical facilitators have responsibilities for facilitating nursing students [28] despite many of these nurses having no preparation for the educative role [29]. The quality of the relationship between the nursing student and the clinical facilitator directly affects the student outcome [30–32].

What Was the Need?

Clinical facilitators usually need as much support as the students, finding it difficult to manage and complete a workload and support student learning [33, 34]. The clinical facilitator role lacks clarity, so the facilitators need to reflect on how they approach facilitation in clinical learning environments [35]. There is also a need to improve consistency in clinical practices between the nursing education institution and the clinical learning environment to support students' adaptation to clinical practice [36]. Clinical facilitators have a significant role in providing effective educational and clinical experiences [37]. Therefore, clinical facilitators must strive to develop their knowledge and clinical educational skills according to student's needs in the clinical settings. Academic, professional preparation for clinical facilitators and good collaboration between faculty and clinical facilitators in the clinical setting should be prioritized to develop clinical facilitating skills [38].

Strategies that will help to develop clinical facilitators' skills and ensure quality clinical experiences for undergraduate nursing students include educational support and mentoring from more experienced clinical facilitators [39]. Important factors identified in effective clinical teaching indicate that facilitators foster meaningful learning using active strategies and meet individual students' needs at each program level [40].

Simulation is a learner-active method that is effective in learning both "technical and non-technical" skills in healthcare [41]. Simulation is defined as "A technique that creates a situation or environment to allow persons to experience a representation of a real event for the purpose of practice, learning, evaluation, testing, or to gain understanding of systems or human actions" [42]. The methods comprise three phases: Briefing, scenario simulation, and debriefing (guided reflection) [43]. To our knowledge, this is the first time that simulation has been used to improve clinical facilitation skills. We developed and evaluated a simulation-based course in clinical facilitation for nursing student facilitators.

What Did We Do?

The simulation-based facilitation course was a one-day (8-h) course based on didactic theory [44] and simulation principles [43]. In the planning phase, the faculty developed the course content, including the following learning objectives:

After completion of the course, the clinical facilitators will:

- Be aware of how facilitation styles influence students' learning in clinical practice
- Reflect on and make changes in one's own facilitation style when supervising nursing students
- Support colleagues in improvement of facilitation of nursing students in clinical practice

Two weeks before the course started, the participants received the course material via email. In the course introduction, a booklet with the Model of Practical Skill Performance [45], Gibb's Reflective cycle [46] and clinical evaluation templates from the University of Stavanger Bachelor of Nursing program was distributed to the participants. On the morning of the course day, the faculty provided a short oral introduction of the educational material and the simulation scenarios. The participants engaged in the following five simulation scenarios during the course:

Table 13.1 Characteristics of the respondents ($N = 29$)

Variable	Category	*n* (%)
Gender		
	Female	29 (100)
Age		
	≤21–30 years	23 (79)
	31–40 years	5 (17)
	≥40 years	1 (3)
Have you previously completed any clinical facilitation courses?		
	Yes	14 (48)
	No	15 (52)
How do you assess your clinical facilitation skills?		
	Slightly good	1 (3)
	Moderately good	17 (60)
	Good	9 (31)
	Very good	1 (3)
	Missing	1 (3)
Experience with clinical facilitation of nursing students?		
	Yes	21 (72)
	No	8 (28)
If "Yes," have you facilitated nursing students within the last 6 months? ($n = 21$)		
	Yes	20 (95)
	No	1 (5)
If "Yes," have you facilitated nursing students in the last year? ($n = 21$)		
	Yes	20 (95)
	No	1 (5)

- The clinical facilitator and the nursing students planning the schedule of the shift
- Facilitation of inserting a urinary catheter into a female patient in bed
- Evaluating the nursing students' skill performance using the Model of Practical Skill Performance [45]
- Facilitation of caring for a female patient in bed
- Evaluating the nursing student's performance during the shift

During the scenarios, the participants rotated as clinical facilitators, nursing students, and observers. The observers were present in the simulation room during the scenarios, observing one learning objective each. The faculty used the Gibb's Reflective cycle [46] as the debriefing model. Gibbs proposes that reflection takes place after an experience and that the cycle provides a structure that generally guides the process of reflecting. Gibb's Reflective cycle consists of cue questions based on key concepts and provides a checklist for learners to work through, answering and considering the cue questioning as they progress [47]. The reflective cycle focuses on learning from experiences by involving feelings, thoughts, and recommendations for future actions. The reflective process follows the six stages of the model (description, feelings, evaluation, analysis, conclusion, and action plan), with each step informing the next.

What Was the Impact?

Evaluation (The Questionnaire)

The didactic model of relation guided the design of the questionnaire [44] (Fig. 13.2). The questionnaire encompassed the six factors described in *the didactic model of relation*: learner expectation and assumptions, learning objectives, content and material, learning process and methods, and assessment. All factors are mutually dependent; changes in one feature will have consequences for the other features. The questionnaire included ten items: eight required a response based on a 5-point Likert scale from 'strongly agree' to 'strongly disagree,' and one item with response options from 'very satisfactory' to 'very unsatisfactory.' The last question included the response option 'yes' or 'no.' The last part of the questionnaire included three open-end questions: (1) What is your experience of attending the clinical facilitation course? (2) What was positive about the course? (3) Do you have any suggestions for improvement of the course? Additionally, background information regarding the clinical facilitators' age, gender, experience with the facilita-

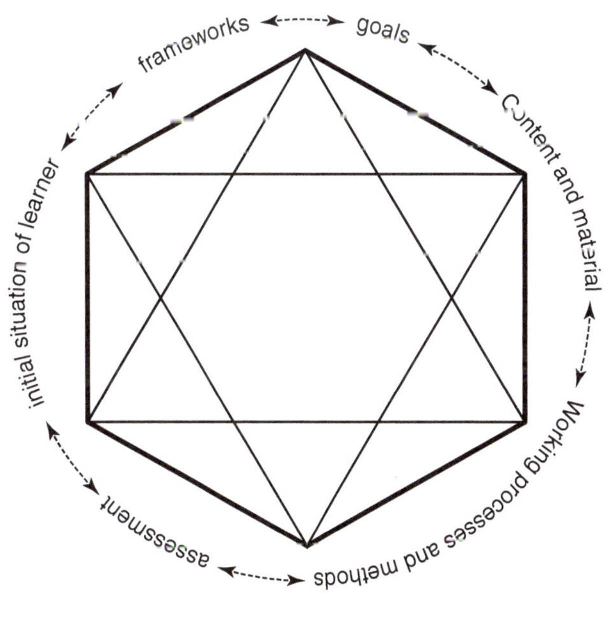

Fig. 13.2 The didactic model of relation [44]—reproduced with permission

tion of nursing students, and their assessment of their own clinical facilitator skills was collected.

Findings and Insights

Characteristics of the nurses. Characteristics of the respondents are shown in Table 13.1. All participants were female nurses, and the majority were between 21 and 30 years. Only half of the nurses had previously attended a clinical facilitation course.

Evaluation Ratings.

The majority of nurses (58.6% strongly agree and 41.4% slightly agree) reported that the facilitator course met their expectations, was motivating (75.9% strongly agree and 24.1% slightly agree), achieved the learning objectives (48.3% strongly agree and 41.4% slightly agree), and the course content was relevant to their role as clinical facilitators (89.7% strongly agree and 10.3% slightly agree) (Table 13.2). The nurses perceived simulation of clinical facilitating situations as an appropriate method (62.1% strongly agree and 37.9% slightly agree) and the discussion and reflection after the simulated facilitation scenarios were very instructive (75.9% strongly agree and 20.7% slightly agree). Additionally, they responded that the course provided several tools that would be useful in facilitation of nursing students (79.3% strongly agree and 20.7% slightly agree) and that the duration and scope of the course was sufficient to learn new facilitation skills (55.2% strongly agree and 37.9% slightly agree). The results also showed that most nurses were satisfied with the course (44.8% very satisfactory and 55.2% satisfactory) and recommended the course to peers (93.1% yes).

Three open-ended questions asked facilitators to express their views about the course. Three themes were revealed: "Instructive and useful," "Joint reflection and discussion," and "Role clarification and too lengthy."

Instructive and Useful

The nurses experienced the clinical facilitator course as a good learning experience, making them think about improving their facilitator skills. One nurse wrote: "Very instructive in relation to how I can improve my facilitator skills. By doing the course through simulation, it helped me highlight the course objectives" (participant 24). The nurses perceived the course as a sufficient basis for clinical facilitation and the tools as useful in facilitating nursing students. For instance,

Table 13.2 Nurses' perspectives of the simulation-based clinical facilitation course ($n = 29$)

Items	Strongly agree (5) %	Slightly agree (4) %	Neither agree nor disagree (3) %	Slightly disagree (2) %	Strongly disagree (1) %	Mean ± SD
1. The clinical facilitation course met my expectations.	58.6	41.4				4.59 ± 0.50
2. It was motivating to attend the clinical facilitation course.	75.9	24.1				4.76 ± 0.43
3. I achieved the learning objectives of the course.	48.3	41.4	10.6			4.38 ± 0.67
4. The content of the course was very relevant to my role as a clinical facilitator.	89.7	10.3				4.90 ± 0.31
5. Simulation of facilitation situations was an appropriate method to use in the course.	62.1	37.9				4.62 ± 0.49
6. The discussion and reflection after the simulated facilitation situations were very instructive for my role as clinical facilitator.	75.9	20.7	3.4			4.72 ± 0.52
7. The clinical facilitator course provided several tools that will be useful when I facilitate nursing students.	79.3	20.7				4.79 ± 0.41
8. The duration and scope of the course were sufficient to learn new clinical facilitation skills.	55.2	37.9	6.9			4.48 ± 0.63
	Very satisfactory (1) %	Satisfactory (2) %	Moderately satisfactory (3) %	Unsatisfactory (2) %	Very unsatisfactory (1) %	
9. How would you evaluate the clinical facilitation course you attended today?	44.8	55.2				4.45 ± 0.50
	Yes %	No %	Missing %			
10. Would you recommend the clinical facilitation course to other nurses?	93.1		6.9			

one nurse stated: "It was useful with tools to evaluate students and that they can evaluate themselves" (participant 41). Some participants experienced the feeling of being in challenging facilitation situations during the scenarios and developing strategies to manage the situations. The introduction of facilitating a pair of students at the same time was new to some participants, as one nurse wrote: "I have been a clinical facilitator for a long time but have not had two students at the same time. In this course, I have learned what it is like to have two students at the same time and how I can guide them" (participant 35).

Joint Reflection and Discussion

Another strength of the course identified by nurses was the opportunity to share their experiences with peers, discuss common challenges in facilitating, and have reflections that provided new insight. One nurse expressed that the course contributed with "A lot of good reflection that has led to better insight into the facilitator role. Several "a-ha" experiences and good faculty of the course" (participant 44). Some participants appreciated the post-scenario reflections where they could pick up good advice from peers and faculty, as expressed by one nurse: "Good reflections, got tips on how to facilitate students" (participant 40). Another nurse wrote: "Fine with good reflections after simulation. Good tips from more experienced clinical facilitators" (participant 15).

Role Clarification and Too Lengthy

The nurses suggested some improvement issues for the course. Their suggestions included more comprehensive instruction before the scenarios regarding the student roles and their level of knowledge and skills, and the post scenario reflections and discussions were too long. They would rather prefer shorter and more scenarios. One nurse wrote: "More short simulations with fast and efficient feedback" (participant 32). When it came to role clarification, several participants experienced that it was difficult to be in the student role and suggested that they should be more prepared before the scenarios, as illustrated in the following quote: "Could have been assigned more specific roles for the students to create better discussions and reflections" (participant 31).

Lessons Learned

The majority of nurses were very satisfied with the clinical facilitation course. Most nurses responded that the course improved their facilitator skills. Combined evaluation feedback revealed that the discussion and reflection after the simulated scenarios were very instructive and useful and that the course provided several tools that would be helpful in facilitation of nursing students. The course also provided new insights into the clinical facilitator role. The course faculty has to consider the nurses' suggestions for improvement regarding student role clarity and the length of the discussions and reflections.

Key Points

- Clinical facilitators need more preparation for the educative role
- Simulation might be an appropriate method to improve clinical facilitation skills
- The evaluation provided promising results that undertaking a clinical facilitator course can improve nurses' ability to facilitate nursing students in clinical practice

Acknowledgments
The author acknowledges Bente D. Rossavik, Head of the Nursing Service, Department of Surgery, clinical facilitator and registered nurse Ellen Synnøve Strandberg, Vibeke Torkelsen, and Hilde Gunn Gjesteland Ims, Stavanger University Hospital, for their contribution to development and implementation of the clinical facilitator course. SEH thanks the nurses who willingly participated in the study.

Case Study: South Korea

Author: Yun Kang
Title: The Interprofessional Team-based High-fidelity Simulation Education
Location: College of Nursing, Taegu Science University, South Korea

Background

In today's constantly changing healthcare environment, patients have complex health-related needs and require collaborative healthcare to address these needs [48]. Interprofessional collaboration can improve care for patients with complex health-related needs, which positively affects their outcomes, such as decreased length of hospital stay, increased satisfaction, and reduced healthcare costs [49, 50]. Despite the benefits of interprofessional collaboration, healthcare professionals lack an understanding of their own and others' roles and do not communicate effectively in providing healthcare [50, 51]. Despite many factors contributing to interprofessional collaboration, the siloed approach in undergraduate health professions education and a lack of training in interprofessional collaboration are considered the foremost factor affecting interprofessional collaboration [52]. Thus, interprofessional education (IPE) among undergraduate health professions students is needed to practice and develop interprofessional competencies for future collaborative healthcare practice before graduation.

IPE in undergraduate health professions programs is the process where two or more professions students learn with, from, and about each other to understand roles and collaboration, enhance communication, and improve patient outcomes [50, 53]. In the United States (U.S.), the Interprofessional Education Collaborative (IPEC) Expert Panel has developed the four core competencies necessary for effective interprofessional collaboration. These include value/ethics for interprofessional practice, roles and responsibilities, interprofessional communication, and teams and teamwork, which needs to be strengthened all together rather than as one of the core competencies of IPE [53, 54].

Recently, simulation education has become a favorite type of IPE [55, 56] in undergraduate health professions programs and helps develop interprofessional teamwork and communication [50, 57]. Interprofessional team-based simulation education can provide a realistic educational approach and standardized experience using simulation modalities and clinical scenarios designed to increase interprofessional collaborative practice [58, 59]. It allows students from two or more health professions to practice together and then reflect on their collaborative practice, such as teamwork and communication skills, by creating clinical situations in a simulated environment [59].

What Was the Need?

The interprofessional simulation-based education (IPSE) in undergraduate health professions programs shows positive outcomes on undergraduate students' interprofessional competencies, such as interprofessional communication and teamwork, and their affective behaviors, such as increased self-efficacy [55]. Despite the rapid increase of the IPSE in Western countries such as the US, Canada, and Australia and these positive findings, IPSE is still relatively new in South Korea.

In South Korea, undergraduate health professions students, particularly nursing students, have increasingly limited practical experience in hospital settings. Due to the legal and safety concerns in hospital settings, they are not encouraged to actively participate in patient care during the clinical practicum and are not directly involved in patient care as a member of healthcare team [55, 56]. Nursing students also have clinical practicums in a hierarchical, medically dominated hospital structure where physicians focus on biomedical treatment, seeing registered nurses (RNs) focus on medical treatment and follow the physician's perspective. In this healthcare management structure, R.N.s at the bedside usually prioritize skilled nursing procedures that support medical treatment and do not have opportunities for participating in clinical decision-making. In addition, nursing has remained a predominantly female occupation, perpetuating societal stereotypes about women. In the traditional patriarchal society of South Korea and other Asian countries, the woman's role is confined to things that are 'soft and mild.' Hence the image of nurses is linked with concepts of love, care and sacrifice. Thus, IPSE in undergraduate health professions programs, particularly nursing, is needed to address these gaps by promoting students' active involvement in patient care and enhancing interprofessional collaboration as a healthcare team member in a realistic, safe, simulated environment.

What Did We Do?

The IPSE program proceeded through five phases: (1) agreement between the College of Nursing Taegu Science University and the School of Medicine, Ajou University; (2) analysis on the education condition; (3) IPSE program design and development; (4) IPSE program implementation; and (5) IPSE program evaluation (Fig. 13.3).

Educational Exchange Agreement

Leadership at the College of Nursing Taegu Science University and School of Medicine, Ajou University recognized the importance of interprofessional collaboration and for their students to receive an IPSE experience in undergraduate health education programs so that they can perform interprofessional collaboration when they enter the workplace. A decision was made to provide IPSE opportunities for their nursing and medical students.

Six months prior to the IPSE program implementation, we signed an educational exchange agreement to prepare for the IPSE program, considering the academic schedule of nursing and medical students. In order to develop the IPSE scenario template, we identified and adopted the framework of the IPEC core competencies [53, 54]. We met to discuss implementing the interprofessional team-based simulation education using high-fidelity simulators. Then we formed three teams (i.e., two nursing and two medicine faculty members per team) to develop three modules.

Analysis of the Education Condition

We examined the existing nursing and medical students' simulation learning experience to serve as a basis for developing the IPSE program. Nursing students experienced three high fidelity simulator (HFS)-based courses and completed a 20-week clinical practicum for adult, child, women's health, mental health and community health nursing. Before this

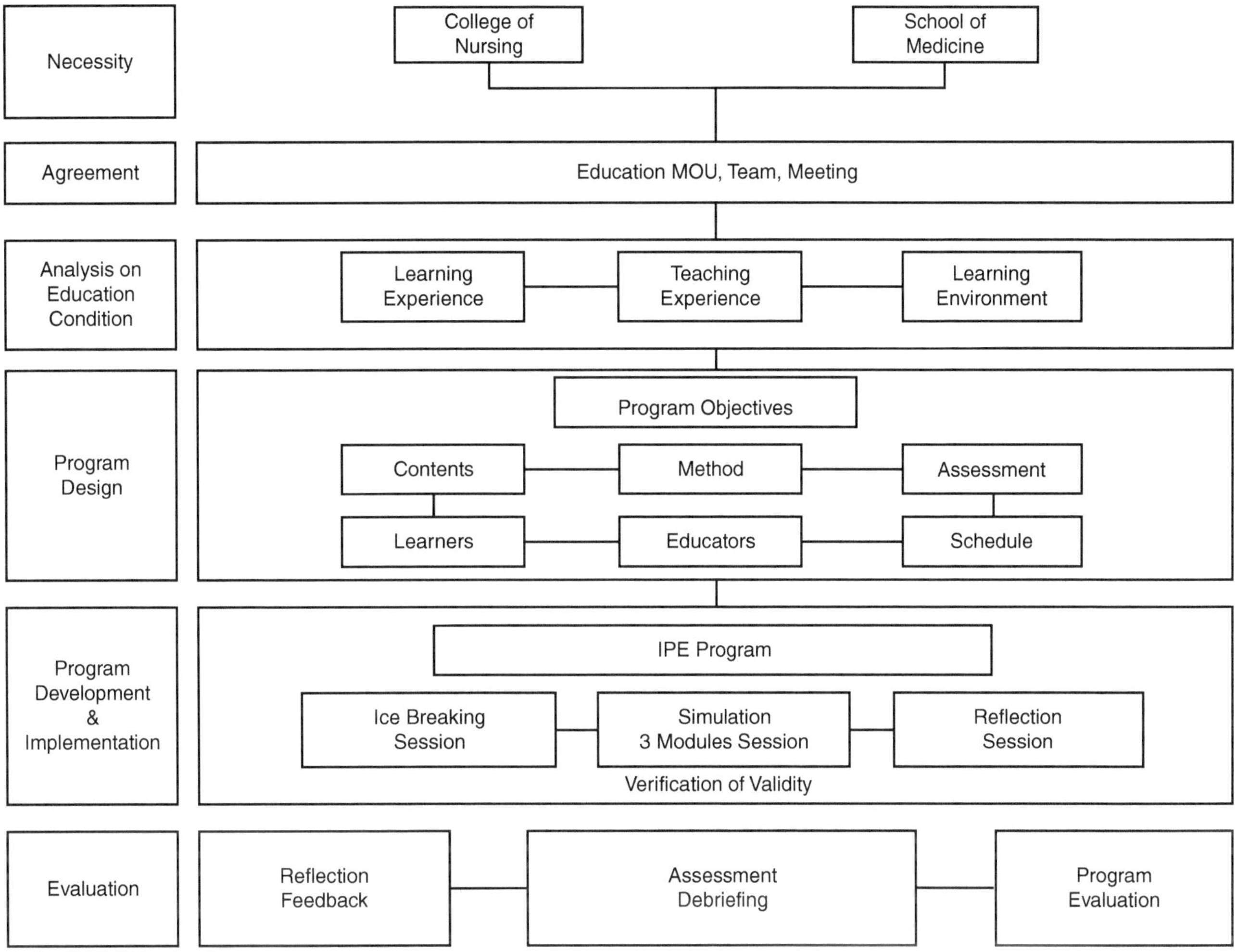

Fig. 13.3 Development and Implementation Process of IPSE Program

program, medical students did not experience HFS-based courses and completed a 36 week clerkship for internal medicine, surgery, pediatrics, obstetrics and gynecology, and psychiatry. Both student groups had not received a formalized IPSE program.

Regarding nursing and medicine faculty facilitators' simulation experiences, all faculty members had more than one semester of simulation experience. One medicine faculty member had simulation experience, and the other five had received formal simulation training. Before implementing the IPSE program, a one-hour facilitator training for the IPSE program was conducted. A guide for facilitators in each IPSE module was provided, including the learning objectives, plan, descriptions of scenarios, and debriefing methods.

Considering adequate rooms and facilities able to accommodate a large number of nursing and medical students, faculty, and staff, it was decided to implement the IPSE program at the nursing simulation center, College of Nursing Taegu Science University.

IPSE Program Design

The IPSE program, specifically designed for undergraduate nursing and medical students, consisted of an introduction, ice breaking and patient safety activities, three IPSE modules, and reflection sessions (Table 13.3).

The program objectives were to develop teamwork and communication skills, increase awareness around healthcare provider error prevention, understand other professional roles, improve interprofessional collaboration and develop clinical performance. Each team discussed the learning objectives for their IPSE module that focused on interprofessional collaborative practice in clinical scenarios regarding deteriorating patients. We created module learning objectives based on three domains of learning: knowledge, skills and attitudes, considering the levels of 4th-year nursing students and 3rd-year medical students. The clinical scenarios consisted of chest pain management in an adult male with acute myocardial infarction, febrile seizure management in a child, and postpartum bleeding management after vaginal delivery using the IPSE scenario template. We then reviewed,

Table 13.3 Design of the program

Session	Session I			Session II	Session III		Session IV	
Method	Puzzle Game	Room of Errors	Reflection	O.T.	Simulation		Reflection	Closing
Online	5 Group X 2Room	4Group X 3Room	Reflection on Session I	Introduction	Module I 4 Group X 2Room Module II	Module I 4 Group X 2Room Module1 II	Reflection on Program	Commencement Ceremony
Pre-requisite Learning	4Group X 3Room	3Group X 4Room			3 Group X 2 Room Module III 4 Group X 2Room	4 Group X 2Room Module III 3 Group X 2Room		
Run time	30 min	30 min	30 min	20 min	240 min	240 min	40 min	20 min

discussed, and refined these scenarios within each module team until an agreement was reached (Table 13.4)

IPSE Program Development and Implementation

The two-day IPSE program was conducted over two days. One week prior to the IPSE program implementation, pre-study resources on three IPSE modules were given to all nursing and medical students. One student group consisted of two nursing students and two medical students, which resulted in a total of 21 groups.

The IPSE program began with the facilitators using introduction and ice-breaking activities to build a sense of community and shared purpose. Ice-breaking activities included puzzle games in which the student group had to find the missing puzzle piece to win the game. Patient safety activities were then provided to the student groups who had to identify risk factors in surgical or medical patients in simulated environments.

During the IPSE session, each student group was led by one nursing facilitator and one medical facilitator. All nursing and medical students in the groups engaged in role-play and then as observers. While one student group (i.e., 2 medical students and 2 nursing students) took the role play at one time, the next student group observed the scene in person. The IPSE session used a five-step model: pre-briefing, pre-scenario activities, task training, simulation running, and debriefing. Each IPSE module session took 4 h, and all students in the groups participated in two IPSE module sessions (Table 13.5).

IPSE Program Evaluation

At the end of the IPSE program, all students gathered together in one place for a more thorough debriefing and reflection session about their IPSE experience that was co-facilitated by nursing and medical faculty.

What Was the Impact?

Nursing and medical students who participated in the IPSE reported positive experiences, positive learning outcomes, and benefits to patients of interprofessional collaborative practice. Nursing students reported that the IPSE experience helped them understand their own and medical professions' roles and responsibilities in providing patient care. As a healthcare team member, it may contribute to interprofessional collaborative practice in providing health care. Medical students expressed the value of simulation activities incorporated into the IPE. Before this program, medical students had not experienced HFS-based courses, although they were in year 3 of their studies. Medical students learned how to work together with other team members in the simulated clinical situations. It allowed them to do hands-on practice of clinical skills in a safe, realistic environment [55, 56]. They could also receive valuable and sincere feedback from nursing and medicine faculty facilitators and peers during the debriefing sessions [60]. These outcomes showed that the use of HFS in IPE provided the benefits of simulation for undergraduate medical and nursing students in our cultural context to learn and practice interprofessional collaboration through hands-on experience.

Nursing and medical students reported collaboration enhancement as positive learning outcomes. A better rapport between nursing and medical students during the interprofessional team-based education led nursing students to perceive the sense of empathy and respect from medical students, which resulted in enhanced collaboration. The team-based HFS education in each module promoted nursing and medical students' active involvement in patient care [55, 56]. It led medical students to understand the importance of good teamwork, which enhanced collaboration.

Table 13.4 Three Interprofessional Team-based High-Fidelity Simulation Module Outline

Module Topic		1. Chest pain management in adult men with acute myocardial infarction		2. Postpartum bleeding management after vaginal delivery		3. Febrile seizure management in child	
Simulation running	Simulator	SimMan3G		SimMom, Noel		SimBaby	
	Running time	30 min		30minutes		30 min	
	Laboratory	E.R.		DR		NICU	
	Roles	Dr. 1, 2, Nr. 1, 2		Dr. 1, 2, Nr. 1, 2		Dr. 1, 2, Nr. 1, 2	
	S.P.	–		–		Mom (family caregiver)	
	Debriefing	Time	40 min	Time	40 min	Time	40 min
		Place	Debriefing room 313B	Place	Debriefing room 320B	Place	Debriefing room 205
	Instructors	4 professors of emergency medicine 2 nursing professors		2 professors of obstetrics and gynecology 2 nursing professors		2 professors of pediatrics 2 nursing professors	
Situation		OO Lee, a 55-year-old man, had been diagnosed with HTN and hyperlipidemia 3 years ago and has been without treatment. He had intermittent chest pain due to heavy work and stress from a week ago. He was admitted to E.R. this morning due to persistent and stiff chest pain.		OO Lee, a 39-week-old pregnant woman, arrived at E.R. last night with regular uterine contractions and a 3 cm open cervix. She was admitted to the maternity ward after a natural amniotic fluid disruption and a fetal heart rate of 140 times/min. After 4 h, she enters the D.R. with the cervix progressing to 8 cm, worrying a lot because it is the first time.		This patient (13M/M) was in an appropriate state of development without any special medical history after birth. He was given antipyretic syrup due to coughing and mild fever on the day of the visit. He has trouble breathing and suddenly droops without energy.	
Clinical skills		• Emergency patient medical history and physical examination • Evaluation of vital signs results • Cardiopulmonary resuscitation • ECG monitoring • Defibrillation application • Airway intubation and BVM application • Drug administration • Oxygen therapy • Handover • Report using SBAR • Therapeutic communication and teamwork		• Deep breathing and pushing encouragement • Electronic fetal monitoring device application • Assessment of the degree and location of uterine contractions • Lower uterine massage education • Identification of risk factors after delivery • Intravenous infusion • Neonatal respiratory maintenance • Neonatal assessment • Apgar score measurement • Umbilical cord ligation • Handover • Report using SBAR • Therapeutic communication and teamwork		• Pediatric physical examination • Measurement of vital signs and evaluation of its results • Oxygen therapy and airway intubation • Drug administration • Handover • Report using SBAR • Therapeutic communication and teamwork	
Assessment		Performance evaluation checklist Learner self-evaluation Learner reflective journal writing		Performance evaluation checklist Learner self-evaluation Learner reflective journal writing		Performance evaluation checklist Learner self-evaluation Learner reflective journal writing	
Debriefing (Self-developed tool)		IPE Core Competencies based debriefing		IPE Core Competencies-based debriefing		IPE Core Competencies-based debriefing	

E.R. Emergency room, *D.R.* Delivery room, *NICU* Neonatal intensive care unit, *HTN* Hypertension, *ECG* Electrocardiogram, *BVM* Bag-valve-mask, *SBAR* Situation-Background-Assessment-Recommendation, *IPE* Interprofessional education

Table 13.5 Process of running IPSE modules

No	Category		Time(min)
1	Pre-requisite learning		1 week before
2	Pre-briefing		20
3	Pre-scenario activities		20
4	Task training		40
5	Simulation running		120
6	Post-scenario activities	Peer evaluation	(30)
		Self-reflection	(20)
7	Debriefing		40
	Total		240

Before the IPSE experience, nursing students perceived the doctor as the person who issues orders, an expert, and a man full of knowledge and authority, while medical students perceived the nurse as someone like Florence Nightingale, a woman with a syringe working within a bullying culture (known in Korean as *them*). The current findings might be explained by the nursing and medical students' clinical practicum experiences in hierarchical, medically-dominated hospitals. Such experiences may have nursing and medical students hold onto misconceptions about each other's health professions. The biomedical perspectives may lead nursing students to perceive the treatment paradigm as all-encompassing and see the doctor as the one who orders and controls all aspects. Medical students may have the stereotypical image that nurses should be compliant, patient, uncomplaining, hardworking, and self-effacing. After the IPSE experience, both student groups viewed each other as colleagues. It is believed that interprofessional team-based simulation education can promote collaborative teamwork, which might result in improving nursing and medical students' attitudes toward each other's health professions.

What Lessons Were Learned?

Despite a one-time IPSE program implementation due to time and resource restraints, nursing and medical students began to enhance interprofessional collaboration. Receiving interprofessional team-based simulation education benefitted participating students in understanding each other's roles and responsibilities. This potentially maximized their learning and clinical performance due to developing a better rapport with the other health professional students and promoting teamwork. For IPSE to be beneficial, simulation-based education must be relevant to all health professions of the participating students. The simulation task can then be tailored towards the learning needs of the participating students to optimize their learning. All health profession faculties of the participating students need to be involved in designing and developing IPSE programs to develop knowledge of each other's curriculum, the depth of roles, and the scope of shared practice. The continuation of these programs is needed to translate these positive practice changes into hospitals to contribute to safe, quality health care in the workplace and ultimately to improve patient outcomes.

Key Points

- Regardless of culture, the one-time IPSE program provided positive learning opportunities for undergraduate nursing and medical students to practice and develop interprofessional collaboration.
- The use of high-fidelity team-based simulation in IPE was effective in developing undergraduate nursing and medical students' interprofessional collaboration through hands-on experience.
- Prior to the IPSE implementation, all health professional faculties need to be involved in designing and developing IPSE programs to develop knowledge of each other's curriculum, the depth of roles, and the scope of shared practice

Acknowledgments
I wish to thank everyone who played a role in this interprofessional team-based high-fidelity simulation education accomplishment. Special thanks go to the Dean of the College of Nursing, Woo Sook (Christina) Lee, who made this interprofessional program possible. Without your leadership and guidance, we could never have reached this current level of success.

Chapter Summary

Within this chapter, a snapshot of case studies from four countries has been showcased to offer insights into the diverse yet similar topics of interest emerging in contemporary simulation-based nursing education. The diversity in topics, in part, reflects the current status of SBE and the priority areas of focus within universities and health service providers in relation to:

- Country-specific or global health priorities
- Addressing gaps in education support strategies or curricula
- Cultural norms and expectations of both students, clinicians and patients, and;
- The expansion of SBE offerings to address fundamentals of practice for novice students.

It is likely there will be similarities in the level of achievement or advancement in the showcased case studies to initiatives from other countries. The activities reported in this chapter provide a glimpse of the diversity and areas under development, which may complement or contrast with SBE activities globally. One aspect evident in two of the case studies is the desire to incorporate I.P. simulation activities within health professions curricula. The final points to consider are the cultural and country-specific nuances regarding the expectations of each other's professional roles of patients towards health services and the fundamental importance of creating simulations that align with local contexts.

References

1. Marken PA, Zimmerman C, Kennedy C, Schremmer R, Smith KV. Human simulators and standardized patients to teach difficult conversations to interprofessional health care teams. Am J Pharm Educ. 2010;74(7):120. https://doi.org/10.5688/aj7407120.
2. World Health Organization: Fact Sheets—obesity and overweight; 2020. https://www.who.int/news-room/fact-sheets/detail/obesity-and-overweight#:~:text=In%202016%2C%20more%20than%201.9%20billion%20adults%20aged%2018%20years,650%20million%20adults%20were%20obese.&text=Overall%2C%20about%2013%25%20of%20the,tripled%20between%201975%20and%202016. Accessed 6 Dec 2020.
3. Dennis DM, Carter V, Trevenen M, Tyler J, Perella L, Lori E, et al. Do acutely hospitalized patients in Australia have a different body mass index (BMI) to the general Australian population: a point prevalence study? Aust Health Rev. 2017;42(2):121–9. https://doi.org/10.1071/AH16171.
4. The Government of Western Australia EOC, Equal Opportunity Act Perth, Western Australia; 1984.
5. Gray CM, Hunt K, Lorimer K, Anderson AS, Benzeval M, Wyke S. Words matter: a qualitative investigation of which weight status terms are acceptable and motivate weight loss when used by health professionals. BMC Public Health. 2011;11:513. https://doi.org/10.1186/1471-2458-11-513.
6. Phelan SM, Burgess DJ, Yeazel MW, Hellerstedt WL, Griffin JM, van Ryn M. Impact of weight bias and stigma on quality of care and outcomes for patients with obesity. Obes Rev. 2015;16(4):319–26. https://doi.org/10.1111/obr.12266.
7. Setchell J, Watson B, Jones L, Gard M, Briffa K. Physiotherapists demonstrate weight stigma: a cross-sectional survey of Australian physiotherapists. J Physiother. 2014;60(3):157–62. https://doi.org/10.1016/j.jphys.2014.06.020.
8. Schwartz M, Chambliss HON, Brownell K, Blair S, Billington C. Weight bias among health professionals specializing in obesity. Obes Res. 2003;11(9):1033–9.
9. Flint S. Obesity stigma: Prevalence and impact in healthcare. Br J Obes. 2015;1(1):1–40.
10. Wear D, Aultman J, Varley J, Zarconi J. Making fun of patients: medical students' perceptions and use of derogatory and cynical humor in clinical settings. Acad Med. 2006;81(5):454–62.
11. Alberga AS, Pickering BJ, Alix Hayden K, Ball GDC, Edwards A, Jelinski S, et al. Weight bias reduction in health professionals: a systematic review. Clin Obes. 2016;6(3):175–88.
12. Nursing & Midwifery Council: future nurse: standards of proficiency for registered nurses; 2018. https://www.nmc.org.uk/standards/standards-for-nurses/standards-of-proficiency-for-registered-nurses/. Accessed 4 Nov 2020.
13. Francis G. Skills and simulation in nursing: a great opportunity or huge challenge? Evid Based Nurs. 2018;21(4):87–8. https://doi.org/10.1136/eb-2018-102979.
14. McNamara N. Preparing students for clinical placements: the student's perspective. Nurse Educ Pract. 2015;15(3):196–202. https://doi.org/10.1016/j.nepr.2014.11.011.
15. Doolen J, Mariani B, Atz T, Horsley L, O'Rourke R, McAfee K, et al. High-fidelity simulation in undergraduate nursing education: a review of simulation reviews. Clin Simul Nurs. 2016;12(7):150–60. https://doi.org/10.1016/j.ecns.2016.01.009.
16. Williams B, Song J. Are simulated patients effective in facilitating development of clinical competence for healthcare students? A scoping review. Adv Simul. 2016;1(6):1–9. https://doi.org/10.1186/s41077-016-0006-1.
17. MacLean S, Kelly M, Geddes F, Della P. Use of simulated patients to develop communication skills in nursing education: an integrative review. Nurse Educ Today. 2017;48:90–8. https://doi.org/10.1016/j.nedt.2016.09.018.
18. Nestel D, Sanko J, McNaughton N. Simulated participant methodologies. In: Nestel D, Kelly M, Jolly B, Watson M, editors. Healthcare simulation education. Chichester: John Wiley and Sons; 2018. p. 45–53.
19. Blows T. The Biological basis of clinical observations. 3rd ed. London: Routledge; 2018.
20. Francis G, O'Brien M. Teaching clinical skills in pre-registration nurse education: value and methods. Br J Nurs. 2019;28(7):452–6. https://doi.org/10.12968/bjon.2019.28.7.452.
21. Kunst EL, Henderson A, Johnston A. A scoping review of the use and contribution of simulation in Australian undergraduate nurse education. Clin Simul Nurs. 2018;19:17–29. https://doi.org/10.1016/j.ecns.2018.03.003.
22. Marshall S. A handbook for teaching and learning in higher education: Enhancing academic practice. 5th ed. London: Routledge; 2019.
23. Bovill C, Jarvis J, Smith K. Co-creating learning and teaching: Towards relational pedagogy in higher education Critical Practice in Higher Education. London: Critical Publishing; 2020.
24. NHS Improvement: SBAR Communication Tool—situation, background, assessment and recommendation; 2017. https://improvement.nhs.uk/documents/2162/sbar-communication-tool.pdf. Accessed 4 Nov 2020.
25. Levett-Jones T, editor. Clinical reasoning: learning to think like a nurse. 2nd ed. Melbourne, Australia: Pearson Australia; 2018.
26. Hunter S, Arthur C. Clinical reasoning of nursing students on clinical placement: clinical educators' perceptions. Nurse Educ Pract. 2016;18:73–9. https://doi.org/10.1016/j.nepr.2016.03.002.
27. O'Regan S, Molloy E, Watterson L, Nestel D. Observer roles that optimize learning in healthcare simulation education: a systematic review. Adv Simul. 2016;1(1):4. https://doi.org/10.1186/s41077-015-0004-8.
28. Ministry of Education: Regulations on national guidelines for nursing education; 2019. https://lovdata.no/dokument/SF/forskrift/2019-03-15-412
29. Phillips N, Duke M, Weerasuriya R. Questioning skills of clinical facilitators supporting undergraduate nursing students. J Clin Nurs. 2017;26(23-24):4344–52. https://doi.org/10.1111/jocn.13761.
30. Haugan G, Aigeltinger E, Sørlie V. The importance of the instructor-student nurse relationship to student nurses in clinical hospital praxis. Sykepleien Forskning. 2012;7(2):152–8. https://doi.org/10.4220/sykepleienf.2012.0083.
31. McGowan B. Who do they think they are? Undergraduate perceptions of the definition of supernumerary status and how it works in practice. J Clin Nurs. 2006;15(9):1099–105. https://doi.org/10.1111/j.1365-2702.2005.01478.x.
32. Lofmark A, Wikblad K. Facilitating and obstructing factors for development of learning in clinical practice: a student perspective. J Adv Nurs. 2001;34(1):43–50. https://doi.org/10.1046/j.1365-2648.2001.3411739.x.
33. McCormack B, Slater P. An evaluation of the role of the clinical education facilitator. J Clin Nurs. 2006;15(2):135–44. https://doi.org/10.1111/j.1365-2702.2006.01275.x.
34. Ramritu P, Barnard A. New nurse graduates' understanding of competence. Int Nurs Rev. 2001;48(1):47–57. https://doi.org/10.1046/j.1466-7657.2001.00048.x.
35. Lambert V, Glacken M. Clinical education facilitators: a literature review. J Clin Nurs. 2005;14(6):664–73. https://doi.org/10.1111/j.1365-2702.2005.01136.x.
36. Muthathi I, Thurling C, Armstrong S. Through the eyes of the student: best practices in clinical facilitation. Curationis. 2017;40(1):e1–8. https://doi.org/10.4102/curationis.v40i1.1787.
37. Esmaeili M, Cheraghi M, Salsali M, Ghiyasvandian S. Nursing students' expectations regarding effective clinical education: a qualitative study. Int J Nurs Pract. 2014;20(5):460–7. https://doi.org/10.1111/ijn.12159.

38. Allari R, Farag M. Nursing students' expectations regarding clinical training: a qualitative study. Int J Nurs Sci. 2017;7(3):63–70. https://doi.org/10.5923/j.nursing.20170703.02.
39. Needham J, McMurray A, Shaban R. Best practice in clinical facilitation of undergraduate nursing students. Nurse Educ Pract. 2016;20:131–8. https://doi.org/10.1016/j.nepr.2016.08.003.
40. Matthew-Maich N, Martin L, Ackerman-Rainville R, Hammond C, Palma A, Sheremet D, et al. Student perceptions of effective nurse educators in clinical practice. Nurs Stand. 2015;29(34):45–58. https://doi.org/10.7748/ns.29.34.45.e9640.
41. Husebø S, Silvennoinen M, Rosqvist E, Masiello I. Status of Nordic research on simulation-based learning in healthcare: an integrative review. Adv Simul. 2018;3(1):12. https://doi.org/10.1186/s41077-018-0071-8.
42. Lioce L, Lopreiato J, Downing D, Chang T, Robertson J, Anderson M, et al. Healthcare simulation dictionary. 2nd ed. Rockville, MD: AHRQ Publication; 2020.
43. Nestel D, Kelly M, Jolly B, Watson M, editors. Healthcare simulation education: evidence, theory, and practice. West Sussex: John Wiley & Sons; 2018.
44. Hiim H, Hippe E. Læring gjennom opplevelse, forståelse og handling: en studiebok i didaktikk [Learning through experience, understanding and action: a textbook in didactics]. 2nd ed. Oslo: Universitetsforlaget; 1998.
45. Bjørk I, Kirkevold M. From simplicity to complexity: developing a model of practical skill performance in nursing. J Clin Nurs. 2000;9(4):620–31. https://doi.org/10.1046/j.1365-2702.2000.00328.x.
46. Gibbs G. Learning by doing: a guide to teaching and learning methods. London: Further Education Unit, Oxford Polytechnic; 1988.
47. Husebø SE, O'Regan S, Nestel D. Reflective practice and its role in simulation. Clin Simul Nurs. 2015;11(8):368–75. https://doi.org/10.1016/j.ecns.2015.04.005.
48. Robben S, Perry M, van Nieuwenhuijzen L, van Achterberg T, Rikkert MO, Schers H, et al. Impact of interprofessional education on collaboration attitudes, skills, and behavior among primary care professionals. J Contin Educ Health Prof. 2012;32(3):196–204. https://doi.org/10.1002/chp.21145.
49. Koo L, Layson-Wolf C, Brandt N, Hammersla M, Idzik S, Rocafort PT, et al. Qualitative evaluation of a standardized patient clinical simulation for nurse practitioner and pharmacy students. Nurse Educ Pract. 2014;14(6):740–6. https://doi.org/10.1016/j.nepr.2014.10.005.
50. World Health Organization: Framework for action on interprofessional education and collaborative practice; 2010. https://www.who.int/hrh/resources/framework_action/en/. Accessed 1 July 2020.
51. Costello M, Prelack K, Faller J, Huddleston J, Adly S, Doolin J. Student experiences of interprofessional simulation: findings from a qualitative study. J Interprof Care. 2018;32(1):95–7. https://doi.org/10.1080/13561820.2017.1356810.
52. Hood K, Cant R, Baulch J, Gilbee A, Leech M, Anderson A, et al. Prior experience of interprofessional learning enhances undergraduate nursing and healthcare students' professional identity and attitudes to teamwork. Nurse Educ Pract. 2014;14(2):117–22. https://doi.org/10.1016/j.nepr.2013.07.013.
53. Interprofessional Education Collaborative Expert Panel. Core competencies for interprofessional collaborative practice: report of an expert panel. Washington D.C.: Interprofessional Education Collaborative; 2011.
54. Interprofessional Education Collaborative. Core competencies for interprofessional collaborative practice: 2016 update. Washington D.C.: Interprofessional Education Collaborative; 2016.
55. Labrague L, McEnroe-Petitte D, Fronda D, Obeidat A. Interprofessional simulation in undergraduate nursing program: an integrative review. Nurse Educ Today. 2018;67:46–55. https://doi.org/10.1016/j.nedt.2018.05.001.
56. Reeves S, van Schaik S. Simulation: a panacea for interprofessional learning? J Interprof Care. 2012;26(3):167–9. https://doi.org/10.3109/13561820.2012.678183.
57. Decker S, Anderson M, Boese T, Epps C, McCarthy J, Motola I, et al. Standards of best practice: simulation standard VIII: Simulation-Enhanced Interprofessional Education (Sim-IPE). Clin Simul Nurs. 2015;11(6):293–7. https://doi.org/10.1016/j.ecns.2015.03.010.
58. Gough S, Hellaby M, Jones N, MacKinnon R. A review of undergraduate interprofessional simulation-based education (IPSE). Collegian. 2012;19(3):153–70. https://doi.org/10.1016/j.colegn.2012.04.004.
59. Sanford PG. Simulation in nursing education: a review of the research. Qualit Rep. 2010;15(4):1006–11.
60. Roberts FE, Goodhand K. Scottish healthcare student's perceptions of an interprofessional ward simulation: an exploratory, descriptive study. Nurs Health Sci. 2018;20(1):107–15. https://doi.org/10.1111/nhs.12393.

Resources

Beyond Blue. Counseling; n.d. https://www.beyondblue.org.au/

Cancer Council of W.A. Resources, advice; n.d. https://www.cancer.org.au/about-cancer/online-resources/

Centrelink. Sickness Allowance payment (currently superseded during COVID-19 with JobKeeper); n.d. https://www.servicesaustralia.gov.au/individuals/services/centrelink/sickness-allowance

Independent Living Centres Australia; n.d. https://ilcaustralia.org.au/

Assessment and Evaluation in Nursing Education: A Simulation Perspective

14

Loretta Garvey and Debra Kiegaldie

Assessment in Undergraduate Nursing Education: A Simulation Perspective

Author: Dr. Loretta Garvey

Background

Assessment As, For, and Of Learning

Traditionally assessment is a measurement tool to quantify what students have learned. In other words, '*assessment of learning*. Traditional assessment is characterized by tests and examinations designed to improve teaching, measure learning, and measure student achievement of learning outcomes [1]. Assessment determines the quantity and quality of student learning, and students structure their learning according to the assessment tasks. This view of assessment sees assessment as independent of learning, as done by teachers to students. Research in Higher Education tells us that '*assessment for learning*' is better for students and that assessment practices, therefore, play a complex and pivotal role in the student experience [2]. Furthermore, if assessment only measures recall and memory, students will adopt a surface approach to learning which is the antithesis to the aims of education. Simulation has progressed the landscape of assessment by moving learners from the simpler knows and knows how the level of Miller's pyramid (Fig. 14.1) to the shows how level [3]. Simulation in nursing provides students the opportunity to demonstrate the behavior of a nurse under supervision, proving that they can use their knowledge while being supervised and observed.

Assessment as learning occurs when students reflect and self-assess their progress to inform their future learning goals (formative assessment). Through this process, students can learn about themselves as learners and become aware of how they learn. Examples of this type of assessment used in the undergraduate nursing space include immersive simulations using manikins or simulated participants. Immersive simulations are commonly used as a learning opportunity in undergraduate education but may only sometimes be considered a form of assessment. However, in considering *assessment as learning* in the formative sense, educators may now reconceptualize immersive simulation as a form of assessment and signpost this opportunity for learners.

Assessment for learning is when teachers use inferences about student progress and learning to inform their teaching (often formative assessment) and usually occurs more than once during the learning period. Students understand exactly what they are to learn and what is expected of them and are given feedback and advice on improving their work. This is interactive with the student and teacher and involves immediate feedback. In nursing, this can include psychomotor skill acquisition in a simulated ward or laboratory environment. Similar to assessment as learning, this type of assessment frequently occurs in undergraduate nursing programs and can be more readily signposted and structured as a formative assessment opportunity emphasizing feedback and the progression of learning.

Assessment of learning happens when teachers use evidence of student learning to make judgments on student achievement against goals and standards and is usually done at the end of the task (summative assessment). Its effectiveness as an opportunity for learning depends on the nature and quality of the feedback. Examples of these assessments in undergraduate nursing include Objective Structured Clinical Examinations (OSCEs) and competency hurdles. The OSCE is a method of assessment where the learner rotates through several scenarios known as stations. OSCEs can be tailored to the course requirements, looking at cognitive, technical,

L. Garvey (✉)
Federation University Australia, University Dr, Mount Helen, VIC, Australia
e-mail: lgarvey@swin.edu.au

D. Kiegaldie
Holmesglen Institute, Healthscope Hospitals, Monash University, Mount Helen, VIC, Australia

J. M. Kutzin et al. (eds.), *Comprehensive Healthcare Simulation: Nursing*, Comprehensive Healthcare Simulation,
https://doi.org/10.1007/978-3-031-31090-4_14

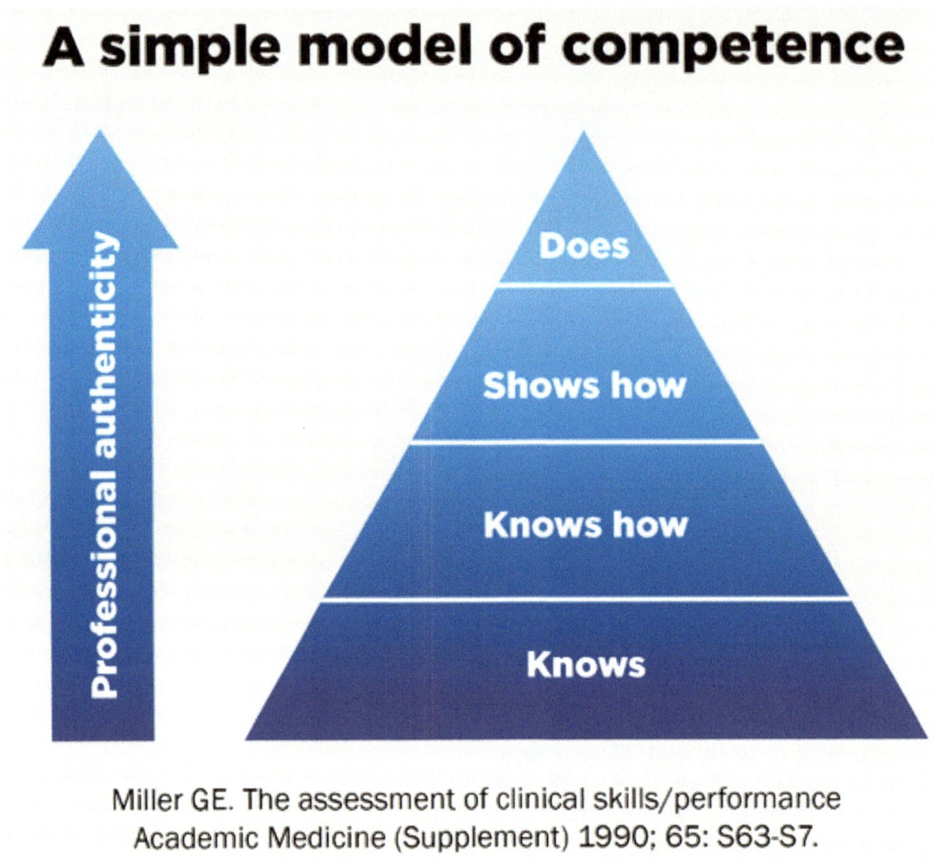

Fig. 14.1 Miller's model of competence

and professional skill levels. This assessment method is widespread throughout health professions training from undergraduate to vocational training assessment, and learners are usually judged on a development scale of performance. OSCE has been proven to be an effective evaluation tool to assess practical skills, particularly with the inclusion of simulated participants to increase authenticity and fidelity. OSCEs have been implemented as a formative assessment in nursing [4] but are more commonly utilized as summative assessment opportunities. Competency hurdles are another example of simulation in the form of assessment of learning commonly found in undergraduate nursing. In contrast to OSCE, competency hurdles can be completed as a single assessment of a particular skill, and learners are deemed to have met the competency standard or not. Like the OSCE, implementation can be with or without the use of simulated participants, depending on the purpose, objectives, budget, and fidelity level required.

Future Uses of Simulated Assessment

Simulation is a complex yet useful form of assessment, it has undergone much change and development since its initial inception, and the opportunities for further improvement seem only limited by educators' imagination. Simulation can be a safe space to assess something difficult or controversial that might not be appropriate or ethical to assess in a real-life situation. Two particular aspects being developed and piloted for future use in undergraduate nursing include interprofessional learning (IPL) and professionalism.

IPL is ongoingly identified as a high-need area in health care to improve healthcare delivery and optimize patient outcomes. This is achieved through appropriate teamwork and understanding of the roles and responsibilities of different health professions. Simulation has emerged as a modality for assessing IPL and teamwork. While outside the scope of this chapter to go into explicit detail, many of the principles identified here are relevant. Consideration is needed in IPL surrounding scheduling, logistics, and learner level for participating professions.

Professionalism is a challenging concept to assess and is often judged through the absence of unprofessional behavior. Including professionalism in the simulation allows one to consider it more positively. Professionalism may be difficult to construct in a simulation as fidelity may be lost in a simulated environment. An idea of how this might be appropriately achieved is the inclusion of interaction with a simulated participant or video clip followed by conversation and questioning from the examiner to discuss the circumstances, options, and potential outcomes. This format could broaden the scope of what can be assessed, allowing the examiner to identify a deeper level of understanding of the learner's perspective by asking the why questions.

Best Practices

In the 1970s and 1980s, new approaches to assessing students in the healthcare professions began developing, and a need for international collaborations to share views and experiences of assessment from different countries was identified. This has subsequently developed into the world-leading conference on the assessment of competence in medicine and the healthcare professions, The Ottawa Conference. This group regularly gathers world-leading experts from different professional backgrounds and experience in assessment to develop a consensus statement and recommendation in relation to the criteria for a good assessment, in other words, best practice. 2018 was the last published version of this statement, with a notable shift from focusing on one assessment to an assessment system where "systems integrate a series of different individual measures assembled for one or more purposes" [5] p 1105. This raises the concept of planning and designing a purposeful program of assessment rather than looking at one assessment in isolation or multiple ones that are not connected.

The 2018 consensus statement includes seven criteria for good assessment. These are guiding principles from development to implementation of all assessments, including simulation.

1. Coherent. The assessment system is composed of multiple, coordinated individual assessments and independent performances that are orderly and aligned around the same purposes.
2. Continuous. The assessment system is ongoing, and individual results contribute cumulatively to the system's purposes.
3. Comprehensive. The assessment system is inclusive and effective, consisting of components that are formative, diagnostic, and/or summative as appropriate to its purposes.
4. Feasible. The assessment system and its components are practical, realistic, efficient, and sensible, given the purposes, stakeholders, and context.
5. Purposes driven. The assessment system supports the purposes for which it was created.
6. Acceptable. Stakeholders in the system find the assessment process and results to be credible and evidence-based.
7. Transparent and free from bias. Stakeholders understand the system's workings, and its unintended consequences are minimized [5].

Appropriate planning of assessments is fundamental to ensuring the development and delivery of quality assessments. The following sections will outline practical ways to plan simulated assessment with specific reference to the above criteria to ensure best practice assessment.

An Example of Integrating Simulation Assessment into Existing Education

Blueprinting—Constructive Alignment

The first step in developing a simulation assessment is to undertake an assessment blueprint, collaborating with key stakeholders in your assessment program. This ensures that the process of assessment is *acceptable* and *transparent*. In undergraduate nursing, it is important to involve both university-based academics and clinical partners in this process, as both are key stakeholders who have an important role in assessing students. Blueprinting is a seamless way of integrating a new simulated assessment into an existing program or reviewing existing assessments to ensure they are constructively aligned. Blueprinting originated in architecture and engineering as a technical drawing or plan for building a structure. It was used to ensure that everyone working on the construction followed the same plan to achieve the desired structural outcome. The same concept applies to the use of blueprinting in assessment. An assessment blueprint facilitates alignment of the desired learning outcomes or competencies with the teaching and learning activities and the assessments, termed constructive alignment [6]. The content and form of assessment need to be aligned with their purpose and desired outcomes [5]. A blueprint can be undertaken at a macro level (a program, course, or unit) and a micro level for individual assessment items. An assessment blueprint ensures that all people involved in the assessment process have a transparent plan about what the desired out comes of that assessment are and how these constructively align to the learning, learning outcomes, and overall program or course. The benefits of a blueprint include enhanced validity and appropriate sampling of content as the assessments are directly mapped to the learning that it intends to measure. In relation to simulated assessments at the item or micro level, blueprints become an efficient tool to begin the construction of the simulation scenario and assessment rubric as it will identify the content (e.g., skill–history taking) and domain (pediatrics) that has been chosen to sample and the level required of the student.

The process of blueprinting can be achieved by following the steps outlined below:

1. Define the broad objective/outcome of your program
   (a) What is it that your program is meant to be achieving?

Table 14.1 Example content matrix undergraduate nursing

Learning Activity & Assessment Key	Topics/Content									
Learning Objectives/Competencies										

Table 14.2 Example content matrix undergraduate nursing

Key Lecture = (L) Tutorial = (T) Clinical Placement = (P) Self-Directed Learning = (S) Simulated Laboratory (SL)	Neurological	Pain	CVS	Respiratory	GIT	Renal	MSK	Endocrine	ENT
Learning Objectives									
1. Demonstrate an understanding of therapeutic communication within the interdisciplinary health care team to enhance the personal interaction involved in assessment;	T S	P	T S	T S	T S	T S	T S	T S	T S
2. Accurately demonstrate comprehensive health and physical assessment skills in simulated and clinical practice environments;	SL P	SL P	SL P	SL P	SL P	SL P	SL P	SL P	SL P
3. Plan, implement, and evaluate nursing care using a person-centered approach cognizant of everyone's autonomy, self-esteem, and dignity;	SL P	SL P	SL P	SL P	SL P	SL P	SL P	SL P	SL P
4. Demonstrate the ability to integrate scientific knowledge with nursing practice;	T	T	T	T	T	T	T	T	T
5. Demonstrate understanding of the basic principles of medication management related to patient safety;	T, SL	T, SL	T, SL	T, SL	T, SL	T, SL	T, SL	T, SL	
6. Demonstrate professional and personal accountability as a novice practitioner when providing nursing care;	P	P	P	P	P	P	P	P	P

2. Create a content matrix (see Tables 14.1 and 14.2)
   (a) Define the purpose and focus of the assessment
      (i) Competencies/learning outcomes
   (b) Define the context, content & scope
      (i) Stage of learning: Year level/semester/stream
      (ii) What are the content area/topics taught
   (c) Blueprint
      (i) Populate your learning activities
3. Create an assessment matrix (see Table 14.3)
   (a) Define the purpose and focus of the assessment
      (i) Competencies/learning outcomes
   (b) Define the context, content & scope
      (i) Year level/semester/stream
      (ii) Content/topics to be assessed
      (iii) What components of the task will be assessed?
   (c) Blueprint
      (i) Populate with your assessment

The final step, populating your assessments, must ensure that you include both formative and summative assessment activities. A color-coded system or key might assist in definitively representing each type. Including both formative and summative assessments allows educators to ensure a *comprehensive* representation of the learning opportunities and aligns with the third criterion for good assessment.

The subsequent tables provide additional examples of blueprints at the micro and macro levels. Table 14.4 exempli-

Table 14.3 Example—assessment matrix (blueprint) undergraduate nursing

Key	**TOPICS**								
Written Assignment = (A) Written Examination = (E) Clinical Placement = (P) Simulated Medication Competency = (M) Formative Quiz = (FQ) Formative Medication competency (FM)	Neurological	Pain	CVS	Respiratory	GIT	Renal	MSK	Endocrine	ENT
Learning Objectives									
1. Demonstrate an understanding of therapeutic communication within the interdisciplinary health care team to enhance the personal interaction involved in assessment;	P	M P FM	P	PM FM	P	P	P	P	P
2. Accurately demonstrate comprehensive health and physical assessment skills in simulated and clinical practice environments;	P E FQ	P	P E FQ	P E	P E	P E FQ	P E	P E FQ	P E
3. Plan, implement, and evaluate nursing care using a person-centered approach cognisant of each individual's autonomy, self-esteem, and dignity;	AE	A	A E	A E	A E	A E	A E	A E	A E
4. Demonstrate the ability to integrate scientific knowledge with nursing practice;	E	E FQ	E	E FQ	E FQ	E	E FQ	E	E FQ
5. Demonstrate understanding of the basic principles of medication management related to patient safety;		M FM		M FM					
6. Demonstrate professional and personal accountability as a novice practitioner when providing nursing care;	P	P	P	P	P	P	P	P	P
7. Discuss the legal and ethical principles surrounding safe care delivery to individuals and the implications to nursing/ midwifery care;		M		M					

Table 14.4 Example—blueprinting assessment tools

Context	Migrant client			Elderly client		
Cognitive /Affective Categories	Language support	Case Planning	Housing support	Home visit	Case Planning	Group Activity
Recall		x			x	
Reasoning			x			
Affect	x			x		
Skill		x		x		x

fies a blueprint at a tool level that measures the cognitive and affective capabilities of the learner with included details of the context for the simulated assessment. Table 14.5 is a complex blueprint of an entire year which includes complex detail of the content (body system), the context of the assessment (problem, practice context, patient age, clinical task), the competency level of Miller's pyramid, and what assessment instrument will be used to assess each aspect. The later example clearly covers the first two criteria for good assessment being *continuous* across the year and *coherent* with varying assessment techniques. These two examples identify that a blueprint can be as complex as is necessitated by your environment to ensure all those contributing to the assessment have a shared mental model about the assessment requirements and standards.

Developing a Simulated Assessment

Working through the developmental process of an assessment may be required if you are looking to improve an existing assessment or construct a new assessment to ensure constructive alignment of your program. The guiding criteria for good assessment are relevant throughout this developmental phase. In the context of simulation, the assessment should be relevant and realistic to what the learners will encounter in the future profession, meeting the guiding principle of the assessment being *purpose driven*. This development process should begin with planning or determining through the work already done on your blueprint: the context, stage of learning, competencies/outcomes, assessment purpose (formative/summative), and method, i.e., simulation. Table 14.6 provides a template on which to record this detail.

Feasibility, the fourth criterion for a good assessment, must be considered when designing your simulated assessment to ensure that it will be possible and practical to implement. The template in Table 14.6 will also assist in documenting these considerations and decisions. A challenge with simulated assessment is often the cost associated with implementing the assessment. Consider the following questions for the assessment you are developing:

Table 14.5 Example—Complex blueprint [7]

What to assess																	How to assess
System	Problem	Practice context		Age			Clinical task						Competency level				Test instrument
		1	2	1	2	3	1	2	3	4	5	6	1	2	3	4	
Gastrointestinal	Upper GI bleeding	x			x				x	x			x				A-type MCQ Key feature question
	Projectile vomiting – pyloric stenosis	x		x			x	x	x	x	x		x	x			A-type MCQ R-type MCQ
	Blood in the stool – rectal cancer		x			x	x	x	x	x	x		x	x	x		MEQ OSCE – X-ray
Cardiovascular	Cardiac arrest	x				x			x		x				x		OSCE – CPR
	Chest pain	x			x		x	x	x	x			x	x	x		Written OSCE – ECG – Simulated patient

Key:

Problem	Practice context	Age	Clinical task	Competency level	Test instrument
Presentation or pathology	1 = Emergency 2 = Non-emergency	1 = Child 2 = Adult 3 = Elderly	1 = History taking 2 = Physical examination 3 = Diagnosis 4 = Investigation 5 = Treatment 6 = Follow-up	1 = Knows 2 = Knows how 3 = Shows how 4 = Does	**1 = Written** a. A-type MCQs b. R-type EMQs c. Key feature questions d. Modified essay question (MEQ) **2 = OSCE**

Table 14.6 Assessment planning template

Context	
Stage of learning	
Competencies/Outcomes	
Assessment Type (formative/summative)	
Method	
Assessors (who & how many)	
Assessor Training/Standardisation	
Time requirement (Date & length)	
Feedback Model	

- How many assessments are required to make a judgment? e.g., How many OSCE stations and competency hurdles?
- How much time will it take for each learner? Is there enough time in their current timetable, or will additional scheduling time and space be required?
- Who will be the assessor/s and simulated participants (if needed)?
- Can this be managed within the current staff workload, or will additional staff be required? If so, is there a budget to facilitate this cost
- When will the assessment occur? Are these assessment hurdles to attending clinical placements?
- Will there be adequate time between testing/learning to improve/perform?

A significant element that requires consideration in developing a simulated assessment is the variables that impact the reliability and validity of an assessment. The human factor, being assessors and simulated participants, is often a substantial influence on these two things. Therefore, training is essential to ensure that you adequately prepare staff who will be involved in the assessment and to ensure that they are all marking to the same standard or benchmark if you have multiple assessors. Standardization can be achieved by ensuring a shared mental model of the desired outcomes or competency between assessors and safeguarding the process is *free from bias*. Training should include details of the assessment (e.g., simulation), what it is assessing (e.g., learning outcomes/competencies), the instructions to students, associated learning that has occurred, the marking criteria/rubric, what each criterion means, and the expected standard. The marking group should collectively work through any misconceptions and agree on a set standard. In simulation, role-playing a practice student with practice assessment is a common way of ensuring the context and requirements are shared between assessors. This can also improve the consistency and, therefore, interrater reliability between assessors. The training should also include the expectations of delivering feedback to learners. The design of the assessment must include time for the provision of feedback (written/verbal). The choice of feedback model should ensure it is constructive for the learner.

Challenges and Solutions—Common Barriers and Successful Solutions

Simulated assessment in undergraduate nursing is an opportunity for students to participate in authentic assessment in a safe environment. However, it has its challenges. It is important when embarking on the development and implementation process to be aware of potential challenges and consider ideas for mitigation. In the earlier sections of this chapter, several challenges have been identified, ensuring the validity and reliability of the assessment and cost associated with simulation. Validity and reliability can largely be managed through the appropriate planning and standardization training identified previously. Additionally, designing user-friendly and consistent marking rubrics (detailed in the subsequent section) will also assist in mitigating this issue.

The fiscal challenges associated with simulated assessment are more often associated with summative assessment as the requirements for standardization of assessors and simulated participants are higher. If the stakes of the assessment are lower, consideration can be given to the use of volunteer simulated participants, which may only bear the cost of time for training and the provision of refreshments. Some identified challenges associated with volunteer simulated participants are that their attendance at the assessment time may be less reliable, and they may not have the acting skills required to meet the needs of the assessment. On a positive note, using volunteers can be an opportunity for community engagement and the ability to build a patient case to the volunteer's background (where appropriate). Another cost saving that can be considered during the developmental stage of the assessment is to determine if a simulated participant is required. Alternatively, can a mannequin meet the intended assessment need, or can another student play the role? Such suggestions are dependent on your program of assessment and what your overarching outcomes are. However, the inclusion of simulated assessment, even without paid actors, may provide a superior assessment opportunity for nursing students compared to other less authentic and less relevant assessment modalities.

The culmination of an undergraduate nursing degree is to progress students along the trajectory to become registered nurses. The learning journey, however, continues beyond this junction. Therefore, part of the responsibility of an undergraduate program is to develop students to become lifelong learners who continually expand their knowledge to stay up to date with best-practices in healthcare. One part of developing life-long learning skills is learning how to self-assess one's own performance and make improvements, which are essential for continuous development. Simulated assessments provide an opportunity for students to practice self-assessment. However, in simulated assessment, challenges with self-assessment exist based on the stakes of the assessment. In formative modalities, self-assessment is key to the learning journey; examples where this is seamlessly achieved, are in high-fidelity simulations through the structured debrief and after singular competency hurdles. The challenge with self-assessment exists in high-stakes summative assessments such as OSCEs or multiple competency hurdles. Two problems arise in this space; first, if students perceive that their self-assessment will impact the final grade awarded by the assessor, this may impact how candid they are in identifying areas requiring improvement. Secondly, suppose multiple assessments occur continuously and students must stop and self-assess at the end of each assessment. In that case, this reflection may lead to distress about their past performance, which may, in turn, affect subsequent performance. A potential solution to these problems can be in the timing of the self-assessment; this could occur as a collective self-assessment at the entire assessment. This may be difficult for the student to remember their performance. However, it could mitigate issues of distress or concern over the disclosure of self-assessment.

The final challenge identified in simulated assessments lies in the ability to authentically and appropriately represent cultural diversity. This challenge extends from assessment development to implementation. If a certain culture is to be included in the context of the simulated assessment, assurances need to be made to either co-create the assessment with a person/s from that group or have it reviewed by a representative of that cultural group. On the implementation side, consideration must be made to the authenticity of representing a cultural group with simulated participants. First, the challenge in findings simulated participants from the appropriate cultural group, and second, what supports are put in place to reduce the burden on the simulated participant to represent their cultural group. An appropriate representation of cultural diversity in simulated assessments is important to ensure assessment mimics the real world where students will be nursing in the future. The key to managing solutions in this space lies in the planning and development stages.

Interface with Regulatory Bodies

Regulating bodies vary worldwide; however, most will require some form of simulated assessment to gain accreditation. It may include a minimum amount of simulation-based assessment with detail around when this should occur, for example, prior to placement to ensure student safety before caring for the public. When planning simulated assessment in undergraduate nursing, it is important to identify these specific parameters for your respective regulatory body. In addition to the inclusion of simulated assessment, there will likely be requirements to outline standardized processes to ensure the validity and reliability of your assessment; once again, these will be specific to each country and body. For example, Australia has national accreditation of undergraduate nursing programs but no national licensing exams. Assessments are specific to each individual course and institution and are determined based on the accreditation cycle. The national standards for accreditation will influence decisions and advice around assessment, and the professional standards for practice inform these standards, as learners are required to meet this upon course completion.

Sample Assessments

Rubrics & Marking Criteria

Simulation cases in undergraduate nursing will vary based on the context, formative or summative nature, and learner level. As identified previously, a fundamental element that should be consistently used are assessment rubrics and marking criteria. High-quality rubrics will assist with marking standardization and improve the assessment's *acceptability* and *transparency*. The assessment instructions must be closely aligned with the rubric and criteria to ensure that the expectations of the assessment are transparent. The communication given to the students must be plain and outline all expectations; no parts should be withheld. In the past, assessment has sometimes been considered an opportunity to "trick" students through a hidden agenda only known to the assessor, resulting in raised levels of student anxiety and the notion of the assessor being the gatekeeper to passing. The assessment should allow the student to display their competence and identify areas of their performance that require improvement. The marking criteria in the assessment rubric should directly reflect the assessment instructions and blueprint about the alignment of outcomes/competencies and learning. When developing the criteria, consider the language used to ensure it has a shared understanding of meaning for the learner and the assessor. Spell out any acronyms or what is meant by expectations to avoid ambiguity in understanding. Specificity and concise writing are essential. The assessment type and context will determine the assessment descriptors. In competency-based simulated assessments, this will likely take the form of a developmental model or the required level of support or supervision. Examples include achieved, not achieved, not applicable or independent, developing, and unsatisfactory. Each descriptor must include a definition for the assessment context. For example: independent—the learner can undertake criteria without supervision or prompting; developing—the learner requires minimal prompting and supervision to undertake criteria; not satisfactory—the learner cannot undertake criteria with prompting or supervision. An example can be viewed in Table 14.7.

Table 14.7 Rubric example—measuring heart rate

Instructions:			
	Descriptors		
Marking Criteria	Independent	Developing	Not satisfactory
Performs hand hygiene			
Communicates with the patient using professional behavior and language			
Places the patient's arm in a relaxed position			
Palpates radial pulse—places the first two fingers over the radial side of the patient's inner wrist.			
Counts HR for 1 min			
Records findings accurately on the observation chart			
Ensures that patient is comfortable and concludes interaction			
Performs hand hygiene			
Discusses findings with the examiner, including normal parameters			

Evaluation of Simulation in Undergraduate Nursing

Author: Professor Debra Kiegaldie

Background

As mentioned in the introduction to this chapter, the terms assessment and evaluation are often used interchangeably in education. This may contribute to the limited scholarly activity on program evaluation [8]. Assessment deals with assessing a learner's skills, knowledge, and attributes. Evaluation measures the effectiveness, process, and outcomes of an educational experience/program. Therefore, evaluation in nursing education is an important consideration as it helps identify the educational impact of learning and provides valuable feedback to educators that can assist with course improvement and future planning [9, 10].

Simulation in undergraduate nursing education can be viewed as a distinct learning experience. A simulation experience may be as small as a single simulation scenario, a series of simulations across a semester of learning, or an entire undergraduate program where simulation is firmly integrated across all stages. All deserve a robust evaluation plan.

In the context of this chapter, evaluation is the process used to assess the design, implementation, improvement, or outcomes of a simulation experience to monitor the quality and effectiveness of the simulation program [8, 11]. In essence, it can be used as a process to make decisions about the value or worth of a simulation program. It is a critical step for continuous quality improvement in nursing to achieve simulation goals.

Historically, contemporary evaluation dates to the late 1960s, but evaluation is as old as the history of human activity [12]. The history of evaluation in education has broadly followed two main streams: the measurement stream that focuses on tests and measurements and the social science stream that focuses on social research methodology (alkin and King). While initially quite distinct in the early evaluation history, these two streams later converged.

Outcomes assessment emerged as the focus of educational evaluation in the 1980s [13], and by the late 1990s, nursing education began to follow higher education trends, with universities placing a greater emphasis on program evaluation.

Best Practice Evaluation of Simulation: Models and Tools

The aim of simulation evaluation is to assess the adequacy of the processes surrounding program implementation and establishment, identify the impact of the program upon students and graduates and compare a new and old program. Best practice approaches of simulation evaluation involve the use of a systematic process of collecting data and information to make educational decisions [8].

Simulation evaluation, therefore, needs to be carried out in four main areas:

- **Processes** surrounding the simulation implementation and design
- **Content** of the simulation and teaching methods used
- **Impact** through assessment of student performance
- **Outcomes** via performance of graduates in the community

The antecedents of evaluation for a simulation include articulating the goals, learning objectives (the knowledge, skills, and abilities that students demonstrate), and simulation approaches to be used. Selecting a specific evaluation model allows faculty to structure their planning and ensure critical information is noticed. In a guide on conducting program evaluation, Frye and Hemmer [9] describe four evaluation models. Two of these models are useful to discuss in the context of simulation evaluation.

Models of Evaluation

Kirkpatrick developed an organizational tool in 1967 [14] that has enjoyed wide popularity in educational evaluation over many years. Kirkpatrick's model is a four-level hierarchy to evaluate outcomes that can be applied in many contexts. Evaluation starts at the first level

Level 1 REACTION: Learner perceptions, satisfaction, or reaction to a program.
Level 2 LEARNING: Measures of learning attributed to the program (e.g., knowledge gained, skills improved, attitudes changed).
Level 3 BEHAVIOUR: Changes in learner behavior in the context of the learning situation.
Level 4 RESULTS: The results on whether the learning transfers to the clinical setting and improves patient and/or organizational outcomes [9, 10].

One of the major criticisms of the Kirkpatrick model has been its propensity towards the use of the lower levels of the model, as the higher levels are more difficult to implement and substantiate [15]. It also tends to be focused on outcomes rather than the process [16]. As a result, a New World Kirkpatrick Model [17] was developed, which enhances these four levels and targets individuals, team behaviors, and processes, and is more aligned to the real-world setting. See Fig. 14.2

The CIPP Model (Context/Input/Process/Product)

The CIPP model uses a set of approaches that focus on program improvement instead of improving something about a program. It provides a theoretical framework to determine the quality and merit of a simulated learning experience [19]. It includes the following aspects.

CONTEXT: Identify and define program goals and priorities by assessing needs, problems, assets, and opportunities. Data collection can include document review, demographic data, interviews, surveys, and focus groups.

INPUT: Feasibility and cost-effectiveness analysis often related to resourcing

PROCESS: The fidelity of implementation including activities, roles, documentation processes, budget considerations, problem identification, views on the quality of the process

PRODUCT: Positive and negative outcomes, short-term implications, effectiveness, sustainability, transferability [9].

Evaluation and Its Interface with Regulatory Bodies

The internal drivers for simulation program evaluation are often based on a desire to strive for excellence in simulation teaching and learning and to ensure the quality of outcomes for graduates [13]. The external drivers for simulation program evaluation often relate to the imposed requirements from external regulatory bodies [9, 13]. Most international

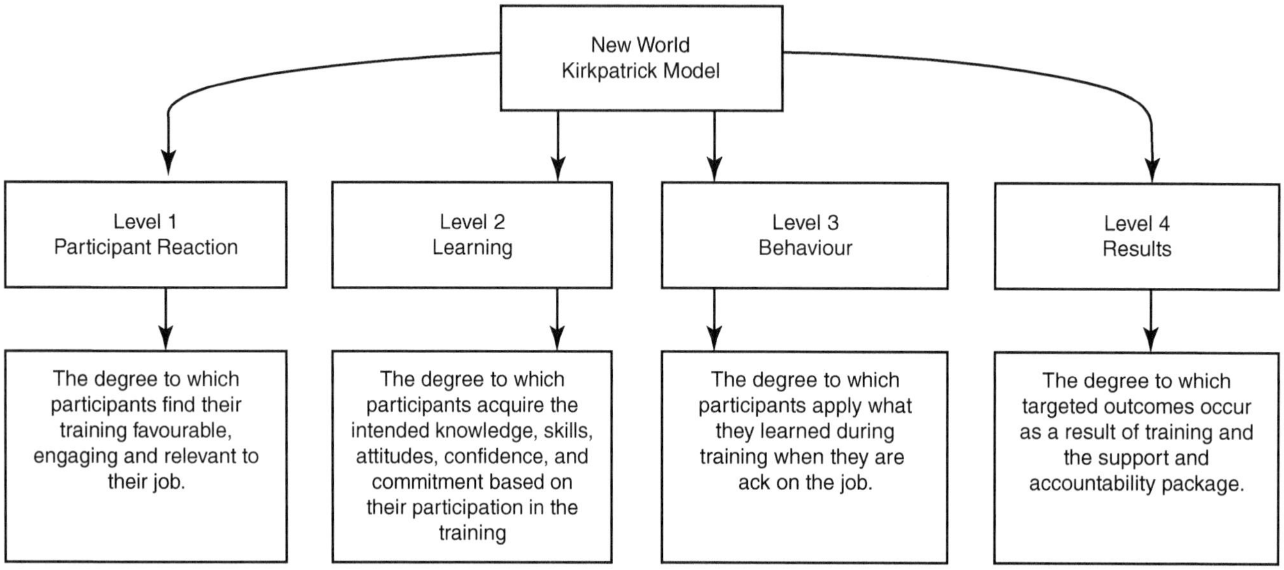

Fig. 14.2 The New World Kirkpatrick Model [18]

accrediting bodies mandate program evaluation (including simulation methods) to meet accreditation standards leading to nursing registration and licensure. A strong program evaluation supports accountability and provides educators with useful knowledge to improve the program. While individual evaluation of simulation is often not an overt requirement in most accreditation processes, evaluation of simulation forms one component of the overall course evaluation process.

Although there are differences in how standards may be worded, simulation evaluation can relate to three areas. Firstly, standards associated with fiscal resources. Simulation is a costly teaching and learning endeavor that requires an organizational commitment to infrastructure and equipment funding. Secondly, standards associated with teaching and learning methods. Key questions include, are simulation teaching methods using best practices? Are scenarios fit for purpose, authentic, and well-designed, do debriefing methods foster engagement and deep learning? Does simulation education contribute to the development of student's knowledge, skills, and professionalism? Third, program effectiveness (Lewallen) about achievement of program outcomes, readiness to practice, and student satisfaction levels.

As a quality improvement exercise, program evaluation can result in positive changes to the simulation design and implementation process to achieve this goal.

Unfortunately, many nursing programs have historically been overly dependent on accreditation processes to drive evaluation efforts, and it is well recognized that this approach may need to include some important elements that contribute towards and influence a program's success. A continuous and comprehensive approach to program evaluation (including simulation evaluation) should be firmly embedded as a routine requirement of curriculum planning at all levels and stages of a course.

Evaluation Instruments

There are a multitude of survey instruments of varying quality that have been reported in the literature that support the process of evaluation of simulation [20]. Tools should only form one part of the evaluation plan and must be selected according to key criteria such as validity, reliability, and feasibility. Reliability refers to the extent that the tool yields the same results over multiple tests, and validity refers to the extent that the instrument measures what it was designed to measure [21]. Feasibility aspects to consider include whether the tool is concrete, usable, understandable, clear, and objective [21, 22]. Further development is needed to design, test and validate the use of evaluation instruments in undergraduate settings. Table 14.8 presents examples of different tools that can be used in nursing. These tools have undergone varying degrees of reliability and validity testing. The selection of instruments should match the evaluation goals, the context of the learning, the simulation modality, and the cohort of students. Of most significance are the tools that the United States National League of Nursing has published.

Table 14.8 Example evaluation instruments

Title of tool	Characteristics	Domains
General simulation evaluation tools		
Educational Practices Questionnaire (Student Version) [23–25]	16 items Validity and reliability data	Educational practices in simulation and their importance. Attitudes towards active learning, collaboration, diverse ways of learning, and high expectations.
Student Satisfaction and Self-Confidence in Learning Scale [23–25]	13 items Validity and reliability data	Student satisfaction and self-confidence in instruction with simulation
Simulation Design Scale [23–25]	20 items Validity and reliability data	Perceptions of objectives, information, support, problem-solving, feedback, and fidelity in simulation
Team-based tools		
Clinical Team Scale [26]	15 items Rating scale (1–10; Poor to perfect) Validity and reliability data	Communication, situational awareness/resource management
The Team Survey & Psychological Contract Scale [27]	43 items 5-point rating scale Validity and reliability data	Team identification, Team potency, Team interaction models, Team models, Metacognition, Communication, Perspectives, Valuing others, Relationship to the team

Conclusion

Assessment and evaluation are two important components of undergraduate nursing education. Simulation plays a significant role in measuring the applied knowledge, skill, and attributes of the student nurse. Evaluation of simulation is equally important in that it helps to identify the impact of simulation. It assists with feedback, quality improvement, and future planning of simulation activity across an entire curriculum. Assessment and evaluation both require the use of evidence-based theoretical models and frameworks, a well-developed plan, and the use of validated, reliable and feasible instruments.

References

1. Masters GN. Reforming Education Assessment: Imperatives, principles, and challenges. Camberwell: ACER Press; 2013.
2. MacLellan E. Assessment for Learning: the differing perceptions of tutors and students. Assess Eval High Educ. 2001;26(4):307–18.
3. Miller GE. The assessment of clinical skills/competence/performance. Acad Med. 1990;65(9):S63–7.
4. Alinier G. Nursing students' and lecturers' perspectives of objective structured clinical examination incorporating simulation. Nurse Educ Today. 2003;23(6):419–26.
5. Norcini J, Anderson MB, Bollela V, Burch V, Costa MJ, Duvivier R, et al. 2018 Consensus framework for good assessment. Med Teach. 2018;40(11):1102–9.
6. Biggs J. Constructive alignment in university teaching: HERDSA. Rev High Educ. 2014;1:5–22.
7. Hamdy H. Blueprinting for the assessment of health care professionals. Clin Teach. 2006;3(3):175–9.
8. Welch S. Program evaluation: a concept analysis. Teach Learn Nurs. 2021;16(1):81–4.
9. Frye AW, Hemmer PA. Program evaluation models and related theories: AMEE Guide No. 67. Med Teach. 2012;34(5): e288–e99.
10. Johnston S, Coyer FM, Nash R. Kirkpatrick's evaluation of simulation and debriefing in health care education: a systematic review. J Nurs Educ. 2018;57(7):393–8.
11. ACGM. Glossary of Terms: Accreditation Council for Graduate Medical Education 2020. https://www.acgme.org/globalassets/pdfs/ab_acgmeglossary.pdf.
12. Shadish WR, Luellen JK. History of evaluation. In: Mathison S, editor. Encyclopedia of evaluation. Sage; 2005. p. 183–6.
13. Lewallen LP. Practical strategies for nursing education program evaluation. J Prof Nurs. 2015;31(2):133–40.
14. Kirkpatrick DL. Evaluation of training. In: Craig RL, Bittel LR, editors. New York: McGraw Hill; 1967.
15. Cahapay M. Kirkpatrick model: its limitations as used in higher education evaluation. Int J Assess Tools Educ. 2021;8(1): 135–44.
16. Yardley S, Dornan T. Kirkpatrick's levels and education 'evidence'. Med Educ. 2012;46(1):97–106.
17. Kirkpatrick J, Kirkpatrick W. An introduction to the new world Kirkpatrick model. Kirkpatrick Partners; 2021.
18. Bhatia M, Stewart AE, Wallace A, Kumar A, Malhotra A. Evaluation of an in-situ neonatal resuscitation simulation program using the new world Kirkpatrick model. Clin Simul Nurs. 2021;50:27–37.
19. Lippe M, Carter P. Using the CIPP model to assess nursing education program quality and merit. Teach Learn Nurs. 2018;13(1) :9–13.
20. Kardong-Edgren S, Adamson KA, Fitzgerald C. A review of currently published evaluation instruments for human patient simulation. Clin Simul Nurs. 2010;6(1):e25–35.
21. Solutions S. Reliability and Validity; 2022
22. Rauta S, Salanterä S, Vahlberg T, Junttila K. The criterion validity, reliability, and feasibility of an instrument for assessing the nursing intensity in perioperative settings. Nurs Res Pract. 2017;2017:1048052.
23. Jeffries PR, Rizzolo MA. Designing and implementing models for the innovative use of simulation to teach nursing care of ill adults and children: a national, multi-site, multi-method study (summary report). Sci Res. 2006;
24. Unver V, Basak T, Watts P, Gaioso V, Moss J, Tastan S, et al. The reliability and validity of three questionnaires: The Student Satisfaction and Self-Confidence in Learning Scale, Simulation Design Scale, and Educational Practices Questionnaire. Contemp Nurse. 2017;53(1):60–74.
25. Franklin AE, Burns P, Lee CS. Psychometric testing on the NLN Student Satisfaction and Self-Confidence in Learning, Simulation Design Scale, and Educational Practices Questionnaire using a sample of pre-licensure novice nurses. Nurse Educ Today. 2014;34(10):1298–304.
26. Guise J-M, Deering SH, Kanki BG, Osterweil P, Li H, Mori M, et al. Validation of a tool to measure and promote clinical teamwork. Simul Healthc. 2008;3(4)
27. Millward LJ, Jeffries N. The team survey: a tool for health care team development. J Adv Nurs. 2001;35(2):276–87.

Part III

Graduate Nursing Education

Simulation Modalities for Graduate Nursing Programs

15

Bernadette Henrichs and John M. O'Donnell

Simulation Modalities for Nursing

Background

Educating students to become successful nurses, specifically advanced practice nurses, is critical for nursing faculty. Graduates must be prepared to take on their new roles in nursing. Because the new nurse's role involves actual patients, nursing faculty need to ensure that graduates can competently care for patients and deliver a high level of care, whether that patient is critically ill or in a stable condition.

Because hands-on education is a vital component in the training of nurses for expanded roles in nursing, faculty have the opportunity to use several simulation modalities to help assure that graduates are prepared with adequate knowledge, skills, and attitudes. Using simulation to teach a concept is an excellent method to help transfer new knowledge and skills to the student. Simulation has been used in aviation since World War II and has now transitioned to nursing education [1]. The National League of Nurses endorsed the use of simulation in 2003 as a method for preparing students in clinical skills, critical thinking skills, and self-reflection [1]. Simulation can be used for teaching clinical and crisis management skills and nontechnical skills such as communication, leadership, and team-building skills. These skills are refined as advanced practice nursing students learn to take charge of life-threatening situations. If confronted with any of these complications in their future practice, it is hoped that the scenario will be familiar to them, and they will have adequate knowledge and skill to effectively address and treat the complication. The simulation environment, including computerized simulators and realistic equipment, can set the stage for learning to manage unusual conditions or complications. For example, many advanced practice nurses (such as Nurse Anesthetists) are unlikely to experience rare critical events such as malignant hyperthermia (MH) during their training. However, properly diagnosing and treating MH if encountered during practice is essential and must be carried out expeditiously, or the patient may not survive. Using simulation to help develop the skills and knowledge necessary to address rare but life-threatening events has two advantages. First, the immersive learning experience is thought to create a more memorable experience that will help nurse anesthetists recall the proper diagnosis, symptom recognition, and treatment methods. Second, it is hoped that these simulation experiences will help to develop providers' confidence in their ability to be successful when faced with critical clinical events.

Simulation poses no risk to an actual patient, even though it provides an enhanced sense of reality. Teaching is accomplished as students learn in a controlled environment where mistakes can be made without harm to the patient. Repeated, deliberate practice can serve as a means to strengthen the learning experience. The simulation environment can be made quite realistic in order to help the students understand how the simulation experience connects to the actual clinical setting. Simulation can improve knowledge, help develop clinical skills, build confidence levels of the learner, and help to develop psychomotor and critical thinking skills [2]. This can reduce the time it takes to reach competency and practice in a real-life setting and a safe manner [3]. Many errors or accidents may be avoided if detected and corrected during a potentially critical situation. Simulation gives instructors the opportunity to teach students how to address serious situations through practice in a simulated, controlled environment. With adequate practice, students will learn to react flawlessly whenever a problem arises. With repetitive teach-

B. Henrichs (✉)
Goldfarb School of Nursing/Barnes-Jewish College, St. Louis, MO, USA

Washington University Department of Anesthesiology, St. Louis, MO, USA
e-mail: bhenrichs@bjc.org, henrichsb@wustl.edu

J. M. O'Donnell
University of Pittsburgh, Pittsburgh, PA, USA

J. M. Kutzin et al. (eds.), *Comprehensive Healthcare Simulation: Nursing*, Comprehensive Healthcare Simulation,
https://doi.org/10.1007/978-3-031-31090-4_15

ing using the simulator, human error will potentially decrease when students care for a real patient in the future.

Training with simulation can help the student retain knowledge by combining "hearing, seeing, and doing" in comparison to only "hearing" information during a traditional lecture. Simulation can also be used to evaluate didactic teaching. Since didactic teaching aims to prepare students for clinical practice, the information should be presented in a *clinically* useful manner. The simulator is a way to present information that will help the student clinically. Students can use the simulator to learn how to conduct a physical examination, perform clinical skills such as arterial catheter placement, detect and correct equipment faults, perform routine procedures, or recognize and respond to critical incidents.

Nursing educators can also use simulation to teach nursing students how to work with patients of diverse cultures that they may encounter in their practice. The simulated patient encounter can be developed to allow students to care for patients of a different race, culture, or group with unique beliefs about their healthcare or with specific challenges to providing care. For example, simulated patients can present as hard of hearing, with visual loss, or speaking an unfamiliar language. Simulation provides an excellent opportunity for nursing educators to address the cultural diversity/sensitivity among our patients. It allows students to practice for these encounters during the simulation. It also offers an opportunity during debriefing to gain a deeper understanding to improve patient care. This is critically important as it has become apparent that patients differing in age, race, gender, sexual orientation, and religious backgrounds have different health beliefs and needs.

Best Practices: Types of Simulation Modalities

Using simulation for nursing education can be carried out in a variety of ways, including the use of manikins and task trainers for teaching clinical skills, standardized patients to improve interaction and communication, computer-based and virtual reality programs for critical thinking and problem-solving, role-playing with a classmate to improve team building, and low and high fidelity simulations to improve knowledge, skills, and attitudes of nurses.

Task Trainers

Task trainers are useful for teaching basic nursing skills such as intravenous insertion, foley catheter placement, nasogastric tube placement, and wound and tracheostomy care. Task trainers are also very helpful in teaching specific advanced skills to advanced practice nurses. The simulator can be used to test the performance of psychomotor skills of advanced practice nurses, such as insertion of a central venous catheter (CVC), arterial catheter placement using a simulated arm with a pulsating artery, intubation and placement of an endotracheal tube, placement of a chest tube into the pleural cavity, or performing a cricothyrotomy, a needle placed into the cricothyroid membrane to emergently establish an airway in a patient who cannot be intubated or ventilated by airway experts. Allowing the student to visually see the demonstration of the skill as it is explained is a successful method for teaching psychomotor skills. The student can then practice the skill as often as he/she wants so that he/she is comfortable completing the clinical task or procedure. This hands-on practice experience enhances the student's preparation and replaces what was used in the past: "See one, then do one" on an actual patient.

Task trainers can provide a method for standardizing testing and demonstrating psychomotor skills. Each student can be presented with an identical situation in the same manner so that the scenario can be standardized. The simulator allows multiple attempts at skills without resultant harm to a patient. The simulation activity should allow time for the instructor to pause the session to teach or talk aloud while demonstrations occur. Immediate feedback can be provided to the student without concern that the patient will hear the instructor during the teaching session. When a student can practice a specific skill with a task trainer, the student is better prepared to complete the skill on a real patient.

Checklists can be combined with task trainers to enhance the performance of the skill and assess whether or not the student is performing the steps of the task appropriately. For example, a student can follow numbered steps in completing a specific skill, assuring that each step is completed. Students can practice these skills with another student, especially when using a checklist. Each step of the task is listed, so if the student does not perform a step, the observer can give feedback to the student completing the task, letting that student know if a step was missed or performed incorrectly. The checklists can be brought with the students to the clinical area and followed step-by-step if a procedure needs to be completed and the student needs to be refreshed on the appropriate steps. For example, when the student learns that he/she needs to place a double-lumen endobronchial tube in the patient and realizes he/she needs to review the steps. The checklist can be reviewed before the procedure, and the steps can be followed when the student performs the procedure. Thus, checklists may reduce errors and improve patient safety [4].

Standardized Patients

Standardized patient utilization for healthcare education was developed in the early 1960s and is an effective method to enhance learning [5]. A standardized patient is a person who is trained to portray a patient with certain comorbidities or an actual person with such comorbidities where the person uses his/her own history and physical exam findings [6]. A disadvantage to a standardized patient who does not have the diagnosis of the simulated patient that he/she is playing is the lack of physical signs and symptoms that correlate to a specific diagnosis [5]. For example, a standardized patient may not have a heart murmur even though the simulated patient that he/she is playing has a heart murmur. However, standardized patients still play an important role in preparing the learner for the clinical experience through role-playing and communication. The realism of the simulated experience is enhanced through the use of a real person that interacts with the student. Perhaps the most realistic component of the standardized patient encounter is the ability to have a relatively normal conversation, something that is difficult when using manikin simulators.

Standardized patients cannot only help teach the learner to develop certain clinical skills, such as physical examination of a patient but also help with performance assessment of the learner. The standardized patient can provide feedback to the student and the instructor after the scenario on how well the learner performed. A standardized patient provided with significant training and preparation can also play several other important roles when educating nurses. This can be accomplished by having the standardized patient play the role of the patient, the family member, or even a fellow healthcare professional. Standardized patients can also be used in combination with task trainers. If a student is being taught how to place a central line, the standardized patient can simulate patient responses. The student can then explain the procedure to the patient, answer questions the patient may have, and obtain consent. The actual task can then be performed on a task trainer that allows for central line placement. This may enhance the educational experience since a task trainer cannot communicate with the learner, but a standardized patient can talk and ask questions. The standardized patient can change his/her personality to the needs of the educational experience. For example, he can be an angry patient, a confused patient, or a very uncooperative patient. Thus, communication skills can be taught, along with specific clinical skills, through the use of standardized patients [7].

Screen-based or Computer Simulations on a Mobile Phone or Desktop

Computer-driven, screen-based programs can be run on a personal computer or a smartphone at the convenience of the trainee. Many students own a laptop computer and/or a smartphone as mobile technology is now a major part of our lives. For students without these devices, faculty can work within their institutions to provide the necessary resources. These programs can also be run on a desktop computer. Combining nursing education with mobile technology is a logical choice. The learner can download the application and can decide when and where he/she wishes to participate in the learning program. The learning can be done nearly anywhere on his/her own time and is helpful for learners whose learning style is visual or kinesthetic [8]. Such smartphones or computer programs can be used to acquire knowledge, build technical skills, assess the competency of knowledge attainment, and evaluate and provide feedback related to clinical knowledge and critical-thinking skills of critical incidents or events [4]. Computer-driven, screen-based programs are an effective training tool for nursing education. In a study by Yoo & Lee in 2015, a mobile application specific to cardiopulmonary assessment education effectively improved knowledge retention and provided clinical assessment skills similar to high-fidelity human patient simulators [9]. Because technology is playing an important role in the education of nurses, nurse educators are "being challenged to integrate technological innovation to assist students in their learning" (p. 1) [10]. In a study by Kim and Park in 2019, learning using a smartphone significantly positively impacted nursing students' knowledge, skills, confidence in performance, and learning attitude [11]. It is important that technological support be available for those who need support in obtaining or implementing the program.

An example of using screen-based simulation on a mobile phone or desktop is basic life support (BLS) or advanced cardiac life support (ACLS) certification that many health care providers complete. After reviewing the information, the student completes the course and then takes an electronic exam through the computer-based program. The student then completes the second session with either an instructor using a task trainer or with an automated feedback task trainer [12]. In both circumstances, the student demonstrates the proper technique for basic life support skills of ventilation and chest compressions for basic life support. For advanced life support, the student demonstrates how to diagnose and treat a scenario such as ventricular tachycardia or asystole. The process involves: educating on the topic through bookwork, demonstrating that the expected knowledge was achieved through an examination, and demonstrating proper psychomotor skills were learned through demonstration-again either with an instructor or using an automated system. Once these steps are completed, the student earns their certifications which are required in order to participate in clinical practice.

Virtual Reality and Visualization

With virtual reality, human immersion in the education of a concept is achieved by using computer technology to create a simulated environment. Virtual reality places the user inside an experience instead of viewing it on a screen. Users are immersed and can interact with 3-dimensional images. Many senses, including vision, hearing, touch, and sometimes smell, can be involved [4]. An example used in healthcare education is virtual reality to teach a student how to place an intravenous catheter or intubate a virtual patient. It may also be used to allow surgeons to practice a specific technique, such as a laparoscopic approach to abdominal surgery. The learner places a head-mounted display on his/her head and visually looks at a simulated, monitored patient through the virtual screen. Both examples help the learner develop psychomotor skills using a virtual environment. Virtual reality simulation can also be used for teaching non-technical skills, specifically teamwork, communication, and situational awareness [13].

Manikin-based Patient Simulation (the Spectrum of Low to High Fidelity)

The use of manikins allows the instructor to present to the student a variety of scenarios where the patient can gather the information and decide how to address the concern. Systems that model the physiologic responses into the manikins can help teach the student more complicated tasks. The term high fidelity with respect to a simulator means that the device more realistically replicates certain human functions (e.g., palpable pulses, the motion of breathing, eye blinking) than more static and thus 'low-fidelity' simulators, making the scenario experience more engaging for the student. Computerized simulators with more functions can support dynamic and interactive instruction and provide considerable variation within the simulated environment. The higher fidelity manikins can be programmed with specific vital sign responses corresponding to a patient story incorporating different weights, ages, or medical problems. For example, a "patient" can be a 70-year-old, 120-kg male with a history of smoking and heart disease presenting to repair an abdominal hernia. The simulator computer program directs the manikin's responses to medications and treatment in a fashion that a real person with similar medical problems would respond to during his anesthesia and surgery.

Crisis resource management skills can also be taught using simulation, a set of nonmedical skills required to address medical emergencies [14]. These nontechnical skills include critical thinking, leadership, problem-solving, situational awareness, resource utilization, and communication skills [14]. These nontechnical skills can be evaluated using checklist or global rating scores for performance evaluation. A study by Kim et al. (2009) demonstrated that both checklists and global rating scores were both valid tools to assess performance; however, users indicated a strong preference for the global rating scale due to its ease of scoring, the ability to obtain an overall score and the potential for formative evaluation [14]. A critical incident can occur, such as a bronchospasm or a pneumothorax, and the student must make a differential diagnosis and appropriately treat the crisis event. The student can attempt different treatment methods to see which treatment is appropriate and effective. The instructor can allow errors in the treatment methods, so the learner can experience the consequences of treating inappropriately without harming an actual patient. Decision-making skills are enhanced as the learner is required to decide how to address life-threatening emergencies. The manikin experience will also help the learner improve communication skills and collaborate with other healthcare team members if other students play different roles in the healthcare team, such as a pharmacist, a respiratory therapist, or a physician [15]. Debriefing and reflective thinking after the scenario can promote communication skills and confidence in nursing [15]. Thus, high-fidelity simulation can be a useful tool for improving knowledge and confidence in critical care nurses [16].

High-fidelity simulation is often used in nurse anesthesia programs to educate students on how to address life-threatening emergencies that may be seen in the operating room when a patient is under anesthesia. Examples of scenarios that nurse anesthesia educators commonly address through simulation are anaphylaxis, pulmonary aspiration, hemorrhage and hypovolemic shock, pneumothorax, cardiac ischemia, hyperkalemia with succinylcholine induction, and cardiac arrhythmias. Although the events rarely occur, the nurse anesthetist must immediately respond and treat the emergency, or the patient may not survive. Simulation can help the nurse anesthesia student diagnose and treat such life-threatening emergencies.

Although high-fidelity simulators can make simulation experiences more realistic because of the physiologic responses, they are more complicated technologically, and resources are needed to support the manikin if it does not function properly. Also, using high-fidelity simulation can be expensive as it is time-consuming and resource-intensive for faculty to run the scenarios [17, 18]. Recognizing this issue, many simulation educators use the strategy of scaffolding learning. This process would include teaching a concept in the classroom, followed by the use of online or mobile technology with a case example or screen-based simulation to reinforce the concept. This could be practiced by the student multiple times. The student could then be brought to the simulation center for hands-on practice with simulation scenarios with the high technology manikin. Using this approach for teaching can maximize efficiency in the use of simulation resources and potentially reduce faculty time in the simulation center because of the increased preparation of the students for the experience.

Problem-based Learning (PBL) and Simulation

Problem-based learning occurs when students are exposed to a specific situation or nursing problem that involves problem-solving skills. It requires both self-directed and collaborative problem-solving, and learning involves making a critical appraisal, processing information, communicating with the group of students involved, and collaborating with teamwork to solve the problem presented to them [19]. Problem-based learning can also be combined with high-fidelity simulation, proven to improve the application of theory in clinical practice, increase learning motivation and enhance the educational activity in class. It can also accelerate the learning progress and enhance student satisfaction [19]. An example of a simulation incorporating problem-based learning is a simulated operating room where the learner is at the head of the bed. The student is presented with a scenario, such as a patient who needs anesthesia due to a motor vehicle accident and is very unstable. The patient may also wear a cervical collar due to a possible neck fracture. The student can discuss the anesthetic plan with the other students, and the instructor can provide feedback on the plan prior to the student administering "anesthesia" to the simulated patient. The clue of the cervical collar should stimulate the student to understand that the patient requires specialized airway management.

Improving Critical Knowledge, Skills, and Attitudes

Using simulation to teach undergraduate and graduate nurses can improve critical knowledge, skills, and attitudes that in the past had to be learned through trial and error in the clinical setting. Simulation has demonstrated that it can successfully achieve these goals if well-designed and thoughtfully implemented. Skills taught using simulation can successfully transfer to the clinical setting, and professional behavior and attitudes can also be taught using simulation [20].

Simulation can also be used to teach students various non-technical skills, including leadership, communication, and differentiating a patient diagnosis. For example, communication failures are the most common root cause of medical errors [21]. However, teaching and assessing communication skills in the clinical environment is challenging. The simulation setting is ideal for developing these skills. For example, a new graduate nurse should be able to call an attending physician at night to bring up a patient concern. The ability to develop a simulation scenario where a 'standardized participant acting as a physician' will ask specific questions about the patient underscores the nurse's importance of gathering and organizing the information before making the call. Furthermore, it can be stress-inducing for a new nurse to realize that he/she is 'waking up' the physician. The simulation encounter is an effective way to help the soon-to-be graduate nurse develop the skill and confidence to engage in this conversation in a real-world setting. Another example is teaching the nurse how to deal with the death of a patient. This can be a very challenging emotional situation, and students need to be informed about the objectives of the simulation and understand the purpose. The student can simulate what actions must occur when a patient dies, including engaging in difficult conversations such as notifying the physician, comforting the family, and being familiar with transferring the body to the morgue. The simulation scenario can also focus on how the nurse can effectively communicate with family members. Some members may be accepted, some may be in denial, and some may be angry. The student can explore methods of communication with the different personalities of family members and gain additional communication skills.

Summary

In summary, using simulation to teach nursing students the knowledge, skills, and attitudes to become successful nurses is an excellent way to prepare future nurses in pre-licensure and advanced practice programs. As described in this chapter, many modes can be used in effective simulation training. Importantly, effective learning through simulation is accomplished by combining the psychomotor and cognitive and affective domains utilized in classroom lectures and examinations [22, 23]. The hands-on training and interactions, whether with part-task trainers, computerized manikins, screen-based programs, and standardized patient encounters, provide a visual route to learning that can complement classroom lectures and discussions. With the ongoing emphasis in the educational community on measurable outcomes and teaching objectives, simulation technology can support the achievement of these educational goals.

Using simulation can decrease stress by increasing confidence as the student becomes familiar with managing patient care while also reinforcing the steps needed to complete specific skills. When confronted with how to communicate or take on a leadership role, simulation is an effective tool to teach such skills, whether the student is an undergraduate student learning basic nursing or an experienced nurse at the graduate level learning an advanced practice role.

Example of a Skills Checklist: Arterial Line Insertion

SKILL	Satisfactory	Unsatisfactory
1. States indications for direct blood pressure monitoring: Such as CABG, major vascular, HD instability, research, pheochromocytoma, controlled hypotension, or multiple ABGs and explains to patient.		
2. Washes hands.		
3. Performs time out and marks site.		
4. Tests collateral blood flow of ulnar artery by performing Allen's test (Controversial since most complications are embolic in nature & Allen's test is of little benefit then)		
5. Wears personal protective gear, including mask, hat, goggles, sterile gloves		
6. Dorsiflexes wrist over roll & secures on arm board; temporarily tapes thumb back to raise artery to surface as needed		
7. Prepares the site by cleansing with Duraprep and placing a sterile drape over the wrist		
8. If the patient is awake, generously inject the site with a local anesthetic to prevent pain and also to prevent vasospasm		
9. Places a small skin incision with a needle at the puncture site to prevent creation of a skin plug on the insertion catheter if indicated		
10. Appropriately locates and cannulates artery using ultrasound by using a 45° angle to insert a 20 g IV catheter-over-the-needle system into the artery (22 or 24 g if pediatrics)		
11. If not using ultrasound, palpates the artery and use a 45° angle to insert a 20 g IV catheter-over-the-needle system into the artery (22 or 24 g if pediatrics)		
12. Once arterial blood flashes back, advances 1 mm, decrease the angle to 30°, and inserts guide wire (if used) gently into the artery and (if or if not used) advance the catheter over the wire/needle into the artery		
13. Removes guide wire or needle		
14. Quickly connects catheter end to short, pressure tubing with stopcock, assuring it is secured tightly		
15. Aspirates all air from tubing and stopcock; confirms arterial pulsatile flow		
16 Flushes with NS and connects to pressurized transducer setup, preventing any air from entering tubing and stopcocks		
17. Sutures catheter securely to skin PRN		
18. Place occlusive, sterile dressing over the site		
19. Properly disposes of equipment and documents procedure		
20. Compares noninvasive blood pressure reading to direct, invasive reading. (Noninvasive should be within 10–20 mmHg lower)		
21. Identifies those at increased risk for ischemic damage: Those with Raynaud's disease, hyperlipidemia, low CO, shock, sepsis, prolonged cannulation >48 h, and those on vasopressors		

______________ ________ __________________

SRNA Signature **Date** **Name/Title of Evaluator**

Example of a Skills Checklist: Insertion of a Double-Lumen Endotracheal Tube (DLT)

SKILL	Satisfactory	Unsatisfactory
1. Checks both cuffs (bronchial & tracheal) before insertion to verify the patency of the cuffs		
2. Lubricates tube & stylet; places stylet in tube		
3. Holds distal concave curvature facing anteriorly		
4. Inserts tube until blue cuff passes cords. (MacIntosh #3 laryngoscope blade recommended)		
5. Removes stylet from endobronchial tube		
6. Turns DLT 90° to the appropriate side (Turn left if left DLT; turn right if right DLT)		
7. Quickly advances as far as possible until moderate resistance is felt. The tip should now be seated in the mainstem bronchus.		
8. Connects opti-port connectors to end of DLT.		
9. Inflates tracheal and bronchial cuffs and checks breath sounds bilaterally. (You should hear equal breath sounds.)		
10. Checks placement with fiberoptic bronchoscope (FOB).		
11. Turns patient operative side up. Rechecks and verifies placement of DLT with FOB.		

SKILL	Satisfactory	Unsatisfactory
12. To initiate one-lung ventilation, clamp either the left or right connecting tube behind the optical port. Clamps left if left lung surgery; clamps right if right lung surgery.		
13. Listens in the axilla to hear breath sounds. (You should hear no breath sounds on the ipsilateral side and clear breath sounds on the contralateral side.		
14. Opens connector port between clamp and DLT to allow deflation of lung		
15. Checks peak airway pressures after clamping; checks placement of DLT using FOB.		
16. If hypoxic, adds the following PRN:		
(a) PEEP to ventilated lung PRN (5–10 cm H_2O)		
(b) CPAP to nonventilated lung PRN 5–10 cm H_2O)		

SRNA Signature **Date** **Name/Title of Evaluator**

References

1. Sanford PG. Simulation in nursing education: a review of the research. Qual Rep. 2010;15(4):1006–11. http://www.nova.edu/ssss/QR/QR15-4/sanford.pdf
2. Cant R, Cooper S. The value of simulation-based learning in pre-licensure nurse education: a state-of-the-art review and meta-analysis. Nurse Educ Pract. 2017;27:45–62.
3. Al-Ghareeb A, Cooper S. Barriers and enablers to the use of high-fidelity patient simulation manikins in nurse education: an integrative review. Nurse Educ Today. 2016;36:281–6.
4. Decker S, Sportsman S, Puetz L, Billings L. The evolution of simulation and its contribution to competency. J Contin Educ Nurs. 2008;39(2):74–80.
5. Kowitlawakul Y, Leng Chow Y, Salam ZHA, Ignacio J. Exploring the use of standardized patients for simulation-based learning in advanced practice nurses. Nurse Educ Today. 2015;35:894–9. https://doi.org/10.1016/j.nedt.2015.03.004.
6. Howley LD, Gliva-McConvey G, Thornton J. Standardized patient practices: initial report on the survey of US and Canadian Medical Schools. Med Educ Online. 2009;14:7. https://www.ncbi.nlm.nih.gov/pmc/articles/PMC2779617/
7. MacLean S, Kelly M, Geddes F, Della P. Use of simulated patients to develop communication skills in nursing education: an integrated review. Nurse Educ Today. 2017;48:90–8.
8. Mann E, Medves J, Vandenkerkohf EG. Accessing best practice resources using mobile technology in an undergraduate nursing program. CIN Comput Inform Nurs. 2015;33(3):122–8. https://doi.org/10.1097/CIN.0000000000000135.
9. Yoo I, Lee Y. The effects of mobile applications in cardiopulmonary assessment education. Nurse Educ Today. 2015;35:e19–23. https://reader.elsevier.com/reader/sd/pii/S0260691714003979?token=77D25E5DE39A8B7615714F33ABC1751E3477021 0E0FEF14DCA85A2B7663CD9A7E398DCF11B58FC6E9CCA4EE1C735E8B3
10. Mackay B, Anderson J, Harding T. Mobile technology in clinical teaching. Nurse Educ Pract. 2017;22:1–6.
11. Kim J, Park H. Effects of smartphone-based mobile learning in nursing education: a systematic review and meta-analysis. Asian Nurs Res. 2019;13:20–9.
12. Cheng A, Mancini MB, Hunt EA, Sinz EH, Merchant RM, Donoghue A, Duff JP, Eppich W, Auerbach M, Bigham BL, Blewer AL, Chan PS, Bhanji F. Resuscitation education science: educational strategies to improve outcomes from cardiac arrest: a scientific statement from the American Heart Association. Circulation. 2018;138(6):e82–e122. https://doi.org/10.1161/CIR.0000000000000583.
13. Bracq M, Michinov E, Jannin P. Virtual reality simulation in non-technical skills training for healthcare professionals. Simul Healthc. 2019;14:188–94.
14. Kim J, Neilipovitz D, Cardinal P, Chiu M. A comparison of global rating scale and checklist scored in the validation of an evaluation tool to assess performance in the resuscitation of critically ill patients during simulated emergencies. Simul Healthc. 2009;4:6–16.
15. Shin S, Park J, Kim J. Effectiveness of patient simulation in nursing education: Meta-analysis. Nurse Educ Today. 2015;35:176–82.
16. Boling B, Hardin-Pierce M. The effect of high-fidelity simulation on knowledge and confidence in critical care training: an integrative review. Nurs Educ Pract. 2016;16:287–93.
17. Henrichs B, Thorn S, Thompson J. Teaching student nurse anesthetists to respond to simulated anesthetic emergencies. Clin Simul Nurs. 2018;17:63–71.
18. Levett-Jones T, Lapkin S, Hoffman A, C. & Roche, J. Examining the impact of high and medium fidelity simulation experiences on nursing students' knowledge acquisition. Nurse Educ Pract. 2011;11:380–3.
19. Kang K, Kim S, Kim S-J, Oh J, Lee M. Comparison of knowledge, confidence in skill performance (CSP) and satisfaction in problem-based learning (PBL) and simulation with PBL educational modalities in caring for children with bronchiolitis. Nurse Educ Today. 2015;35:315–21.
20. O'Donnell J, Goode J, Henker R, Kelsey S, Bircher N, Peele P, Bradley J, Close J, Engberg R, Sutton-Tyrrell K. Effect of a simulation educational intervention on knowledge, attitude, and patient transfer skills: from the simulation laboratory to the clinical setting. Simul Healthc. 2011;6(2):84–93.
21. The Joint Commission: about our standards. https://www.jointcommission.org/standards/about-our-standards/
22. Anderson LW, Sosniak LA, editors. Bloom's taxonomy: A forty-year retrospective. National Study for the Study of Education Yearbooks; 1994.
23. Krathwohl DR, Bloom BS, Masia BB. Taxonomy of educational objectives: the classification of educational goals, Handbook II: Affective domain. New York: David Mckay Company Incorporated; 1964.

16 Writing Clinical Simulations for Advanced Practice Registered Nurse Education

Sabrina Beroz

Introduction

The use of simulation in undergraduate education has grown at a staggering rate as a profound and effective teaching-learning methodology. In the education of advanced practice registered nurses (APRN), the use of simulation is gaining momentum. The events of the COVID-19 pandemic 'shined a light' on the importance of simulation in the education of nurses at all levels. However, there is a need for evidence to explore how simulation can enhance the development and mastery of skills in APRN education. Thoughtful integration, administrative support, and trained simulation educators provide high-quality simulation experiences – each important factors in meeting learner outcomes. This chapter focuses on advanced practice simulation and best practices, curriculum integration, challenges, and solutions for writing clinical simulations in graduate nursing education. Highlights include theory, standards, competencies, and curriculum models in APRN programs.

Background

Many Advanced Practice Registered Nurse (APRN) students come to graduate education with experience in simulation and know its effectiveness in augmenting clinical practice [1]. Unfortunately, the National Organization of Nurse Practitioner Faculty (NONPF) and the National Task Force on Quality NP Education continue to require 750 clinical hours in direct patient care and are adamant that these hours cannot be substituted with simulation [2, 3]. Advanced practice students are finding clinical sites insufficient for readiness to practice because the quality of the experience and preceptor vary [4, 5]. In one study, 65% of clinical time was unaccounted for at clinical practice sites [6]. Nye et al. found that 98% of APRN programs use simulation at levels above the required clinical hours, with 77% supporting the replacement of a percentage of clinical hours with simulation [7]. Research found improved confidence and satisfaction in learning with simulation [8] and improvement in communication skills [9]; however, there needs to be more quality studies on student behavioral changes, competency, and clinical performance [10]. Some APRN programs found simulation was effective in educating about case management [11] and differential diagnosis [12]. Recognizing the value of simulation in NP education, the NONPF Board of Directors appointed a 17-member committee to create simulation guidelines and resources for NP educators [13]. This living document incorporates existing theories, standards, and guidelines with application to NP education and simulation activities [13]. Although simulation is in use in APRN education, high-quality, multi-site research is necessary to support these findings and provide evidence to regulatory bodies.

Best Practices: Theory, Standards, Competencies, and Certification

Best practices in simulation-based experiences, whether face-to-face or virtual, begin with the identification of an educational theory to underpin the program. Selection of the theory must align with the vision and mission of the nursing program and parent institution. There are several theories for consideration—constructivism, experiential learning, reflective practice, adult learning principles, novice to expert, and the National League for Nursing (NLN) Jeffries Simulation Theory.

Theory

Constructivism is a theory recognizing that learning is a process of constructing meaning to make sense out of an experience [14]. Experiential learning describes a progression

S. Beroz (✉)
School of Nursing, Montgomery College, Takoma Park, MD, USA

J. M. Kutzin et al. (eds.), *Comprehensive Healthcare Simulation: Nursing*, Comprehensive Healthcare Simulation,
https://doi.org/10.1007/978-3-031-31090-4_16

where knowledge is gained from one experience, becoming the tool for action in new situations [15]. Kolb [16] created the learning cycle, further defining how the transformation of experience leads to changes in behavior. The cycle as it relates to mastery learning through simulation starts with the concrete experience (scenario), followed by reflective observation and abstract conceptualization (debriefing), ending with active experimentation.

Other theories relevant to best practices for simulation-based education include reflective practice and adult learning principles. When writing clinical simulations for graduate education, both constructivism and experiential learning support the notion of reflective practice. Learning takes place during the debriefing phase of a simulation experience to uncover the assumptions or mental models which drove the decision-making process [17] (see Chap. 3, Debriefing). And foundational to graduate education is the concept of adult learning principles, otherwise known as andragogy, which provides educators with tools for understanding how age, maturity, and life experience influence adult learning—the simulation experience (scenario) must be relevant and readily applicable for the learner [18]. Adults are partial toward independent learning, and simulation supports the adult learner through a facilitated process.

Graduate education, much like undergraduate education, takes the learner across a continuum from novice to expert. The Theory of Novice to Expert aids in leveling the simulation scenario to the knowledge, skills, and attitudes of the learner to promote consistent programmatic outcomes [19, 20]. All the aforementioned theories work in concert to provide a theoretical framework underpinning the NLN Jeffries Simulation Theory.

The NLN Jeffries Simulation Theory [21] is essential for developing simulation experiences. It describes concepts that frame simulation-based education at all levels of nursing preparation. The concepts include an overall context influencing the background and design of the simulation, the facilitator, the participant, and the outcomes. Context guides the general purpose of the simulation with a predetermined level of evaluation—formative or summative/high-stakes [20]. It is important to plan the experience with the end in mind. The background provides context for curriculum alignment and the design of the simulation. The design of the simulation includes outcomes and objectives leveled to the knowledge of the participant. The creation of physical, conceptual, and psychological fidelity is necessary to support realism and is relevant to the concept of adult learning principles. The scenario progression defines expected performance and strategies inherent in the evaluation of learner performance. The simulation experience, characterized as learner-focused, collaborative, experiential, and interactive, happens within an environment of trust. Furthermore, facilitator and educational strategies describe the dynamic relationship between the facilitator and the participant (learner). The participant brings life experiences and attributes such as age, gender, and self-confidence—all affecting the facilitator-participant relationship. Lastly, there are three levels of outcomes important to simulation-based education, the participant, the patient, and the healthcare system.

In addition to defining a theory to underpin your simulation program, standards provide guidance in the development of high-quality simulation scenarios based on the latest evidence.

Standards

The Healthcare Simulation Standards of Best Practice™ [20] offer 11 standards for best practices in simulation education. The standards, written on a common template, define the evidence for each standard and criteria with corresponding elements to meet the standard. The standards are not standalone and are to be used as a collective whole. Successful undergraduate and graduate programs use the standards across the curriculum when developing a simulation portfolio. While all standards are paramount for integration, one stands out for writing clinical simulation scenarios: The Healthcare Simulation Standard of Best Practice™ (HSSOBP) Simulation Design.

The HSSOBP™ Simulation Design begins with a statement of the standard stating: "Simulation-based experiences are purposely designed to meet identified objectives and optimize achievement of expected outcomes."([20], p. 14) The design should follow the criteria set out for consideration in order to meet the expected outcomes. Consequences of not using the criteria include ineffective evaluation of learner performance and inability to meet the outcomes and objectives—all necessary for student learning. Table 16.1 provides the eleven criteria (the what) and elements (the how) to meet the Simulation Design standard [20]. Keep in mind that prewritten scenarios can be reviewed against the Simulation Design standard.

The Simulation Design standard gives the simulationist reference to the other standards for further in-depth information. The HSSOBP™ Professional Development supports initial and ongoing professional development across the simulationists career [20]. The HSSOBP™ Outcomes and Objectives requires all simulation experiences to be written using SMART objectives to achieve expected outcomes [20]. The HSSOBP™ Facilitation describes the design of the facilitation method to be congruent with the outcomes and objectives of the case [20]. Although outside the scope of this chapter, it is imperative to understand that the facilitator has full responsibility and oversight of the simulation experience and, thus, must be knowledgeable in the facilitative process. The HSSOBP™ Prebriefing:

Table 16.1 Healthcare Simulation Standards of Best Practice™ Simulation Design

Criteria (What)	Elements (How) with Select Measures (as applicable)
Criterion 1. Design simulation-based experiences in consultation with content experts and simulationists knowledgeable in best practices in simulation education, pedagogy and practice.	Review stakeholder surveys, outcome data, and standards from regulatory bodies and/or clinical practice guidelines. Include patient safety goals, end-of-program competencies, and programmatic evaluations. Use the analysis to build scenarios and develop simulation-specific objectives.
Criterion 2. Perform a needs assessment to provide the foundational evidence of the need for a well-designed simulation-based experience.	Develop a blueprint for the scenario using broad and specific objectives. Objectives are specific, measurable, attainable, realistic, and time-phased (SMART). Define which objectives to share with the participants in preparatory work. Key to learning is the facilitator's use of the objectives to guide the simulation experience.
Criterion 3. Construct measurable objectives.	Select the modality appropriate for the simulation (virtual, face-to-face, in situ, level of manikin, OSCE, etc.). Design the scenario progression from start to participant performance expectations to the end-point. Determine the length of the scenario.
Criterion 4. Build the simulation-based experience to align modality with objectives.	Use a template to ensure consistency across the curriculum. Develop a patient backstory, the clinical progression, and time frames. Develop a scenario for consistency/repeatability according to the objectives. Determine performance measures (expected outcomes) (see APRN Simulation Template Considerations [13].
Criterion 5. Design a scenario or case to provide the context for the simulation-based experience.	Design or review the three levels of fidelity. Physically relates to props and environment; conceptual refers to how the scenario realistically runs (vital signs change in context to the scenario), and psychological refers to the feeling of realism.
Criterion 6. Use various types of fidelity to create the required perception of realism.	Select the level of facilitation needed for each scenario. Train all facilitators for a consistent approach. Ensure all facilitators have simulation knowledge. Measures: Facilitator Competency Rubric [22]
Criterion 7. Maintain a facilitative approach that is participant-centered and driven by the objectives, participant's knowledge or level of experience, and the expected outcomes.	Develop preparatory work for the participant such as readings or case studies for example and a structured briefing script to include conduct during the experience, professional integrity, review of objectives, and orientation to the room (onsite) or technical requirements (virtual).
Criterion 8. Create a prebriefing plan to include preparatory work and a briefing to guide participant success during the simulation-based experience.	Identify debriefing or feedback method, length of time, and synchronous or self-debrief process (virtual). Measures: Debriefing Assessment for Simulation in Healthcare (DASH) [23]
Criterion 9. Create a debriefing or feedback session to follow the simulation-based experiences.	Develop an evaluation process for the effectiveness of the simulation scenario, facilitator competency, and level of participant evaluation. Measures: Simulation Design Scale [24]; Simulation Effectiveness Tool-Modified [25]
Criterion 10. Develop a plan of evaluation for the participant(s), facilitator(s), the simulation-based experience, the facility, and the support team.	Simulation designers should have formal or informal education in simulation pedagogy and practice such as conference attendance, certificate programs, workshops and mentorship to name a few.
Criterion 11. Pilot test simulation-based experiences before full implementation.	Pilot test the scenario with an audience similar to the target population. Use a valid/reliable evaluation instrument.

Preparation and Briefing ensures participants are prepared for the experience enhancing psychological safety; while, the HSSOBP™ The Debriefing Process describes the importance of selecting the theory-based debriefing method best suited for the scenario [20]. As stated above, the HSSOBP™ Evaluation of Learning and Performance asks the simulationist to determine the level of evaluation based on the needs assessment and outcome and objectives when beginning to write the scenario [20]. When writing interprofessional simulations for APRN learners, the HSSOBP™ Simulation-Enhanced Interprofessional Education (SimIPE) offers criteria for the need of a theoretical framework and recognition of barriers to implementation [20]. Interprofessional education is a key domain in APRN education. Lastly, the HSSOBP™ Professional Integrity, Glossary, and Operations provide guidance for ethics, common language, and capacity considerations when developing simulation scenarios [20].

APRN learners use standardized patients in simulation-based experiences—most often during objective structured clinical examinations commonly referred to as OSCEs. The Association for Standardized Patient Educators (ASPE) focuses on standardized patient (SP) methodology and established standards of best practice intended to be used in conjunction with the HSSOBP™ [26]. The ASPE standards are organized into five domains—safe work environment, case development, SP training, program management, and professional development—informed by five underlying values—safety, quality, professionalism, accountability, and collaboration [26].

APRN Competencies

The American Association of Colleges of Nursing [27] created competencies for expected levels of achievement in doctoral-level APRN students across eight domains. These competencies, designed to be observable, realistic, and measurable, provide two distinct progression indicators—at the start of the first clinical experience (Time 1) and at program completion (Time 2). They are written to be easily understood by educators, preceptors, and learners. Ultimately, these competencies can be used to design, scaffold and integrate simulation experiences across the continuum of education.

Certification

The Society for Simulation in Healthcare [28], an international and interprofessional organization, offers two levels of certification for the simulation educator as recognition of simulation proficiency—Certified Healthcare Simulation Educator (CHSE) and Certified Healthcare Simulation Educator- Advanced (CHSE-A). A second certification is offered for operations specialists at a proficient and advanced level.

Curriculum Integration and Curriculum Models

Curriculum Integration

The first step, as described in the Simulation Design standard, is a needs assessment to identify curricular gaps where simulation is the best teaching-learning strategy to achieve learner outcomes. Simulation is no longer tangential. It is a sophisticated methodology requiring simulationists to write simulation scenarios at the knowledge, skill, and ability of the graduate-level learner and thoughtfully embed them into the curriculum. Curriculum integration is a linear process starting with program outcomes followed by course outcomes/objectives, concepts, and simulation objectives. An alignment grid, commonly known as a curriculum map, is used to integrate simulation across a program of study Consideration of the complexity of the simulation and the learner's cognitive load are important for the learner when designing experiences [29]. Cognitive load theory (CLT) postulates the learner perceives new information through a formal process that has discrete limitations on how much information can be taken in at one time. The magic number is seven pieces of information a person can manage at any one time [29]. CLT is helpful when designing simulation scenarios and determining the level and number of objectives in each scenario – CLT informs simulation design!

Curriculum Models

Online ARNP programs with onsite simulation experiences. Simulation scenarios offer an opportunity for APRN students to learn clinical decision-making, diagnosis, and prescription in preparation for practicums. They also give faculty the ability to evaluate end-of-program readiness for practice. There are several models for the integration of simulation into the curriculum. Writing scenarios for APRN education depends on the model, placement within the curriculum, and expected outcomes. Most APRN programs are online with a face-to-face requirement. The frequency, length, and context of the onsite experience are determined by the university. Simulation is part of the face-to-face encounter. Keep in mind the COVID-19 pandemic has altered the implementation of simulation models, moving them to virtual experiences. Faculty need to evaluate the impact of virtual simulation in APRN education - what went well and what to improve.

At the George Washington University School of Nursing [30], the APRN online program requires students to come to campus three times for skills acquisition and simulation experiences. The sessions are:

1. Comprehensive Learning and Skill Intensive (CLASI) is the first simulation event integrated into the Health Assessment course. This is a two-day experience where students practice with faculty on day one. On day two, the student is expected to perform a physical assessment to standard in preparation for clinical with a preceptor. During COVID-19, the students submit physical exams remotely and upload the video for faculty review.
2. Objective Structured Clinical Exam I (OCSE I) is a four-step process where students provide a primary care visit for an SP with a simulated medical problem (see Fig. 16.1).
3. OSCE II (Patient Test Out) is integrated into the end of the ARNP program. The process is similar to OSCE I with different cases.

Likewise, Athabasca University in Alberta, Canada, has a requirement for APRN students to attend a one-week on-

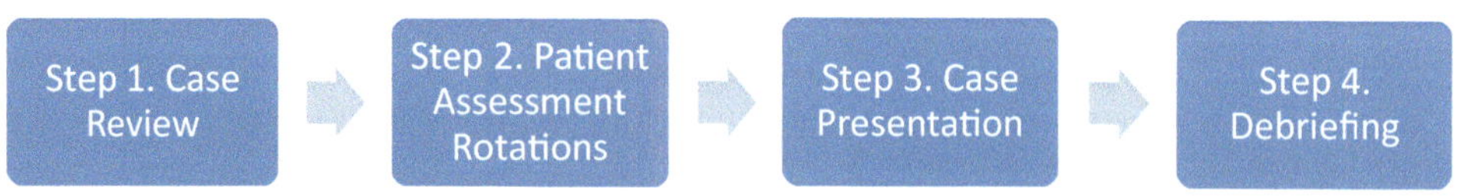

Fig. 16.1 Four-step OSCE experience

campus component inclusive of simulation education [31]. The experience is a pre-program residency prior to the start of the online coursework. These are two examples of how APRN students in online programs utilize simulation in preparation for patient-facing clinical experiences.

Scaffolding. Schneidereith and Daniels [32] from the University of Maryland Debra L. Spunt Clinical Simulation Labs demonstrated the integration of simulation by scaffolding concepts across an adult-gerontology acute care curriculum. They describe scenarios for students enrolled in diagnosis and management courses using high-fidelity manikins. Some of the scenarios used standardized patients in the role of family members. Scenario objectives were developed across five semesters and leveled to the learner (scaffolded) to meet APRN competencies. Scenarios were built using the Simulation Module for Assessment of Resident's Targeted Event Responses (SMARTER) tool [33].

Furthermore, Bauman [34] describes a layered learning model where virtual learning and technology precede and does not replace traditional didactic teaching. It serves as a cognitive aid leveled to face-to-face simulation and gives support to future clinical practice. The virtual experiences, whether games, interactive applications, or virtual environments, all map back to curricular objectives and outcomes.

Virtual simulation curriculum. The use of virtual simulation has expanded in APRN programs due to the greater availability of patient scenarios. These screen-based and virtual platforms are interactive, asynchronous, or synchronous and implemented as a group or independently. Screen-based scenarios provide the learner with decision-making opportunities and metrics on performance. The learner can return to the scene as often as necessary to improve care management. The HSSOBP™ Simulation Design is important for evaluating virtual scenarios. Additionally, the same standards apply to virtual experiences as face-to-face. All sessions should provide preparatory work followed by a briefing session. Built into the simulation orientation should be a technology check ensuring the participant's ability to participate in the experience. Participant metrics from the virtual scenario provide the basis for debriefing. Verkuyl et al. [35] recommend self-debriefing followed by a synchronous debriefing with a facilitator for best practice and optimal outcomes.

Telehealth. NONPF supports the use of telehealth in APRN education, describing telehealth as supporting technical competencies [2]. Telehealth is a viable option for online clinical learning. NONPF counts telehealth as part of the 750 required direct patient care clinical hours. Ainslie & Bragdon [36] introduced telemedicine with scenarios including virtual standardized patients. They found encounters with human standardized patient simulations using telemedicine to be a promising modality for clinical competency assessment [36]. Scenarios can be developed to hone health assessment, communication, and interprofessional skills.

Deliberate practice. Deliberate practice is training focused on improving a particular task aimed toward training and assessment. There are four conditions associated with improved performance that are necessary for success: (1) well-defined goals, (2) internal motivation, (3) immediate feedback, and (4) ample repetition to refine performance [37]. Skills acquisition in ARNP education, such as suturing or central line placement, requires deliberate practice. Scenarios and checklists accompany the experience.

Challenges and Solutions

Simulation in Nurse Practitioner Education Consortium

The George Washington University School of Nursing collaborated with NONPF to hold a national summit to discuss simulation in ARNP education in January 2019 [5]. In attendance were thought leaders from NONPF, NLN, American Association of Nurse Practitioners, AACN, and National Council State Boards of Nursing (NCSBN). The focus was threefold: (1) current research in simulation for ARNP education and gaps in the evidence, (2) opportunities and challenges in the use of simulation in ARNP education, and (3) potential for a multisite study to examine the effectiveness of simulation achievement of clinical competencies. The attendees were charged with identifying enablers and inhibitors in the use of simulation [5]. The top enablers and inhibitors for the use of simulation to meet APRN competencies are listed in Table 16.2.

Summit attendees called to action the need for more evidence on the use of simulation in ARNP education and standardization on the modality best suited for advanced practice both online and face-to-face. The Simulation in Nurse Practitioner Education Consortium [38] was formed to meet the charge. Below, faculty workload will be addressed as other inhibitors have been discussed earlier in the chapter.

Table 16.2 Top enablers and inhibitors to simulation ([5], p. 629)

Enablers	Inhibitors
Generational Learners	Resource and Equity
Cost efficiency/quality	Faculty competency
Need for competency-based movement	Gaps in the literature
Standardization	Resistance to change
Increasing expectations of employers/public	Lack of standardization/ outcomes measures
Limited resources	Multiple regulatory body expectations
Need to address the complexity of care	Workload allocation

Faculty Workload

Often, faculty workload for simulation-based education is not counted in workload calculations, and workload for those in simulation education varies among institutions. Depending on the setting and workload structure, faculty in academia may have additional workload requirements, such as teaching assignments. This impacts the writing of quality scenarios. Blodgett et al. [39] found six determinants informing the development of a simulation faculty workload model: simulation to clinical hour ratio, length of time during the simulation, faculty preparation for simulation, coordinator/director role, the substitution of clinical with simulation, and faculty to student ratio. All factor into writing scenarios thoughtfully for curriculum integration!

Essential Components for Simulation Cases

The following chapters provide case-specific scenarios. Here we offer the essential components for developing scenarios to ensure consistency across the curriculum and participant experience [40]. A sample scenario template is included in the appendix.

1. Patient Name and Demographics
2. Patient's chief complaint and history of present illness
3. Past medical and social history
4. Handoff script if necessary
5. Scenario objectives and level of learner
6. The role will be primary care provider (PCP)
7. ASPE template for SP script development (if using one) ASPE [41]
8. Run time: Prebrief, scenario, and debrief
9. Fidelity: Physical, conceptual, and psychological
10. Select debriefing method
11. Scenario progression

Summary

In summary, writing simulation scenarios for ARNP learners requires a knowledgeable educator in the pedagogy of simulation. Best practices necessitate the simulation educator to use theory, standards, competencies, and certification to develop high-quality simulation scenarios. Simulation educators must identify curricular gaps where simulation is the best strategy for meeting program outcomes. Integrating scenarios into the curriculum requires strategic planning to scaffold and level simulation across the continuum of education. NONPF supports the use of simulation above the mandatory 750 hours of direct patient contact—they do not endorse the substitution of clinical hours for simulation. Unfortunately, many clinical sites are insufficient to meet clinical learning outcomes. It is incumbent upon ARNPs, stakeholders, and regulatory bodies to conduct research on the efficacy of simulation as a substitute for a portion of ARNP clinical hours.

References

1. Hayden J, Smiley R, Alexander M, Kardong-Edgren S, Jeffries P. NCSBN national simulation study: a longitudinal, randomized, controlled study replacing clinical hours with simulation in prelicensure nursing education. JNR. 2014;5:S1–S64.
2. National Organization of Nurse Practitioner Faculties [Internet]. The leader in nurse practitioner education; Washington, DC; 2020 [cited 2020 October 4]. https://www.nonpf.org/#
3. National Task Force on Quality Nurse Practitioner Education. Standards for quality nurse practitioner education: A report of the National Task Force on quality nurse practitioner education. 6th edition. Washington, DC: NONPF; 2022.
4. Hart AM, Bowen A. New nurse practitioners' perceptions of preparedness for and transition into practice. J Nurse Pract. 2016;12(8):545–52. https://doi.org/10.5480/10-465.
5. Jeffries PR, Bigley MB, McNelis AM, Cartier JM, Pintz C, Slaven-Lee PW, Zychowicz ME. A call to action: building evidence for use of simulation in nurse practitioner education. J Am Assoc Nurse Pract. 2019;31(11):627–32. https://doi.org/10.1097/xx.0000000000000335.
6. Fulton CR, Clark C, Dickinson S. Clinical hours in nurse practitioner programs equals competence: Fact or misnomer? Nurse Educ. 2017;42(4):195–8. https://doi.org/10.1097/NNE.0000000000000346.
7. Nye C, Campbell SH, Hebert SH, Short C, Thomas M. Simulation in advanced practice nursing programs: A North-American survey. Clin Simul Nurs. 2019;26(C):3–10. https://doi.org/10.1016/j.ecns.2018.09.005.
8. Warren J, Luctkar-Flude M, Godfrey C, Lukewich J. A systematic review of the effectiveness of simulation-based education on satisfaction and learning outcomes in nurse practitioner programs. Nurse Educ Today. 2016;46:99–108. https://doi.org/10.1016/j.nedt.2016.08.023.
9. Koo LW, Idzik SR, Hammersla MB, Windemuth BF. Developing standardized patient clinical simulations to apply concepts of interdisciplinary collaboration. J Nurs Educ. 2013;52(12):705–8. https://doi.org/10.3928/01484834-20131121-04.
10. Rutherford-Hemming T, Nye C, Coram C. Using simulation for clinical practice hours in nurse practitioner education in the United States: a systematic review. Nurse Educ Today. 2016;37:128–35. https://doi.org/10.1016/j.nedt.2015.11.006.
11. Kesten KS, Brown HS, Meeker MC. Assessment of ARNP competency using simulation: a pilot study. Nurs Educ Perspect. 2015;36:332–5.
12. Harris J, Shoemaker K, Johnson K, Tompkins-Dobbs K, Domian E. Qualitative descriptive study of family nurse practitioner student experiences using high-fidelity simulation. Kans Nurse. 2016;91:12–5.
13. Lioce L, Cornelius J, Brown K, Schneidereith T, Nye C, Weston C, Bigley M. Simulation guidelines and best practices for nurse practitioner programs. Washington DC: National Organization of Nurse Practitioner Faculties; 2020.
14. Bruner J. The act of discovery. Harv Educ Rev. 1961;31:21–32.
15. Dewey J. Experience and education. New York: Macmillan; 1938.
16. Kolb D. Experiential learning: experience as the source of learning and development. New Jersey: Prentice-Hall; 1984.

17. Argyris C, Schon D. Organizational learning: a theory of action perspective. Revista Española de Investigaciones Sociológicas. 1997:345–8.
18. Knowles M. The adult learner: a neglected species. 3rd ed. Texas: Gulf; 1984.
19. Benner P. From novice to expert: excellence and power in clinical nursing practice. Boston: Addison-Wesley; 1984.
20. INACSL Standards Committee. Healthcare Simulation Standards of Best Practice™. Clin Simul Nurs. 2021; 58:1–65.
21. Jeffries PR. The NLN Jeffries simulation theory. Philadelphia: Wolters Kluwer; 2016.
22. Leighton K, Mudra V, Gilbert G. Facilitator Competency Rubric. 2020 [Cited 2018]. https://sites.google.com/view/evaluatinghealthcaresimulation/fcr
23. Center for Medical Simulation. Debriefing assessment for simulation in healthcare: Student and instructor versions; 2020 [cited 2011]. www.harvardmedsim.org
24. National League for Nursing. Simulation Design Scale; 2020 [cited 2005]. http://www.nln.org/professional-development-programs/research/tools-and-instruments/descriptions-of-available-instrument
25. Leighton K, Ravert P, Mudra V, Macintosh C. Updating the simulation effectiveness tool: item modification and reevaluation of psychometric properties. Nurs Educ Perspect. 2015;36(5):317–23.
26. Lewis KL, Bohnert CA, Gammon WL, Holzer H, Lyman L, Smith C, Thompson TM, Wallace A, Gliva-McConvey G. The Association of Standardized Patient Educators (ASPE) Standards of Best Practice (SOBP). Adv Simul. 2017;2(1) https://doi.org/10.1186/s41077-017-0043-4.
27. American Association of Colleges of Nursing. Common Advanced Practice Registered Nurse Doctoral-Level Competencies; 2020 [cited 2017 October]. https://www.aacnnursing.org/Portals/42/AcademicNursing/pdf/Common-APRN-Doctoral-Competencies.pdf
28. Society for Simulation in Healthcare. SSH Certifications; 2020 [cited 2020]. https://www.ssih.org/Credentialing/Certification
29. Reedy GB. Using cognitive load theory to inform simulation design and practice. Clin Simul Nurs. 2015;11(8):355–60. https://doi.org/10.1016/j.ecns.2015.05.004.
30. George Washington School of Nursing. Master of Science in Nursing; 2020 [cited 2020]. https://nursing.gwu.edu/master-science-nursing
31. Athabasca University. Master of Science in Nursing; 2020 [cited 2020]. http://fhd.athabascau.ca/programs/grad/mn/
32. Schneidereith T, Daniels A. Integration of simulation to prepare adult gerontology acute care nurse practitioners. Clin Simul Nurs. 2019;26(C):18–23. https://doi.org/10.1016/j.ecns.2018.10.009.
33. Rosen M, Salas E, Silvestri S, Wu T, Lazarra E. A measurement tool for simulation-based training in emergency medicine: the simulation module for assessment of resident targeted event responses (SMARTER) approach. Simul Healthc. 2008;3(3):170–9.
34. Bauman E. Games, virtual environments, mobile applications, and a futurist's crystal ball. Clin Simul Nurs. 2016;12(4):109–14.
35. Verkuyl M, Lapum JL, St-Amant O, Hughes M, Romaniuk D, McCulloch T. Exploring debriefing combinations after a virtual simulation. Clin Simul Nurs. 2020;40(C):36–42. https://doi.org/10.1016/j.ecns.2019.12.002.
36. Ainslie M, Bragdon C. Telemedicine simulation in online family nurse practitioner education: clinical competency and technology integration. J Am Assoc Nurse Pract. 2018;30(8):430–4.
37. Ericsson KA. Deliberate practice and the acquisition and maintenance of expert performance in medicine and related domains. Acad Med. 2004;79(10):S70–81.
38. George Washington University School of Nursing. Simulation in nurse practitioner education consortium; 2020 [cited 2020]. https://nursing.gwu.edu/simulation-consortium
39. Blodgett NP, Blodgett T, Kardong-Edgren SE. A proposed model for simulation faculty workload determination. Clin Simul Nurs. 2018;18:20–7. https://doi.org/10.1016/j.ecns.2018.01.003.
40. National League for Nursing. Simulation design template; 2020 [cited 2019]. http://www.nln.org/sirc/sirc-resources/sirc-tools-and-tips
41. Association for Standardized Patient Educators. Case development template; 2020 [cited 2017]. https://www.aspeducators.org/

Simulation in Family Nurse Practitioner Education

17

Jo Loomis

Simulation has been used for decades to train medical practitioners and is used extensively in undergraduate nursing education. The large-scale simulation study by the National Council of State Boards of Nursing (NCSBN) in 2014 supported the use of up to 50% of simulation as part of prelicensure nursing student clinical education [1]. This use of simulation has improved nursing education and thus impacts and improves patient health and safety.

Nurse practitioners (NP) as advanced practice registered nurses (APRNs) provide care in primary, acute, or specialty care areas for patients across the lifespan. Providing clinical education to prepare students for their NP role is increasingly complex. Competition for clinical education sites and shortages of experienced and available preceptors have driven faculty to explore alternate clinical training experiences for students. Unlike the use of simulation at the undergraduate level, there is currently no standard for the use of simulation to replace graduate-level clinical hours in NP education [2]. The National Organization for Nurse Practitioner Faculties (NONPF) issued a statement on March 23, 2020, reiterating the requirements for clinical training hours [3]. This statement was supported by accrediting and certifying bodies of nurse practitioner education, indicating that for eligibility to sit for the initial NP certification examinations

> "All nurse practitioner (NP) students are required to complete a minimum of 500 supervised direct patient care clinical hours over the course of the NP program. In addition, clinical hours are distributed to support competency development that represents the needs of the chosen population. If additional clinical hours are required by the institution or a certification organization (above the minimum 500 supervised direct patient care clinical hours), these additional hours may be completed as simulation if students have completed the direct patient care clinical hours that are necessary and required for them to be fully prepared to practice as an NP in the population focus area." [3, 4]

This statement goes on to cite the National Task Force on Quality Nurse Practitioner Education (5th Ed., Criterion III.E., NTFC p. 12)

> "Simulation is recommended to augment the clinical learning experiences, particularly to address the high-risk low-frequency incidents; however, simulation experiences may only be counted as clinical hours over and above the minimum 500 direct patient care clinical hours. Programs are encouraged to track the use of simulation to enhance the clinical experience." [4]

What is needed to move towards the development of standards for the use of simulation to be counted as clinical hours is the publication of rigorous high-quality studies [2, 5]. Research into the use of simulation at the graduate level, especially for NP education, is still in its infancy. Despite the lack of high-quality studies supporting the use of simulation as a replacement for clinical experiences in graduate nursing education, recent surveys have indicated that faculty are using simulation and incorporating it into Nurse Practitioner curriculum. Hawkins-Walsh in 2011 noted that 85% of pediatric nurse practitioner (PNP) programs surveyed across the country indicated some use of simulation, and seven years later, the Nye et al. study, a descriptive survey on the use of simulation in advanced practice nursing (APN) educational programs in the United States and Canada, found that 98% of respondents indicated they were using simulation in some form in their programs [6, 7].

Recognizing the need for guidelines for the use of simulation in nurse practitioner programs, NONPF published *Simulation Guidelines & Best Practices for Nurse Practitioner Programs* [8]. This "living document" provides guidance and support for faculty developing simulations for use in the NP curriculum above and beyond the current requirements for direct patient care clinical hours. The NONPF Simulation Committee also created a simulation portal on the NONPF website that is continuously updated with resources and tools to support NP faculty [8].

J. Loomis (✉)
University of San Francisco, School of Nursing and Health Professions, San Francisco, CA, USA
e-mail: jaloomis2@usfca.edu

J. M. Kutzin et al. (eds.), *Comprehensive Healthcare Simulation: Nursing*, Comprehensive Healthcare Simulation,
https://doi.org/10.1007/978-3-031-31090-4_17

Simulation methodology can create clinical experiences that mirror aspects of real-world experiences. Community-based clinical experiences may be increasingly difficult to secure and difficult to ensure standard educational experiences. Simulation as a pedagogy allows for specific, planned, and standardized clinical experiences, especially those that might not be readily available in the real clinical setting, such as practicing for 'never events.' These experiences should be portrayed in an authentic and realistic manner [9]. The term *fidelity* describes the degree of realism and includes the domains of the physical, conceptual, and psychological [10]. Safe and effective simulations should be designed and conducted according to the standards developed by the International Nursing Association for Clinical Simulation and Learning (INACSL) Standards of Best Practice: Simulation^{SM} and if using human simulated patients, also by the use of the Association of Standardized Patient Educators (ASPE) Standards of Best Practice (SOBP) [10, 11].

Types of Simulation Delivery

Simulation exercises can be carried out in a spacious, well-designed laboratory that is set up to look like the clinical setting it is intended to simulate, whether that is an emergency room, a primary care clinic exam room, or a patient's home. The more realistic the look, function, feel, and even smell of the room, the higher the *fidelity* or degree of realism [9]. Computer-controlled manikins or humans playing the part of patients, called standardized or simulated patients (SP), can be trained to portray disease conditions, with the help of a script and moulage, in the form of silicone molds, wigs, and makeup.

Lower levels of fidelity, such as role-playing in a scenario or reading a case study, are also effective types of simulation. This type of clinical experience can be carried out in a classroom setting with two chairs at the front of the room. An unfolding case study with several 'scenes' can be presented during one class period or allowed to unfold across the semester as students interact with the "patient" for several patient encounters. Students ask questions of the patient, a paid actor, or a scripted student volunteer, with help from the instructor as needed, and then present the case to their classmates, who will also have opportunities to question the patient.

Task trainers, or partial trainers, are models of a particular part or region of the body [9]. They are often the safest way to teach invasive skills that require repetitive practice. These can be combined with case studies or other simulation experiences to increase the fidelity if required by the goals and objectives of the curriculum.

Computer (web-based) technology is used to provide simulation remotely, with either the instructor, the learners, or both separated from each other in different locations [8]. This is also called distance learning or telepresence [9]. Web conferencing tools and video are used to facilitate communication between simulated patients and providers. This type of remote simulation is often used by NP programs that have distance learners. Telehealth visits are a type of remote access environment that provide needed clinical experience in this rapidly growing clinical area.

Computer technology, or screen-based simulation, also can create a "virtual environment" with a three-dimensional quality [10]. Virtual reality often involves the use of special equipment for vision and hearing interfaces that connect the physical with the virtual world. Augmented reality has been described as "a technology that overlays digital computer-generated information on objects or places in the real world for the purpose of enhancing the user experience." ([9], p. 9) Virtual patients can be created that can dialog with participants with a range of preset responses. There are many commercially available software programs that will provide learning experiences for NP students, from teaching health history acquisition and physical examination skills to opportunities for exercises that develop critical diagnostic thinking.

Integrating Simulation into the Curriculum

The Flipped Classroom

Simulation experiences can be included in the existing curriculum with the goal of supporting the NP competencies defined by the American Association for Colleges of Nurses (AACN) and the National Organization of Nurse Practitioner Faculties (NONPF) [12, 13]. The increasing volume of information required by nurse practitioners can be overwhelming to students. Flipping the classroom is an instructional design concept that has been used since 2007 that organizes curriculum so that the content for student learning is typically presented in an online pre-class assignment format asynchronously, rather than in-person lecture format, allowing for higher order learning functions to be explored during in-class, face to face time [14]. Students study textbook content and other written material, as well as recorded lectures and videos covering the increasingly complex information required for nurse practitioner knowledge in today's clinical settings [15]. This study can be guided so that students have activities to perform while reading to help them organize their reading and develop a framework for their learning. Some ideas for this scaffolding include requirements for taking a pre-class quiz, guided outlining of chapters and other published materials, working through case studies, development of care plans, or the development of a diagnosis-based learning notebook.

Besides clinical knowledge, nurse practitioners must also possess critical thinking skills and ultimately be able to demonstrate competency for graduation. Following adult learning theory, this requires a real partnership where the graduate student shares responsibility for learning and becomes an active learner and participant in the knowledge translation. Under the flipped classroom concept, with lectures moved to the pre-class preparation time frame, time is available for experiences during in-class or synchronous class time that more closely resemble real clinical practice where faculty take on the role of clinical instructor rather than lecturer. Simulation during class time provides opportunities for students to develop their clinical reasoning skills and for faculty evaluation and fortification of those skills [15].

Formative learning experiences during synchronous class time, using case-based simulation, can prepare students for OSCE high-stakes exams and reduce test-taking anxiety. This type of evaluation also offers opportunities for faculty to make corrective interventions while students have time to learn and improve their skills prior to the end of the semester.

Replacing Clinical Experiences with Simulation

While NP programs are required to incorporate a minimum of 500 supervised direct patient care hours into their curricular development, clinical hours over and above those specified may be used in the simulation [3]. An ideal use of simulation is for the teaching of history-taking and physical assessment skills [16]. Securing appropriate community-based clinical sites for student practice of these basic skills is difficult. Students often spend more time shadowing rather than practicing these skills and don't have the ability to contribute to the clinic workload at this point in their education. Learning and practicing health history taking and physical assessment skills with SP in the simulation laboratory, along with cases coordinated to didactic lessons, will reinforce the material and allow faculty to help students who might be struggling with certain skills and ensure they have a solid foundation with which to begin clinical training in the community.

Formative Simulation

Simulation, using high-fidelity manikins or standardized or simulated human patients (SPs), can be used to teach beginning skills such as history taking. Nurse practitioner faculty use simulation to teach more invasive hands-on skills such as suturing and toenail removal that increase student competence and confidence while supporting the role transition from RN to APRN [17]. Simulation also allows for the practice of skills such as the use of telehealth equipment, role playing on-call or after-hours decision-making, and interprofessional experiences such as making a referral or transporting a patient [18, 19].

Teaching a wide array of communication and clinical decision-making skills in the simulation setting allows for deliberate practice with the opportunity for faculty input and guidance. Scenarios and case studies closely aligned with the goals and objectives of the curriculum provide opportunities to evaluate and correct student understanding of the material while providing opportunities to build on that understanding.

Summative Simulation

Competency-based education is replacing content-based education in the nurse practitioner curriculum [20, 21]. This shift moves the focus from the content delivered over time in the educational process to the outcomes demonstrated by the student [17, 18].

This learner-focused change has implications for the evaluation of student learning [20]. The multiple-choice exam, commonly used as an evaluation tool for student knowledge, does not adequately assess competencies and clinical skills [15]. The challenge for educators is creating an evaluation process that is standardized and fair for every student, efficient for faculty, and allows for timely evaluation of student skills and competencies.

The Objective Structured Clinical Examination (OSCE) has been used as an evaluation component of medical education for decades and is now being used to evaluate nursing students at the undergraduate and graduate levels [22]. This methodology allows faculty to observe student performance of competencies either face-to-face within the laboratory setting or remotely via telecommunication. The OSCE can be skills-focused, with multiple short stations testing specific competencies, or it can involve one or more stations with simulated office-based or acute care-based case scenarios that feature the student in the provider role with a standardized or simulated patient (SP). Faculty observe the student performance, either directly or remotely, synchronously or asynchronously. The student is evaluated by faculty and sometimes by the trained SP according to previously developed checklists and rubrics coordinated with outcome competencies for the profession [11]. The OSCE can be used either as a formative teaching method or for summative, high-stakes evaluations. Cases are developed to elicit the competencies taught throughout each clinical semester. This clinical appraisal can evaluate the student's readiness for clinical practice (Time One) or the student's clinical competencies at the completion of the educational program (Time Two) [12]. While faculty-student visits in other clinical settings may vary, an OSCE is a type of simulated clinical experience where the expectations for the clinical visit, the patient, the case, the setting, and the method of evaluation are standardized across all students. Students are prebriefed with these expectations, with the grading rubric, and with the setting, they will encounter during the OSCE exam.

Face-to-Face and Remote Simulation

Simulation can be performed face-to-face within the simulation laboratory or classroom, with the SP providing the opportunity for a hands-on physical examination as part of the scenario. However, increasingly, NP programs are faced with the necessity to utilize distance simulation technology, with online video conferencing platforms such as Zoom, to connect students, faculty, and SPs who may all be in different locations. A remotely held OSCE, for instance, will require that the student be provided with the specific goals and objectives of the simulation experience, the grading rubric if used, and reminded to verbalize any assessments that they would like to perform. Students can be taught techniques for telehealth assessment of patients and talk the SP through the process that will help them reveal details of the physical examination. Instead of physical 'cue cards' with examination findings and photos, written cues can be passed to the NP student through the conferencing text functions. The SP can be taught to verbalize the important details of the case and should be given a script that describes body language, attitude, and manner of speech to help in portraying the patient depicted in the case. Remotely held simulations can be recorded for offline review by faculty and to provide students with a visual way of assessing their own performance.

Barriers to Simulation Use

One of the perceived barriers to the use of simulation in the nurse practitioner curriculum is a lack of faculty workload provision for the development and implementation of simulation experiences into the curriculum [7, 23]. There is no simple solution to this issue. As the use of simulation, both for formative and summative evaluations, becomes more frequently used, faculty and students will begin to see the value and demand more time spent on this type of teaching method. Invested faculty often spend donated time to develop these experiences into the curriculum.

The creation, development, management, and evaluation of simulation-based high-stakes exams, such as OSCEs, are time and resource-intensive endeavors. The cases must be written and validated, often requiring the support of multiple faculty or even reaching out to national experts for collaboration. Scheduling time for the exams with faculty needed for grading, scheduling lab, and debriefing space in an impacted lab adds to the time and stress levels of faculty. Determining remediation procedures, which may involve additional and repeat simulation, adds to this burden and must be part of the costs counted for this process as well as faculty release time.

Lack of financial support for simulation, lack of support staff, and lack of faculty knowledge and comfort in the use of simulation at this level are other common barriers to the use of simulation in NP programs. The NONPF, INACSL, ASPE, and SSH annual conferences are beginning to offer more instructional support for NP faculty for the development and advanced execution of simulation at the graduate level.

Cases suitable for formative and summative OSCE simulation are available in publications for NP faculty and with many online sources. A resource page is available on the NONPF website with many suggested sites listed. (10) Faculty often write case scenarios from their own practice experience. The cases should be evidence-based, use a standardized format, and be validated by content experts [24]. The INACSL Standards of Simulation Design and the ASPE Standards of Best Practices provide support and guidance for simulation case design [10, 11].

Exemplar Cases

Nurse practitioner students enrolled in the family nurse practitioner track of the Doctor of Nursing Practice program in a private university in the Pacific West Coast experience a series of simulations, and case studies for formative and summative simulation experiences that help faculty evaluate student learning and readiness for clinical practice or for end of semester high stakes evaluation.

Identification of Sex Trafficking Victim Scenario

An example of a scenario for formative teaching during the physical assessment course is a case depicting an adolescent female who presents to the simulated clinic along with her "boyfriend," presenting with a chief complaint of pain during urination. This case is used during the week that the genitourinary system is discussed in didactic classes. Health assessment goals are to take a general health history and sexual health history, assess the patient and formulate differential diagnoses related to the chief complaint. A young female actor or student volunteer is recruited as SP and prepared with the script for the case, along with a slightly older male actor or volunteer SP. The male SP is coached to respond to questions directed at the female patient and to appear protective and overbearing. The goals for the NP student are to ask the male 'boyfriend' to leave the room and to assess the young patient for potential infection and sexual abuse. The case, as written, does not include invasive physical examinations such as a pelvic exam but could if using trained pelvic educators as SP. This case provides the NP student with the opportunity to practice "phone calls" to law enforcement officers and the National Human Trafficking Resource Center Hotline. The debriefing with the NP student health assessment class includes a discussion of the role of NP in assessing adolescent sexual behavior, state laws related to the age of consent for sexual activity and for medical care, and assessment of patients with sexually transmitted infections. The emotions, personal feelings, and beliefs of the individual NP related to this issue are also explored during the debriefing session.

Precipitous Labor Scenario

A formative simulation case used during the reproductive and child health promotion course revolves around the topic of precipitous birth. An SP actor or student volunteer is prepared ahead of time using an externally worn body suit and silicone "baby bump" that appears to be of 9 months gestation, an externally worn nursing bra with silicone breast inserts, and a stretchy maternity dress. A ball is used under the silicone "tummy" at the umbilicus for the purpose of practicing assessing the uterine fundus. A baby manikin is used along with a silicone placenta and umbilical cord. "Blood" used for this simulation can be a commercial product or as simple as water and food coloring cooked with a small amount of corn starch for 'body' or more to simulate blood clots. Crushed iron tablets can be added to increase the fidelity of the smell of fresh blood. The scene is set, and the NP student is sent into the room to assess a patient with a chief complaint of abdominal pain and uterine cramping. The goals for this student simulation are for the student to call for help, assess the immediate postpartum mother and newborn and provide a handoff report. Cue cards are provided for the student with the mother and newborn vital signs. This scenario could also include the opportunity to collaborate with students from emergency medical services (EMS) and practice a handoff, providing interprofessional experiences. Debriefing includes a discussion of emergency maternal and child assessment and care during precipitous community-based childbirth. If this is used as an interprofessional experience, the debrief could also include a discussion of NP and EMS roles.

OSCE Summative Case Scenario Finding a Breast Lump

For a high-stakes summative OSCE, cases should provide the opportunity for faculty to assess student competencies taught during the course. For this university, a checklist has been developed that is keyed to NONPF and AACN DNP program outcome competencies [12, 13]. A case used for the reproductive and child health promotion final OSCE involves a woman who has found a lump in the upper outer quadrant of her left breast while showering. The case focuses on clinical breast assessment and discussion of diagnostic options with a patient who has a family history of breast cancer. Relationship development with an anxious patient is an important expectation. Debriefing for an OSCE is different than for a formative simulation as the goal is the evaluation of student competencies rather that fostering student learning at this endpoint in the course. The student is given an opportunity to provide an oral presentation and a SOAP note for the simulated patient visit, and the faculty then provides feedback according to the grading rubric on the student's performance during the simulation and oral presentation.

Simulation is becoming an integral part of nurse practitioner education. This clinical experience adds value to the educational process and helps prepare students for the transition to graduate nurse practitioner. Evidence-based and validated case design and evidence-based facilitation are important considerations. Faculty should be supported in this process.

Appendices: Exemplar Cases

Appendix 1: Identification of Sex Trafficking Victim

Section I: Scenario Overview

Scenario Title:	Tina Lane Case: Identifying Sex Trafficking Victim	
Original Scenario Developer(s):	Jo Loomis DNP, FNP-C, CHSE	
Date - original scenario 10/13/2012, revised 8/16/2019	Validation: 12/2020	Pilot testing: 11/16/19
Estimated Scenario Time: 15 minutes	Debriefing time: 30 min	
Target group: Nurse Practitioner Students enrolled in Advanced Physical Assessment (first clinical course)		
Core case: Identification of Sex Trafficking Victim, assessment of adolescent with urinary tract infection and pelvic inflammatory disease (PID).		
Brief Summary of Case: Adolescent female is brought to the clinic with a chief complaint of pain during urination. She is accompanied by an older male identified as a 'boyfriend' who is overbearing in his behavior to the patient. NP students in the role of provider must recognize the need to separate patients and perform physical and sexual health assessments, provide treatment plans, and contact proper authorities.		
QSEN Competencies & Team*STEPPS* Competencies		
❑ X Patient-Centered Care ❑ X Patient Safety ❑ X Teamwork and Collaboration	❑ Informatics, ❑ Quality Improvement ❑ X Evidence-Based Practice	

EVIDENCE BASE / REFERENCES (APA Format)
National Human Trafficking Resource Center (2020). Identifying Victims of Human Trafficking Fact Sheet. US Department of Health and Human Services. https://www.acf.hhs.gov/sites/default/files/orr/fact_sheet_identifying_victims_of_human_trafficking.pdf
Ernewin, C. & Nieves, R. (2015). Human Sex Trafficking: Recognition, Treatment, and Referral of Pediatric Victims. *Journal for Nurse Practitioners. 11*,8. 797-803.
Iman, T. (2020). Bacterial urinary tract infections *Merck Manual (*online) https://www.merckmanuals.com/professional/genitourinary-disorders/urinary-tract-infections-utis/bacterial-urinary-tract-infections
Goje, O. (2019) Pelvic Inflammatory Disease, *Merck Manual (online) https://www.merckmanuals.com/professional/gynecology-and-obstetrics/vaginitis,-cervicitis,-and-pelvic-inflammatory-disease-pid/pelvic-inflammatory-disease-pid*
Photo Credit CNN https://www.napnappartners.org/tattoos-human-trafficking-victims

Section II: Curriculum Integration

A. SCENARIO LEARNING OBJECTIVES

Critical Learner Actions

1. Wash hands and introduce yourself to the patient.
2. Take patient history, focusing on the chief complaint
3. Perform physical exam
4. Develop differential diagnoses list

B. PRE-SCENARIO LEARNER ACTIVITIES

Prerequisite Competencies	
Knowledge	**Skills/ Attitudes**
1. Sexual health history assessment	1. Taking a sexual health history
2. Physical examination	2. Performing a physical examination
3. Sexually transmitted disease assessment	3. Performing a pelvic examination
4. Recognition of potential sex trafficking	4. Making an agency referral

SECTION III: SCENARIO SCRIPT

A. Case Summary

This case is designed to focus on the beginning skills of performing a sexual health history but could be expanded to include the physical skill of performing a pelvic examination. This would require a specific arrangement with the SP/actress for this case. As written, it is considered a non-invasive physical examination case. The pelvic exam findings are provided for the NP student in the form of 'cue cards.'

B. Key contextual details

Setting: Primary Care Clinic room in Simulation Laboratory

C. Scenario Cast

Patient	❑ High fidelity simulator	❑ Mid-level simulator	X Standardized Patient
	❑ Task trainer	❑ Hybrid (Blended simulator)	❑

Participants/Role	Brief Descriptor (Optional)	Embedded Participant (IP) or Learner (L)
Patient	Youthful female actor (SP)	
	Male companion actor (SP)	
Provider	Nurse Practitioner Student	
	NP Faculty as Preceptor	

D. Patient/Client Profile

Last name: Lane	First name: Tina	Gender: Female	Age: 15	Spiritual Practice:	unknown
Ethnicity: Caucasian	Language: English	Vital Signs: T 100.8^0 P 92, R 18	BP 110/75 Ht. 5'5' Wt. 108 lb. BMI 17.5		

1. Chief complaint

Pain on urination. I feel like I'm peeing all the time, and it burns. I will reluctantly admit it hurts to have intercourse if asked. `

Personality/Emotional tone/ Approach: *Tina is shy and hesitant to speak in Bobby's presence. Bobby is defensive and pushy.*

History of Present Illness: Pain on urination for the past week.

Past Medical/surgical history: No significant past medical or surgical history.

OB/GYN history: Menarche age 11, regular monthly periods since then. Sexually active for the past 6 months with multiple male partners daily. Two medical abortions in the past 6 months.

Social History: Tina left school in Houston and has been exchanging sexual activity for money for the past six months for her pimp and boyfriend Bobby. Tina is a US citizen, having been born in Texas. Her parents are unaware of where she is or that she has been taken to San Francisco to work.

Family Health History: Unknown

Diet History: Mostly fast food

Current Medications: None

Medication allergies:	NKDA	Reaction:	
Food/other allergies:	No known allergies.	Reaction:	

Physical Exam: (Each component of the exam is provided for NP students in the form of 'cue cards' after the student performs or describes the examination process.)	Thin, anxious-looking young woman scantily dressed. HEENT: WNL Heart: S1, S2 with no adventitious sounds. Lungs: Clear to auscultation. Skin: Tattoo on chest depicting crown and initials. Abdomen: Tender to palpation in both lower quadrants. Pelvic exam: Mucopurulent cervicitis with positive cervical motion tenderness.

4. Laboratory, Diagnostic Study Results (List significant labs, & diagnostic test results)

UA per dipstick: Bacteria present, > 1+ RBCs, positive leukocytes and positive nitrites (cue card)

HealthImpact
Optimizing health through nursing

CSA template (abbreviated) 03/2020; MMiller, MA, RN, CHSE

ALL DATA IN THIS SCENARIO IS FICTITIOUS

Sim Set-up card		
Patient Information	**Set-Up / Moulage**	**Equipment/Supplies**
Tina has a $1,000 quota per night that she must earn for Bobby. He tells her he is saving money for them to buy a house. Tina is often scared while out on the streets, but Bobby reminds her that she is making money for their future and that the situation is only temporary. Bobby has other girls who work on the streets for him, but Tina knows that she is special to him because Bobby does not hit her like he does the others. Tina has developed pain when she urinates and sees bright red blood in the toilet after she urinates. She also has pain deep in her abdomen. Bobby brings her into the clinic and is hovering over her, defensively answering all the questions for her. If the NP questions Tina further, she may disclose that she is often afraid on the street and has 6-10 customers per night with unprotected sex. She has burning and pain when she	The actress/SP is scantily dressed, wearing exaggerated facial makeup. Tattoo (moulage) on the chest below left clavicle depicting crown and initials. Present photo on cue card.	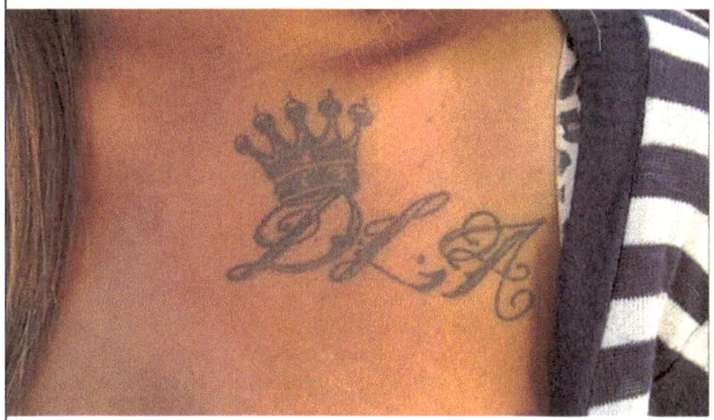 Image: CNN https://www.napnappartners.org/tattoos-human-trafficking-victims
urinates and sees bright red blood sometimes in the toilet bowl. She has mild pain when the NP presses on her lower abdomen. She has had two medical abortions in the past 6 months with pills that Bobby provides for her.		

Case Flow / Triggers/ Scenario Development States
Initiation of Scenario: Patient and 'boyfriend' are waiting in a simulated clinic examination room setting when an NP student arrives.
The patient is sitting on the exam table, 'boyfriend' actor is hovering over her.

State / Patient Status	**Desired learner actions & triggers to move to the next stage**		
Baseline	**Operator**	**Learner Actions**	**Debriefing Points:**
NP student introduces self and begins assessing the patient. 'Bobby' answers for the patient. NP student asks Bobby to leave the room, and after arguing briefly, he does leave the room. NP student continues to elicit health history and then proceeds to conduct a physical	 **Triggers** Overbearing male SP answers questions for the female SP	NP student asks Bobby to leave the room so that the student may examine the patient in private. After arguing briefly, he does leave the room. NP student discusses options with faculty preceptor and then with SP. NP student	Discuss privacy for adolescents during sexual health assessment. Appendix A includes assessment points for bacterial urinary tract infection and pelvic inflammatory disease and for assessment of a potential victim of sexual trafficking.

CSA template (abbreviated) 03/2020; MMiller, MA, RN, CHSE

ALL DATA IN THIS SCENARIO IS FICTITIOUS

examination of the patient.	Once alone, the female SP discloses her situation to the NP student.	conducts health assessment and physical examination. NP student develops three differential diagnoses: bacterial urinary tract infection, possible pelvic inflammatory disease, and possible victim of human sex trafficking.	
Scenario End Point: NP Student wraps up the visit with a treatment plan and discussion with the patient about options, including a call to the national human trafficking hotline or referral to a local county law enforcement agency.			

CSA template (abbreviated) 03/2020; MMiller, MA, RN, CHSE

HealthImpact

ALL DATA IN THIS SCENARIO IS FICTITIOUS

Differential Diagnoses and Debrief: Important Take-Home Points to discuss post case:

Urinary Tract Infection:

Symptoms:

- Frequency
- Urgency
- Burning on urination
- Suprapubic pain
- Low back pain

Diagnosis laboratory tests:

- Urinalysis
- Urine culture

Treatment:

- Antibiotics "Choice of antibiotic should be based on the patient's allergy and adherence history, local resistance patterns (if known), antibiotic availability and cost, and patient and provider tolerance for risk of treatment failure" (Merck Manual Online)
- Phenazopyridine, if desired, for dysuria

Pelvic Inflammatory Disease:

When symptoms are present, the most common symptoms of PID are

- Lower abdominal pain
- Mild pelvic pain
- Increased vaginal discharge
- Irregular menstrual bleeding
- Fever (>38° C)
- Pain with intercourse
- Painful and frequent urination
- Abdominal tenderness
- Pelvic organ tenderness
- Uterine tenderness (along with endometriosis)
- Adnexal tenderness (along with salpingitis)
- Cervical motion tenderness
- Inflammation

Diagnosis:

- A high index of suspicion
- Polymerase chain reaction (PCR)
- Pregnancy test

Treatment:

- Antibiotics appropriate for *N. gonorrhoeae*, *C. trachomatis*
- HIV testing

Human trafficking victims:

- Are involved in domestic, sex, or farm work and multiple other types of service jobs.
- Are drawn into the work by means of force, fraud, or coercion.
- Maybe minors in the U.S. under the age of 18 involved in commercial sex acts.
- They are not the same as persons who are smuggled.
- Are primarily women and children.
- They are often kept in isolation and may adapt to the situation.
- Are likely not to be identified by healthcare providers.
- Have access to health and legal interventions when identified.
- May benefit from interventions based on the stage of trafficking they are in when identified; and,
- They are burdened for a lifetime with physical and mental health effects.

Red flags for providers

- Discrepancies in behavior and reported age
- Evidence of sexual trauma
- Multiple or frequent sexually transmitted infections
- Excessively large number of pregnancies
- Tattoos or other types of branding
- Use of slang relating to involvement in prostitution
- Evidence of controlling or dominant relationship
- Malnourishment or generally poor health

The National Human Trafficking Hotline connects victims and survivors of sex and labor trafficking with services and supports to get help and stay safe. The Trafficking Hotline also receives tips about potential situations of sex and labor trafficking and facilitates reporting that information to the appropriate authorities in certain cases. Phone: 1-888-373-7888

Appendix 2: Precipitous Birth Case

Section I: Scenario Overview

California Simulation Alliance
a program of HealthImpact

Scenario Title: Precipitous Labor Scenario		
Original Scenario Developer(s): Jo Loomis		
Date - original scenario 11/15/2016	Validation: Spring 2017	Pilot testing: 11/15/2016
Estimated Scenario Time: 15 minutes	Debriefing time: 30 min	
Target group: Nurse Practitioner Students during first clinical course—Advanced Physical Assessment		
Core case: A woman experiences a precipitous birth, and NP students must assess a newly postpartum woman and her neonate.		
Brief Summary of Case: An 19-year-old woman comes to the urgent care center complaining of acute abdominal pain. Before the NP student steps into the exam room, the patient cries out for help. The NP student rushes into the room and sees a lustily crying neonate kicking and waving his arms on the exam table between the legs of a distressed woman. This case offers the NP student the opportunity to assess an immediate postpartum women and a neonate. The student also has the opportunity to practice a handoff with EMR personnel. It may be used in a collaborative interprofessional scenario with EMR students.		
QSEN Competencies & Team*STEPPS* Competencies		
X Patient-Centered Care X Patient Safety X Teamwork and Collaboration	❑ Informatics, ❑ Quality Improvement X Evidence-Based Practice	

EVIDENCE BASE / REFERENCES (APA Format)
Shunji Suzuki (2015). Clinical significance of precipitous labor. J Clin Med Res., 7(3): 150–153. Published online 2014 Dec 29. doi: 10.14740/jocmr2058w
World Health Organization (2015). Pregnancy, childbirth, postpartum and newborn care: A guide for essential practice. 3rd. Ed. https://www.ncbi.nlm.nih.gov/books/NBK326674/
Schorn, M. & Wilbeck, J. (2009). Unexpected Birth in the Emergency Department: The Role of the Advanced Practice Nurse. Advanced Emergency Nursing Journal, 31, 170-177. https://doi.org/10.1097/TME.0b013e3181a4154e

CSA template (abbreviated) 03/2020, MMiller, MA, RN, CHSE

HealthImpact
Optimizing health through nursing

Section II: Curriculum Integration

California Simulation Alliance
a program of HealthImpact

SECTION II: CURRICULUM INTEGRATION

A. SCENARIO LEARNING OBJECTIVES

Critical Learner Actions

5. Assess postpartum mother
6. Assess newborn
7. Facilitate bonding and promote safety
8. Prepare mother and neonate for transfer to local hospital/report off to EMR personnel

B. PRE-SCENARIO LEARNER ACTIVITIES	
Prerequisite Competencies	
Knowledge	**Skills/ Attitudes**
5. Understand postpartum care needs	5. Postpartum care assessment
6. Understand newborn assessment needs	6. Newborn care assessment
7.	7. Leadership and teamwork
8.	8. Handoff report to EMR personnel

SECTION III: SCENARIO SCRIPT

B. Case Summary

A 19-year-old woman comes to the urgent care center complaining of acute abdominal pain. Before the NP student steps into the exam room, the patient cries out for help. The NP student rushes into the room and sees a lustily crying neonate kicking and waving his arms on the exam table between the legs of a distressed woman. This case offers the NP student the opportunity to assess an immediately postpartum woman and a neonate. The student also has the opportunity to practice a handoff with EMT personnel. It may be used in a collaborative interprofessional scenario with EMT students and their faculty.

B. Key contextual details

Setting: Simulated primary/urgent care clinic

C. Scenario Cast

Patient	❑ High fidelity simulator	❑ Mid-level simulator	X Standardized Patient
	❑ Task trainer	❑ Hybrid (Blended simulator)	❑

Participants/Role	**Brief Descriptor (Optional)**	**Embedded Participant (IP) or Learner (L)**
Patient	Young female actor	
Provider	Nurse Practitioner Student	
	NP Faculty in preceptor role	
	EMT students and faculty	

HealthImpact
Optimizing health through nursing

CSA template (abbreviated) 03/2020; MMiller, MA, RN, CHSE

ALL DATA IN THIS SCENARIO IS FICTITIOUS

California Simulation Alliance
a program of HealthImpact

D. Patient/Client Profile					
Last name: O'Leary	First name: Jenny	Gender: F	Age: 19		
Spiritual Practice: unknown	Ethnicity: White	Language: English			
Vital Signs: T 98.6^0 P 110	BP 100/60	R 20 b/m	Ht. 5' 3" Wt. 145 lbs. (Prepregnancy wt. 125 lbs.)		

Chief complaint
Sharp lower abdominal pain and pain in the lower back, intermittent, now about every 1-2 minutes.
Personality/Emotional tone/ Approach Scared, anxious and uncomfortable
History of Present Illness: Pain began "all of a sudden" about three hours ago. He has had some diarrhea and saw some red blood in the toilet, and it scared you.
Past Medical/surgical history: She broke her right arm when she was 7 years old, and fell out of a tree.
OB/GYN history: First menstrual period was age 14, regular every month since then until about 9 months ago. " I just never got around to going to the clinic. Never had morning sickness, so at first just hoped I wasn't pregnant." G1P1A0
Social history: Parents live in Ohio, and a 16-year-old brother is still at home. She lived with their parents until she graduated from high school. Parents have a rule that their children must move out of the house when they turn 18. Jenny moved out and came to California looking for work. She met a boy and moved in with him for a while, but he left about 4 months ago. Jenny works part-time in a shop sewing uniforms with 5 other girls. She tried to hide the pregnancy and worried now that she'd lose her job.
Family health history: Parents and brother were in good health when she left home.
Diet history: Whatever she can get at the soup kitchen around the corner and what she can manage to buy on her meager salary.
Current Medications: None, no prenatal vitamins

Medication allergies:	None	Reaction:	
Food/other allergies:	None	Reaction:	
Review of Systems:	Denies headache, vision change, upper abdominal pain		
	Experiences diarrhea, lower abdominal and back pain.		
Physical Exam Findings:	General: Surprised and slightly anxious young woman crouching on the exam table, yelling with crying, and kicking baby on the table between her legs. Approx. 300 ml. blood covering baby and exam table. Uterine fundus firm, midline, and at the umbilicus Perineum intact		

HealthImpact
Optimizing health through nursing

	Moderate rubra lochia Breasts soft with colostrum Newborn male, pink overall with slightly blue extremities, some vernix, crying vigorously, rapidly moving arms and legs APGAR 9 and 10 Heart rate 150 bpm Respiration 45, clear to auscultation Weight 2500 gm Length 48.26 cm

California Simulation Alliance
a program of HealthImpact

4. Laboratory, Diagnostic Study Results (List significant labs,& diagnostic test results)		
Sim Set-up card		
Patient Information	Set-Up / Moulage	Medications/Equipment/Supplies
Young female patient actor briefed with the script. If EMT students collaborate, they and their faculty will be prepared with the script.	The female actor is wearing: Silicone breast inserts in a nursing bra worn over a body suit, silicone belly, 9 months gestation also strapped over the body suit. A soft ball is placed at the actor's umbilicus under the silicone belly. Loose-fitting street clothes over all. Life-like silicone baby model, weighed 5 pounds, is covered with simulated blood. Placenta and umbilical cord silicone model. Cued when NP student "calls" 911.	Simulated blood recipe: Water Red Food Coloring A drop of black food coloring Corn starch for thickening (May stain manikins, clothing, hair, skin.) Use commercial theatrical blood. EMT students bring a gurney to the simulation lab and take reports from NP students.

Case Flow / Triggers/ Scenario Development States			
Initiation of Scenario :			
Patient (actor) is shown into the simulated clinic exam room at beginning of the scenario. Student NP is told that the patient's chief complaint is acute abdominal pain. Baby and simulated blood are arranged on the exam table between the actor's legs. The camera in the exam room is turned off. The actor must be cued to yell out just as the NP student is moving into the exam room. The camera can be turned on at this time for observers.			
State / Patient Status	Desired learner actions & triggers to move to the next stage		
Baseline	Operator	Learner Actions	Debriefing Points:

CSA template (abbreviated) 03/2020, MMiller, MA, RN, CHSE

HealthImpact
Optimizing health through nursing

California Simulation Alliance
a program of HealthImpact

		NP student must walk into the exam room, assess the need for another support person, and call for help (another NP student ask someone to call 911).	Advocacy/Inquiry model Plus/Delta debriefing (what went well/ what could be changed/done differently
	Triggers		
	SP yells for help at the beginning of the scenario		
State / Patient Status	Desired actions & triggers to move to the next stage		
Frame 2	Operator	Learner Actions:	Debriefing Points:
		EMT student responds to call and brings practice gurney to simulation lab	
	Triggers:		
	NP student, with guidance from NP faculty preceptor, calls for EMT personnel through 911 call.		
Scenario End Point: NP student completes an assessment of mother and neonate, calls 911, and provides handoff report.			
Suggestions to <u>decrease</u> complexity: Suggestions to <u>increase</u> complexity: The addition of EMT students will create an interprofessional experience for both NP and EMT students.			
Notes for future sessions:			

CSA template (abbreviated) 03/2020, MMiller, MA, RN, CHSE

HealthImpact
Optimizing health through nursing

Use this chart for women and newborns during the first hour after complete delivery of the placenta. https://www.ncbi.nlm.nih.gov/books/NBK326674/#childbirth.s23

California Simulation Alliance
a program of HealthImpact

MONITOR MOTHER EVERY 15 MINUTES:	**MONITOR BABY EVERY 15 MINUTES:**
▪ For emergency signs, using rapid assessment (RAM) ▪ Feel if the uterus is hard and round. ▪ Record findings, treatments, and procedures ▪ Keep mother and baby in the delivery room - **do not separate them.** ▪ **Never leave the woman and newborn alone.**	▪ Breathing: listen for grunting, look for chest in-drawing and fast breathing ▪ Warmth: check to see if feet are cold to touch
CARE OF MOTHER AND NEWBORN	**INTERVENTIONS, IF REQUIRED**
WOMAN ▪ Assess the amount of vaginal bleeding. ▪ Encourage the woman to eat and drink. ▪ Ask the companion to stay with the mother. ▪ Encourage the woman to pass urine.	▪ If the pad is soaked in less than 5 minutes or constant trickle of blood, manage ▪ If the uterus is soft, manage. Place a cupped palm on the uterine fundus and feel for a state of contraction. ▪ Massage the fundus in a circular motion with a cupped palm until uterus is well contracted. ▪ When well contracted, place fingers behind the fundus and push down in one swift action to expel clots. ▪ Collect blood in a container placed close to the vulva. Measure or estimate blood loss and record. ▪ If bleeding from a perineal tear, **refer to the hospital.**
NEWBORN ▪ Wipe the eyes. ▪ If blood or meconium, wipe off with a wet cloth and dry. ▪ DO NOT remove vernix or bathe the baby. ▪ Continue keeping the baby warm and in skin-to-skin contact with the mother. ▪ Encourage the mother to initiate breastfeeding when the baby shows signs of readiness. Offer her help. ▪ DO NOT give artificial teats or pre-lacteal feeds to the newborn: no water, sugar water, or local feeds.	▪ If breathing with difficulty — grunting, chest in-drawing, or fast breathing, examine the baby ▪ If feet are cold to touch or mother and baby are separated: ▪ Ensure the room is warm. Cover mother and baby with a blanket → Reassess in 1 hour. If still cold, measure the temperature. ▪ If unable to initiate breastfeeding (mother has complications):
MONITOR MOTHER EVERY 15 MINUTES:	**MONITOR BABY EVERY 15 MINUTES:**
▪ Examine the mother and newborn one hour after delivery of placenta.	▪ **Refer to the hospital** now if the woman had serious complications at admission or during delivery but was in late labor.

CSA template (abbreviated) 03/2020, MMiller, MA, RN, CHSE

HealthImpact
Optimizing health through nursing

Appendix 3: Finding a Breast Lump OSCE Case

Section I: Scenario Overview

California Simulation Alliance
a program of HealthImpact

Appendix C: Finding a Breast Lump OSCE Case

SECTION I: SCENARIO OVERVIEW

Scenario Title: Nellie Marcos Case: Finding a Breast Lump		
Original Scenario Developer(s):	Jo Loomis, DNP, FNP, CHSE, and Cathy Coleman, DNP, CNL, CPHQ	
Date - original scenario 4/30/14	Validation: Summer 2019	Pilot testing: Summer 2019
Estimated Scenario Time : 20 minutes	Debriefing time: 30 min	
Target group: Nurse Practitioner Students enrolled in Reproductive and Child Health Promotion (third clinical semester.)		
Chief Complaint: I found a lump under my left arm when taking a shower last night.		
Brief Summary of Case: • A woman with a family history of breast cancer finds a lump under her arm while showering. • She is anxious and seeks advice from her primary care provider.		
QSEN Competencies & Team*STEPPS* Competencies		
X Patient-Centered Care X Patient Safety ❑ Teamwork and Collaboration	❑ Informatics, ❑ Quality Improvement X Evidence-Based Practice	

EVIDENCE BASE / REFERENCES (APA Format)
Sabel, S. (2020) Clinical manifestations, differential diagnosis, and clinical evaluation of a palpable breast mass Up to Date https://www.uptodate.com/contents/clinical-manifestations-and-diagnosis-of-a-palpable-breast-mass?search=fibroadenoma%20breast&source=search_result&selectedTitle=3~14&usage_type=default&display_rank=3
Clemons M, Goss P. Estrogen and the risk of breast cancer. N Engl J Med 2001; 344:276.
https://www.uptodate.com/contents/clinical-manifestations-and-diagnosis-of-a-palpable-breast-mass?search=fibroadenoma%20breast&source=search_result&selectedTitle=3~14&usage_type=default&display_rank–3

Section II: Curriculum Integration

California Simulation Alliance
a program of HealthImpact

Appendix C: Finding a Breast Lump OSCE Case

SECTION I: SCENARIO OVERVIEW

Scenario Title:	Nellie Marcos Case: Finding a Breast Lump	
Original Scenario Developer(s):	Jo Loomis, DNP, FNP, CHSE, and Cathy Coleman, DNP, CNL, CPHQ	
Date - original scenario 4/30/14	Validation: Summer 2019	Pilot testing: Summer 2019
Estimated Scenario Time : 20 minutes	Debriefing time: 30 min	
Target group: Nurse Practitioner Students enrolled in Reproductive and Child Health Promotion (third clinical semester.)		
Chief Complaint: I found a lump under my left arm when taking a shower last night.		
Brief Summary of Case: • A woman with a family history of breast cancer finds a lump under her arm while showering. • She is anxious and seeks advice from her primary care provider.		
QSEN Competencies & Team*STEPPS* Competencies		
X Patient-Centered Care X Patient Safety ❑ Teamwork and Collaboration	❑ Informatics, ❑ Quality Improvement X Evidence-Based Practice	

EVIDENCE BASE / REFERENCES (APA Format)
Sabel, S. (2020) Clinical manifestations, differential diagnosis, and clinical evaluation of a palpable breast mass Up to Date https://www.uptodate.com/contents/clinical-manifestations-and-diagnosis-of-a-palpable-breast-mass?search=fibroadenoma%20breast&source=search_result&selectedTitle=3~14&usage_type=default&display_rank=3
Clemons M, Goss P. Estrogen and the risk of breast cancer. N Engl J Med 2001; 344:276.
https://www.uptodate.com/contents/clinical-manifestations-and-diagnosis-of-a-palpable-breast-mass?search=fibroadenoma%20breast&source=search_result&selectedTitle=3~14&usage_type=default&display_rank=3

CSA template (abbreviated) 03/2020, MMiller, MA, RN, CHSE

HealthImpact
Optimizing health through nursing

D. Patient/Client Profile				
Last name: Marcos	First name: Nellie	Gender: F	Age: 42	
Spiritual Practice: Catholic	Ethnicity: Hispanic	Language: English		
Vitals: T: 98.4 P: 80	R: 20 O2 Sat 98%	BP: 124/82	Ht: 5' 1" Wt: 105 BMI 19.8	

1. Chief complaint

- I found a lump under my left arm when I was taking a shower last night.
- Felt well until last night when I found the lump.
- No discharge, no pulling or puckering of the skin, no difference in size or shape of the breasts
- The lump is about the size and shape of an almond, no redness, no pain.
- Lump is moveable, well-defined borders

Assessment Data

Social History: Lives with husband and two sons, 10 and 12 years old, in a rented 3- bedroom house in Pacifica. She works as a secretary in an accounting firm, and their husband Tomas works in a camera shop nearby. Married to Tomas for 16 years, in a loving, monogamous relationship.

Personality:

- (key emotional tone and approach to responses): Panicky, scared, worried about the possibility of having breast cancer, knowing that mother and grandmother died of breast cancer. "I'm so afraid that I'll die too! I have young boys at home! "
- Appear anxious; may tear up at times. Worried that your young sons may lose their mother? Last night when you were taking a shower, you noticed a lump the size of an almond under your left arm.
- Hoping it is nothing because it doesn't hurt and isn't red or irritated-looking

Past Medical History (past illnesses including surgical or psychiatric conditions):

- The appendix was removed at age 15
- Head cold last month, but it went away after two weeks.

OB/GYN History:

- Menarche at age 10, regular periods every 28 days since then except when pregnant.
- My last menstrual period 3 and a half weeks ago.
- G2P2A0
- Two-term pregnancies with spontaneous vaginal deliveries. Breastfed both sons until they were each 1-year-old.
- Last mammogram 8 months ago, normal findings

Family Medical History:

- Maternal Grandmother died of breast CA at age 48. She was ill for less than 2 years and refused treatment.
- Maternal Grandfather died at age 68 CVA
- Mother died from breast CA, age 65, one year ago. You were very close to your mother, and her death is a real loss to you.
- Father alive, age 70 HTN
- Sister 38 AW

California Simulation Alliance
a program of HealthImpact

• Sons 12 and 10 AW			
Medications: Oral birth control pills for the past 9 years. Occasional Tylenol for headache.			
Medication allergies:	None	Reaction:	
Food/other allergies:	None	Reaction:	
Diet history	Caffeine: Coffee for breakfast, occasional "Coke" in the afternoon Exercise: Walks 4 blocks to school back and forth with sons.		
Social history	Nellie is a secretary in an accounting firm, and her husband Tomas works in a camera shop nearby. Married to Tomas for 16 years; it's a loving, monogamous relationship.		
Vital signs for this visit	Vitals: T: 98.4 P: 80 R: 20 BP: 124/82 O2 Sat 98% Ht: 5' 1" Wt: 105 BMI 19.8		
Physical Exam:	General Exam: Healthy, alert woman appears stated age. The patient looks worried and nervous, chewing her lip HEENT: WNL, Neck supple, smooth Skin: Clear, warm to touch Cardiac/Heart: S_1 S_2 no adventitious sounds Lung/Respiratory: Clear to auscultation Abdominal: WNL Breasts: On inspection, breasts are symmetrical and equal in size and shape. Skin intact, no edema, puckering, or dimpling noted. Slight striae on the upper, and outer aspects. No discharge was noted from the nipples. Nipples erect. Symmetrical areolae, dark color consistent with previous pregnancies. On palpation, the skin is warm, smooth, and elastic; no axillary, infraclavicular, or supraclavicular lymphadenopathy. One smooth, round well-circumscribed mobile lump of about 1.5 cm length at 2 o'clock on the left breast, 5 cm distance from the nipple. Slightly tender to palpation. Pelvic: Deferred Rectal: Deferred		

4. Laboratory, Diagnostic Study Results (List significant labs,& diagnostic test results)

Sim Set-up card		
Patient Information	**Set-Up / Moulage**	**Medications/Equipment/Supplies**
The patient is given a script with the above information related to the case.	The patient is seated on the exam table of the simulation laboratory primary care clinic room.	

HealthImpact
Optimizing health through nursing

CSA template (abbreviated) 03/2020; MMiller, MA, RN, CHSE

ALL DATA IN THIS SCENARIO IS FICTITIOUS

California Simulation Alliance
a program of HealthImpact

Case Flow / Triggers/ Scenario Development States			
Initiation of Scenario :			
SP Actress is seated on an examination table in the simulation laboratory primary care clinic room. She appears anxious.			
State / Patient Status	**Desired learner actions & triggers to move to the next stage**		
Baseline	**Operator**	**Learner Actions**	**Debriefing Points:**
		NP student enters the room. Washes hands and introduces self. Asks how the patient would like to be called.	Personal, professional presentation
		NP student responds to patient's anxiety and speaks in a soothing tone.	Relationship building skills
	Triggers	After eliciting a pertinent history and performing a physical examination, the NP student discusses treatment options and next steps with the patient.	History taking skills Physical examination skills
	Cue cards are given for each component of the physical exam that the student describes/mentions.		
Scenario End Point: NP student discusses treatment plan with the patient and when to return to the clinic.			
Suggestions to <u>decrease</u> complexity: Suggestions to <u>increase</u> complexity: Add in the expectation of performing a clinical breast examination. Prepare the SP ahead of time for this skills practice and add 15 minutes to the scenario time expectation.			
Notes for future sessions:			

HealthImpact
Optimizing health through nursing

CSA template (abbreviated) 03/2020; MMiller, MA, RN, CHSE

ALL DATA IN THIS SCENARIO IS FICTITIOUS

References

1. Hayden JK, Smiley RA, Alexander M, Kardong-Edgren S, Jeffries PR. The NCSBN national simulation study: a longitudinal, randomized, controlled study replacing clinical hours with simulation in prelicensure nursing education. Journal of Nursing Regulation [Internet]. 2014;5(2):S3–40. https://search.ebscohost.com/login.aspx?direct=true&AuthType=sso&db=ccm&AN=144224957&site=ehost-live&scope=site
2. Jeffries PR, Bigley MB, McNelis AM, Cartier JM, Williams DB, Pintz C, et al. A call to action: building evidence for use of simulation in nurse practitioner education. 2019;31(11):627–32. http://search.ebscohost.com/login.aspx?direct=true&AuthType=sso&db=ccm&AN=139637839&site=ehost-live&scope=site&custid=s3818721
3. Statement Regarding Nurse Practitioner Students and Direct Care Clinical Hours Released March 23, 2020
4. National Task Force. The National Task Force on quality nurse practitioner education, criteria for evaluation of nurse practitioner programs, 5th ed. Washington, DC; 2016. https://www.nonpf.org/page/14.
5. Rutherford-Hemming T, Nye C, Coram C. Using simulation for clinical practice hours in nurse practitioner education in the United States: a systematic review. 2016;37:128–35. http://www.sciencedirect.com/science/article/pii/S0260691715004633
6. Hawkins-Walsh E, Berg M, Docherty S, Lindeke L, Gaylord N, Osborn K. A national survey of the primary and acute care pediatric nurse practitioner educational preparation. 2011;25(1):5–15. http://www.sciencedirect.com/science/article/pii/S0891524510001458
7. Nye C, Campbell SH, Hebert SH, Short C, Thomas M. Simulation in advanced practice nursing programs: a North American survey. 2019;26:3–10. http://search.ebscohost.com/login.aspx?direct=true&AuthType=sso&db=ccm&AN=133643494&site=ehost-live&scope=site&custid=s3818721
8. Lioce L, Cornelius J, Brown K, Schneidereith T, Nye C, Weston C, Bigley M. Simulation guidelines and best practices for nurse practitioner programs. Washington, DC: National Organization of Nurse Practitioner Faculties; 2020.
9. Lioce L. (Ed.), Lopreiato J. (Founding Ed.), Downing D., Chang T.P., Robertson J.M., Anderson M., Diaz D.A., and Spain A.E. (Assoc. Eds.) and the Terminology and Concepts Working Group (2020), Healthcare Simulation Dictionary, 2nd ed. Rockville, MD: Agency for Healthcare Research and Quality; September 2020. AHRQ Publication No. 20-0019. doi: https://doi.org/10.23970/simulationv2.
10. INACSL Standards of Best Practice: SimulationSM Simulation Design. 2016;12: S5. http://www.sciencedirect.com/science/article/pii/S1876139916301268
11. Lewis KL, Bohnert CA, Gammon WL, Hölzer H, Lyman L, Smith C, Thompson T, Wallace A, Gliva-McConvey G. The Association of Standardized Patient Educators (ASPE) Standards of Best Practice (SOBP). Adv Simul. 2017;2(1):10. https://doi.org/10.1186/s41077-017-0043-4.
12. APRN Doctoral-Level Competencies Work Group Common Advanced Practice Registered Nurse Doctoral-Level Competencies October 2017 https://cdn.ymaws.com/www.nonpf.org/resource/resmgr/competencies/common-aprn-doctoral-compete.pdf
13. NONPF. Nurse practitioner core competencies content; 2017. https://cdn.ymaws.com/nonpf.site-ym.com/resource/resmgr/competencies/20170516_NPCoreCompsContentF.pdf
14. Oliver R, Luther L. Flipping the graduate nursing classroom: an integrative review. 2020;59(6):305–10. http://search.ebscohost.com/login.aspx?direct=true&AuthType=sso&db=ccm&AN=143590852&site=ehost-live&scope=site&custid=s3818721
15. Bristol T. Flipping the classroom. 2014;9(1):43–6. http://www.sciencedirect.com/science/article/pii/S155730871300108X
16. Loomis J. Expanding the use of simulation in Nurse Practitioner education: a new model for teaching physical assessment. J Nurse Practition. 2016;12(4):e151–7.
17. Avadhani A. Should procedural skills be a part of the Acute Care Nurse Practitioner curriculum? 2017; 50:115–8. http://search.ebscohost.com/login.aspx?direct=true&AuthType=sso&db=ccm&AN=120672402&site=ehost-live&scope=site&custid=s3818721
18. Knight EP, Prettyman AV. Rural telehealth team education for baccalaureate and nurse practitioner students. 2020;59(5):274–7. http://search.ebscohost.com/login.aspx?direct=true&AuthType=sso&db=ccm&AN=143003961&site=ehost-live&scope=site&custid=s3818721
19. Kelly MM, Blunt E. Nestor K. After-hours/on-call experience during primary care nurse practitioner education utilizing standard scenarios and simulated patients. 2017;29(12):725–32. http://search.ebscohost.com/login.aspx?direct=true&AuthType=sso&db=ccm&AN=126965214&site=ehost-live&scope=site&custid=s3818721
20. Gruppen LD, Burkhardt JC, Fitzgerald JT, Funnell M, Haftel HM, Lypson ML, et al. Competency-based education: program design and challenges to implementation. 2016;50(5):532–9. http://search.ebscohost.com/login.aspx?direct=true&AuthType=sso&db=ccm&AN=114490780&site=ehost-live&scope=site&custid=s3818721
21. Hodges AL, Konicki AJ, Talley MH, Bordelon CJ, Holland AC. Galin FS. Competency-based education in transitioning nurse practitioner students from education into practice. 2019;31(11):675–83. https://search.ebscohost.com/login.aspx?direct=true&AuthType=sso&db=ccm&AN=139637840&site=ehost-live&scope=site&custid=s3818721
22. Harden RM, Stevenson M, Downie WW, Wilson GM. Assessment of clinical competence using objective structured examination. Br Med J. 1975;1:447–51.
23. Blodgett NP, Blodgett T, Kardong-Edgren SE. a proposed model for simulation faculty workload determination. 2018;18:20–7. http://www.sciencedirect.com/science/article/pii/S1876139917302153
24. Waxman KT. The development of evidence-based clinical simulation scenarios: guidelines for nurse educators. 2010;49(1):29–35. http://search.ebscohost.com/login.aspx?direct=true&AuthType=ss o&db=ccm&AN=105291741&site=ehost-live&scope=site&custid=s3818721

Acute Care Nurse Practitioner

18

Mary K. Donnelly

Background

Innovative models of nurse practitioner clinical education are needed to advance the preparation of acute care nurse practitioners to provide high-quality care in our evolving and complex healthcare system and must be designed in an environment characterized by significant shortages of clinical sites, clinical preceptors, and substantial financial challenges. According to the Society for Simulation in Healthcare (SSH), simulation can enhance education, assessment, research, and health system integration [1]. Simulation exercises are most successful when they become part of the standard curriculum. The need to focus on the preparation of Acute Care Nurse Practitioners (ACNPs) has become more apparent as the employment of ACNPs has grown in recent years. The use of ACNPs practicing in inpatient settings continues to increase because the number of hours that residents work has been regulated and decreased (as mandated by the Accreditation Council for Graduate Medical Education), the proven efficacy of ACNPs in reducing the length of stay and cost of care and increasing patient satisfaction with care [2].

Best Practices

The literature on simulation in healthcare has gradually evolved from evaluations of individuals to evaluations of teams [3]. Teamwork and communication are identified as critical components of safe healthcare systems. The importance of multidisciplinary teamwork is now reflected in the simulation literature [3]. The direct involvement of healthcare providers across disciplines benefits the goal of improving patient outcomes. When participants are invested in the process of organizational change and feel encouraged to communicate system-level issues, issues identified by the interdisciplinary team members during the debriefings can be processed and solutions implemented. The value of interdisciplinary training and discussion of social dynamics is also recognized in these simulations through the identification of latent safety threats at the system level. System-based threats to patient safety can materialize at any time and can be unrecognized at the time by healthcare providers. Collaboration among interdisciplinary team members can catalyze a shift in culture that emphasizes safety and breaks down implicit authority gradients. During debriefings, discussions should include the times when team members did not feel comfortable addressing communication or collaboration issues despite knowing mistakes were being performed. Communication issues should be addressed as a potential safety threat to patient outcomes. The role of the debriefing process is not only focused on skill-based improvement but also on the acquisition of a shared mental model. A shared mental model among interdisciplinary team members is one of the focal concepts of quality improvement efforts. A multidisciplinary simulation is an opportunity to discuss social dynamics, hierarchy, power relations, and other factors affecting inter-professional teamwork

Integration into Existing Curriculum

A recent descriptive study of 133 advanced practice nursing (APN) programs reported that almost all (98%) used simulation as a teaching pedagogy, using a variety of modalities, including standardized patients, unfolding case studies, role play, mannequins, virtual simulations, task trainers, video recording, and telehealth [4]. Nye et al. examined the use of the International Nursing Association for Clinical Simulation and Learning (INACSL) Standards in APN simulations and found that 83% reported aligning simulation objectives with program outcomes, and 71% reported aligning learning objectives to National Organization of Nurse Practitioner Faculty (NONPF) competencies [4]. In Nurse Practitioner

M. K. Donnelly (✉)
VA Northern California Health Care System, Mather, CA, USA
e-mail: Mary.Donnelly@va.gov

J. M. Kutzin et al. (eds.), *Comprehensive Healthcare Simulation: Nursing*, Comprehensive Healthcare Simulation,
https://doi.org/10.1007/978-3-031-31090-4_18

(NP) educational programs, simulation has been shown to affect time in assessing and measuring case management competencies [5], development of differential diagnoses [6], and interdisciplinary learning [7]. Members of the 2019 NONPF summit meeting recommended new models of NP education that include using clinical simulations to standardize and measure learner clinical competencies, using a known framework and national standards [8].

Continuing Education

Adult Gerontological Acute Care Nurse Practitioners (AGACNP), in order to practice in the inpatient setting, need to be credentialed and privileged through their individual institutions. Credentialing is the process by which a provider's license, certificate, and education are authenticated by an institution. Privileging is the process of authorizing a provider to perform specific clinical duties, including diagnostic testing, treatment, invasive testing, and invasive procedures within a particular healthcare setting. Individual states in which the AGACNPs practice set the general requirements, regulations, and scope of practice required to work within the state. Each state mandates that providers be credentialed and privileged after a defined period of time, usually between two and three years after the original appointment. For privileges, an organization must adopt its own policy that outlines the specifics. The most common method of privileging for invasive procedures is proctoring by a supervising physician [9].

Challenges and Solutions

Nursing workforce shortages, generation workforce concerns, changing delivery systems, and increasing clinical practice complexity within the health environment has accentuated the fragmentation in care that accompanies the delivery of episodic, specialized care across the continuum of emergent, acute, and chronic care services. Limited access to care, the aging of the population, chronicity, and dependence on medical technology across the lifespan contribute to the number of vulnerable populations. Management of stable and progressive chronic illness in an acute care setting where episodic care is provided often results in a lack of continuity and increases patient vulnerability to poor outcomes. Patient needs are often unmet when care is limited to specialty treatment of an acute care illness, resulting in the lack of attention to comorbidities and chronic health conditions or the recognition and minimization of physiologic, psychologic, and iatrogenic risks. Significant resources are expended for specialized, focused care, both inpatient and outpatient, which again affects the continuity of care. The result is an environment of uncoordinated high resource utilization and poorly defined holistic patient outcomes. What has emerged is a need for a provider with unique knowledge, skills, and abilities to manage a patient's care across the full continuum of acuity and care services. Acute Care Nurse Practitioners (ACNPs) are uniquely prepared to meet this need and collaborate with their healthcare colleagues to achieve continuity for effective patient- and family-centered care. Providing simulation experiences during the ACNP training or within the work setting are both options to provide practice experiences to attain competency in interprofessional communication, collaboration, and clinical skills.

Regulatory Bodies

Depending on their patient population focus, nurse practitioners can seek national certification through one of the following organizations: the American Nurses Credentialing Center (ANCC), the American Academy of Nurse Practitioners Certification Board (AANPCB), the American Association of Critical Care Nurses (AACN), the Pediatric Certification Nursing Board (PCNB), or the National Certification Corporation (NCC). There are two exam options for national board certification as an AG-ACNP: One organization offering the exam is the American Nurses Credentialing Center (ANCC), while the other is the American Association of Critical Care Nurses (AACN). The ANCC uses the acronym AG-ACNP for "adult-gerontology acute care nurse practitioner," while the AACN uses the acronym ACNPC-AG® for "acute care nurse practitioner certified in adult-gerontology [10]". All 50 state boards of nursing (SBON) and employers accept both certificates and certification exams. The adult-gerontology acute care nurse practitioner (ACNP) is a registered nurse educated at the graduate level to provide continuous and comprehensive advanced nursing care to acutely ill adult-gerontology patients (young adults, older adults, and frail elderly) experiencing episodic illness, exacerbation of chronic illness or terminal illness. The practice of the adult-gerontology ACNP is determined by the acuity of patient needs rather than by the setting. The ACNP practices in any setting in which patient care requirements include complex monitoring and therapies, high-intensity nursing intervention, or continuous nursing vigilance within the range of high-acuity care. While ACNPs may traditionally practice in acute care and hospital-based settings, including subacute care, emergency care, and intensive care, the continuum of acute care services spans the geographic settings of home, ambulatory care, urgent care, and rehabilitative care. The practice environment extends into the mobile environment, including advanced air and ground ambulances, virtual locations, such as tele-intensive care units (tele-ICUs), and areas using telehealth. The scope and standards of practice, specialty certification, and nurse practice acts with rules and regulations, institutional policies and procedures, and self-determination serve as regulators of ACNP practice. The American Nurses Association Nursing Scope and Standards of Practice [11] provides the foundation for specialty organizations to define practice for the specialty and population served. The AACN Scope and Standards for acute and critical care nursing practice [10] provides an additional definition of foundational practice for clinicians caring for acutely and critically ill patients. Licensure at the state level is an external regulator of ACNP practice. State governments ensure public safety through regulations. Requirements for the recognition and practice vary among the States. An exception to state regulation is within the Veterans Health Administration system. Institutional policies and procedures and medical staff bylaws define practice within institutions. To maximize the impact that the ACNP has on patient outcomes, they participate in peer review and regular external performance evaluations. Lastly, the final regulation of the ACNP is accomplished by ACNPs exercising autonomy within their scope of practice. Expert knowledge and the willingness to commit to self-regulation and accountability for practice are the foundations for ACNP autonomy.

Sample Case Discussion

Simulation scenarios are often focused on high-risk, low-frequency situations such as cardiac arrest, pulmonary emergencies, septic shock, or other rapidly deteriorating patient care situations that require nurse interventions [12]. Conducting (Adapted from Willhaus, [13, 14]) a high-fidelity simulation requires sufficient and appropriate resources [15]. The simulation facilitator should identify available resources early on in the development and implementation phase of each scenario. The first step is to determine whether a high-fidelity simulator, part-task trainer, a standardized patient, or a combination of simulators will be used. A manikin (male and female), such as the Laerdal SimMan with technical manipulation using SimManSoftware version 3.3.1(Laerdal et al.), are examples of high-fidelity simulators and were used in the Pascual et al. study [16]. Video cameras capable of capturing high-fidelity video and audio performance are used to review during debriefings and in the evaluation phase.

Live actors may serve as standardized patients, family members, and team members. Engagement with a live person allows the learner to identify a spectrum of verbal and nonverbal cues in the scenario. Standardized participants need training for their roles and training on how to participate in the debriefing. Employing standardized patients may be less expensive than the cost of equipment, maintenance, and storage of manikins. Some potential sources of standardized patients include the student body, faculty, or volunteers. Care must be taken to ensure that invasive physical procedures should not be performed on role players. "Partial task trainers" are components that imitate portions of human anatomy and can be used to practice a procedural skill. Huang [17] defines fidelity as the degree to which a simulation resembles reality. A partial task trainer can be substituted for initiating an invasive procedure on the standardized patient if required by the scenario's objectives [17].

Recordings of the simulations serve many purposes. Punitive reprisals should not be a part of the debriefings. A review of a recorded scenario can reveal potential concerns or improvements related to patient safety. During the debriefing, participants review key learning points to help learners recall thoughts or perceptions during specific moments. Facilities that record simulations should prepare and adopt a policy specifying how recordings are stored and used before any simulation activities begin.

Both in situ and dedicated space training locations have advantages and disadvantages. Advantages for participants taking part in an in-situ training include familiarity with the environment and equipment and a decrease in travel time. Disadvantages include canceling or rescheduling if space or rooms are not available. The advantages of conducting training in a Simulation center include a more controlled setting away from the work setting, but adversely, participants may be unfamiliar with the equipment and environment and the required expenditures needed to maintain a Simulation center.

Facilitator Preparation is another aspect of a well-run simulation. The simulation facilitator should adhere to the following three steps:

1. Reviews the Scenario Overview, Learning Objectives, Scenario Script, and Sim setup card.
2. Tests all systems used, such as computers, audio/visual equipment, and mannequin, and practice operating all equipment if needed.
3. Prepare learners by providing any materials before simulation, including orienting learners to the environment and equipment, assigning roles, setting expectations, and pre-briefing learners. Reviewing the Agency for Healthcare Research and Quality website at https://www.ahrq.gov/sites/default/files/wysiwyg/teamstepps-program/teamstepps-pocket-guide.pdf is an excellent resource for educators to address TeamSTEPPS competencies prior to the simulation

Surgical intensivists proposed the following five scenarios for training acute care practitioners (AP) [16] as priority subjects for learners to practice skills and obtain competencies. These scenarios are relatively uncommon (but not rare) emergent occurrences requiring a rapid response call or an intervention in the ICU.

Scenarios:

Anaphylaxis with tension pneumothorax
Septic shock from Clostridium difficile colitis
Myocardial infarction with diabetic ketoacidosis
Hemorrhagic shock with abdominal compartment syndrome
Deteriorating traumatic brain injury with status epilepticus

Pascual et al. [16] also suggested four areas of distinct clinical environment subtypes for acute care simulations:

Emergency Department /Trauma Bay
Operating Room
Intensive Care Unit (ICU)—adult, pediatric, cardiac, surgical
Interprofessional simulation-based training before implementation of prone position ventilation
Inpatient Ad Hoc Resuscitation Team/Code Team

There are many challenges when attempting to conduct simulation training for acute care nurse practitioners. High-fidelity human patient simulator training (HPS) offers the advantage of perspective and reported experiential learning in select short-duration scenarios providing a limitless opportunity to practice margin high-stakes events in a risk-free environment. A first priority is ensuring that appropriate educational personnel are available and trained in simulation. It is vital that the educators involved with the program be knowledgeable in the topics being taught and skilled in debriefing and facilitating. In addition, it is important to involve current emergency department leaders and educators in the program so that current evidence-based practice (as well as facility specifics) can be discussed. Although most simulation training in critical care has centered on procedural

skill acquisition, there is much evidence to suggest that the focus should be on cognitive and leadership skills that are of paramount importance when caring for critically ill patients with time-sensitive conditions [15, 16, 18–20].

Secondly, when conducting simulations in a simulation center, getting protected time for staff is necessary. Often, staff time is not dedicated to simulation training, and staff is instead "released from clinical responsibilities" for the predetermined time. If their time is not protected and dedicated to training, it can be challenging for participants to be fully engaged if they are preoccupied with their assigned patient responsibilities.

Conclusion

Our present clinical, educational model faces ongoing challenges and requires new thinking. There is a need for more evidence on the use of clinical simulation as an educational intervention to assess clinical competencies. There are many barriers as well as opportunities for educators to develop new models capitalizing on a strong tradition of precepted clinical experiences. In the clinical environment, we find significant shortages of clinical sites, clinical preceptors, and the lack of financial resources to support innovative nurse practitioner education. We have the opportunity to leverage innovative, evidence-based simulations that meet national competencies as we prepare acute care nurse practitioner (ACNP) students for practice as well as practicing NPs.

References

1. Society for Simulation in Healthcare (SSH). About SSH; 2021. https://www.ssih.org/About-SSH
2. Newhouse RP, Stanik-Hutt J, White KM, Johantgen M, Bass EB, Zangaro G, et al. Advanced practice nurse outcomes 1990-2008: a systematic review. Nurs Econ. 2011;29(5):230–50. https://pubmed.ncbi.nlm.nih.gov/22372080/
3. Armenia S, Thangamathesvaran L, Caine AD, King N, Kunac A, Merchant AM. The role of high-fidelity team-based simulation in acute care settings: a systematic review. Surg J. 2018;4(3):e136–51. https://doi.org/10.1055/s-0038-1667315.
4. Nye C, Campbell SH, Hebert SH, Short C, Thomas M. Simulation in advanced practice nursing programs: a North-American survey. Clin Simul Nurs. 2019;26:3–10. https://doi.org/10.1016/j.ecns.2018.09.005.
5. Kesten KS, Brown HF, Meeker MC. Assessment of APRN competency using simulation: a pilot study. Nurs Educ Perspect. 2015;36(5):332–5. https://doi.org/10.5480/15-1649.
6. Harris J, Shoemaker K, Johnson K, Tompkins-Dobbs K, Domian E. Qualitative descriptive study of family nurse practitioner student experiences using high-fidelity simulation. Kansas Nurs. 2016;91(2):12–5. https://search.proquest.com/openview/9b0409c36f1b8dc95fff704dbef0068e/1.pdf?pq-origsite=gschoar&cbl=48934
7. Koo L, Layson-Wolf C, Brandt N, Hammersla M, Idzik S, Rocafort PT, et al. Qualitative evaluation of a standardized patient clinical simulation for nurse practitioner and pharmacy students. Nurse Educ Pract. 2014;14(6):740–6. https://doi.org/10.1016/j.nepr.2014.10.005. Epub 2014 Oct 23.
8. Jeffries PR, Bigley MB, McNelis AM, Cartier JM, Pintz C, Slaven-Lee PW, Zychowicz ME. A call to action: building evidence for use of simulation in nurse practitioner education. J Am Assoc Nurse Pract. 2019;31(11):627–32. https://doi.org/10.1097/JXX.0000000000000335.
9. Jalloh F, Tadlock MD, Cantwell S, Rausch T, Aksoy H, Frankel H. Credentialing and privileging of acute care nurse practitioners to do invasive procedures: a statewide survey. Am J Crit Care. 2016;25(4):357–61. https://doi.org/10.4037/ajcc2016118.
10. Bell L, editor. AACN scope and standards for acute and critical care nursing practice. American Association of Critical-Care Nurses; 2017.
11. American Nurses Association. Nursing scope and standards of practice, 3rd ed.; 2015. nursebooks.org
12. Lewis KA, Ricks TN, Rowin A, Ndlovu C, Goldstein L, McElvogue C. Does simulation training for acute care nurses improve patient safety outcomes: a systematic review to inform evidence-based practice. Worldviews on Evid Based Nurs. 2019;16(5):389–96. https://doi.org/10.1111/wvn.12396.
13. Willhaus J. Simulation basics: how to conduct a high-fidelity simulation. Adv Crit Care. 2016;27(1):71–7. https://doi.org/10.4037/aacnacc2016569.

14. Carey JM, Rossler K. The how when why of high fidelity simulation. In: StatPearls. Treasure Island (FL): StatPearls Publishing; 2023.
15. Keiser MM, Turkelson C. Using simulation to evaluate clinical performance and reasoning in adult-geriatric acute care nurse practitioner students. J Nurs Educ. 2019;58(10):599–603. https://doi.org/10.3928/01484834-20190923-08.
16. Pascual JL, Holena DN, Vella MA, Palmiere J, Sicoutris C, Selvan B, et al. Short simulation training improves objective skills in established advanced practitioners managing emergencies on the ward and surgical intensive care unit. J Trauma. 2011;7(2):330–7; discussion 337–338. https://doi.org/10.1097/TA.0b013e31821f4721.
17. Huang YM, Rice J, Spain A, Palaganas JC. Terms of reference. In: Palaganas J, Maxworthy J, Epps C, editors. Defining excellence in simulation programs. Lippincott Wolters Kluwer; 2015.
18. Carman M, Xu S, Rushton S, Smallheer BA, Williams D, Amarasekara S, Oermann NM. Use of a virtual learning platform for distance-based simulation in an acute care nurse practitioner curriculum. Dimens Crit Care Nurs. 2017;36(5):284–9. https://doi.org/10.1097/DCC.0000000000000259.
19. Barndt SN. Death in trauma: the role of the ACNP in patient advocacy and familial support in end-of-life care decision-making. J Trauma Nurs. 2018;25(3):171–6. https://doi.org/10.1097/JTN.0000000000000363.
20. Holliday A, Samanta D, Budinger J, Hardway J, Bethea A. An outcome analysis of nurse practitioners in acute care trauma services. J Trauma Nurs. 2017;24(6):365–70. https://doi.org/10.1097/JTN.000000000000032.

Psychiatric Mental Health Nurse Practitioner

19

Joan Fraino

Background

Due to the expansion of healthcare reform and coverage, a growing need for community providers exists [1]. Healthcare shortages are prevalent, and nurse practitioners (NP) continue to demonstrate their expertise and necessity in addressing the existing healthcare gaps.

The role of the NP is to deliver medical care in the area of specialty where they receive training. Nurse practitioners can provide primary and/or specialty care. The role of a nurse practitioner includes but is not limited to the following areas: pediatrics, adult medicine, family medicine, occupational medicine, cardiology, women's health, pain management, and psychiatry.

The Role of the Psychiatric Mental Health Nurse Practitioner

There is a growing need for healthcare services and providers to meet the challenges of those with psychiatric needs. Particularly with the recent COVID-19 pandemic, mental health facilities and providers are being called upon to care for those impacted by the current crisis and its impact on the mental health of individuals due to feelings of loss, uncertainty, and widespread fear.

The role of the Psychiatric Mental Health Nurse Practitioner (PMHNP) was created to bridge the gap of services in mental health, which oftentimes fell upon primary care providers to include the Family Nurse Practitioner (FNP). There are similarities between the role of the PMHNP to that of the FNP. Both roles require advanced degrees and training at the graduate level. The FNP may function and treat those with mental health needs in the primary care setting with medications that the PMHNP may also prescribe. Often times this occurs due to a lack of a PMHNP in their primary care setting. The responsibility for the mental health needs of patients may fall upon the hands of the FNP. Having a PMHNP present to address the psychiatric needs of individuals is extremely valuable in primary care. Many FNPs, as well as primary care providers (PCPs), find it challenging to address the psychiatric complexities of patients who present in primary care settings. It was noted that several FNP graduates went back to obtain their certification as PMHNPs to serve the rural areas better [2]. This additional certification helped to expand their expertise in patients who presented with comorbid psychiatric conditions.

The PMHNP must envelop the core competencies of the NP in addition to the PMHNP competencies. PMHNPs have advanced graduate degrees and training in the behavioral healthcare field. PMHNPs provide specialty care to individuals, families, groups, and communities with psychiatric conditions. These specialists apply the nursing process through diagnostic assessment, psychotherapeutic and psychopharmacological treatment, and evaluation of care [3]. The fundamental role of the PMHNP cannot be overemphasized as these advanced specialists can be uniquely placed in all areas where behavioral health services are in demand. However, the estimation is that there are at most 50–75 graduates per year in this field, below the demand needed to treat individuals [3].

PMHNPs specialize in addressing behavioral health issues such as schizophrenia, bipolar, or attention deficit hyperactivity disorder that cannot be addressed by many primary care providers. PMHNPs must be knowledgeable in the intricacies involved in diagnosing individuals who may be overlooked or undertreated by other health professionals due to a lack of knowledge or expertise. Individuals

Supplementary Information The online version contains supplementary material available at https://doi.org/10.1007/978-3-031-31090-4_19.

J. Fraino (✉)
Psychiatric Nurse Practitioner, Pleasanton, CA, USA
e-mail: jafraino@usfca.edu

J. M. Kutzin et al. (eds.), *Comprehensive Healthcare Simulation: Nursing*, Comprehensive Healthcare Simulation,
https://doi.org/10.1007/978-3-031-31090-4_19

that require psychotherapeutic interventions are best suited for the PMHNP who is trained to deliver these specific modalities.

Educational Opportunities to Build the Foundation of the PMHNP

Education for the PMHNP begins with the foundation of nursing practice that nurses already possess. PMHNPs have a foundation in nursing and are well-equipped to provide holistic approaches that meet the biopsychosocial needs of their patient. As advanced nurse practitioners, they must also be well-versed in diagnosing, interpreting labs, and prescribing medications. Building from this foundation and knowledge allows the practitioner to expand upon their field of expertise. Academic institutions must create opportunities for learning with a well-rounded educational program to facilitate the growth of the advanced nurse practitioner to meet the complexities of today's patients.

The need for educational opportunities and preparation for students to practice as PMHNPs is paramount. The PMHNP program should encompass intensive education in the development of physical and mental health assessment, diagnosis of mental health conditions, integration and implementation of care, psychopharmacology, psychotherapy, practice evaluation, consultation, and liaison [4]. An opportunity exists for faculty with this advanced degree to share their expertise with students as they embark on their graduate journey.

For the PMHNP, the psychiatric mental health building blocks are identified in academia through didactic courses that successfully build upon one another. As the student progresses through the expected sequences to meet the core competencies of the psychiatric nurse practitioner, so will their level of knowledge and skill. There is a movement in healthcare to standardize competency-based educational frameworks from the conventional content-based curriculum toward a competency education curriculum. According to Schumacher and Risco [5], current standards of education have typically encompassed clinical hours in combination with the completion of specified coursework.

However, a movement toward competency-based education focuses on patient outcomes and offers the opportunity to meet measurable or observable performance goals, thus improving patient outcomes. Transitioning from a focus on instructor requirements, the competency curriculum is designed around nationally standardized NP competencies. The core competencies have been revised and expanded to emphasize the need for lifespan focus which includes children, adolescents, adults, and geriatrics, specifically in rural areas [6]. Focusing on these core competencies takes into account the importance of a comprehensive approach to meeting individuals from childhood to the older adult that may be struggling with psychiatric illness.

Simulation

Simulation experiences allow students a venue to practice skills in a controlled setting. Through simulation, students implement teaching, apply skills taught, and receive feedback. Simulation for FNPs exists in most teaching institutions. However, psychiatric simulation has yet to be well developed for the PMHNP student. This is a fundamental part of complementing the learning and skills required of the PMHNP student. Future clinicians that specialize in psychiatry are needed to meet the mental health challenges that are present today. Without adequate opportunities to engage in meaningful experiences in classroom and clinical settings, they may be ill-prepared for the challenges they face as specialists in their field. The value of simulation allows students to have a variety of different scenarios to encounter and work through in preparation for potential situations that may occur in the clinical setting.

Given the current state of affairs, educational institutions have largely gone with remote learning. This can pose some problems with the delivery of education, particularly in graduate programs such as PMHNP programs. Through this type of educational avenue, students will receive support and guidance to hone their skills, allowing them to feel more competent when transitioning to clinical practicum. Learning institutions are called upon to create diverse and creative pathways in the delivery of education, particularly through remote teaching.

Simulation is a useful teaching tool to build competencies in learners by creating real patient scenarios in a controlled setting. They are allowed to make errors in the simulation settings, learn how to handle difficult or unfamiliar situations, receive feedback, and practice skills for clinical situations [7].

Simulation offers a platform to deliver education through remote learning. Specifically, in psychiatry, telepsychiatry is widely used to reach those that cannot come into the office for face-to-face assessments and treatment. Even before the COVID-19 pandemic, mental health providers were able to deliver psychiatric care effectively to these individuals, only able to receive care remotely. Preparing the PMHNP for this widely used delivery platform is imperative in educational institutions. Thus, simulation opportunities support PMHNP education.

Opportunities for simulation exist where various psychiatric scenarios that can occur in actual clinical situations are presented to the PMHP student. As students become exposed to the different simulated scenarios that can occur in clinical settings, they become more confident in their skills while still feeling safe. A variety of clinical experiences can and should be embedded in the PMHNP program. These may include in-person visits with standardized patients, computerized simulations, telepsychiatry platform simulations, and collaborative provider simulations.

One Minute Preceptor Model

Hickey, Kelly, and Nash [8] offer a methodology for teaching the "One-Minute Preceptor Model" popularized by Neher, Gordon, Meyer & Stevens [9]. This framework for simulation employs short films/vignettes of different psychiatric scenarios. Through the use of this model, students are given the availability to view, discuss, and receive feedback from seasoned clinicians/preceptors. This allows students to discuss films viewed, discuss alternative scenarios, and re-enact simulations with new lenses.

Various simulations can be developed from actual to potential cases that students may encounter in their clinic settings. These simulations should include scenarios with children, adolescents, adults, and geriatrics. It will give students the ability to test different therapeutic schemas and receive feedback from peers and faculty. The simulation also allows students to practice using screening tools specific to psychiatry. These include depression, anxiety, attention deficit hyperactivity disorder, and drug and alcohol screenings. Utilizing and analyzing psychiatric tools helps students gain familiarity, thus preparing them to administer these tests in their practicum settings comfortably.

Collaboration Scenarios Through Simulation

Ideally, providers should collaborate care with mutual patients. However, FNPs and PMHNPs rarely collaborate with care once in practice. Providing simulation experiences that promote collaboration can not only give students experiences with working together with other specialists but also provides an opportunity for each specialty nursing student to experience the different approaches each specialist utilizes for the same scenario. This can increase their knowledge as well as allow each specialist to see how important collaboration is in the clinical setting.

According to Woroch et al. [7], a telephone simulation program was instituted with FNP and PMHNP students on effectively managing a patient requesting a refill on a benzodiazepine. This particular scenario afforded the FNP and PMHNP the opportunity to explore different ways of handling a situation with a patient on controlled medication asking for a refill. It reinforced the importance of monitoring the providers previously and or currently prescribing the medication, the potential for doctor shopping in which the patient may be trying to abuse the medication by using various providers, as well as overall management of this scenario. FNPs understood the value of seeking consultation from a PMHNP as well as understanding how they themselves could handle such a case in the future despite its focus on psychiatry.

Telephone triage simulations can be implemented by different students for the same case, and this can be discussed in case conferences. This particular high-risk scenario can allow students to practice skills and implement knowledge of treatment strategies they will utilize in actual practice while being in a safe environment through simulation. Students will rely on skills learned in didactic courses as well as the skills of the clinician they are working with and receive immediate feedback from faculty monitoring the simulation. Through this simulation, students relied on the skill sets of one another, and collaboration proved useful in handling such a scenario.

High Fidelity Simulation

Combining a high-fidelity simulator with a standardized patient (SP) is a strategy that can be used in the classroom setting to support the learning of the advanced nurse practitioner, such as the PMHNP. It allows live interaction with an actor posing as a patient with realistic clinical scenarios that allow the student to work through the simulation, in turn developing cognitive, affective, and psychomotor skills through practice [10].

Abram & Forbes use Kolb's Experiential Learning theory [11] to allow students a full experience that includes: converging, diverging, assimilation, and accommodation. Using this model allows students a rich experience through a variety of measures that will support their learning in theory and apply them to skill practice. Simulation provides the students with a safe environment where they can interact with standardized patients and feel relatively safe. Faculty can monitor students in simulation settings and address safety concerns that may occur should they have been in actual practice settings.

Since actual clinical settings provided to patients may only provide some scenarios that PMHNPs will encounter in their practice, simulation provides an opportunity for PMHNP students to get exposed to these different scenarios they may not otherwise encounter in their clinical settings. The ability to apply theories learned in didactic courses also improves the confidence of students to utilize what they have learned in theory.

Opportunities for Integration into Existing Education

Preparing the FNP/PMHNP by combing the educational program to remove redundancies that may occur at both programs that can rather be addressed through the development and implementation of a combination of preparation courses was done.

A Health Resource and Services Administration grant was awarded to the University of Nebraska Medical Center for the development and integration of FNP and PMHNP practice skills [2]. The preceptor responsible for developing this model had to be certified in both family and mental health. This ensured that someone knowledgeable was addressing the needs of education for both specialties.

Examples of case studies to support an integrated process included anxiety, insomnia, fatigue, headaches, weakness, and forgetfulness to stimulate critical thinking and draw on skills from both specialties [2]. Other case studies can be created within the educational curriculum that supports the various psychiatric conditions that PMHNPs will encounter in their clinical settings as well as their future professional settings. New directions should continue to focus on distance learning options to enhance skills and knowledge of specialty practices such as the PMHNP.

Examples of PMHNP simulation scenarios: See Electronic Supplementary Material.

References

1. Forsberg I, Swartwout K, Murphy M, Danko K, Delaney KR. Nurse practitioner education: Greater demand, reduced training opportunities. J Amer Assoc Nurse Pract. 2015;27(2):66–71. https://doi.org/10.1002/2327-6924.12175.
2. Hulme PA, Houfek JF, Fiandt K, Barron C, Muhlbauer S. Educating integrated family/psychiatric–mental health nurse practitioners: program development and evaluation. J Nurs Educ. 2015;54(9):493–9.
3. Chapman SA, Phoenix BJ, Hahn TE, Strod DC. Utilization and economic contribution of psychiatric mental health nurse practitioners in public behavioral health services. Amer J Prevent Med. 2018;54(6):S243–9.
4. American Psychiatric Nurses Association. APRN consensus mode; 2008. https://www.apna.org/i4a/pages/index.cfm?pageID=4387
5. Schumacher G, Risco K. Competency-based nurse practitioner education: an overview for the preceptor. J Nurs Pract. 2017;13(9):596–602. https://doi.org/10.1016/j.nurpra.2017.07.020.
6. Hubbard G, Woods-Giscombe CL, Hageman A, Vimba N. Innovative clinical training site for psychiatric mental health nurse practitioner students: elementary school-based group therapy (Manuscript ID UMHN-2017-0143). Iss Ment Heal Nurs. 2018;39(4):357–61.
7. Woroch RA, Alvarez DV, Yingling CT, Handrup C. T Family nurse practitioner/psychiatric mental health nurse practitioner collaboration in drug-seeking telephone triage simulation in an advanced practice registered nurse curriculum. Clin Simul Nurs. 2018;18:14–9.
8. Hickie C, Kelly B, Nash L. Development and use of scripted filmed scenarios to teach the One-Minute Preceptor model. Acad Psych. 2017;41(1):110–3.
9. Neher JO, Gordon KC, Meyer B, Stevens N. A five-step "micro-skills" model of clinical teaching. J Am Board Fam Pract. 1992;5:419–24.
10. Abram MD, Forbes MO. High-fidelity simulation: an application to psychopharmacological training for the psychiatric nurse practitioner student. Iss Ment Health Nurse. 2019;40(3):260–7.
11. Kolb DA. Experiential learning: experience as the source of learning and development. Englewood Cliffs, N.J: Prentice-Hall; 1984.

Primary Care Pediatric Nurse Practitioner Simulation Techniques

20

Ruth K. Rosenblum and Julianne Doucette

Background

In 2008, the National Organization of Nurse Practitioner Faculties (NONPF) developed the APRN Consensus Model: Licensure, Accreditation, Certification, and Education [1]. NONPF developed the Primary Care Pediatric Nurse Practitioner Competencies within the Population-Focused Nurse Practitioner Competencies, updated in 2013, which describes competencies that build on core knowledge. The expectation is that entry-level nurse practitioners will be competent in various knowledge and skills by graduation. The categories of competency include Scientific Foundation, Leadership, Quality, Practice Inquiry, Technology and Information Literacy, Policy, Health Delivery System, Ethics, and Independent Practice [1]. The first step in developing a simulation curriculum is to align the objectives of the simulation experience with the American Nurses Credentialing Center (ANCC), NONPF, and Pediatric Nursing Certification Board (PNCB) recommendations and competencies.

The pediatric population-focused competencies build on the core knowledge that all nurse practitioners should achieve. The role of the primary care pediatric nurse practitioner (PNP) is to provide care to children from birth through young adults with in-depth knowledge, experience, and skill in pediatric primary health care. This may include well child care, prevention/management of common pediatric acute illnesses and chronic conditions, and may also expand into specialty practice such as neurology, pulmonary, and gastrointestinal, in the outpatient or inpatient setting, depending on the needs of the patient and the ecosystem in which the PNP functions. PNPs foster the health of children within the context of their family, community, and environmental setting.

R. K. Rosenblum · J. Doucette (✉)
Rush University College of Nursing, Chicago, IL, USA
e-mail: ruth.rosenblum@sjsu.edu; Julianne_Doucette@Rush.edu

Doucette et al. (2018) asked, "Does consistent evaluation of clinical progress and attainment of the recommended skills and competencies occur in the clinical setting?" with factors including varied clinical opportunities, sites and preceptors, and faculty evaluation nearly always limited to reliance on preceptor evaluation of students' patient care skills [2]. This is especially true in online APRN programs where students are often in a different state than faculty. To ameliorate this concern, Doucette et al. used simulation as a method of consistent evaluation of PNP primary care student mastery of clinical competencies and selected skills. Using the NONPF competencies, multiple/serial simulation skills labs, and Objective Structured Clinical Exams (OSCE) were developed and implemented. Finally, the evaluation of clinical progress and attainment of NONPF competencies was assessed using a faculty-developed rubric. The evaluation was consistent with the use of the simulation lab and OSCEs, and student learning was enhanced. A challenge that remains for PNP faculty and students, and likely all areas of practice, is translating performance in skills and simulation and OSCEs to actual practice and patients.

In another instance, Borgmeyer et al. (2017) explored the effectiveness of PNPs in teaching providers how to implement the Asthma Action Plan (AAP) using simulation [3]. In this PNP-led class, resident physician knowledge of the AAP and confidence in teaching families improved significantly pre- and post-simulation. While simulation is used frequently for attaining procedural skills, these authors suggest that it can be effective also as a method to improve communication and teaching strategies amongst varied members of the healthcare team for a variety of settings and diagnoses.

Caring for healthy or ill children can be challenging. Using simulation as a method of education offers PNP primary care students a venue where they can improve their skills, knowledge, and communication in a safe and supportive environment. While there is no substitute for an actual child and their caregiver, high or low-fidelity simulation of a specific diagnosis can effectively mimic an encounter and

J. M. Kutzin et al. (eds.), *Comprehensive Healthcare Simulation: Nursing*, Comprehensive Healthcare Simulation,
https://doi.org/10.1007/978-3-031-31090-4_20

provide the student and faculty with valuable information for future teaching and learning. Acquisition of skills and competencies specific to pediatrics can be effectively accomplished in the simulation skills lab with the added benefit of consistent evaluation of clinical progress and competency acquisition. Kinesthetic skills may include nasal or ear foreign body removal, splinting, spirometry, diagnostic testing, nebulizers, spacer usage, etc. Simulation of skills like those noted here, along with exhibiting age-appropriate patient and family-centered communication skills, can also be accomplished via a robust simulation plan. Finally, in their systematic review, Rutherford-Hemming et al. (2016) identified a lack of empirical evidence in the literature to support using simulation in lieu of direct patient care clinical hours in NP education and recommended further rigorous scientific, quantitative data to support it [4]. Further research is required to improve current simulation curriculums, develop validated assessment tools, and demonstrate improved clinical outcomes after simulation-based training.

Best Practices

When implementing simulation in PNP education as a learning modality, several points must be considered. These include the *pediatric physical exam* and other nuances of pediatric care (e.g., non-invasive to invasive during an exam of an infant or toddler). Will the NP be doing a standard exam vs. a focused examination, and which is appropriate under various circumstances? Other nuances to consider include, formulation of *differential diagnosis* and development of critical thinking skills for the student who will be caring for the child and family unit. Additionally, best practices in the adult setting using *Standardized Patients* (SP) cannot easily be implemented in pediatrics due to potential legal and ethical limitations, especially for the younger child. SPs can effectively 'be' adolescent patients, but the scenario may be less authentic if an adult SP portrays a younger child. The use of simulation for *formative and summative evaluation* via OSCE and the lack of universally accepted standard evaluation tools is a limitation in the discussion of best practices. OSCEs are used internationally, but Johnston et al. (2017) reiterate that there is no validated, reliable tool for student perception that could be applied across facilities [5]. Further, they state recommendations include the need for an evidence-based form of assessment of both students and outcomes. In primary care PNP education, this is true, and there are even fewer evidence-based assessments.

The pediatric physical exam can be practiced on a manikin that has the capability to mirror the physiologic parameters and medical responses of an infant or child. PNP students can acquire diagnostic skills and practice medical procedures that vary widely in complexity. Assessment skills of an infant or child can be perfected, and diagnostic skills can be learned by varying the underlying physiologic status of the manikin. Haut et al. (2014) used high-fidelity simulation (infant with sepsis) to teach acute care PNP students [6]. Students responded positively, though the study did not show statistical significance of before- and after-knowledge. Medical education best practices have evolved to employ simulation in high-risk, low-volume 'uncommon' situations such as resuscitation and stabilization of pediatric trauma. The spacing effect, referring to educational encounters spaced and repeated over time (spaced distribution), may result in more efficient and improved retention of learning compared with more concentrated educational encounters. This strategy has yet to be reviewed in PNP education, though anecdotally, it has been done and has been successful with regard to both skill acquisition and critical thinking.

When determining the differential diagnosis of a pediatric patient, several studies have used simulation-based assessment tools and have found that the simulation-based assessments are valid and reliable measures of clinical performance and competency. Faculty who implement simulation into PNP curricula must determine if the goal of the simulation is a standard or focused examination. Simulation of a standard exam may provide students with a basic understanding of how to approach history-taking and examining a child, likely eliciting information from the child's caregiver and interacting with a young child, which may be a new experience for the student. The use of simulation for a focused examination, for example, as noted above, resuscitation, has promising possibilities from work that has been done to date, though evidence of improved clinical outcomes after simulation-based training has not been determined. The clinical significance of measured performance in a simulated setting remains uncertain.

The use of Standardized Patients (SP) has gained a following in simulation-based education. As noted above, SPs can more readily mimic adolescents rather than infants or young children. Schram and Mudd (2015) state that a pilot study experience using SPs in a graduate APRN program was shown to be an effective learning strategy to promote an engaging context for learning and student performance improvement [7]. However, these were FNP graduate students, not PNP, and the use of SPs in PNP education remains a newer modality with unique challenges. Barber (2018) also implemented SPs in an FNP simulation program [8]. In an Ethics Rounds article, Khoo et al. (2017) discuss ethical concerns when minors act as SPs [9]. This practice can raise a number of unique ethical issues. Can minors consent to be teaching tools in medical education? Are there certain practices that could cause harm for the children who decide, or whose parents decide, to go this route? Child labor laws, parental and child consent, and beneficence vs. nonmaleficence are all issues that arise when considering the use of children as SPs. Other more pragmatic concerns arise, such as—Can the child maintain the 'story' consistently? What if the child becomes 'bored' or loses interest or patience? And if an incidental finding is determined, what are the next steps for that child? The welfare of the child must remain paramount, and every effort must be made to minimize potential harm to the child during the SP process. Other issues to be considered include recruitment, training, and compensation. Importantly, any assessment of pediatric clinical skills must examine balancing the parent–child–pediatric provider triangle and the physical examination of younger children and newborns [10]. Adult or young adult SPs are commonly used in the role of child/adolescent. Acting or drama students can enhance this due to their ability to inhabit a 'character' or age, though some reality must be suspended if the SP is a very small or young child. Finally, adult SPs can easily act as parents or caregivers, especially with regard to history taking, education, things to watch for, and procedural teaching, e.g., insulin administration.

Formative and summative evaluations are the basis of any learning plan. OSCEs are one method of accomplishing this. However, there are many more ways for evaluation to occur. In addition to formative and summative evaluations, the determination of processes and outcomes must also be addressed. Process evaluation may include how the OSCE was done; outcome evaluation would be whether the OSCE or other method did what it set out to do, i.e., was there an appropriate scenario for students to prepare, participate, and debrief? Formative and summative evaluations are similar; however, the emphasis should be focused on competency, i.e., did students respond to the scenario properly and appropriately and determine the correct differential diagnosis (or whatever topic/case was under study?) In their 2017 article, Aronowitz et al. postulate that students can simulate practice and be evaluated within their NP role in a safe, controlled environment [11]. They further add that the use of OSCEs as a simulation tool in an advanced practice curriculum can be both an evaluative and pedagogical tool. As cases become more complex, over time, critical thinking and formulation of differential diagnoses can take place. OSCEs offer uniform evaluations of all students and are easily inserted into each semester's curriculum. Additionally, OSCEs and other forms of formative and summative evaluations can offer the opportunity for complex case management and diagnostic questions along with opportunities for child and family communication. This can all be done in an educational, safe, 'low stakes,' non-threatening environment. This information is general and not PNP-focused; however, concepts can be transferred to the PNP educational setting. Lee et al. (2018) found a Mock OSCE (MOSCE), with upper-level students teaching newer students, to be a feasible and acceptable means of providing additional OSCE practice to students prior to higher-stakes evaluation [12]. While not pediatric-focused, this learning methodology would benefit students in all roles in a PNP program, as both teachers and learners.

Sample Curriculum

The ultimate goal of graduate-level nurse practitioner education is to prepare nurses to practice at a higher level of critical thinking and decision-making as they transition from the RN role to the APRN role. Throughout the graduate program, the didactic courses provide the foundational knowledge and background information to prepare students for clinical experiences. The National Organization of Nurse Practitioner Faculties (NONPF) has established standards for Core Competencies and Population-Focused Nurse Practitioner Competencies that pediatric nurse practitioner students must master prior to graduation (Core Competencies for Nurse Practitioners 2022) [1]. Developing a curriculum that seamlessly integrates simulation, indirect, and direct clinical experiences focused on the attainment of the NONPF competencies is the goal of graduate programs. The development of the curriculum should be intentional and follow a stepwise approach.

Furthermore, simulation can be used as a tool for acquiring clinical competence/confidence prior to direct clinical experiences or as an evaluation tool as students progress through direct clinical experiences. Evaluation of students in both scenarios will ensure progress towards the acquisition of required competencies set by both NONPF and certification boards. These formative and summative experiences provide faculty with the opportunity to both educate and evaluate competence in a uniform environment.

The Pediatric Nursing Certification Board (PNCB) outlines procedures nurse practitioner students should be com petent in performing before sitting for the national certification exam [13]. Providing practice completing procedures that are unique to pediatrics should guide faculty in developing simulation scenarios. One of the recommended procedures includes cerumen removal from the ear canal. Since infants and young children have small ear canals, even a small amount of cerumen can obstruct the view of the tympanic membranes. A practitioner who is efficient at removing cerumen can visualize the tympanic membranes to rule out otitis media. This procedure, along with foreign body removal from the ear and nose, fluorescein staining of the eye, and rapid tests such as influenza, strep, and the mono spot, could be taught in a simulation skills lab with some equipment such as a task trainer model head with realistic ear, eye, nose, and mouth. Techniques for careful examination of the tympanic membrane of a crying and moving child using an otoscope upside down with the hand resting on the child's head to prevent penetration of the tip into the canal can also be practiced in the simulation setting. The simulation skills lab could also provide practice in completing a newborn nursery examination, umbilical cord cauterization, and identification of a patent ductus arteriosus heart murmur. Some pediatric outpatient offices have spirometry or pulmonary function tests available; therefore, teaching students how to perform these diagnostic tests are of value during simulation. Another procedure specific to pediatrics PNCB recommends students practice is the reduction of nurse maid's elbow. Reduction of this common condition in pediatrics can be practiced on a manikin, especially if a homemade manikin is created for this purpose. Common pediatric simulation scenarios can be devised based on meeting the clinical competencies, as well as attaining competency in performing procedures. Furthermore, the scenarios can include both expected encounters all nurse practitioner students should have in clinical practice, as well as incorporate aspects of pediatric care that students may not be exposed to in direct clinical on a routine basis. Learning objectives can be tailored to the specific scenario.

In general, the simulations should involve all body systems to ensure faculty are evaluating student progress towards mastery of the comprehensive pediatric history, physical exam, development of a problem list, differentials, a management plan, education plan, and follow-up plan of various conditions. In the pediatric population, the history varies by age, and the anticipatory guidance provided by the PNP student varies according to developmental stage. Often students struggle to learn the appropriate development by age and the associated anticipatory guidance for teaching parents. Teaching differences in development by age during simulation can assist the student in retaining knowledge of the various stages and pediatric milestones. In terms of the history, pediatric-specific questions such as prenatal history, birth complications, any early hospitalizations for conditions such as bronchiolitis, or emergency room visits should be reviewed. Immunization and allergy history are important for infants and children, as well as separation anxiety, teething, sleep issues, and toilet training. Including some of these history components unique to pediatrics during the simulation, scenario helps students to retain the information for future use in practice. In terms of the physical exam, there are also variations specific to pediatrics that could be incorporated into the simulation. Teaching students that respirations and heart rate parameters change according to age can be incorporated into the simulation experience. A very common innocent pediatric heart murmur could be simulated so students recognize Still's murmur and can differentiate it from ominous heart murmurs using a simulation stethoscope capable of producing instructor-determined sounds and a manikin.

Developing the scenario keeping in mind pediatric variations may involve the following steps: select or develop the evaluation tool (will you evaluate the simulation experience of the student, student knowledge attainment, and/or student confidence with skills and procedures), schedule the SPs, develop the SP script in detail, develop the student simulation schedule and assigned faculty, provide an orientation for the faculty and SPs. Scham and Mudd describe scheduling a 30-min one-on-one simulation experience between the student and the SP and a 30-min block between the student and faculty in a debriefing session [7]. Doucette et al. planned a simulation for more students; therefore, the total individual session was 20 min between the student and the SP and 10 min for debriefing with a longer debriefing session with the whole group of students at the end of the simulation day for about 30 min to review the entire scenario [2]. According to Ballman et al. (2016), the use of a Standardized Patient who is educated on the nuances of the scenario with a detailed script prior to the actual encounter ensures "consistent evaluation" of each student's performance during the simulation experience [14].

Many pediatric patients visit the outpatient pediatric office for respiratory concerns; therefore, including a respiratory scenario is advantageous to student learning. Common differentials in pediatrics include the common cold, asthma, allergic rhinitis, viral upper respiratory illnesses, croup, bronchiolitis, community-acquired pneumonia, etc.; therefore, working knowledge of the respiratory exam, diagnoses and management is important. To incorporate many of the recommended skills suggested by NONPF, a scenario that involves obtaining pulse oximetry, spirometry, administering a nebulizer, reassessing respiratory status, possibly ordering and interpreting a chest x-ray, and providing inhaler teaching with spacer devices all provide practice with attaining recommended competencies (https://cdn.ymaws.com/www.nonpf.org/resource/resmgr/Competencies/CompilationPopFocusComps2013.pdf) [15]. The first step in developing the scenario is creating the learning objectives for the students. The learning objectives of this scenario could include:

1. obtaining a comprehensive respiratory history including immunization status, allergies, pertinent past medical history, and family history of asthma or atopy;
2. performing a focused respiratory exam; identifying and managing signs of respiratory distress, including ordering tests and lab work;
3. developing, implementing, and discussing a management plan; implementing nonpharmacologic and pharmacologic methods to improve respiratory status;
4. evaluating the effectiveness of treatment interventions; and
5. demonstrating appropriate patient-centered communication skills with patients and families.

Schram and Mudd (2015) describe using the Association of Standardized Patient Educators Simulation Scenarios Development guidelines to develop the simulation scenarios [7]. In general, faculty can follow this guide to develop the scenarios using their own clinical expertise in pediatrics. Schram and Mudd (2015) describe initiating a simulation scenario after students have received information related to the scenario in didactic coursework. They describe the simulation as occurring at the end of the first clinical management course [7]. Ideally, the first simulation would take place after didactic information was provided to the students but before the student attended clinical.

Securing and scheduling SPs for the scenario is variable across NP programs. Some larger universities have access to a Simulation Center where staff has a pool of SPs and sign the SPs up for the simulation experience. Other universities may need access to a simulation center and must secure their own SPs or use faculty members as the SPs. Simulation centers can utilize the Association of Standardized Patient Educators Case Development Template to provide the SPs with pertinent information related to the pediatric case. The SPs should have training as actors able to imitate a child or adolescent for the scenario to be realistic.

Evaluation tools for simulation exist, but many need to be more specific to graduate-level nursing or pediatrics. Often faculty develop their own evaluation checklist based on their developed scenarios. Some validated tools to use as a guide for developing the pediatric scenario include instruments developed by the National League for Nursing. The Student Satisfaction and Self-Confidence in Learning Instrument is a 13-item questionnaire that uses a five-point Likert scale to obtain information related to the student's satisfaction with the simulation experience, including the teaching materials and how the instructor taught the simulation is easy to use as a quick evaluation from the student perspective (NLN 2005) [16]. The NLN also developed the Educational Practices Questionnaire (Student Version), a 16-item questionnaire using a five-point Likert scale to measure if best practices are being used in the simulation from the perspective of the student. These two tools are useful for student evaluation of the simulation experience. In terms of the faculty evaluation of the student, the Creighton Simulation Evaluation Instrument is one option as a competency-based qualitative evaluation tool focusing on the four main areas of assessment, communication, critical thinking, and technical skills (Hayden et al. 2014) [17]. This tool was updated to the Creighton Competency Evaluation Instrument. The Lasater Clinical Judgement Rubric focuses more on judgment, communication, and demeanor during patient interaction and may not be as comprehensive as necessary when evaluating graduate-level pediatric nurse practitioner students (Adamson et al. 2013) [18]. The Clinical Simulation Evaluation Tool (CSET) developed by the University of Massachusetts is described by Radhakrishnan et al. (2007) as an evaluation designed to evaluate students using patient simulators including assessment skills, safety, prioritization, problem-focused assessment, interventions, delegation, and communication skills [19]. This tool could be adapted for the evaluation of pediatric nurse practitioner students. In addition, the Objective Structured Clinical Examination (OSCE) is often used in medical education as an assessment of student clinical skills and knowledge using an objective checklist and is an excellent option for graduate pediatric nursing simulations [11, 20]. Typically, the student interviews and assesses one standardized patient (SP) who can provide valuable feedback about communication skills [11]. Doucette et al. developed the Pediatric Focused Respiratory OSCE Evaluation Tool related to the sample pediatric OSCE simulation scenario below in the sample cases section. (See Appendix A).

Integrating into Existing Education

Most primary care pediatric nurse practitioner programs provide didactic core courses followed by specialty courses and clinical courses. An appropriate place in the program for simulation may vary by program; however, providing the simulation experience prior to direct clinical experiences has been recommended in the literature [19]. This approach allows for faculty to provide similar initial clinical skills or experiences in a controlled environment to all students with the goal of increasing confidence and exposure to pediatric-specific skills and techniques prior to real-life experiences in direct clinical. Since clinical sites are becoming more difficult to obtain student's initial clinical experiences can be achieved via simulated cases. Simulated computerized plat forms can provide beginning pediatric nurse practitioner students with practice before a simulated experience in the simulation lab. One example is Aquifer, an online simulation software program that provides clinical cases for students to review and interactively participate in quizzes and knowledge checks. The purpose of the platform is to provide practice with clinical decision-making skills http://www.aquifer.org [21]. Aquifer is particularly suited for use with beginning nurse practitioner students since the pediatric cases are thorough, evidence-based, and do not require a high level of critical thinking. Reeldx is another option as a virtual platform that provides "real" patient encounter videos to introduce a case https://www.reeldx.com [22]. The video is a short one-minute snapshot of a patient visit with a pediatric provider where a description of the presenting symptoms of the patient is revealed. The student is then given the task of determining the differentials and problem list, ordering laboratory tests or images, diagnosing, and developing a management plan. The higher level of critical thinking involved with Reeldx allows for more experienced students to expand their simulation practice.

In addition, simulation can be useful throughout the program as a touchpoint with students who participate in direct clinical experience in varied clinical sites. Many programs educate students at a distance, and clinical oversight by faculty is difficult when the student lives and completes clinical experiences in another state. In addition, clinical sites will not provide the exact same experience for each student; therefore, evaluation of the attainment of the skills and competencies expected by graduation in the simulation lab allows for interventions throughout the program to ensure all students obtain the level of mastery required to practice as pediatric nurse practitioners after graduation. Although outcomes related to the integration of simulation at the graduate level are scarce, Schwindt and McNeils (2015) describe the feasibility of integrating into a psychiatric mental health nurse practitioner program and student outcomes such as increased confidence and motivation, as well as clinical self-evaluation through reflection [23]. If students receive feedback and can self-reflect on their performance or mastery of competencies, then new clinical goals could be set and positive improvements expected.

The Nursing Education Simulation Framework can be used as a guide to incorporating simulation into pediatric nurse practitioner education. Jefferies et al. (2015) describes the five aspects of the framework, including the facilitator (faculty), the participant (student), educational practices to include in the simulation, simulation design, and expected participant outcomes. This model suggests that faculty must be an integral aspect of the simulation planning. Meetings to discuss the objectives, pediatric content, flow of the simulation scenario, and practice evaluation of students help faculty become more comfortable conducting the simulation with students [24]. Providing explicit instructions for faculty, students, and SPs provides for a more organized simulation experience. A script for SPs to follow or "learn" prior to the actual scenario is helpful for a more authentic interaction with the student.

Challenges and Solutions

There are many challenges with the use of simulation in PNP education. Generally, the broad categories of challenges are divided in two. First are technology or 'hardware' challenges. This may include infant and child manikins, high or low fidelity, and the 'fidelity' with which physiologic responses can be replicated in a skills/sim lab. For example, a crying, fussy infant who is pushing the examiner away as ears are attempted to be examined cannot realistically be replicated on a manikin. Second are the challenges surrounding the child and family. This can further be stratified into direct child/family issues and secondary challenges involving the use of children in simulation, which may include legal, language, and issues of cost, space, and time.

Infant manikins can be used to teach PNP students about a complete newborn exam; this can be basic or enhanced depending on the fidelity and technology present. For example, newborn heart sounds or abnormal heart sounds consistent with congenital heart disease may be possible on an appropriate manikin. Since pediatric parents can be patients too, and the family unit is the patient, simulation in PNP programs can be used to show students and/or parents (and teach students how to teach parents) elements of caring for a newborn e.g., milia, stool expectations. More importantly, simulation in a PNP program can offer students a safe place to have 'mock' conversations with parents about potentially sensitive topics; these might include: postpartum depression, vaccine-hesitant parents, etc. Certainly, the PNP caring for an older child can benefit from simulation for a variety of topics, including toddler through adolescent well-child exams, sports physicals, asthma exacerbation, concussion evaluation, and many more. Much of this (with an older child) adapts well for online or distance learning or for the introduction of telehealth into a PNP curriculum. Finally, the PNP could benefit from simulation in implementing/grading the Ages and Stages questionnaire and MCHAT autism evaluation tool.

Other challenges exist when planning simulation experiences for PNP students. As stated above, the parent-child dyad is the patient, so communication must be directed at and appropriate for both, keeping the age of the child and level of understanding in mind. Other challenges that arise are the assessment and diagnosis of various dermatologic disorders or the red reflex in patients with darker skin tones. This might be more difficult for PNPs and also less amenable to simulation. However, simulation could provide a venue for this information to be discussed, especially if culturally appropriate manikins can be used. Additionally, as stated above, Khoo et al. (2017) discuss ethical concerns when minors act as SPs [9]. Although not often used as true SPs, children may be used as patient models for skills practice or for assessment of normal and/or abnormal findings. Certainly, a child should not be used as a model or standardized patient for painful or embarrassing procedures, and assent should be attained (along with parental consent) for the child to participate. Child labor laws in entertainment exist because it is understood that the work that a child actor does (i.e., playing the part of a child) cannot be done by an adult [25]. However, it is unlikely that a pediatric SP would need to be absent from school or work away from home to the extent and frequency that a child actor might.

Finally, costs, space, and time may be challenging for pediatric simulation for PNP students. Simulation lab personnel, payment or incentives for child standardized patients/parents, and completing the simulation at a convenient time for all (i.e. not during school hours) must be explored. Simulation, in general, is time and equipment intensive for students and faculty. Including child-standardized patients adds another level of complexity and time constraints to the equation. Long-term sustainability of any plan involving children would need to be examined, and thoughts about a 'pipeline' of potential standardized patients could be considered.

Regulatory Bodies

Research needs to include more on the use and effectiveness of simulation in primary care NP education, and especially in specialty PNP education. Further research and determination of best practices, as well as the development of valid and reliable tools to measure clinical performance and clinical reasoning skills, must occur in order to maximize the use of simulation as an effective tool in education. Simulation using SPs may be a useful addition to traditional precepted experiences for reinforcing student knowledge, skills, and attitudes in a PNP program. What remains unclear, however, is whether learning in a simulated environment transfers to effective clinical practice. While simulation is useful in assisting students in meeting course and program learning outcomes, it is still being determined if simulation, OSCEs, and related techniques will serve to ensure that these PNP students become safe and effective providers [8]. Rutherford-Hemming and Jennrich (2013) are looking at the transfer of learning from a sim lab to a clinical setting, asking the following questions [26]:

(a) Does the clinical competency of students in a standardized patient setting differ from their clinical competency in a clinical setting (that is, does competency transfer from the simulated to the clinical setting)?
(b) How do students describe the effect of a standardized patient simulation on their clinical competence?
(c) Does clinical self-efficacy change among students who participate in a standardized patient simulation?
(d) How do students describe the effect of a standardized patient simulation on their clinical self-efficacy?
(e) What is the relationship between clinical competency and clinical self-efficacy of students who participate in a standardized patient simulation?

Finally, Rutherford-Hemming et al. (2016) and Schram and Mudd (2015) identify that there needs to be more empirical evidence in the literature to support using simulation in lieu of direct patient care clinical hours in NP education [4, 7]. While they did not examine PNP education, certainly primary care pediatrics presents more complex challenges, as discussed here.

Accreditation and credentialing organizations such as NONPF and PCNB supported the transition and facilitated a revision of their nurse practitioner (NP) core and population-focused competencies to support the integrated DNP NP curriculum (2015). PNPs may be certified either by PNCB or AACN [27]. The purpose of certification is to validate the knowledge and entry-level clinical skills that are linked to competent PNP practice and achieved through completion of an accredited graduate PNP educational program.

Every primary care NP program/track, including pediatric primary care, has a minimum of 500 supervised direct patient care clinical hours overall. As per the AACN regulatory organization, simulation is recommended to augment the clinical learning experiences, particularly to address high-risk, low-frequency incidents; however, simulation experiences may only be counted as clinical hours over and above the minimum 500 direct patient care clinical hours. Programs are encouraged to track the use of simulation to enhance the clinical experience. https://www.aacnnursing.org/Portals/42/AcademicNursing/pdf/Criteria-Evaluation-NP-2016.pdf.

NONPF has a robust simulation portal, though states no policy or restrictions/regulations on the use of simulation beyond those of AACN noted above. NONPF's goal is to support faculty in implementing quality simulation for NPs, and, in their portal, provides links to many simulation-related organizations and entities, though they do not recommend or associate with any in particular. There is a special interest group (SIG) that was developed in response to member discussion about supporting the use of simulation-based strategies in NP education.

Finally, the NCSBN has exhaustively examined the use of simulation in prelicensure programs and sanctions the use of high-quality simulations for up to half of traditional clinical hours in prelicensure undergraduate nursing programs in some states, evidence from graduate advanced practice nursing education programs is not present [28]. A recent systematic review compared high-fidelity simulation to online or traditional classroom lectures and noted limited evidence to support the use of simulation within nurse practitioner programs [29].

References

1. Consensus model for APRN regulation: licensure, accreditation, certification & education. APRN Joint Dialogue Group Report [Internet]. 2008 [cited 17 September 2020]. https://cdn.ymaws.com/www.nonpf.org/resource/resmgr/consensus_model/aprnconsensusmodelfinal09.pdf.
2. Doucette J, Manion A, Odiaga J. Promoting excellence in clinical practice: the use of simulation to evaluate doctor of nursing practice

nurse practitioner competencies. 2018. http://dnpconferenceaudio.s3.amazonaws.com/2018/DoucetteJ_2018DNPConf_Poster.pdf.
3. Borgmeyer A, Gyr P, Ahmad E, Ercole P, Balakas K. Pediatric nurse practitioners effective in teaching providers the asthma action plan using simulation. J Pediatr Nurs. 2017;34:53–7.
4. Rutherford-Hemming T, Nye C, Coram C. Using simulation for clinical practice hours in nurse practitioner education in the United States: a systematic review. Nurse Educ Today. 2016;37:128–35.
5. Johnston A, Weeks B, Shuker M, Coyne E, Niall H, Mitchell M, et al. Nursing students' perceptions of the objective structured clinical examination: an integrative review. Clin Simul Nurs. 2017;13(3):127–42.
6. Haut C, Fey M, Akintade B, Klepper M. Using high-fidelity simulation to teach acute care pediatric nurse practitioner students. J Nurse Pract. 2014;10(10):87–91.
7. Schram A, Mudd S. Implementing standardized patients within simulation in a nurse practitioner program. Clin Simul Nurs. 2015;11(4):208–13.
8. Barber L, Schuessler J. Standardized patient simulation for a graduate nursing program. J Nurse Pract. 2018;14(1):e5–e11.
9. Khoo E, Schremmer R, Diekema D, Lantos J. Ethical concerns when minors act as standardized patients. Pediatrics. 2017;139(3):e20162795.
10. Stollar F, Cerutti B, Aujesky S, Nendaz M, Galetto-Lacour A. Evaluation of a best practice approach to assess undergraduate clinical skills in pediatrics. BMC Med Educ. 2020;20(1):46.
11. Aronowitz T, Aronowitz S, Mardin-Small J, Kim B. Using objective structured clinical examination (OSCE) as education in advanced practice registered nursing education. J Prof Nurs. 2017;33(2):119–25.
12. Lee C, Madrazo L, Khan U, Thangarasa T, McConnell M, Khamisa K. A student-initiated objective structured clinical examination as a sustainable cost-effective learning experience. Med Educ Online. 2018;23(1):1440111.
13. Pediatric Nursing Certification Board [Internet]. 2020 [cited 26 September 2020]. https://www.pncb.org.
14. Ballman K, Garritano N, Beery T. Broadening the reach of standardized patients in nurse practitioner education to include the distance learner. Nurse Educ. 2016;41(5):230–3.
15. Thomas A. Population focused nurse practitioner competencies: family/across the lifespan, neonatal, acute care pediatric, primary care pediatric, psychiatric-mental health, & women's health/gender-related. population-focused nurse practitioner competencies. 2013. https://cdn.ymaws.com/www.nonpf.org/resource/resmgr/Competencies/CompilationPopFocusComps2013.pdf.
16. National League of Nursing. Descriptions of available instruments [Internet]. 2020 [cited 27 September 2020]. http://www.nln.org/professional-development-programs/research/tools-and-instruments/descriptions-of-available-instruments.
17. Hayden J, Keegan M, Kardong-Edgren S, Smiley RA. Reliability and validity testing of the Creighton competency evaluation instrument for use in the NCSBN National Simulation Study. Nurs Educ Perspect. 2014;35(4):244–52.
18. Adamson KA, Kardong-Edgren S, Willhaus J. An updated review of published simulation evaluation instruments. Clin Simul Nurs. 2013;9(9):e393–400.
19. Radhakrishnan K, Roche JP, Cunningham H. Measuring clinical practice parameters with human patient simulation: a pilot study. Int J Nurs Educ Scholarsh. 2007;4(1):8.
20. Cant R, Cooper S. Simulation-based learning in nurse education: systematic review. J Adv Nurs. 2010;66(1):3–15.
21. Aquifer: your trusted source for clinical learning [Internet]. 2020 [cited 27 September 2020]. https://aquifer.org.
22. ReelDx: transforming medical education with real patient video cases [Internet]. 2020 [cited 27 September 2020]. https://reeldx.com.
23. Schwindt R, McNelis A. Integrating simulation into a reflection-centered graduate psychiatric/mental health nursing curriculum. Nurs Educ Perspect. 2015;36(5):326–8.
24. Jeffries R, Dreifuerst T, Kardong-Edgren S, Hayden J. Faculty development when initiating simulation programs: lessons learned from the National Simulation Study. J Nurs Regul. 2015;5(4):17–23.
25. Child Entertainment Laws: U.S. Department of Labor [Internet]. 2020 [cited 17 September 2020]. https://www.dol.gov/agencies/whd/state/child-labor/entertainment.
26. Rutherford-Hemming T, Jennrich J. Using standardized patients to strengthen nurse practitioner competency in the clinical setting. Nurs Educ Perspect. 2013;34(2):118–21.
27. American Association of College of Nursing [Internet]. 2020 [cited 17 September 2020]. https://www.aacnnursing.org/Education-Resources/Curriculum-Guidelines.
28. Alexander M, Durham C, Hooper J, Jeffries P, Goldman N, Kardong-Edgren S, et al. NCSBN simulation guidelines for prelicensure nursing programs. J Nurs Regul. 2015;6(3):39–42.
29. Warren J, Luctkar-Flude M, Godfrey C, Lukewich J. A systematic review of the effectiveness of simulation-based education on satisfaction and learning outcomes in nurse practitioner programs. Nurse Educ Today. 2016;46:99–108.

Simulation for Certified Nurse-Midwifery and Women's and Gender-Related Health Care Nurse Practitioner Students

21

Nancy Selix and Justin Waryold

Introduction

Simulation is an evidence-based learning strategy for student nurse practitioners (NPs) and nurse-midwives (CNMs). It has been used to teach about the birthing process, normal and complicated deliveries, post-partum care, and other gynecological and obstetrical topics to medical students, residents, and midwifery and women's health nurse practitioner students for many years. This chapter is going to focus on using simulation to teach CNM and NP students about the transgender and gender noncofirming (TGNC) population they may encounter. The use of high-fidelity simulation scenarios using standardized patients (SP) can increase the application of skills learned in didactic formats and may more readily transfer knowledge, skills, and attitudes to actual clinical TGNC patients. The use of simulation provides an opportunity for students to access patient populations that they may not readily encounter in rural or underserved clinical sites. Additionally, the use of simulation modalities for clinical learning provides protection from psychological harm for TGNC patients while CNM and NP students gain skills in communication, cultural humility, and care for this population [1].

Transgender and gender nonconforming (TGNC) individuals are those whose gender identity does not align with the sex assigned at birth. Transmen are those who are assigned female sex at birth but embrace a more masculine representation. Transwomen are those who are assigned male sex at birth but embody a more feminine gender expression. It is critical to note that gender is not binary. There are numerous expressions of gender identity besides transmen and transwomen, but the authors will use the abbreviation TGNC to describe this population. Factors such as fear of identification, lack of nonbinary gender choices on government forms such as the US Census, and obtaining accurate numbers of those within the TGNC population are problematic. However, the best estimates indicate approximately 1.4 million TGNC individuals in the US as of 2016 [2].

Few TGNC patients seek primary care or preventive health services due to barriers to care that increase health disparities and shorten the lifespan of this population. NPs and CNMs often provide primary care services. They are poised to address the TGNC population's needs in all healthcare areas, including preventive health services, gender-related care, and treatment of acute and chronic illness. NPs and CNMs approach care from a nursing framework in which the patient's values, goals, and needs are paramount. Because NPs and CNMs are educated within such a framework, they are especially attuned to the TGNC population's needs. However, additional instruction and changes in curriculum for CNM and NP students regarding the unique cultural aspects of the TGNC population will enhance the services provided, and the care received and ultimately improve healthcare outcomes.

Many transgender individuals experience prejudice and discrimination almost daily. Threats of violence and harassment, actual violence, and homicide are common in this population. Because TGNC individuals live outside of societal binary gender norms, they are especially susceptible to violence perpetrated upon them by others. Individuals who are members of racial or ethnic minority groups may experience additional stressors and health disparities due to the intersectionality of socioeconomic and demographic factors described by Meyer [3]. Healthcare providers may possess biases toward the TGNC population. They may perpetuate discrimination and health disparities by their lack of understanding and knowledge about this population's unique healthcare, cultural, and social needs.

When providing care to TGNC patients, it is imperative to examine this population's needs and improve healthcare providers' cultural humility. By offering training in cultural sensitivity and awareness of implicit bias, NP and CNM students can gain skills in administering services that meet the physical, emotional, mental, spiritual, and intellectual needs of TGNC patients. Applying cultural humility confers a sense of acceptance and improves bi-directional communi-

N. Selix (✉) · J. Waryold
University of San Francisco (USF), San Francisco, CA, USA
e-mail: nwselix@usfca.edu

J. M. Kutzin et al. (eds.), *Comprehensive Healthcare Simulation: Nursing*, Comprehensive Healthcare Simulation,
https://doi.org/10.1007/978-3-031-31090-4_21

cation between care recipients and providers. Simple modifications in the language used and approaches to these patients confer much-needed sensitivity, and providing appropriate care services leads to optimal care outcomes.

No one is ever entirely culturally competent because it is impossible to share the same worldview and experience through the lens of one who has had a life of discrimination and prejudice. An individual cannot gain humility through awareness and applying knowledge of another person's lived experience and awareness of one's limitations to fully embrace the culture of the TGNC patient. However, attempting to understand such experiences and how those experiences shape one's perceptions helps the care provider understand the meaning from the care recipient's point of view. Applying aspects of cultural humility to design and implement healthcare service systems and educational programs that prepare CBM and NP students further reduces stigmatization, barriers to care, and health disparities, ultimately leading to improved overall health for the TGNC population. Possessing cultural humility extends beyond knowledge attainment and includes applying principles learned in the provision of clinical care and the development of healthcare delivery models that address these issues.

The National Organization of Nurse Practitioner Faculties (NONPF) found core competencies utilized by all NP programs illustrating proficiency in areas needed for independent practice. These competencies are demonstrated upon graduation regardless of the program's population focus, allowing entry-level NPs to meet the complex challenges of ever-rapidly expanding knowledge into practice and function in a constantly changing healthcare environment [4]. In observation of individuals self-identifying as TGNC, the Sexual and Reproductive Health Special Interest Group of NONPF authored the *Patient-Centered Transgender Care: A Toolkit for Nurse Practitioner Faculty and Clinicians* to assist both faculty and providers in meeting the needs of this population [5]. Within this toolkit, specific core competencies are identified and crosswalked through a suggested curriculum with related resources.

The American College of Nurse-Midwives (ACNM) has created *Core Competencies for Basic Midwifery Practice* [6]. These competencies were revised in 2020 to reflect midwives' roles in caring for TGNC individuals and to incorporate more inclusive language regarding midwifery care recipients. ACNM has adopted a philosophy founded on the belief that all people have the right to culturally appropriate health care surrounding childbearing, access to reproductive care, and sexual health. Additionally, various terms for care recipients have expanded to include the terms "women, transgender, gender non-conforming, and intersex" to reflect the variety of gender expressions that individuals may possess. These core competencies may be exercised within simulation training in the care of the TGNC patient.

Using simulation scenarios allows NP and CNM student participants to practice cultural humility and clinical skills while avoiding harm to patients and reducing implicit biases toward the TGNC patient. Additionally, cultural humility skills learned in simulation reduce stigmatization of marginalized populations, which promotes access to care. One of the unique aspects of simulation learning is that TGNC-standardized patients use improves simulation scenario fidelity and enhances participant engagement, knowledge retention, and application of skills attained.

Understanding the Unique Needs of the TGNC Population in the Healthcare Setting

Sexuality and gender identity are two vastly different phenomena that are not interrelated. One may be a transwoman or transman or another gender and be sexually attracted to any number of individuals at any given time. Additionally, sexual attraction is a fluid phenomenon that may change throughout an individual's life course based on various factors. Asking about an individual's sexual preference and sexual activity must only be done within the evaluation of related health problems such as sexually transmitted infections, erectile dysfunction, rule out pregnancy, or other such issues. Providers must never assume to know an individual's sexual preference based on gender expression.

The terminology used in working with the TGNC population is of utmost importance. As with anything in today's society, terminology is fluid and may change based on culture, environment, and perception. It is imperative to respect the individual as they are given that point in time using their preferred name, pronouns, and other terminology that speaks to them as a person. See Table 21.1 for a list of commonly used terms regarding the TGNC population. Many individuals in this population have a name different from those on their birth certificates or legal documents. The choice of pronouns is equally crucial as the person's self-described gender. The provider must avoid misgendering the patient or calling the patient by a name other than what they desire.

Additionally, studies have shown that TGNC individuals may have been a victim of sexual trauma. Regardless of this history, TGNC patients may be especially sensitive about body parts' appearance. The provider should avoid uncovering sensitive areas, especially the genitals or breast and chest areas, unless needed for an appropriate evaluation. When it is necessary to uncover these areas, the use of transitional phrases such as provide instruction such as,

"Now I need to uncover your chest area to check your dressing," or "Because you are experiencing pain in your genital area, I need to uncover this area briefly so that I can examine that body part." The use of transitional phrases, as demonstrated, confers the reason for the examination while providing time for the patient to consider the need for such an exam.

Table 21.1 Common terms and definitions used in caring for the TGNC population

Term	Definition
Cisgender	An individual whose gender identity aligns with the sex assigned at birth; a non-transgender person
Gender dysphoria	The distress and unease experienced if gender identity and designated gender are not entirely congruent
Gender expression	Refers to the external appearance expressed through name, pronoun, clothing, behavior, or body characteristics
Gender identity	One's internal, deeply held sense of gender. Unlike gender expression, gender identity is not visible to others
Gender reassignment	Treatment for individuals wanting to adapt their bodies to the experienced gender through hormones and/or surgery. Not all transgender individuals seek reassignment
Gender-confirming or gender-affirming surgery	Refers only to the surgical portion of confirming/gender-affirming treatment
Sex designated at birth.	Refers to sex assignment at birth, usually based on an objective view of genitalia
Transgender	An umbrella term for people whose gender identity and/or gender expression differs from what is typically associated with their sex designated at birth
Transman or Transgender male	An individual whose gender identifies as a male and assigned female sex at birth
Trans woman or transgender female	An individual whose gender identifies as a female and assigned male sex at birth
Gender nonconforming or Genderqueer	An individual whose gender identity differs from that which was assigned at birth but may be more complex, fluid, multifaceted, or otherwise less clearly defined than a transgender individual
Non-binary	An individual whose gender identity and/or gender expression differs from what is typically associated with the designated gender
Hormone therapy	Use of hormones as a medical treatment option for feminization or masculinization of the body

Adapted [8]

Creating a Simulation Scenario for Examination of the TGNC Patient

The use of simulation to prepare healthcare providers for clinical care is well documented. When learning skills needed to care for the TGNC patient, simulation training is particularly useful to avoid physical or psychological harm. This type of interaction allows for applying new skills and deep learning through application and feedback from the TGNC standardized patient (SP) and clinical observers (faculty or simulationist) in a hospital setting. Additionally, simulation learning allows access to patient populations that student CNMs and NPs may not encounter in various geographic regions where clinical training sites are located.

The Scenario

When creating the scenario, learning objectives should include obtaining a detailed health history and the experience of bidirectional communication skills with the TGNC-SP. Including learning objectives on cultural humility, the person's approach, not just the situation, and inclusion of primary prevention measures in addition to acute care needs is key to a successful learning experience. Careful selection of the individual from the TGNC community interested in student skill acquisition or locating an individual who plays the SP role is essential to improve fidelity and create realism in the scenario. The SP must "fit the part" when playing the role of the patient. Ensuring that the SP's age and ethnicity are congruent with the scenario, if part of the scenario, further adds to the fidelity. The script must be crafted to include correct terminology often used in the TGNC population and common health problems encountered by TGNC patients to attain further fidelity. The use of guidelines for sexual health history taking may provide additional resources for the scenario creation. The Fenway Institute has created such guidelines for use with the TGNC population when asking sexual health history questions.

Enacting the Scenario (Example in Appendix)

Introduction and Acknowledgment of the Patient

Introduce the provider to the patient. Verify patient identity and ask about preferred name and pronouns. Ask the chief complaint for a visit.

Pre-briefing

Providing participants with learning experiences in cultural humility, uncovering and diffusing implicit bias, and interviewing skills will promote early skill acquisition. These skills may be provided by an online learning module that is completed days before or in an in-person format just before the simulation scenario is conducted. There are online courses that can be completed that are about these topics in general and not specific to the TGNC population. See Table 21.2 for resources. Participants may apply these newly acquired skills in the simulation environment. Information on obtaining a detailed sexual health history that includes the sexual practices involved in sexual encounters, the number

Table 21.2 Resources for training on implicit bias

Website and organization	Content
American Academy of Family Physicians https://www.aafp.org/dam/AAFP/documents/patient_care/health_equity/implicit-bias-training-facilitator-guide.pdf	Implicit Bias Training facilitator guide
Harvard University Project Implicit Bias https://implicit.harvard.edu/implicit/takeatest.html	Self-assessment test for determining bias
Lawrence Berkeley National Laboratory (Berkeley Lab) https://ideas-in-action.lbl.gov/topics/implicit-bias/implicit-bias-learning-resources	Six-course online training series
The Kirwan Institute for the Study of Race and Ethnicity; The Ohio State University http://kirwaninstitute.osu.edu/implicit-bias-training/	Four modules on implicit bias-free
University of California at Los Angeles Equity, Diversity, and Inclusion https://equity.ucla.edu/know/implicit-bias/	Training videos, guides, and reports on implicit bias-free
University of California https://ucnet.universityofcalifornia.edu/working-at-uc/your-career/talent-management/professional-development/managing-implicit-bias.html	Six-course online training on bias-free

of partners, infection protection strategies used, history of sexually transmitted infections, plans for pregnancy or pregnancy prevention [7]. These concepts must be included in pre-learning.

Obtaining Health History

Begin data collection regarding health history or the reason for the encounter.

Set the stage, ask screening questions, determine if there is a need for more details for health history (multiple partners, long-term monogamous partner, not sexually active - including reasons -no partner, pain, erectile dysfunction, or anorgasmia).

Key points in determining success in meeting learning objectives:

Healthcare Provider:

- Asks the patient's preferred name and pronoun
- Listens and pays attention to the patient
- Body posture and eye contact consistent with attending behaviors
- It avoids "talking down" to patient
- Avoids technical terms
- Explains the reason for the encounter and the health questions
- Encourages the patient to "tell the story."
- Uses open-ended phrases and avoids yes or no questions
- Does not interrupt the patient
- Collects data in an organized manner
- Uses statements of empathy and support
- Uses nonverbal behaviors that conveyed support – nodding, smiling, eye contact, leaning forward when seated
- Displays unconditional positive regard toward the patient regardless of the health complaint
- Offers a summary of the visit and assessed patient understanding
- Explains which body parts need to be examined and why
- Provides an opportunity for the patient to ask questions and clarify misinformation
- Offers a return visit

Standardized Patient

- Remains in the role and follows the script closely, avoiding varying away from scripted language
- Physical presentation is congruent with the scripted scenario
- Provide feedback to the participant on the simulated experience

Debriefing

The debriefing process should be conducted separately for both the SP and the participant to discover perceptions and experiences during the scenario. Debriefing questions for the SP may include some of the following, as they pertain to communication from the participant toward the SP: verbal and nonverbal communication experiences; the presence of medical jargon or confusing language; and fluency of history collection in a logically organized manner. For the participant, debriefing questions may include communication techniques used; screening tests offered related to epidemiology, pathology, clinical presentation; and self-reflection on the interaction and communication strategies.

Post-scenario Evaluation of Learning

It is of great value to obtain a pretest and post-test to compare participant knowledge and skill before and after the debriefing. This information can assist the simulationist in modifications needed for the scenario and SP training and provide insight into the participants' knowledge. This type of data is useful for organizations and individuals to demonstrate competency in meeting the scenario's learning objectives.

References

1. Grabenski A, Chuisano S, Strock K, Zielinski R, Anderson O, Sadovnikova A. A pilot study to evaluate the effect of classroom-based high-fidelity simulation on nurse-midwifery students' self-efficacy in clinical lactation and perceived translation of skills to the care of the breastfeeding mother-infant dyad. Midwifery. 2021;102:103078.
2. Flores AR, Herman JL, Gates GJ, Brown TNT. How many adults identified as transgender in the United States. Los Angeles, CA: Williams Institute; 2016.
3. Meyer IH. Prejudice, social stress, and mental health in lesbian, gay, and bisexual populations: conceptual issues and research evidence. Psychol Bull. 2003;129(5):674.
4. Thomas A, Crabtree MK, Delaney K, Dumas MA, Kleinpell R, Marfell J, et al. Nurse practitioner core competencies content. The National Organization of Nurse Practitioner Faculties; 2017.
5. National Organization of Nurse Practitioner Faculties. Patient-centered transgender care: a toolkit for nurse practitioner faculty and clinicians. J Nurse Pract. 2019;15(7):502–5.
6. American College of Nurse-Midwives. Core competencies for basic midwifery practice 2020. Available from: https://www.midwife.org/acnm/files/acnmlibrarydata/uploadfilename/000000000050/ACNMCoreCompetenciesMar2020_final.pdf.
7. Center for Disease Control and Prevention. A guide to taking a sexual history. 2015.
8. Hembree WC, Cohen-Kettenis PT, Gooren L, Hannema SE, Meyer WJ, Murad MH, et al. Endocrine treatment of gender-dysphoric/gender-incongruent persons: an endocrine society clinical practice guideline. J Clin Endocrinol Metab. 2017;102(11):3869–903.

22 Simulation in Nurse Anesthesia Education

John M. O'Donnell and Bernadette Henrichs

Background and Historical Perspective

There is a significant history of simulation use in Nurse Anesthesia Education. The integration of simulation into Nurse Anesthesia educational programs was first reported by Dr. Joanne Fletcher in 1995 at the University of Pittsburgh [1]. This was presented in the Journal of the American Association of Nurse Anesthetists as a 'journal course' for continuing education credit. Later in 1995, Dr. Fletcher and Dr. John O'Donnell (also from the University of Pittsburgh) presented the first documented faculty development course in the use of simulation at the University of Buffalo, and Dr. Alfred Lupien opened the first Nurse Anesthesia simulation center at the Medical College of Georgia. In 1996, Dr. Lupien, Dr. O'Donnell, and Dr. Fletcher, along with Dr. David Gaba (Stanford University), presented the first live high-fidelity simulation demonstration to more than 1500 CRNAs at the AANA Annual Congress in Philadelphia, PA. Since this initial presentation, every US Nurse Anesthesia program has developed simulation educational offerings for their students ranging from simulation as a component of required BLS, ACLS, and PALS training to complex clinical scenarios requiring the implementation of critical thinking, team skills, and crisis management behaviors. The first paper reporting on the development of a formal Anesthesia Crisis Management Course in Nurse Anesthesia education was published by O'Donnell et al. in 1998 [2]. Over the intervening two decades, many programs have adopted this format to prepare students for rare but critical events that cannot be reliably offered as a clinical experience in the course of a typical anesthesia educational program. Interest in this area is widespread in Nurse Anesthesia education, with numerous authors exploring alternative approaches. For example, Henrichs et al. (2018) reported the use of repeated crisis management scenarios on student performance outcomes demonstrating that repetition is an important factor in the development of these skills [3].

In 2007, the Council on Accreditation of Nurse Anesthesia Educational Programs, Practice Doctorate Commission announced that by 2022, all US Nurse Anesthesia Programs were required to convert to a practice doctorate entry level (from the masters level), and the process to develop appropriate doctoral level standards and guidelines was initiated with the first draft of the trial standards published in 2014 followed by the final Standards being published in January 2015 [4]. The most recent version of the master's accreditation standards does *not* include the requirement that simulation education be a part of every nurse anesthesia program curriculum; however, in the Clinical Case Requirements Appendix, the requirements for three technical procedures (endoscopic techniques, central venous catheter insertion, and peripheral nerve blocks) can be partially met through simulation and one technique (fiberoptic bronchoscopy) can be fully met using simulation [5]. The rationale for allowing these clinical procedures to be met through simulation is two-fold. First, in many practices, CRNAs are not permitted to participate in these techniques due to practice restrictions. Secondly, some of these techniques have greatly diminished in clinical use due to evolving technology. For example, fiberoptic bronchoscopy use has greatly diminished in many anesthesia practices due to the widespread adoption of videolaryngoscopy devices such as the Glidescope (Verathon Inc., Bothell, WA).

The Standards for Accreditation of Nurse Anesthesia Programs, Practice Doctorate *does* require the integration of simulation into all Nurse Anesthesia educational programs offer-

J. M. O'Donnell (✉)
Department of Nurse Anesthesia, University of Pittsburgh, Pittsburgh, PA, USA

Winter Institute for Simulation Education and Research (WISER), University of Pittsburgh, Pittsburgh, PA, USA
e-mail: jod01@pitt.edu

B. Henrichs
Goldfarb School of Nursing, Barnes-Jewish College, St Louis, MO, USA

Department of Anesthesiology, Washington University in St Louis, St. Louis, MO, USA

J. M. Kutzin et al. (eds.), *Comprehensive Healthcare Simulation: Nursing*, Comprehensive Healthcare Simulation,
https://doi.org/10.1007/978-3-031-31090-4_22

Table 22.1 Council on Accreditation of Nurse Anesthesia Educational Programs

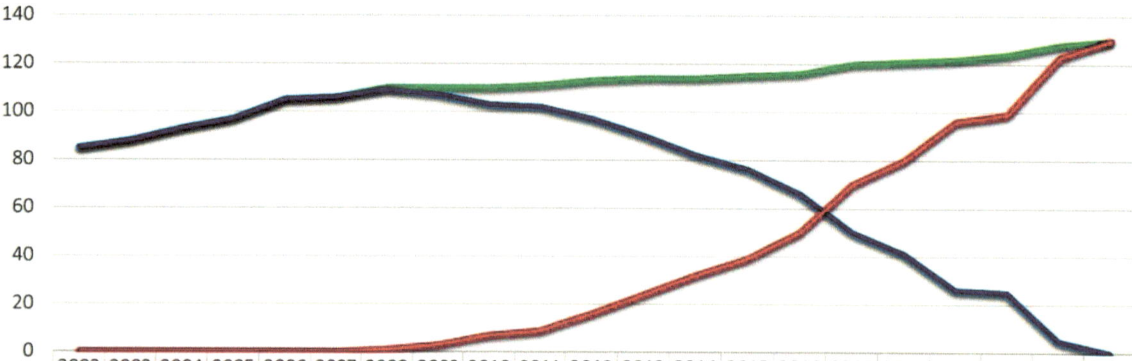

	2002	2003	2004	2005	2006	2007	2008	2009	2010	2011	2012	2013	2014	2015	2016	2017	2018	2019	2020	2021	2022
Total	85	88	93	97	105	106	110	110	110	111	113	114	114	115	116	120	121	122	124	128	130
Masters	85	88	93	97	105	106	109	107	103	102	97	90	82	76	66	50	41	26	25	5	0
Doctoral	0	0	0	0	0	0	1	3	7	9	16	24	32	39	50	70	80	96	99	123	130

ing a doctoral degree (i.e., Doctor of Nursing Practice [DNP] or Doctor of Nurse Anesthesia Practice [DNAP]). As of December 2020, 103 of the 124 US Nurse Anesthesia Programs have successfully transitioned to offering a doctoral degree, with 21 programs required to transition by January 2022 [6] (Table 22.1).

Because of this transition, these programs are now required to adhere to Doctoral Standard E. Curriculum Standards, 11. which states: "Simulated clinical experiences are incorporated in the curriculum" [7]. Simulated clinical experiences are defined in the Accreditation Glossary as "learning experiences involving the imitation or representation of clinical activities that are designed for competency attainment, competency assessment, or competency maintenance. Simulation involves a wide range of options including but not limited to standardized patients, web-based simulation, computer-based simulation, manikin-based technologies ranging from low- to high-fidelity, task trainers, and holodecks. These clinical learning experiences are intended to help bridge didactic learning with safe and effective patient care delivery". While this is certainly a comprehensive definition, it must be clarified that the requirements for students are very similar to the COA Masters' Standards and that "simple models and simulated experiences may be used to satisfy part of this [clinical] requirement. No clinical experiences can be obtained by simulation alone" [7]. This requirement helps to ensure that students have the opportunity to translate simulation learning into actual clinical practice applications.

Curricular Integration in Nurse Anesthesia Education

One problem faced by many Nurse Anesthesia Programs is that of curricular compression. In 1998, Nurse Anesthesia Programs were required to transition to offering a graduate degree. In transitioning from the certificate to graduate framework, program designs were robust, often including between 50–100 credits over a 28-month program. Given the ever-expanding knowledge base needed for safe and effective anesthesia practice, advances in technology and technique, and the requirement to adhere to numerous accreditation organization guidelines, it is difficult to plan and implement new simulation offerings within a curriculum- especially in light of new doctoral accreditation standards. Therefore, it is important that nurse anesthesia educators are aware of existing best practices and standards in the literature that can inform the design of simulation activities within a curriculum.

Table 22.2 Simulation Education Best Practices (BPs)

1.	Feedback
2.	Deliberate practice
3.	Curriculum Integration
4.	Outcome measurement
5.	Simulation fidelity
6.	Skill acquisition and maintenance
7.	Mastery learning
8.	Transfer to practice
9.	Team training
10.	High-stakes testing
11.	Instructor training
12.	Educational and professional context

Several reviews of simulation educational approaches have identified simulation best practices (BPs) and their impact on outcomes [8–12]. The most cited works are review papers by Issenberg et al. (2005) and McGaghie et al. (2010), which critically reviewed the available simulation literature to identify the most frequently incorporated educational approaches [10, 11]. These 'best practices' remain relevant today despite the intervening years (Table 22.2).

Note that best practice number 3 is Curriculum Integration, and that number 12 is Educational and Professional Context. One approach utilized at the University of Pittsburgh Nurse Anesthesia Program over the past two decades is to develop a curricular integration plan contextualized for anesthesia providers and include all simulation activities within the program (Table 22.3). The entire plan is organized within the existing program course structure. Another approach utilized

Table 22.3 University of Pittsburgh Curriculum Integration Plan

Part or full task workshops	Course placement	Primary objective-students will:	Simulator (s) used	Hours/ student	Prep/ turnover	Students/ session (pre-COVID)	Faculty: student ratio (pre-Covid)	Evaluation data: knowledge, skill attitude (KSA)	Formative or summative evaluation (F/S)	GAS Debrief	Assessment Instrument
Basic principles of airway management	Basic principles of anesthesia	Demonstrate standardized approach to airway management using a variety of approaches	Laerdal™ Intubation Training Heads-Adult and Pediatric	4	3	20	1:5	K, S	S	No	Checklist
IV Insertion workshop	Basic principles of anesthesia	Demonstrate standardized IV insertion skills	NASCO™ IV line insertion trainer and Laerdal VirIV	3	2	10	1:5	K, S	F/S	No	Checklist
Arterial line insertion workshop	Basic principles of anesthesia	Demonstrate standardized arterial line insertion skills	NASCO™ arterial line insertion trainer	3	2	10	1:5	K, S	F/S	No	Checklist
Patient positioning lab	Basic principles of anesthesia	Demonstrate competency in safe patient positioning and use of the operating room table	Standardized Patient (SP) or Nurse Anne™	3	2	7	1:3.5	K, S	F	No	n/a
Mock induction workshop	Basic principles of anesthesia	Demonstrate skills in anesthesia care plan development, induction of anesthesia and complication management	Laerdal SimMan™ Laerdal 3G™	8	3	7	1:3.5	K,S, A	F/S	Yes	Checklist, exam
Mock induction—emergence sessions	Basic principles of anesthesia	Demonstrate skills in emergence from anesthesia	Laerdal SimMan™ Laerdal 3G™	3	2	7	1:3.5	K, S	F/S	Yes	Checklist/ exam
Mock induction-practice sessions	Basic principles of anesthesia	Participate in deliberate practice in anesthesia care plan development, induction of anesthesia and complication management	Laerdal SimMan™ Laerdal 3G™	4	2	3	1:3	K, S, A	F	Yes	n/a
Sterile technique, spinal, US practice	Basic principles of anesthesia	Demonstrate competency in sterile technique (gloves, kits), spinal insertion and basic principles of ultrasound examination	NASCO™ Spinal simulator Standardized Patient (SP)	3	2	8	1:2	K,S,A	F/S	No	Checklists/ exam
Medication safety workshop	Basic principles of anesthesia	Demonstrate competency in drug calculation, safe medication administration and error mitigation	Lumis Corp. InSight™ platform	2	2	10	1:10	K, S, A	F/S	No	Checklist/ exam
AGM checkout and troubleshooting	Chemistry and physics in anesthesia	Demonstrate competency in anesthesia gas machine (AGM) checkout and troubleshooting and use of the	Laerdal SimMan™ Laerdal 3G™	4	2	4	1:4	K, S	F/S	No	Checklist, exam

(continued)

Table 22.3 (continued)

Part or full task workshops	Course placement	Primary objective-students will:	Simulator (s) used	Hours/ student	Prep/ turnover	Students/ session (pre-COVID)	Faculty: student ratio (pre-Covid)	Evaluation data: knowledge, skill attitude (KSA)	Formative or summative evaluation (F/S)	GAS Debrief	Assessment Instrument
Problem based simulation adult	Applied anatomy, physiology and pathophysiology 1	Demonstrate anesthesia management skills integrated with course content to address scenario-based anesthesia critical events (e.g. autonomic dysreflexia, bronchospasm, hemorrhage, elevated ICP, myocardial depression)	Laerdal SimMan™ or 3G™	8	2	12	1:6	K, S, A	F/S	Yes	Checklist, survey, exam
Standardized patient exams	Physical diagnosis clinical	Demonstrate skills in cardiac auscultation, palpation and diagnosis of cardiopulmonary findings as well as interview and interaction with SPs for H and P purposes	Harvey Cardiopulmonary Simulator™ Standardized Patient (SP)	8	2	8	1:2	K, S, A	F/S	No	Checklist/ survey/exam
Pediatric anesthesia simulation for SRNAs (PASS)	Pediatric clinical rotation (just in time training)	Demonstrate skill in pediatric anesthesia set-up, drug calculation, induction of anesthesia, problem identification and management	Laerdal SimBaby™ Laerdal SimMan™ or 3G™ Laerdal Megacode Kid™	4	2	12	1:3	K, S, A	F/S	Yes	Checklist/ survey/exam
Fiberoptic bronchoscopy workshop	Pediatric clinical rotation (just in time training)	Demonstrate competency in fiberoptic bronchoscopy through deliberate practice	Laerdal Airman™	1.5	2	6	1:2	K, S, A	F/S	Yes	Mastery checklist
Regional anesthesia workshop (including US practice)	Advanced principles of anesthesia 1	Demonstrate skill in administration of regional anesthetic techniques including spinal, epidural, airway and peripheral nerve blocks	Standardized Patient (SP) NASCO™ Spinal and Simulab Epidural Simulator Cadaver	6	2	20	1:4	K,S	F/S	No	Checklist, exam
Double lumen endobronchial tube placement	Advanced principles of anesthesia 2	Demonstrate skill in double lumen endobronchial tube placement, trouble-shooting and fiberoptic lung examination	Laerdal AirMan™	2	1	5	1:5	K, S	F/S	No	Exam

Jet ventilation workshop	Advanced principles of anesthesia 2	Demonstrate familiarity with high frequency jet ventilation skills including airway exchange catheters, insufflation catheters, various adaptors and troubleshooting strategies	Laerdal SimMan™ Laerdal 3G™	2	1	5	1:5	K, S	F/S	No	Exam
Central venous catheter (CVC) insertion	Advanced principles of anesthesia 2	Demonstrate skill in placement of central venous catheters including internal jugular and subclavian	Laerdal CVC™ Trainer	2	1	20	1:10	S	F	No	n/a
Difficult airway management	Advanced principles of anesthesia 3	Demonstrate skills in assessment, triage and management of the difficult airway according to the ASA difficult airway algorithm	Laerdal SimMan™	4	1	8	1:4	K, S, A	S	Yes	Survey, exam, performance exam
Anesthesia crisis leadership Training (SRNA + Resident)	Advanced principles of Anesthesia 3	Demonstrate skills in assessment, triage and management of anesthesia crisis events in an interprofessional education (IPE) setting	Laerdal SimMan™ Laerdal 3G™ Laerdal SimMom™	4	1	8	1:2	K, S, A	F	Yes	Checklist/ survey/exam
TEAMSTEPPS exercise	Team training in patient safety	Demonstrate TEAMSTEPPS skills during immersive team based scenarios	Laerdal SimMan™ Laerdal 3G™ Laerdal SimMom™	2	1	40	1:20	K, S, A	F/S	Yes	Exam
ACLS/PALS/BLS bundle course	Across curriculum	Demonstrate competence in management of adult and pediatric resuscitation through immersive, contextualized simulation scenarios	Laerdal SimBaby™ Laerdal SimMan™ Laerdal 3G™ Laerdal Megacode Kid™	8	2	16	1:4	K, S, A	F/S	Yes	Checklist/ survey/exam
Anesthesia crisis resource management (SRNA only)	CRNA role seminar	Demonstrate skills in assessment, triage and management of anesthesia crisis events focusing on crew resource management skills	Laerdal SimMan™ Laerdal 3G™	8	1	10	1:5	K, S, A	F	Yes	Checklist/ survey/exam

(continued)

Table 22.3 (continued)

Part or full task workshops	Course placement	Primary objective-students will:	Simulator (s) used	Hours/student	Prep/turnover	Students/session (pre-COVID)	Faculty: student ratio (pre-Covid)	Evaluation data: knowledge, skill attitude (KSA)	Formative or summative evaluation (F/S)	GAS Debrief	Assessment Instrument
Mentored student simulation teaching experience for graduate students	Basic principles of anesthesia sequence FOB course US course Regional anesthesia course Problem based anesthesia course Physical diagnosis course Undergraduate honors course	Demonstrate skills in simulation teaching, facilitation and debriefing through mentored experiences in immersive simulation training	Laerdal SimBaby™ Laerdal SimMan™ Laerdal Megacode Kid™ Gaumard Birthing Simulator Standardized Patient (SP)	8–16+	n/a	varies	varies	K, S, A	F	Yes	Survey Debriefing
Undergraduate honors student simulation instruction experience for graduate students	Professional issues in advanced practice nursing: nurse anesthesia	Demonstrate skills in simulation teaching, facilitation and debriefing through mentored simulation teaching experiences	Laerdal SimBaby™ Laerdal SimMan™ Laerdal 3G™	4	2	8	1:2	K, S	F	Yes	Checklist Debriefing

Simulation events are integrated throughout the 86 credit curriculum. The average student experiences ~110 direct contact hours in simulation. Students may also choose to register for independent study in simulation with development of higher level skills in debriefing, assessment and curricular design. Two primary simulation facilities are used; the School of Nursing Skills and Simulation Suite and the Winter Institute for Simulation, Education and Research (WISER). More than 30 full body simulators are available across 14 simulation training areas. Standardized patients are oriented to their roles and responsibilities prior to each course. A wide array of part task trainers are available and are integrated throughout the curriculum

Table 22.4 Design features which have significant impact on learning outcomes

1.	Range of difficulty
2.	Repetitive practice (at one time)
3.	Distributed practice (across time)
4.	Cognitive interactivity
5.	Multiple learning strategies
6.	Individualized learning
7.	Mastery learning (to a particular standard)
8.	Feedback
9.	Longer training time

Table 22.5 INACSL Standards of Best Practice: Simulation©

1.	Simulation design
2.	Outcomes and objectives
3.	Facilitation
4.	Debriefing
5.	Participant evaluation
6.	Professional integrity
7.	Simulation-enhanced interprofessional education
8.	Simulation glossary
9.	Operations

is to ensure that formative or summative assessment strategies and outcomes are clearly identified (BP 4, 6, 10) and that feedback (BP 1) is delivered during both skill training (typically continuous) or after scenario-based events (typically as a debriefing or through an assessment process). Simulation fidelity (BP 5) is addressed by the selection of appropriate simulation devices or standardized patients depending on the objectives and design of the activity. Mastery learning and deliberate practices (BP 2 and 7) are incorporated where possible, as these have been identified as powerful educational interventions relative to outcomes.

It is also important that Nurse Anesthesia educators are aware of the evidence basis for particular design features. A series of systematic reviews and meta-analyses have been conducted looking at simulation education head-to-head with standard education, the translational impact of simulation (BP 8), and the importance of feedback (including debriefing), as well as other design features [12–14]. Cook et al. (2011) reported that when compared to no intervention, simulation approaches were associated with large outcomes for knowledge, skill, and behavior and moderate effects for patient-related outcomes [15].' These authors went on to identify the impact of specific educational design features with significant learning impact, which parallel the best practices identified above (Table 22.4).

In developing a curricular integration plan, it is important to consider the impact of several of these features which differ from the best practices list, such as range of difficulty, multiple learning strategies, individualized learning, and longer training time which can have a significant impact on the time required for activities, allocation of faculty and overall resource utilization.

Application of Simulation Standards in Nurse Anesthesia Education

The International Nursing Association for Simulation and Clinical Learning (INACSL) utilized best practice resources among other publications to develop standards for nursing simulation educators in 2010. These were most recently revised in 2016–2017 and, while primarily focused on undergraduate education, are also relevant to graduate education in Nurse Anesthesia. Each of these INACSL standards is carefully defined and includes criteria for performance as well as specific instructional elements (Table 22.5) [16].

These standards have been embraced by the National Councils of State Boards of Nursing (NCSBN), and Simulation Guidelines for Prelicensure Nursing Programs have been disseminated [17]. No companion document for advanced practice nurses has been published, although this is not surprising given the great variability in clinical requirements and responsibilities between the various advanced practice specialties. Further, in many states, Nurse Anesthesia educational programs are not regulated by the State Boards of Nursing, who instead defer to the AANA COA for oversight.

Nurse Anesthesia Simulation Examples

Example 1 *University of Pittsburgh Fiberoptic Intubation (FOI) Skill Training integrated with Pediatric Anesthetic Simulation for SRNAs (PASS) Course.*

This course has been developed over more than a 15-year period of time. The course originated because the Council on Accreditation of Nurse Anesthesia Education Programs required in 2005 that students have fiberoptic and endoscopic experiences while in their training program [4, 7]. Through collaboration with Dr. Lawrence Borland, an internationally renowned expert in pediatric airway management, the course was designed to offer student anesthetists the necessary knowledge and skill to participate in fiberoptic bronchoscopy and intubation. The course is held at the Winter Institute for Simulation Education and Research (WISER) and was positioned in the curriculum to coincide with Pediatric Anesthetic Simulation for SRNAs (PASS) which is a scenario-based course designed to prepare students for key pediatric anesthetic management prior to their rotation to the Children's Hospital of Pittsburgh (CHP) of the UPMC (Table 22.3).

The PASS course is designed to allow students to deliberately and repetitively practice standardized scenarios requiring pediatric drug calculation, administration, induction of anesthesia, and problem management (e.g., laryngospasm) for patients of various ages. Subject matter experts (SMEs) who are pediatric CRNAs from CHP serve as the in-room facilitators, with Nurse Anesthesia program faculty serving as out-of-room facilitators and course directors. All faculty have access to both student course material and faculty instructions via the WISER Learning Management System in preparation for the course.

The course is operationalized in the following manner. Each day of implementation (Just in Time training four times per year prior to the pediatric rotation), a pre-course huddle is held with faculty prior to and after each session to clarify objectives and expectations. Faculty communicate with SMEs via a walkie-talkie system, and feedback is provided to participants throughout the experience (formative) as well as at the end of each session (summative). Nine to twelve second-year nurse anesthesia students rotate through a total of four clinical scenarios as well as the nasal fiberoptic intubation station for a total of 3–4 students per station. Students take pre-course and post-course knowledge exams and surveys (assessing perceptions regarding the course and confidence) via the WISER Simulation Information Management System or SIMS (Fig. 22.1). Instructors can access student knowledge and survey responses pre and post-course and can thus adjust their instruction to address participant deficits and for the purpose of future course improvements.

The fiberoptic intubation component of the course focuses on a scaffolding approach to the development of skills in this domain. While the fiberoptic skills appear to be generalizable to the adult population (according to student feedback and Typhon™ data from student clinical practice), the specific target of the course is pediatric nasal intubation. The primary clinical need is for nasal fiberoptic intubation of children ages 5–8 undergoing a complete oral restoration procedure (COR) due to severe dental caries. In the clinical setting, these patients undergo an inhalation anesthesia induction, receive an IV, have an occlusive dressing placed over the mouth, and have a nasal airway with a 15 mm adapter inserted in one nare (through which spontaneous ventilation and anesthetic agent delivery occurs) and are intubated via the fiberoptic approach through the other nare. The rationale for this approach is to avoid damage and displacement of diseased teeth during oral intubation. The risk of infected teeth being dislodged and lost in the distal airway during traditional oral laryngoscopy has thus been avoided,

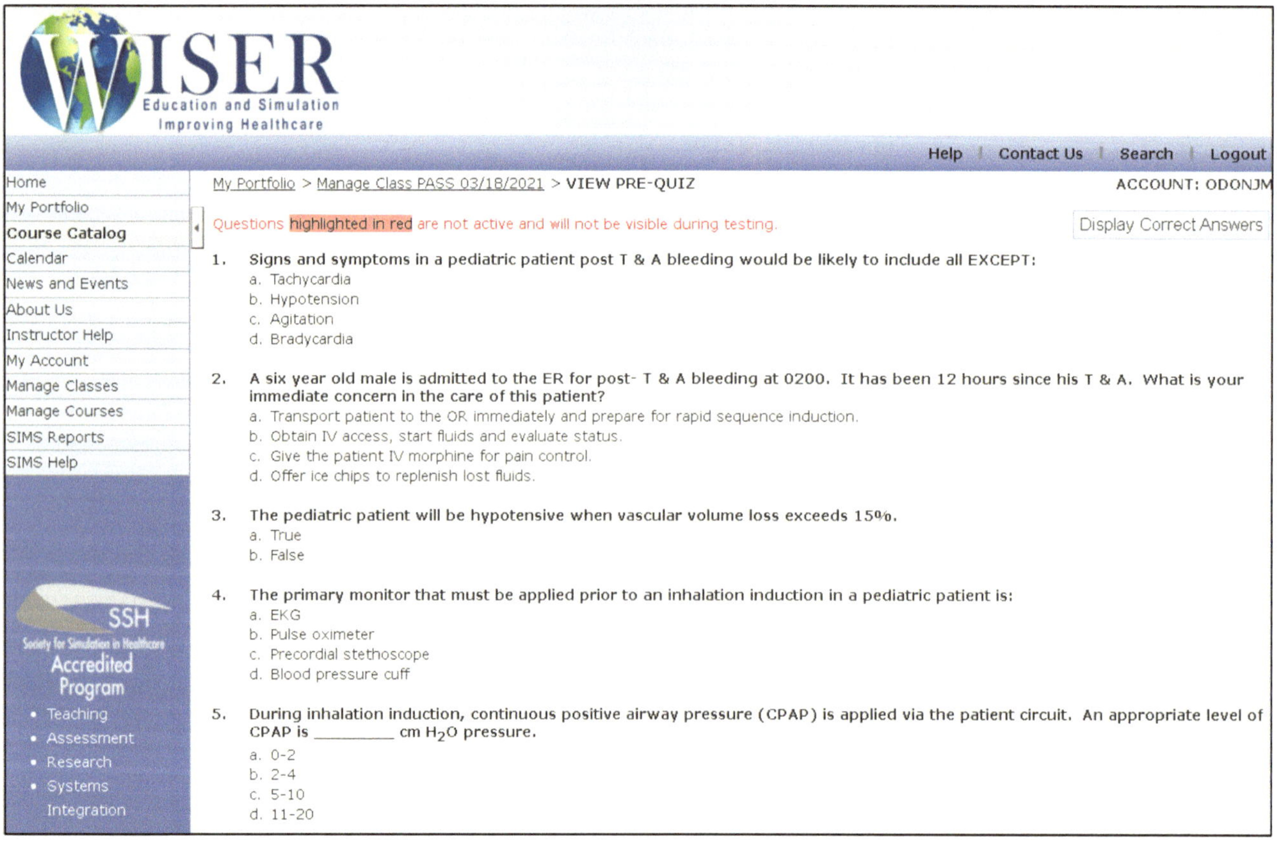

Fig. 22.1 Simulation Information Management System Knowledge Exam for the Pediatric Anesthesia Simulation for SRNAs (PASS) course (with permission, WISER)

with the technique being used safely at CHP for more than 15 years.

This simulation-based fiberoptic intubation training program requires students to participate in and complete an online course prior to attending the program. This online course includes an overview of objectives, an instructional video of the actual FOI process in the clinical setting, a review of the fiberoptic bronchoscope components, standardized guidelines for manipulating the fiberoptic scope (FOS), anatomy and landmarks for fiberoptic use, steps for nasal fiberoptic bronchoscopy (FOB) in the simulation setting and review of a 25-step protocol for nasal FOB at CHP based on a task analysis conducted in the clinical setting (Fig. 22.2). This simulation course was designed to incorporate simulation best practices and includes facilitator training, clinical contextualization, skill scaffolding (using the clock-face simulator—Fig. 22.3), deliberate practice, frequent formative evaluation feedback, clinical variation (we utilize three different Laerdal Airman™ simulators, which vary in clinical presentation and difficulty—Fig. 22.4) and a summative mastery assessment.

Upon arrival to the simulation course, students are offered a standardized curriculum consisting of:

1. Review of fiberoptic scope (FOS) components
2. Review of the guidelines for handling and advancing the FOS
3. Review of an intubation video of the entire process of nasal FOI in the CHP population (de-identified patient)
4. Review of the 25-step protocol for nasal FOB at CHP developed through iterative task analysis conducted through a series of direct observations at the site (Fig. 22.5)
5. Demonstration of ability to master 360-degree FOS manipulation using a simple task trainer (Fig. 22.3)
6. Completion of a minimum of 40 nasal FIOs on the Laerdal™ AirMan mannequin (Laerdal Inc. Stavanger, Norway) (Fig. 22.4) in a deliberate practice model with formative feedback. (40 nasal FIO attempts were based on SME input from an expert panel as well as literature regarding anesthesia skill acquisition [15–17])
7. Completion of a mastery level checklist, including a 'test-out' nasal FOI (Fig. 22.5)

Example 2 *Simulation workshops Co-Sponsored by the Goldfarb School of Nursing at Barnes-Jewish College Nurse Anesthesia Program and Webster University Nurse Anesthesia Program (St. Louis, MO.).*

Two nurse anesthesia programs in the St. Louis area have collaborated for several years on co-sponsoring workshops for their students to help increase their knowledge level of intubation skills and specific anesthesia-related tasks such as arterial catheter placement, regional anesthesia techniques, and central venous catheter (CVC) placement. These workshops are held annually and often in the spring. Each annual workshop includes all three levels of nurse anesthesia students from both programs: first-year, second-year, and third-

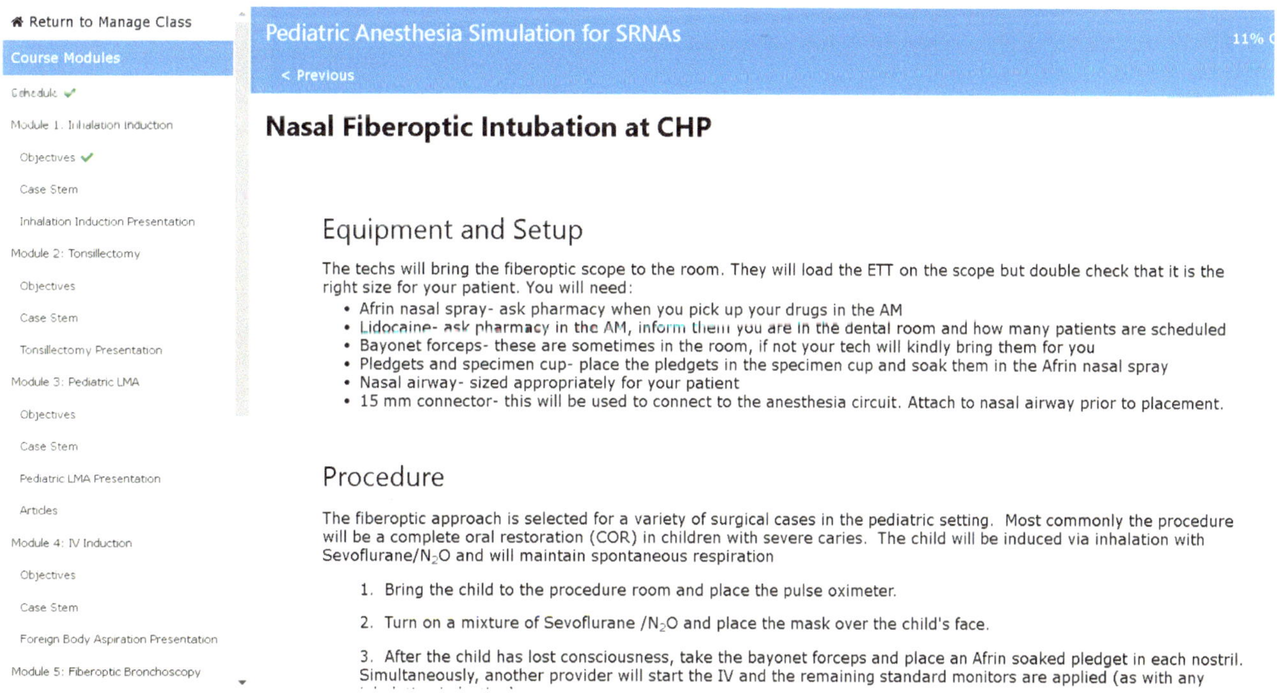

Fig. 22.2 Nasal fiberoptic simulation checklist for the pediatric setting based on iterative task analysis (with permission, WISER)

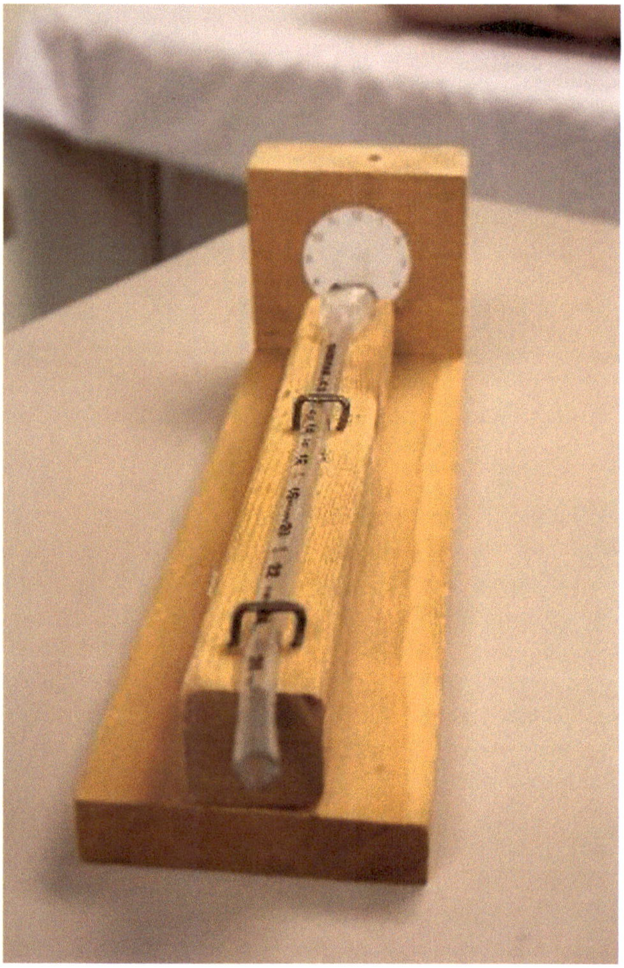

Fig. 22.3 Fiberoptic intubation simple part-task trainer allowing participants to demonstrate articulation of the fiberoptic scope in 360° by identifying each number on the associated clock face (with permission, WISER)

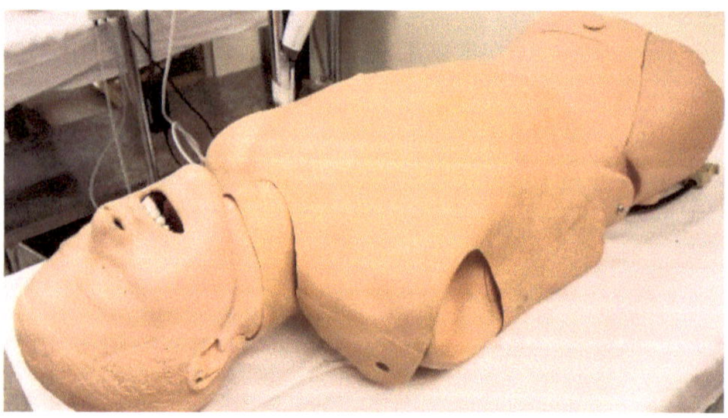

Fig. 22.4 Laerdal Airman™ Simulator which incorporates a realistic lung model for fiberoptic intubation training

year students. The workshops are held to offer new information and skill practice for inexperienced students and to provide information reinforcement and additional clinical skill practice for experienced students. Additionally, the more experienced students are encouraged to teach and mentor the less experienced students, which has the benefit of enhancing professional socialization. The objectives for the workshop include:

1. Discuss local anesthetic type and dosage for neuraxial anesthesia.
2. Using task trainers, review the steps to performing arterial catheter placement and place an arterial catheter under the guidance of an instructor. Use a checklist to ensure all steps are completed.
3. Using task trainers, review the steps to performing a subarachnoid block and epidural block and place the two blocks under the guidance of an instructor. Use a checklist to ensure all steps are completed.
4. Using task trainers, review the steps to inserting a central venous catheter using ultrasound and place the central catheter under the guidance of an instructor. Use a checklist to ensure all steps are completed.
5. Discuss the preparation needed for intubation of a predicted difficult airway.
6. Using airway mannequins and airway devices, place an airway device from a variety of different devices such as multiple styles of laryngeal mask airways (LMA), a fiberoptic scope for intubation, an AirTraq®, a video laryngoscopy, retrograde intubation, a double lumen endotracheal tube, a bronchial blocker, and a cricothyroidotomy.
7. Using a simulated intubation task trainer, follow the steps via a checklist to place a double-lumen tube and bronchial blocker.
8. Using a specialized mannequin, perform a cricothyroidotomy safely, assuring all steps are followed using a checklist.
9. Describe local anesthetics used for a variety of peripheral nerve blocks.
10. Using ultrasound and a volunteer student, describe landmarks for a specific regional anesthesia block technique. Show ultrasound images on the placement of the local anesthetic for that specific block.

Prior to the workshop, students are asked to complete precourse preparation. This includes a review of text resources, topically oriented videos, and classroom notes on the various procedures as well as a variety of articles specific to the topics. These articles include information on the following: Practice guidelines for central venous catheter placement, proper arterial catheter insertion, management of unanticipated difficult intubation, and procedural information on common regional anesthesia techniques administered by anesthesia providers.

On the day of the workshop, students are divided into groups, with approximately 15 students in each group. The

Student ____ Pass/Fail ______ (instructor initials)

Objectives Fiberoptic Bronchoscopy-students will:

1. Demonstrate component knowledge through completion of assigned learning activities and assessments
2. Verbalize the 5 golden guidelines
3. Identify components and function of all aspects of the FO bronchoscope
4. Demonstrate ability to manipulate FO scope in 360 degrees
5. Correctly perform at minimum 40 nasal fiberoptic intubations
6. Perform a test intubation in less than 60 seconds and with acceptable technique

Checklist

Component Knowledge Acquisition	Y	N	Comments
Reviewed video of actual nasal FO intubation in the clinical setting			Pre-course and also during course
Completed pre-course materials			Verified through SIMS tracking of page completion
Completed knowledge and attitude assessments on-line			Verified through SIMS dashboard
Recites 5 'golden guidelines' • Left hand on rigid, right hand on felxible • Do not bend the scope excessively • keep tip elevated when approaching glottis • Maintain central view • Do not advance without visualization			Guidelines based on expert panel review and validated through more than 3000 actual nasal fiberoptic intubations since the course began
Component Skill Acquisition			
Demonstrate scope parts and functions			
Demonstrate ability to 'look' in a 360 degree arc			Using the clock-face fiberoptic simulator
Minimum of 40 intubations (monitored)			Total number of intubations determined empirically through evaluation of skill attainment via an IRB approved study
Skill verification (instructor)			Through both formative and summative mechanisms
Timing **under 60 seconds** for verification intubation			Explain full process of nasal FOB at clinical site Timing starts with FOB entering nare Timing ends with inflation of ETT cuff and one successful ventilation Sixty second threshold established through review of an expert panel

Fig. 22.5 University of Pittsburgh Nasal Fiberoptic Intubation Mastery Checklist (with permission, WISER)

group consists of a mix of students from both nurse anesthesia programs and of different graduate year levels (first-year, second-year, and third-year students). The senior-level students are encouraged to mentor the less experienced students through deliberate practice of skills until they are able to successfully complete the tasks at each station under the guidance of a faculty member. Completion of each skill is determined by the CRNA faculty using checklists referenced to standardized texts and validated by clinical faculty from both programs for content and to ensure that the processes duplicate what is done in practice in order to provide clinical contextualization. This is a great teaching opportunity for the more experienced students and also meets the requirements for 'teaching others' in the COA Doctoral Standards. The students follow a schedule where they rotate from one anesthesia skills station to the next and are required to achieve competence at each station as assessed through the associated checklists (Fig. 22.6). Each station has multiple task

Insertion of a Bronchial Blocker Tube

A single lumen tube with a small lumen along the anterior concave side of the tube. (This small lumen contains a small, hallow lumen catheter that has a cuff at the end of it which serves as a bronchial blocker when the cuff is inflated.)

SKILL	Satisfactory	Unsatisfactory
1. Checks both cuffs (bronchial blocker & tracheal) before insertion to verify patency of cuffs)		
2. Lubricates tube & stylet; places stylet in tube		
3. Holds distal concave curvature facing anteriorly		
4. Inserts the single lumen tube and the bronchial blocker as a unit into the trachea until the tracheal cuff passes cords.		
5. Removes stylet from endobronchial tube (if used).		
6. Inflates tracheal cuff and checks breath sounds bilaterally. (You should hear equal breath sounds.)		
7. Connects elbow connector with a self-sealing diaphragm to the end of the endotracheal tube.		
8. Inserts a fiberoptic scope through self-sealing diaphragm.		
9. Maintains ventilation around the FOB but within the single-lumen tube.		
10. With FOB, identifies right and left mainstem bronchi by noting the relationship of the mainstem bronchi to the posterior membrane and the anterior cartilaginous rings.		
11. Locates the tube of the bronchial blocker by moving the bronchial blocker in and out just beyond the end of its own and the main lumens of the bronchial blocker tube.		
12. Turns the main single lumen tube so that the concavity of the tube is facing the side to be blocked.		
13. To initiate one-lung ventilation, advances the bronchial blocker into the mainstem bronchus under direct vision and inflates the balloon until the cephalad surface of the balloon is just below the tracheal carina.		
14. Withdraws the FOB.		
15. Listens in axilla to hear breath sounds. (You should hear no breath sounds on ipsilateral (bronchial blocker) side and clear breath sounds on contralateral side.		

SRNA Signature **Date** **Name/Title of Evaluator**

Fig. 22.6 Bronchial Blocker Insertion Checklist (with permission, Dr. Bernadette Henrichs, Director, Nurse Anesthesia Program at Goldfarb School of Nursing/Barnes-Jewish College)

trainers and/or devices with 3–4 CRNA faculty who have been prepared to teach and assess each group of students as they rotate throughout the different stations. Students spend approximately 45 min at each station before rotating to the next station. Stations include:

1. Arterial catheter and central catheter placement
2. Upper extremity blocks
3. Lower extremity blocks
4. Airway devices and fiberoptic intubation
5. Airway devices, including completion of a cricothyrotomy on pig tracheas
6. Subarachnoid and epidural blocks
7. Other types of regional blocks (e.g., Transverse abdominal planus (TAP) block)

The programs invite representatives from a variety of airway device companies as well as those that supply ultrasound machines. The sales representatives play an active role in participating in the workshops by displaying various devices and demonstrating the functions and capabilities of the systems. The workshop is an all-day event that starts early at 7:00 am with breakfast and lasts until about 4:00 pm. Breakfast and lunch are normally sponsored by the different companies participating in the event.

The workshop is often held in the spring during the end of the academic year. When held during this time, all students have some awareness and exposure to the topics being taught. Students are required to fill out an evaluation at the end of the day. The students have always evaluated the event very positively, rating their learning experience very highly. The workshop increases their knowledge of the different topics and also improves their skills in performing the different clinical tasks in the actual clinical setting. The students follow a schedule where they rotate from one anesthesia station to the next. The workshop also gives them the opportunity to meet students from the other program, which often leads to ongoing, collegial professional relationships.

This workshop contains many elements identified across the best practices and standards references previously cited. These include the assignment of pre-course material, sharing of the objectives for the overall workshop and for each station with the learners ahead of time, training of facilitators, use of deliberate practice toward skill attainment, integration of both formative and summative evaluation elements (outcome measurement), use of subject matter experts (SMEs) to provide educational and professional context, cognitive interactivity prior to and during the workshop and individualized learning.

Conclusion

There is a long history of simulation use in nurse anesthesia education which is highly likely to increase because of several important reasons. First, students in Nurse Anesthesia programs are anxious to gain skills and knowledge of clinical procedures and processes but equally anxious to avoid patient mishaps. Simulation can help to address this anxiety by helping them to gain skills and knowledge in the management of simple, mundane procedures to incredibly complex clinical management situations in a psychologically safe setting. Further, simulation is now a required component in nurse anesthesia education according to the Standards for Accreditation overseen by the primary accrediting body, the Council on Accreditation of Nurse Anesthesia Education Programs. Finally, the interest in simulation in the nurse anesthesia profession has increased substantially, as evidenced by the formation in 2019 of the AANA Simulation Subcommittee, which reports to the AANA Education Committee [18].

Nurse anesthesia simulation design efforts can be greatly facilitated through the adoption of best educational practices, specific educational approaches which have been shown to improve outcomes, and the modification of the INACSL Standards for application to advanced practice education. We have provided several examples here of simulation activities within several programs that speak to many of these best practices and standards. Finally, the development of a curriculum integration plan allows faculty to gain a much deeper understanding of the role simulation plays within their specific nurse anesthesia programs and helps to quantify both the quantity and quality of the student experience.

References

1. Fletcher JL. AANA journal course: update for nurse anesthetists—anesthesia simulation: a tool for learning and research. AANA J. 1995;63(1):61–7.
2. O'Donnell JM, Fletcher J, Dixon B, Palmer L. Planning and implementing an anesthesia crisis resource management course for student nurse anesthetists. CRNA. 1998;9(2):50–8.
3. Henrichs B, Thorn S, Thompson J. Teaching student nurse anesthetists to respond to simulated anesthetic emergencies. Clin Simul Nurs. 2018;17:63–71.
4. COA. Council on Accreditation of Nurse Anesthesia Educational Programs, History of Nurse Anesthesia Accreditation. 2015, pp. 1–6.
5. COA. Council on Accreditation of Nurse Anesthesia Educational Programs Standards for Accreditation of Nurse Anesthesia Programs (revised 2019), 2004, pp. 1–52.
6. COA. Council on Accreditation of Nurse Anesthesia educational Programs. Program Directors Update. 2020;(86):1–10.

7. COA. Council on Accreditation of Nurse Anesthesia Educational Programs Standards for Accreditation of Nurse Anesthesia Programs, Practice Doctorate (revised 2019). 2015, pp. 1–47.
8. Salas E, Klein C, King H, et al. Debriefing medical teams: 12 evidence-based best practices and tips. Jt Comm J Qual Patient Saf. 2008;34(9):518–27.
9. Bremner MN, Aduddell K, Bennett DN, VanGeest JB. The use of human patient simulators: best practices with novice nursing students. Nurse Educ. 2006;31(4):170–4.
10. McGaghie WC, Issenberg SB, Petrusa ER, Scalese RJ. A critical review of simulation-based medical education research: 2003–2009. Med Educ. 2010;44(1):50–63.
11. Issenberg SB, McGaghie WC, Petrusa ER, Lee Gordon D, Scalese RJ. Features and uses of high-fidelity medical simulations that lead to effective learning: a BEME systematic review. Med Teach. 2005;27(1):10–28.
12. Cook DA, Hamstra SJ, Brydges R, et al. Comparative effectiveness of instructional design features in simulation-based education: systematic review and meta-analysis. Med Teacher. 2013;35(1):e867–98.
13. Cook DA, Brydges R, Zendejas B, Hamstra SJ, Hatala R. Technology-enhanced simulation to assess health professionals: a systematic review of validity evidence, research methods, and reporting quality. Acad Med. 2013;88(6):872–83.
14. Cook DA, Brydges R, Hamstra SJ, et al. Comparative effectiveness of technology-enhanced simulation versus other instructional methods: a systematic review and meta-analysis. Simul Healthc. 2013;7(5):308–20.
15. Cook DA, Hatala R, Brydges R, et al. Technology-enhanced simulation for health professions education: a systematic review and meta-analysis. J Am Med Assoc. 2011;306(9):978–88.
16. Committee IS. INACSL standards of best practice: Simulation©. Clin Simul Nurs. 2016;12:S48–50.
17. Alexander M, Durham CF, Hooper JI, et al. NCSBN Simulation guidelines for prelicensure nursing programs. J Nurs Regul. 2015;6(3):39–42.
18. AANA. AANA Simulation Sub-Committee. Published 2020. Accessed January 5, 2021.

Using Simulation with Master's Entry to the Profession of Nursing Students (MEPN)

23

Amy Nichols and Laura L. Van Auker

Introduction

Master's Entry to the Profession of Nursing (MEPN) programs have, for over 20 years now, been an option for students interested in taking the registered nurse (RN) licensing exam in the course of attaining a master's degree. Developed for those with either a bachelor's degree or a graduate degree in a discipline other than nursing, entry-level master's degrees are also referred to as generic or accelerated programs. These offerings usually take 18–36 months to finish, with baccalaureate-level content and initial RN licensure typically completed within the first year. Paced for students who have shown an ability to succeed at a 4-year college or university, such programs often produce Clinical Nurse Leaders while increasing diversity within the RN workforce and enabling more practitioners to earn advanced degrees. The IOM 2011 report, "The Future of Nursing" [1], challenged the nursing profession to, by 2020, increase the number of nurses with a bachelor's degree to 80%, while doubling the number of nurses holding a doctorate—training that would, in the latter case, prepare these individuals to assume faculty positions in newly proposed accelerated training initiatives, such as MEPN programs. Fast forward to 2023, the IOM realized that the 80% threshold was a lofty goal, and still wants nursing to push forward with increasing the number nurses with bachelor's degrees. While such goals would seem to encourage programs to actively pursue such potential students, many schools of nursing have not tailored their curricular offerings to meet the needs and expectations of this richly experienced population [2].

As opposed to their counterparts in bachelor's-level nursing programs, MEPN students tend to be adult learners whose education is colored by a variety of life experiences and who already exhibit a high degree of self-motivation; to best serve these students, a curriculum and its supporting pedagogy must recognize and incorporate such life experiences, varied educational backgrounds, and socioeconomic and/or demographic characteristics. Those pursuing a MEPN degree expect more from their nursing school experience, often exhibiting little tolerance for busy work, challenging faculty, and demanding the most current and demonstrated teaching methodologies. At the same time, these accelerated students tend to acknowledge the limits of their experience prior to entry into the program and thus desire greater clinical time and more meaningful clinical experiences within and outside the classroom—experiences that are uniquely suited to simulation-based training.

Although simulation-based training has been recognized as beneficial and has been increasingly integrated into nursing education programs, researchers need to pay more attention to *why* such an approach works and which characteristics make simulations the optimal pedagogical technique for MEPN students pursuing knowledge and skill acquisition. This chapter will highlight the motivation for using simulation-based learning for MEPN students and will explain why simulations are best suited to transfer learning to clinical practice for students of this ilk. In doing so, we will contemplate demographic factors and characteristics unique to MEPN students, experiential learning based on a MEPN curriculum, and faculty perceptions and challenges of teaching MEPN students.

Characteristics of MEPN Students

MEPN students are diverse and varied in terms of gender, age, and ethnicity, as well as the focus of their first degree and their experience in the workforce (which is often unrelated to health care) [3]. The motivation of these students to enter the nursing profession and their academic background are gener-

A. Nichols (✉) · L. L. Van Auker
UC Davis Betty Irene Moore School of Nursing, Sacramento, CA, USA
e-mail: aanichols@ucdavis.edu

J. M. Kutzin et al. (eds.), *Comprehensive Healthcare Simulation: Nursing*, Comprehensive Healthcare Simulation,
https://doi.org/10.1007/978-3-031-31090-4_23

ally less traditional, with matriculants having majored in disciplines such as business, psychology, and engineering, as well as having studied in healthcare-related fields like physical therapy, speech and language, and social work.

The increased diversity of MEPN students has been influenced, in the United States, by the targeted efforts of the New Careers in Nursing (NCIN) program, which was designed to recruit minority and disadvantaged populations through scholarship incentives [4]. Sponsored by the Robert Wood Johnson Foundation and the American Association of Colleges of Nursing (AACN) from 2008–2016, the NCIN program provided students and schools with scholarships and grants to help nursing better reflect the changing demographic nature of a diverse nation while also meeting objectives recommended by the IOM [1], specifically regarding the increased professionalization of the nursing workforce through advanced degrees and leadership education [5]. Already having completed a bachelor's degree in a field other than nursing, second-degree MEPN students were the perfect sort of applicants to increase the level of education within the nursing workforce. Scholarship incentives allowing a return to school for a second degree reduced barriers for applicants from minority and lower economic populations, and the ability to exit with a master's degree rather than simply a second bachelor's degree has been especially appealing for students looking for rapid advancement to leadership positions and enhanced salaries. These programs can expeditiously leverage students' previous exposure to mentoring and leadership while repurposing their experiences to fit the professional nursing role [6]. Having already participated in the workforce, MEPN applicants seek accelerated program formats that allow a relatively rapid entry into nursing, a profession offering heightened job security and stability, improved benefits, leadership advancement, and, in many cases, increased income. For some MEPN students, entering nursing has been a dream long delayed; for others, the transition might represent a more recent desire to secure meaningful work in a caring profession that makes a difference in society [7, 8].

Personal or family experiences in or with the healthcare system often have prompted students to consider joining the nursing profession. McKenna et al. [9] surveyed initial perspectives on nursing among graduate-entry nurses and found that MEPN programs attracted individuals with a wide variety of backgrounds, first-degree majors, and work experiences, while also noting that these individuals' perceptions of the nursing profession were based largely on media representations or personal experiences. This disconnect suggests a continued need for public education regarding nursing roles to better recruit non-traditional nursing students, especially men. While data show that male nurses hold a greater percentage of higher paying and managerial positions in the nursing workforce, men in the profession are still distinguished by the additional moniker being a "male nurse" as opposed to a "nurse." Simulation may be an especially apt method for helping diverse nursing students of all kinds support their self-image as professionals and facilitate team-focused care in a safe environment. Capturing demographic data for MEPN students remains a challenge because national databases do not discriminate between pre-licensure students and RN master's-degree students [10]. Better data exist comparing traditional and second-degree graduates of Bachelor of Science in Nursing (BSN) programs, allowing for demographic comparisons between the two cohorts; from this, we can speculate that second-degree BSN accelerated students may align more with MEPN students in that those in the latter group bear less resemblance to traditional students.

The gap in data on the characteristics of MEPN students requires that we consider second-degree, pre-licensure students in accelerated BSN programs who may demonstrate many of the characteristics of MEPN students. These students in accelerated programs tend, for example, to be older, with a median age of 33, as opposed to 25, which is the mean age of traditional BSN graduates. In a figure consistent with that of traditional BSN programs, 78–93% of students in accelerated programs are white [11], with several studies reporting that Black students represent 7–15% of such students (compared to only 6% of students in traditional programs). Meanwhile, Asian-American students now constitute almost 10% of the population in second-degree programs, a rate that has doubled, while students of Hispanic descent remain around 8% of the population in second-degree programs, compared to 11% in traditional BSN programs—a number that has increased recently. This uptick in interest in traditional BSN programs among Hispanic students likely reflects strong recruitment of bilingual Spanish-speaking students from high schools in states with large Hispanic populations. While it is difficult to assess data limited to MEPN programs, in that the AACN combines bachelor's- and master's-level data for ethnic groups in nursing programs, states with larger Hispanic populations report greater enrollment of Hispanic students (e.g., California at 59.9%, Texas at 47.3%, and New Mexico at 53.6%), [12].

Combined data of all diverse students enrolled in nursing programs show higher numbers enrolled in master's level programs compared to undergraduate nursing programs, although these data do not distinguish MEPN students from RNs returning for a traditional master's degree [13]. Women continue to be overrepresented in both traditional and MEPN programs, but MEPN accelerated programs show an enrollment of 12% men, a rate that has doubled. Because they are often older, second-degree MEPN students are more likely to be married (55% vs. 35%) and are more inclined to report having a working spouse—so, too, do they often assume they can successfully continue working despite recommendations of accelerated programs to the contrary. Finally, regarding the complexity of balancing family obligations with educational ambitions, 31% of second-degree students report having at least one child in the home, compared to only 16% of traditional students [14].

Some international second-degree entry programs report higher levels of foreign-born or English-as-a-second language (ESL) students, and data from BSN and MEPN programs indicate higher rates of ESL and foreign-born students in second-degree programs compared to students in traditional undergraduate nursing programs. Meanwhile, anecdotal evidence indicates that students who are refugees or immigrants, many of whom hold advanced degrees and have worked in medicine, nursing, or pharmacy in their homeland, desire MEPN accelerated entry into the professional nursing workforce due to its expedited nature and cost-effectiveness. These foreign-trained healthcare professionals in MEPN programs often enter with years of experience in health-related professions, a significant distinction from traditional entry students; they are, therefore, less focused on—and less in need of—core nursing content and more inclined to apply their knowledge toward and become oriented within their new professional setting. In this regard, McNeisch explained how second-degree students can feel as if they are tourists, traveling through new land and looking for familiar landmarks [15].

As a technique, simulation is well-suited to acclimate both healthcare novices and experienced foreign-trained providers by strategically placing these individuals within a case-based scenario, even to the point of stratifying difficulty in clinical decision-making [16]. Such opportunities offer trainees experiential learning based on peer expertise that enriches the simulation for all parties involved. Simulation can also be individualized, allowing similar experiences to be clustered—and it is particularly good at generating immediate feedback and identifying areas of strength while revealing specifics of prior training that do not align with current practice in the United States. For ESL learners, the opportunity to demonstrate decision-making or knowledge through simulations may enhance student confidence as these individuals become more comfortable with English, as opposed to relying on the "Describe first what you will do"-approach common in the clinical environment. Even more, foreign-trained health professionals can learn from their domestic peers, drawing on social, cultural, and language translation and interpretation assistance within the structured simulation environment. Here, the faculty facilitator must conscientiously monitor experienced foreign-trained healthcare professionals, particularly in adapting and integrating norms related to nursing scope of practice. It can be tempting to defer to the knowledge and experience of an anesthesiologist or neurosurgeon from a developing nation in this respect, but acculturation of professional nursing standards in the United States must be ensured—and such insistence is easier realized within a simulation environment than it is within a clinical setting.

Adult Learners, Andragogy, the MEPN Student and Choosing Simulation to Educate

MEPN students arrive as experienced and successful learners with expectations for what they should receive from their program and faculty. These students must progress from an undergraduate level of learning and need to reach the heightened expectations of an accelerated graduate program while applying contemporary educational strategies such as the "flipped classroom" [17]. While MEPN students have prior academic exposure and workforce credentials, several studies suggest these learners require facilitation into professional nursing for a successful transition, regardless of their prior experience within a health or social health–related field. Often, such facilitation takes the form of "coaching," as opposed to the traditional pedagogies relied on in pre-licensure programs [18]. These students see their success tied to their ability to apply prior life experiences while efficiently developing applicable skills and knowledge; such expectations thus make them more inclined to convey their needs.

To meet the above-described expectations, MEPN programs and faculty must be well-versed in andragogy, the teaching of adults, as opposed to the pedagogy embraced by traditional pre-licensure programs. Applying andragogy as opposed to pedagogy has been recognized as essential by the United Nations because educational programs must be designed to prepare future workforces best to solve complex problems and provide a common level of communication between countries. Applying andragogy using adult learning methods has been deemed a critical facet in the larger endeavor to address global illiteracy and to emancipate women, both of which are concerns that, throughout the world, have too often been excluded from educational opportunities during childhood. Fundamentally, andragogy proffers that adults learn most successfully when they are motivated to pursue and retain knowledge that affects their life goals. Malcolm Knowles, an American educator, has set forth andragogy's six basic principles, which include: (1) Need to know, (2) Experience, (3) Self-concept, (4) Readiness, (5) Problem orientation, and (6) Intrinsic motivation. Within nursing education, these principles, discussed in more detail below, provide a framework for developing structured learning through simulation, a teaching and learning tactic originally developed for use by the military and later adopted in engineering that mimics real-world experiences, offering a variety of models to apply what is known or what is desired. This emphasis on intentional real-world experience meshes well with the adult-learning needs and diverse characteristics of MEPN students described in this chapter.

1. **Need to know** expresses the MEPN student's understanding of the necessity and advantage of learning as a motivating factor for integrating knowledge. Put simply, will this learning improve quality of life or be crucial to work performance or patient care in the future? MEPN students expect relevant experiential learning and show less tolerance for busy work or what they do not perceive to be relevant content. A traditional written exam, for example, can be used to gauge a student's ability to memorize a list of cardiac resuscitation medications for use during a code blue. However, if the goal of assessment is to determine the student's ability to "know how" and understand what "to do" while facilitating a successful cardiac resuscitation, simulation seems better suited to the task, in that it can replicate a high-stakes environment where students appreciate the "need to know" correct medications, doses, and drug mechanisms from memory.
2. **Experience** of MEPN students, especially the way they might integrate their personal identity into this new role of professional nursing, is essential to their success. These students frequently require assistance applying their prior knowledge and competencies because experience, while often a positive value, can also lead to a kind of mental rigidity that could inhibit adaptation to the nursing role [19]. This effect may be particularly salient in the case of students whose identity is strongly associated with their mastery in a prior career, especially those learners with years of healthcare-related experiences, such as foreign-trained physicians or nurses, who may feel vulnerable returning to a comparative novice role as a learner. Confidence motivates professional nursing role development and promotes mastery through simulations that encourage students to leverage their prior successes in problem-solving, communication, and team-leading, encourages these learners to envision themselves as a competent nurse ready, willing, and able to acquire skills and knowledge. An identified characteristic of MEPN students is their recognition of the seriousness of their nursing responsibility to patients and the life-or-death implications of their conduct and decision-making. The life experience of these learners informs them that their actions and omissions have consequences, making them more keenly aware of what they do *not* know, as well as the pathway to mastery requiring of them a commitment of time and effort.
3. **Self-concept** in adult learners recognizes acquired self-awareness and the expectation of maintaining autonomy achieved through maturation. In training settings, these students must perceive their education as having some aspect of independence, offering the ability to make choices within the learning process. In MEPN students, this notion is expressed as a desire for self-paced or independent learning opportunities; under such circumstances, gaming is a form of simulation likely to be well-received.
4. **Readiness** refers to adult learners' inclination to see their training as useful and immediately applicable to solving the day-to-day problems encountered as a nurse. These students will be motivated to learn contingent upon the immediacy of application, suggesting that the timing of content should, for optimal success, match the timing of clinical experiences. Providing active-learning and simulation experiences offers the reality of required readiness amid these learners' real-world clinical training [20].
5. **Problem orientation** focuses on the MEPN student beyond the content itself, scaffolding the educational process by placing learning in the context of building competencies, knowledge, and abilities. Here, the willingness to learn content is demonstrated in advancing levels of competency, from novice to advanced beginner. Simulation meets the MEPN student's need to measure progression to mastery, and Miller's prism of clinical competence models the problem-oriented, scaffolded learning facilitated so well by simulation exercises [21, 22]. The student enters at the fact-gathering level, providing the "knows" that typically are offered in pre-simulation educational content, while the second tier of the exercise, "knows how," can be demonstrated through case presentations, essays, and multiple-choice questions. This is often developed in the introduction to the case-based scenario at the beginning of the simulation. The team discusses plans for its first approach to the simulation, where students will both "show" their knowledge and demonstrate the "does"-element of their understanding. In a rewarding way, this integrates cognitive development and knowledge with enhanced abilities and the building of competency. MEPN adult learners value this demonstrated progression, helping them pass post-graduation licensure examinations before securing employment as a professional nurse, thereby realizing the financial security and life stability that were likely their reasons for enrolling in a MEPN program.
6. **Intrinsic motivation** expresses the characteristics of the adult learner to acquire understanding from internal (intrinsic) motivators as opposed to extrinsic forces provided by educators and others. Educators must know how to trigger intrinsic motivation and should not replace it with extrinsic motivators. Respecting intrinsic motivation recognizes that adult learners have self-determination and acknowledges that innate needs of competency and the ability to relate to a situation are

necessary precursors to change and growth. In this regard, faculty should act as a facilitator and allow students to self-motivate, a process that can be especially challenging for returning students who often learned amid a pedagogy whereby discrete content was "spoon-fed" and where rote knowledge was regurgitated during examinations. Difficulties of this variety often manifest during the first term of a program and should be quickly addressed with adult adjustment to the required learning outcomes. Faculty must clearly articulate expectations for such students and must frame the adjustment process for these learners as akin to the lifelong learning undertaken by professional nurses.

Faculty Skillset for Andragogy-Based Learning and Simulation with MEPN Students

As more faculty teach in accelerated master's entry programs, they should understand how best to approach the challenge of teaching these unique students. Because MEPN programs are designed to expedite the education of individuals already possessing a degree, associated faculty must tailor their approach to best meet the educational needs of this cohort. Unfortunately, faculty are often ill-equipped to handle this crucial step in successfully training MEPN students, although evidence points to several tactics that have demonstrated promise and that have indicated potential [23–25]. Extreme organization, engaging students via life/work experiences tied to learning, effective pedagogy adaptations, and early immersion with case-based learning, for example, are several important elements to consider when designing simulation experiences for accelerated students.

Extreme organization is particularly important for accelerated students who have no time for ambiguity. These students tend to be very well-prepared, tech-savvy, and adept at linking concepts—so much so that faculty must prepare even more diligently to meet their needs. Ideally, classroom experiences should be redesigned, meeting the needs of adult learners by using cutting-edge technologies to bring clinical expertise into the classroom and by integrating simulations into the MEPN curriculum. Successful simulation experiences take a considerable amount of planning and tremendous organization on the part of faculty and those involved with the learning experience; faculty development is, therefore, central to the endeavor, allowing teachers to receive their own education and training necessary to conceive of and implement these crucial exercises.

Acknowledging and encouraging accelerated students to share their prior experiences in work and life is important. Students are more engaged when drawing on experiences that acknowledge their expertise and varied strengths. In the ideal learning environment, essential content should be identified, and strategies should be designed that require students to engage in the learning process, actively applying information within the context of the practice environment. Simulation learning experiences are adept at facilitating the active application of information within a fixed clinical setting; they are also well-suited to help students retain the greatest level of knowledge and skill. If faculty are experienced, they can manage these situations by tapping into students' expertise, acknowledging such facility in adult learners, and drawing on this rich potential during class discussions. Creating simulations that link life and work experiences, allowing students to connect new information to prior knowledge, is a vital but challenging task for simulation educators. Incorporating experiences in the simulation classroom can enrich learning and help students build confidence—and taking the time to thoroughly debrief and discuss the exercise after a simulation can help these individuals internalize what they have learned while applying their knowledge and developing the skillset to future experiences.

In the case of MEPN students, in particular, it is essential that faculty stay current on emerging technologies and deploy a variety of innovative teaching methodologies, such as simulation, case-based learning, and online discussion forums. While all nursing students could benefit from such methods, these options seem especially apt for faculty working with an accelerated cohort. The interest of MEPN students can be maintained by using a variety of simulation-based learning technologies; the key is to link "real-life" learning to theoretical content and thus transfer learning from the confines of the classroom to the clinical mindset. When faculty are innovative and consider the ways accelerated students learn best, they are more likely to meet learning objectives. Faculty must be intentional and systematic about selecting teaching strategies to encourage learning. In this regard, experiential learning is especially effective for MEPN students; simulation exercises inspire students to act and think like nurses. Because of the brief amount of time that MEPN students spend in their programs, they must be immersed in their eventual nursing role as early as possible, allowing them to "learn by doing" and enabling the process by which they can efficiently connect bits of information. From the start of a program, simulation is the perfect means by which to transition students from acting like a nurse to *being* a nurse. Along the way, faculty will need to abandon dated teacher-centric methods in favor of active-learning techniques and emerging technologies. Being well-prepared and organized is crucial for any simulation activity. Faculty development, then, is essential to transforming classroom education through case-based learning, scenario development, evaluation, and post-simulation debriefing—each of which is time- and labor-intensive but also particularly well-suited to adult learners.

Transition of MEPN Students to Postgraduate Practice and Its Implications for Simulation Learning

MEPN students perform especially well on the NCLEX licensure exam and are preferred by employers for their demonstrated leadership, maturity, and critical-thinking skills. For these reasons, they tend to be paid more while also transitioning sooner into leadership positions; that said, their success comes with its own burdens. Engaging MEPN students in simulations prior to their transition to clinical practice can help these learners anticipate many of the challenges of navigating a new position as an RN. As students matriculate through an accelerated program, they must focus all their time and training in total immersion with little opportunity to gain experience working in a health setting—a reality presenting additional challenges for students in accelerated nursing programs. For example, traditional students acquire valuable skills while working as a nursing assistant, an experience that they can then transfer to a future nursing position, whereas the more compressed schedule of MEPN students does not allow these individuals the same opportunity for training and thereby compounds the stress they tend to feel regarding hiring expectations once they go on to seek postgraduate employment.

Registered nurses who have recently graduated with a master's degree face an additional burden; while these new nurses are relatively novice in terms of their clinical skills, their graduate degree tends to signify a level of experience and exposure that they have yet to attain in a practice setting. Consequently, these newly minted graduates do not receive enough time to learn on the job—to be a novice, in other words, among more experienced nurses. Even worse, MEPN graduates just starting out are often paired with a preceptor who has only a bachelor's degree in nursing, creating an interesting power dynamic in that the preceptor is the one essentially supervising while at the same time possessing a lesser academic degree than the recent graduate whose work is being observed. In this way and under such circumstances, new MEPN graduates are often bullied or subject to microaggressions. For example, a preceptor might make a comment like, "Well, you should know how to do that. After all, you have a graduate degree, right?" Alternatively, it could be that unit nurses, talking amongst themselves, openly wonder why recent graduates in their midst function like a novice when they should be operating at a level commensurate with their advanced graduate training. Preparing MEPN students to enter the workforce with the tools to handle situations like these is crucial; creating transition-to-practice simulations in the final quarter or semester and allowing students to work through circumstances they might encounter would reduce the above-described stress by raising the awareness of these recent graduates regarding these and other challenging situations that could be encountered in the workplace.

An additional challenge MEPN graduates face is that they tend to forgo self-care while accommodating the expectations of their patient-care workload. So, too, do they tend not to engage with colleagues in settings outside of work, preferring, instead, to manage the stress of transition by heading home after work to find succor in more familiar social relationships and preexisting support systems. When these graduates do opt to socialize with co-workers, especially as their new colleagues understand better than anyone else the demands of nursing, they are often disappointed by the prevalence of gossip within their units, presumptively about them—the recent graduates—and their adjustment process, further limiting the ability of these individuals to develop healthy social capital with their co-workers [26]. Diminished attachment within the work setting engenders poor communication, inspires conflict, creates frustration, or encourages questions about the fitness of new graduates within the unit. While nursing school is stressful, and self-care strategies are often perceived to be busy work rather than essential to thriving in future practice, simulation can encourage attention to individual health and well-being as a cross-check (there are two patients for each simulation, the patient and the nurse) and can be a part of post-simulation reflection assignments.

Faculty should acknowledge that students of diversity may face additional stressors. For example, male student nurses may experience the above tensions more so than their female colleagues, given that nursing is still, traditionally, a job performed by women [27]. The nursing role, predicated on values of nurturing and care, is often not seen as requiring highly technical professional training in the form of knowledge regarding complex physiologic systems of health and disease. Male graduate-entry nursing students, without a male nursing role model, may be new to the concept of a nursing career; they could also lack the passion for nursing seen in females who have often engaged in progressive work exposure in the healthcare system through volunteerism or by attaining certified nursing assistant positions. The accelerated nature of MEPN programs does not allow time for this added healthcare experience in a lower-responsibility patient-care role. Moreover, the potential for role-transition stress and conflict can be exacerbated if the male nurse experiences bias from faculty, employers, or co-workers. This bias may be positive or negative, creating either facilitators of or barriers to the confidence that a male nurse requires to develop and transition effectively into professional nursing—and this phenomenon could be further pronounced in the case of accelerated graduate-entry program nurses, where higher-level performance expectations are based on a level of degree, greater maturity, and demonstrated leadership and critical-thinking skills [26].

Students and new nurses are especially cognizant of their own inexperience and deficiencies, an effect amplified by gender bias among faculty and employers, which presents men as naturally stronger leaders with greater confidence and better crisis-management and problem-solving skills. Due to this bias, a male student or new graduate experiences greater stress than would be felt by a recent female graduate as he struggles to manage the burden of high expectations and the need to maintain patient safety while, at the same time, lacking the hours in clinical care necessary to establish concomitant confidence in skill-based care. This stress, anxiety, and social stigma have been found to be greater amid the transition of those emerging from graduate-entry programs, such as MEPN programs, as opposed to those graduating from traditional nursing programs. The characteristic identified as a contributor for these students has been the tendency for MEPN students not to socialize with co-workers, a reticence that inhibits the social-support system necessary to modulate the stress, workload, and anxiety felt by a new nurse. This effect is exacerbated in the case of a male nurse who might feel rejected by both patients and nursing co-workers due to biases against care by men or even on account of resentment regarding leadership assignments seen as being doled out to men under a dictate by management. Conditions like these can often result in a hostile environment on the floor and a fear of "set-up" failure for the new nurse, thereby aggravating transition stress and ultimately encouraging nursing burnout.

The role of the male nursing student is an uncultivated area of focus with respect to simulation, especially in that the stigma of entering a female-dominated profession and the experience of bias, facilitating and obstructing transition, have yet to be traditionally addressed in nursing programs. The effects of these factors are heightened for male MEPN students, who may experience greater stress during simulation activities. A shortage of male faculty in nursing schools provides little opportunity for male mentors as simulation facilitators; at the same time, studies have documented the bias that faculty display in selecting male students as group leaders and knowledge holders over their female counterparts. Recognizing this bias is essential to developing purposeful simulations and assigned roles; it is also vital that faculty recognize the stubborn stigma that remains within society and the nursing profession as a whole while drawing on this awareness to craft simulations that address issues male students might face. For example, a simulation might involve a female patient who has refused care from a male nurse, providing a team-wide opportunity to resolve the conflict by supporting the male student and interrogating stereotypes associated with gender identity and attendant capacity for care. Faculty can further enhance this simulation experience by inviting male nurses from clinical partner agencies to mentor the team as it navigates this common sort of scenario; integrating clinical partners into such simulations promotes a wider discussion across entities, encourages greater communications, and builds networks of opportunity for nursing students transitioning into postgraduate work environments.

Recommendations

The lack of evidence in the literature regarding the implementation, time of training, the focus of learning goals, faculty proficiency in use, and outcomes of simulation tactics for educating MEPN students remains the greatest challenge to evaluating such a learning technique in this context. The mixing of data between all master's-level students, whether pre-licensure MEPN students or returning professional RNs seeking an advanced degree or working toward the advanced practice nursing role, is also a significant barrier. This mixing of data occurs, as well, in baccalaureate-level programs, where information from traditional and accelerated second-degree programs is often combined, further confounding the addition of RN to BSN programs catering to the experienced RN returning for the baccalaureate degree. Evidence is also lacking with respect to the institution of accelerated formats appealing to second-degree entry students at either the baccalaureate or master's-entry level regarding the use of simulation and its benefits for adult learners. While demographics in these two populations of second-degree entry-level students may have commonalities, what role do faculty play in applying simulation targeted at the learning preferences of these life-experienced learners in master's-entry programs as opposed to traditional BSN educational environments? What preparation and faculty development in adult-learning theory and its application to simulation-based education is required for teaching in accelerated MEPN programs?

As best practices in simulation-based learning in nursing education are established, the role of simulation in MEPN programs with largely accelerated formats must address the unique learning needs and preferences of the second-degree learner. MEPN learners prefer experiential learning that aligns with the goals of simulation-based education; however, does the requisite suspension of reality in simulation require the highest level of fidelity to motivate these students to learn, or do their broad life experiences enable them to engage in low-fidelity, tabletop, case-based learning with reflective writing? Given the increased student diversity in ethnicity, gender, language, work, education, and life experiences for MEPN students upon entry, how can simulation best address nursing competency goals while integrating and retaining these novice nurses during their career transition into professional nursing?

MEPN students bring with them rich life experiences and diverse needs that may challenge faculty in terms of both curriculum development and the importance of support regarding the balancing of family, work, and education. Faculty identifying as mentors, facilitators, and coaches require the blessing of and nurturing by administration leadership, as well as preparation in best-practice simulation for andragogy focused on adult learning. Schools of nursing should review faculty onboarding practices and professional development programs to prepare faculty to meet the needs of accelerated students. To be successful in their positions, faculty may require support while learning and adjusting to the condensed timeframe; they will also need assistance planning how to cover the same amount of course material in less time and how to most efficiently use technology in the classroom. While many faculty members possess a PhD, only if they possess a doctoral degree (EdD, DNP) especially involving curriculum development and design, most of these educators will struggle with education andragogy, wondering how to create a learning environment with different learners, particularly accelerated students. Certification as a Healthcare Simulation Educator (CHSE) is recommended. Simulation is well-suited in the circumstances such as these, where integrating the prior experiences of the learner is both essential and enriching. Student questioning of content relevance or scenario outcomes in simulations allows for guided insight toward competency and the development of the nursing role in the hands of a faculty member skilled in facilitating simulations.

References

1. Institute of Medicine, Committee on the Robert Wood Johnson Foundation Initiative on the Future of Nursing, at the Institute of Medicine. The future of nursing: leading change, advancing health. Washington, DC: National Academies Press; 2011. https://doi.org/10.17226/12956.
2. McNiesh SG. The lived experience of students in an accelerated nursing program: intersecting factors that influence experiential learning. J Nurs Educ. 2011;50(4):197–203. https://doi.org/10.3928/01484834-20101029-03.
3. Everett B, Salamonson Y, Trajkovski S, Fernandez R. Demographic and academic-related differences between standard-entry and graduate-entry nursing students: a prospective correlational survey. Nurse Educ Today. 2013;33(7):709–13.
4. DeWitty VP, Huerta CG, Downing CA. New careers in nursing: optimizing diversity and student success for the future of nursing. J Prof Nurs. 2016;32(5S):S4–13.
5. Kershaw B. The future of nursing—leading change, advancing Health The future of nursing—leading change, advancing health. Nurs Stand. 2011;26(7):31.
6. Tabloski PA. Setting the stage for success: mentoring and leadership development. J Prof Nurs. 2016;32(5S):S54–8.
7. Moore LW, Kelly CW, Schmidt S, Miller M, Reynolds M. Second degree prelicensure master's graduates: what attracts them to nursing, their views on the profession, and their contributions. J Prof Nurs. 2011;27(1):19–27.
8. Raines DA. What attracts second-degree students to a career in nursing? Online J Issues Nurs. 2010;16(1):8.
9. McKenna L, Vanderheide R, Brooks I. Is graduate entry education a solution to increasing numbers of men in nursing? Nurse Educ Pract. 2016;17:74–7.
10. United States Census Bureau. QuickFacts: United States. 2015 [cited 2021 Mar 17]. Available from: https://www.census.gov/quickfacts/fact/table/US/PST045219.2015.
11. Pellico LH, Terrill E, White P, Rico J. Integrative review of graduate entry programs in nursing. J Nurs Educ. 2012;51(1):29–37.
12. Accelerated baccalaureate and master's degrees in nursing. Aacnnursing.org. [cited 2021 Mar 26]. Available from: https://www.aacnnursing.org/Nursing-Education-Programs/Accelerated-Programs.
13. Accelerated programs: The fast track to careers in nursing. Aacnnursing.org. [cited 2021 Mar 26]. Available from: https://www.aacnnursing.org/nursing-education/accelerated-programs/fast-track.
14. Brewer CS, Kovner CT, Poornima S, Fairchild S, Kim H, Djukic M. A comparison of second-degree baccalaureate and traditional-baccalaureate new graduate RNs: implications for the workforce. J Prof Nurs. 2009;25(1):5–14.
15. McNiesh SG. The lived experience of students in an accelerated nursing program: intersecting factors that influence experiential learning. J Nurs Educ. 2011;50(4):197–203. https://doi.org/10.3928/01484384-20101029-03.
16. Alexander E. Purposeful simulation role assignment. Clin Simul Nurs. 2020;48:1–7.
17. El-Banna MM, Tebbenhoff B, Whitlow M, Wyche KF. Motivated strategies for learning in accelerated second-degree nursing students. Nurse Educ. 2017;42(6):308–12.
18. Bowie BH, Carr KC. From coach to colleague: adjusting pedagogical approaches and attitudes in accelerated nursing programs. J Prof Nurs. 2013;29(6):395–401.
19. Cruz FA, Farr S, Klakovich MD, Esslinger P. Facilitating the career transition of second-career students into professional nursing. Nurs Educ Perspect. 2013;34(1):12–7.
20. Brown J, Kelly MA, McGough S, Fagence A, Bosco AM, Mason J, et al. The impact of simulation on graduate entry master's students' confidence to provide safe patient care: a longitudinal study. Clin Simul Nurs. 2020;45:6–15.
21. Sullivan N, Swoboda SM, Breymier T, Lucas L, Sarasnick J, Rutherford-Hemming T, et al. Emerging evidence toward a 2:1 clinical to simulation ratio: a study comparing the traditional clinical and simulation settings. Clin Simul Nurs. 2019;30:34–41.
22. Gerzina HA, Stovsky E. Standardized patient assessment of learners in medical simulation. In: StatPearls. Treasure Island (FL): StatPearls Publishing; 2020.
23. Christoffersen JE. Teaching accelerated second-degree nursing students: educators from across the United States share their wisdom: teaching ASD students. Nurs Forum. 2017;52(2):111–7. https://doi.org/10.1111/nuf.12174.
24. Rutherford-Hemming T. Simulation methodology in nursing education and adult learning theory. Adult Learn. 2012;23(3):129–37.
25. Clapper TC. Beyond knowles: what those conducting simulation need to know about adult learning theory. Clin Simul Nurs. 2010;6(1):e7–14.
26. Rainbow JG, Steege LM. Transition to practice experiences of first- and second-career nurses: a mixed-methods study. J Clin Nurs. 2019;28(7–8):1193–204.
27. Hoffart N, McCoy TP, Lewallen LP, Thorpe S. Differences in gender-related profile characteristics, perceptions, and outcomes of accelerated second-degree nursing students. J Prof Nurs. 2019;35(2):93–100.

Leading a Multidisciplinary Team to Develop and Implement Interprofessional Education (IPE) Simulation

24

Dayna L. Herrera and Sarah E. Pearce

Background

In 2000, the U.S. Institute of Medicine (IOM) released "To Err is Human: Building a Safer Health System" [1], which called for the development of interdisciplinary teams to increase healthcare quality and safety. In 2015 the IOM and the World Health Organization (WHO) [2] reiterated the link between interdisciplinary teamwork and healthcare quality. They urged educators in health professions to incorporate interprofessional education (IPE) routinely into their curricula. Interprofessional education refers to occasions when students from two or more professions in health and social care learn together during all or part of their professional training to cultivate collaborative practice in providing patient-centered care. The goal of interprofessional education is to prepare health professional students with the knowledge, skills, and attitudes necessary for collaborative interprofessional practice [3] Interprofessional education (IPE) and interprofessional collaborative practice (IPCP) continue to evolve, with a growing body of evidence demonstrating a positive impact on practice and patient outcomes [4]. As a result of the call to action and evidence base, which supports the idea that interprofessional practice (IP) is an effective method of improving efficiency, many health profession programs now require IPE integration to meet accreditation standards. Simulation-enhanced interprofessional education is an active learning strategy that can improve patient and community care outcomes, engage learners to be collaborative practice ready, and meet standards. The purpose of this chapter is to provide insight into necessary components, obstacles, and factors that influence the success of IPE simulation curriculum development. These insights align with the Society for Simulation in Healthcare's (SSH) Accreditation Standards [5] while integrating and referencing the Interprofessional Education Collaborative Core Competencies (IPEC) [3] as demonstrated in theoretical content and clinically simulated environments across health-related disciplines.

Components

Simulation-enhanced interprofessional education is defined as participants and facilitators from two or more professions engaging in simulated healthcare experiences to achieve shared or linked objectives and outcomes [6]. Despite the call to action, many graduate programs still need to offer a comprehensive, integrated IPE curriculum involving multiple healthcare programs and or community partners. Many obstacles and challenges are associated with building and implementing the necessary components of a robust, fully integrated IPE curriculum across multiple programs or even a single integrated IPE simulation. The components of successful implementation begin with leading multidiscipline faculty champions through a process of engagement, training, and mentoring to develop and implement meaningful and successful IPE simulation (Fig. 24.1).

Engagement

Within the IPE literature, there is general recognition that skilled and knowledgeable faculty are required to implement IPE and simulation successfully. These faculty mem-

Supplementary Information The online version contains supplementary material available at https://doi.org/10.1007/978-3-031-31090-4_24.

D. L. Herrera
Learning Environment & Innovation, California Baptist University College of Nursing, Riverside, CA, USA
e-mail: dherrera@calbaptist.edu

S. E. Pearce
Simulation and Standardized Patient Program, California Baptist University, College of Nursing,
Riverside, CA, USA
e-mail: spearce@calbaptist.edu

J. M. Kutzin et al. (eds.), *Comprehensive Healthcare Simulation: Nursing*, Comprehensive Healthcare Simulation,
https://doi.org/10.1007/978-3-031-31090-4_24

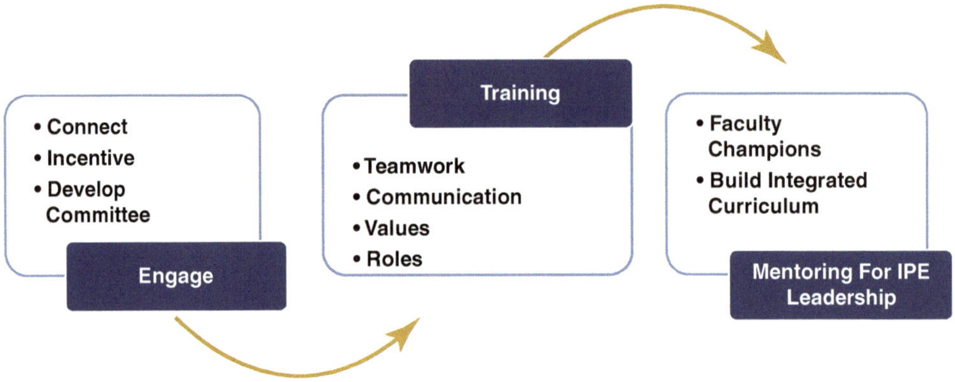

Fig. 24.1 Model for faculty development in IPE & simulation [7] ©Herrera (2014)

bers, in turn, promote collaborative practice and foster graduates who are better prepared to work in healthcare teams. Most literature supports the argument that faculty development is a key element in the successful development of IPE and simulation. Chappell et al. [8] agree that simply bringing faculty members from different healthcare disciplines into the same classroom or another learning environment should not be assumed to result in a beneficial IPE experience for healthcare students. It is essential for collaborating faculty from different disciplines to work as a team within their organization and in conjunction with other healthcare educators and healthcare community partners to integrate and support faculty development programs in IPE, as well as put into place systems and integrated curricula aligned to key IPEC elements, which additionally focus on developing and integrating IPEC aligned simulation-based learning activities [3]. Watts et al. [8] identify the development of skilled educators as a critical, evolutionary process that should be based on educating collaborative, reflective faculty capable of functioning effectively in an interdisciplinary team.

Training

To sustain an integrated IPE simulation program, faculty development in interprofessional competencies and simulation areas is critical [9]. Faculty facilitators must be prepared and trained for the simulation to ensure consistency across multiple disciplines and programs. Faculty development may include formal training courses thru organizations such as IPEC and SSH. Faculty development programs should incorporate components of informal but structured formats thru a train-the-trainer approach while additionally adhering to the IPEC competencies and simulation guidelines. Through the development of these types of faculty development programs, which utilize a variety of formal and informal strategies, programs can maximize resources and increase efficiency in faculty development related to IPE and simulation while additionally creating opportunities to identify potential faculty champions from multiple healthcare professions. A long-term mentoring approach can begin by identifying and selecting faculty champions. Through this approach, continued faculty development can occur in the area of design, development, and integration of IPE curriculum and simulation-based learning activities across multiple programs.

Mentoring

A dedicated team of faculty champions requires complete buy-in and determination from the entire team for the IPE team to succeed as they continually maintain the collective goals of simulation-based learning activities, which align with the IPE competency approach. A suggested approach for finding success in this area is through the formation of a multidiscipline faculty advisory board dedicated to the following goals:

- Working collaboratively to establish meaningful and realistic goals
- Supporting both simulation and IPE initiatives through the sharing of knowledge, standards, and skills
- Supporting the professional and scholarly development of faculty colleagues
- Refining continued to mentor and facilitator debrief skills
- Development of simulation-based learning activities which align with standards of best practice according to SSH accreditation standards and IPEC competencies
- Remaining dedicated to providing a valuable service to the College while meeting multiple programs' accreditation standards

The overall purpose of ongoing mentoring amongst IPE faculty is to provide leadership and insight into the necessary components of IPE Simulation and curricular development and to identify and overcome potential barriers to successful implementation while additionally working to improve overall collaborative relationships and practice.

Curriculum -Simulation Development/ Implementation

Designing an interprofessional education-oriented simulation curriculum can have its challenges; however, according to the International Nursing Association for Clinical Simulation and Learning (INACSL) standards committee, "the complex healthcare needs of today's society require healthcare professionals to work as a collaborative team" [10]. The INACSL standards committee defines "Sim-IPE" as the "overlap of the pedagogy of simulation and interprofessional education, providing a collaborative approach for developing and mastering interprofessional practice competencies" [11]. Building an IPE simulation presents the sometimes-complex process of designing simulation-based learning activities that meet the needs of two or more different disciplines. Differences in languaging, program objectives, faculty perspectives, knowledge base, required student learning outcomes, and accrediting standards can all present unique challenges for individuals on the team responsible for designing an IPE simulation-based learning activity.

According to Watts et al. [6], some initial insights and reflections related to avoiding unnecessary complications during the design process can include gaining institutional support, developing an overall needs assessment and interprofessional curricular plan, designing a faculty development plan, developing interprofessional relationships to promote a collaborative schedule, pre-aligning the level of learners for the appropriate interprofessional team, integrating team concepts into the development of the simulation from the beginning, and developing a detailed and structured implementation plan using the IPE faculty collaborative team. If you know where you are going and have a solid foundation and structure for getting there, the journey to completion can be less complex.

In 2021 the INACSL standards committee published an eleven-criterion model of simulation design which includes eleven linear steps for simulation best practice design. This eleven-criterion design process includes [10]: 9

Criterion 1: Designed in Consultation with Content Experts and Simulationists
- Simulation activities should be designed in collaboration with content experts and simulation experts.

Criterion 2: Needs Assessment
- A needs assessment can include various types of analysis both formal and informal to identify an educational gap across disciplines.

Criterion 3: Constructing Measurable Objectives
- Measurable objectives should be developed which target the identified educational gap discovered during the need's assessment.

Criterion 4: Align the Modality with the Objectives
- The simulation modality should be aligned with the content expert and simulation expert designed learning objectives for the simulation case.

Criterion 5: Designing a Scenario or Case
- The simulation scenario or case should provide context for the simulation-based learning experience.

Criterion 6: Fidelity
- Simulation fidelity (realism) should include aspects of physical or environmental fidelity, conceptual fidelity, and psychological fidelity.

Criterion 7: Facilitative Approach
- Simulation learning activities should be based on a facilitative model and should avoid traditional didactic styles.

Criterion 8: Pre-briefing
- Should be standardized across the curriculum and should set the stage for learning.

Criterion 9: Debriefing
- Should include components of reflection and targeted feedback as well as maintaining standardization across the program.

Criterion 10: Evaluation
- An evaluation framework should be developed and integrated to ensure the quality and effectiveness of simulation-based learning experiences.

Criterion 11: Pilot Test
- A simulation pilot test should be conducted to help refine and identify potential gaps, errors, and or distractions to completion of the simulation-based learning activities. Participants of the pilot test should be from the same or similar population as the learners for whom the simulation is being designed.

The INACSL Standards of Best Practice (2016) eleven-criterion model can be utilized in conjunction with the INACSL Standards of Best Practice for Simulation-Enhanced IPE (Sim-IPE (INACSL Standards Committee, 2016) to design an IPE simulation-based learning activity within a program. In this model, four criteria are outlined and include [11]:

Criterion 1: Conduct Sim-IPE Based on a Theoretical or Conceptual Framework

Criterion 2: Utilization of Best Practices Simulation Design (*eleven-criterion model described above*)

Criterion 3: Recognize and Address Potential Barriers

Criterion 4: Develop an Evaluation Plan

While developing an IPE-based simulation learning activity can be complex and, at times, challenging, the above tools can be utilized to assist in guiding the process while reducing the risk of error and increasing the opportunity for multiple disciplines to benefit from this valuable and vital type of simulation-based learning. An additional tool in the process of IPE simulation-based learning activity development has been included below, containing a sample "IPE Simulation Case Development Template."

Insights

Insights from experienced IPE faculty can be extremely beneficial in avoiding common pitfalls and barriers to IPE simulation and curriculum development. Authors' experience building and implementing a faculty development program resulted in the following:

- A board of key faculty champions from seven graduate healthcare programs and community partners
- University-wide IPE disaster-focused simulation with over 500 participants (20 Community Embedded Participants (e.g., local fire department), 200 Learners, 250 Standardized Patients, and 50 Multidisciplinary Facilitators) from multiple disciplines across the university and the local community
- Nine fully integrated IPE simulation-based learning activities supporting multiple programs
  - Scenarios Include:
    - Mental Health simulation scenario based on non-compliance in medication administration and including Behavioral Science (MFT, LPCC, and Social Work) and Pre-Licensure Nursing Students.
    - The nutrition simulation scenario focused on an eating disorder in a student volleyball player. It included Athletic Training, Physician Assistant, Family Nurse Practitioner, and Behavioral Science (MFT, LPCC, and Social Work) students.
    - Syncopal episode simulation scenario including Athletic Training, Family Nurse Practitioner, and Physician Assistant students.
    - Six Community Health simulation scenarios focus on substance abuse, suicidal ideation, blood pressure management, non-compliant diabetic minor, end-of-life care, and risky behavior with a VP shunt. Including Pre-Licensure Nursing and Behavioral Science (MFT, LPCC, and Social Work) students.
- Fully integrated simulation faculty development training modules which include components of IPE competencies and simulation standards of best practice
  - **Simulation Training Modules Objectives:**
    - Module 1: Why is Simulation Important
      - After completing module 1, learners will reflect on the importance of healthcare simulation within healthcare education.
    - Module 2: History of Simulation
      - After completing module 2, learners will be able to articulate and define the history of healthcare simulation. 3.
    - Module 3: Andragogy of Simulation
      - After completing module 3, learners will be able to articulate and define Andragogy and its relationship to healthcare simulation.
    - Module 4: Best Practices in Simulation
      - After completing module 4, learners will be able to define the standards of best practice simulation as outlined by the Society for Simulation in Healthcare (SSH).
    - Module 5: Simulation Development
      - After completing module 5, learners will be able to articulate the process of best practice healthcare simulation design and incorporate that design into the development of future healthcare simulations.
    - Module 6: Simulation at CBU
      - After completing module 6, learners will be able to identify and articulate the parameters of simulation at California Baptist University (CBU).
    - Module 7: Pre-Briefing and Debriefing
      - After completing module 7, learners will be able to articulate, define, and utilize appropriate methods of pre-brief and debriefing in the development and facilitation of healthcare simulation.
    - Module 8: Evaluation and Data Collection
      - After completing module 8, learners will be able to articulate and define the importance of evaluation and data collection related to best practice simulation design.
  - **Simulation Training Modules Lessons Learned:**
    - These modules have worked well to provide asynchronous simulation training to both current and incoming faculty.

- The ability to offer Continuing Education Units (CEUs) has led to the success of creating incentives for faculty to complete the modules. However, in recent years the decision has been made to require the modules to be completed by all new incoming faculty as part of their process. CEUs are still provided, but the modules are now a requirement.
- A negative of the training modules is that they have to be periodically updated to reflect current trends and changes in simulation-based education. These new updates must be disseminated to faculty who have already completed the modules; this can be a lengthy and sometimes difficult process to track.
- Creating incentives for non-nursing faculty who participate in IPE simulation-based learning activities within the program has been difficult, as CEUs can only be offered to Registered Nurses (RN) within the program. Working with the collaborating disciplines program leads early in the process of new IPE integrations and development of simulation activities to create incentives and expectations has helped to mitigate this difficulty and provide IPE faculty with appropriate and supportive simulation training prior to leading IPE simulation-based learning activities with their students.

- A fully integrated IPE curriculum across seven graduate healthcare programs consisting of 3 courses that are taken within their individual program. Each course program may insert its students at slightly different intervals while meeting the requirements of the curriculum. The three courses are IPE Exposure, IPE Immersion, and IPE Competence. The curriculum is aligned with the IPEC competency domains and is reviewed annually by the multidisciplined IPE faculty committee.

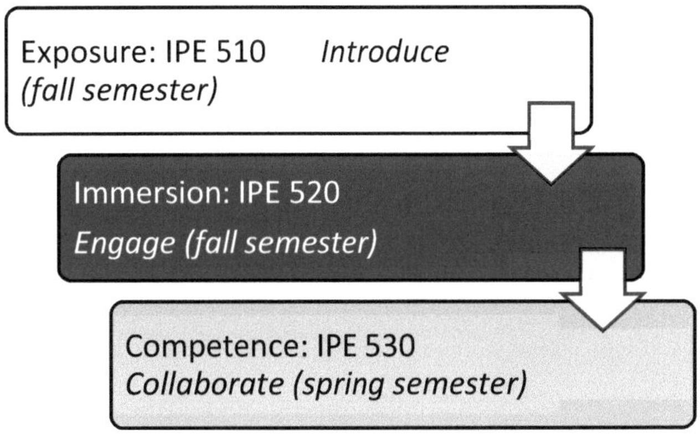

- IPE Immersion course is designed to engage intermediate learners in activities that continue to build upon the IPE competencies while integrating multifaceted active teaching methods such as various interprofessional simulations, community-based projects, service learning, and other IPE activities.

– See IPE Curriculum Framework Below:

Framework for Interprofessional Education Curriculum and Core Competencies

	IPE Student Teams		
	Exposure: Introduction	**Immersion:** Development	**Competence:** Entry-to-Practice
Curriculum	Introduce learners early in their educational programs to engage in activities that offer knowledge-based information, focused on "describing roles and responsibilities" and "demonstrating awareness of interprofessional (IP) communication and teamwork in the context of shared curricular topics required across health professions. An introductory level hybrid course of Inter-Professional Education Collaborative (IPEC) competencies and an end-of-course seminar for all students will be required.	Engage intermediate learners in their educational program together through their own programs activities that provide opportunities to continue to build upon IPE competencies. Programs will integrate multifaceted active teaching methods such as simulation, problem-based learning, clinical practicum, community–based projects, service-learning, and other IPE activities.	Integrate advanced learners to work collaboratively as appropriate, to assess, plan, provide care/intervention, and make decisions to optimize client/patient, family, and community health outcomes and improve quality of care through a university-wide IPE simulation. Students will draw upon previously learned knowledge, skills, and attitudes related to the four domains of IPE education to effectively apply leadership qualities that support collaborative practice, and team effectiveness.
Competency Domain 1: Values and Ethics for Interprofessional Practice	**Knowledge** • Describe IP team dynamics as they relate to individual team members' values and the impact on team functioning in ethical dilemmas. • Describe the nature of IP ethical reasoning and justification. **Skill / Behavior** • Identify IP ethical issues within a team context. • Utilize the basic skills of reasoning and justification as it relates to identified ethical issues within an IP team. **Attitude** • Reflect on own values, personal and professional, and respect those of other IP team members/clients/families. • Clarify values including accountability, respect, confidentiality, trust, integrity, honesty and ethical behavior, equity as it relates to IP team functioning to maximize quality, safe patient care.	**Skill / Behavior** • Contribute to IPE ethical reasoning and decision-making. **Attitude** • Illustrate respect for values that facilitate ethical behavior as it relates to IP team functioning to maximize quality, safe patient care.	**Skill / Behavior** • Practice ethically in an IP team environment. **Attitude** • Demonstrate an integration of respect and value for the IP team contributions inpatient/client, family, community-centered care.

Faculty insights include but are not limited to the following:

Competency Domain 2: Roles and Responsibilities	**Knowledge** Describe own role, responsibilities, values, and scope of practice effectively to clients/patients/families and other professionals.	**Skill / Behavior** • Accurately describe the roles, responsibilities, and scopes of practice of other professions. Contribute to: - Involving other professions in client/patient, family, and community care appropriate to their roles and responsibilities.	**Skill** • Utilize the full scope of knowledge, skills, and abilities of available health professionals and healthcare workers to provide care that is safe, timely, efficient, effective, and equitable.
Competency Domain 3: Communication	**Knowledge** • Recognize and understand how one's own uniqueness, including power and hierarchy within the IP team, contributes to communication effectiveness.	**Skill/Behavior** • Contribute to effective IP team communication, including: - Giving and receiving feedback, - Addressing conflict or difference of opinions, - Self-reflection. **Attitude** • Awareness of and openness to utilize and develop effective IP team communication	**Skill / Behavior** • Communicate effectively, including giving and receiving feedback. • Apply one's own uniqueness, including experience level, expertise, culture, power, and hierarchy within the healthcare team, contributes to effective communication, conflict resolution, and positive IP working relationships.
Competency Domain 4: Teams and Teamwork	**Knowledge** Describe IP practice with respect to the science and theories behind teamwork. Describe the culture of the IP team that facilitates or inhibits collaboration, and its constraints. Identify instances where IP care will improve client/patient, family, community outcomes.	**Skill** Effective decision-making in IP teamwork utilizing judgment and critical thinking. - Team effectiveness through reflection on IP team function.	**Skill / Behavior** • Collaborate with others, as appropriate, to assess, plan, provide care/intervention and make decisions to optimize client/patient, family, and community health outcomes. • Apply leadership practices that support IP team collaboration and effectiveness. **Attitude** •Focus on patients, populations and communities to deliver effective health care. •Advocate for the health of patients and communities.

- IPE simulation development should begin early (e.g., 5–6 months in advance of planned implementation/integration)
- Involvement and participation of lead faculty from each program from the beginning of the development process
- Starting with the establishment of shared objectives across disciplines for the simulation-based learning activity
- Formal and ongoing evaluation of the simulation activity to ensure alignment with program and curriculum objectives and participant outcomes. *(An evidenced based and validated tool should be chosen for the evaluation process, which aligns with SSH accreditation standards and IPEC competencies)*
- Appropriate faculty development for all lead simulation faculty
- Maintaining certification and accreditation through SSH
- Early cultivation of shared understanding and respect for the roles and responsibilities of the team members involved
- Early mapping of simulation activity to the appropriate IPEC competency (see Template)

Conclusion

Interprofessional education, which integrates IPE-based simulation learning activities, is a valuable and vital component of any healthcare professional education program. Through the use of the IPE model of faculty development related to engaging, training, and mentoring, programs can advocate for the development of faculty who feel that they are a valuable member of the team, have a voice, and are able to utilize various tools and methodologies to meet IPE related program accreditation standards. Faculty can utilize the eleven-criterion INACSL simulation design standards of best practice and Sim-IPE four-criterion simulation design process to develop IPE simulation-based learning activities, which support overarching program goals and accreditation standards. With the recognition that all graduate healthcare programs differ and are related to an organization's individual resources, mission, and needs, there is the understanding of a common core set of curricular components required for the successful implementation of any IPE program. Through the utilization of simulation best practice standards and IPEC competencies, programs can develop and integrate IPE simulation-based learning activities and curricula, which supports the development and graduation of collaborative practice-ready healthcare professionals.

References

1. Kohn LT, Corrigan JM, Donaldson MS. Institute of Medicine (US) Committee on Quality of Health Care in America. In: To err is human: building a safer health system. Washington, DC: National Academies Press (US); 2000.
2. Committee on Measuring the Impact of Interprofessional Education on Collaborative Practice and Patient Outcomes, Board on Global Health, Institute of Medicine. Measuring the impact of interprofessional education on collaborative practice and patient outcomes. Washington (DC): National Academies Press (US); 2015.
3. Interprofessional Education Collaborative Expert Panel. Core competencies for interprofessional collaborative practice: report of an expert panel. Washington, DC: Interprofessional Education Collaborative; 2011.
4. Reeves S. Ideas for the development of the interprofessional education and practice field: an update. J Interprof Care. 2016;30(4):405–7. https://doi.org/10.1080/13561820.2016.1197735.
5. Society for Simulation in Healthcare. Society for Simulation in Healthcare (SSH) accreditation CORE standards and measurement criteria. 2016, May. Retrieved April 12, 2021, from https://www.ssih.org/Portals/48/Accreditation/2016%20Standards%20and%20Docs/Core%20Standards%20and%20Criteria.pdf.
6. Watts PI, Peterson T, Brown M, Peterson DT, White T, Epps C, White ML. Faculty reflections on effective strategies utilized to implement simulation-enhanced IPE for future health care providers. Clin Simul Nurs. 2020;46(1):22–9. https://doi.org/10.1016/j.ecns.2020.03.005.
7. Herrera, D. Called2Collaborate: Interprofessional Education (IPE) Faculty Development Program [Doctoral dissertation], 2014.
8. Chappell K, Regnier K, Travlos DV. Leading by example: the role of accreditors in promoting interprofessional collaborative practice. J Interprof Care. 2018;32(4):404–6.
9. Xavier N, Brown MR. Interprofessional education in a simulation setting [Updated 2020 May 31]. In: StatPearls. Treasure Island (FL): StatPearls Publishing; 2021. Available from: https://www.ncbi.nlm.nih.gov/books/NBK557471/.
10. Watts PI, McDermott DS, Alinier G, Charnetski M, Ludlow J, Horsley E, Meakim C, Nawathe P. Healthcare simulation standards of best PracticeTM. Clin Simul Nurs. 2021;58:14–21. https://doi.org/10.1016/j.ecns.2021.08.018
11. INACSL Standards Committee. INACSL standards of best practice: Simulation[SM] simulation-enhanced interprofessional education (Sim-IPE). Clin Simul Nurs. 2016;12:S34–8. https://doi.org/10.1016/j.ecns.2016.09.011.

25 Assessing Learning in Graduate Education Simulation

Garrett K. Chan

Background

Nursing education is at a crossroads. Dr. Patricia Benner and colleagues [1] called for a radical transformation in nursing education. One of the major paradigm shifts in the radical transformation is moving teaching and learning away from abstract theoretical classroom teaching and applying that theory and change to teaching for a sense of salience and situated knowledge use. Said in another way, teaching and learning should reinforce an interpretive, dialogical use of theory **in** practice. The Macy Foundation [2] convened an expert panel to advocate for the health professions to move to a competency-based, time-variable curriculum that supports successful practice development and the American Association of Colleges of Nursing [3] revised the Essentials for professional nursing education. These new essentials focus on competency development as the foundation of nursing curricula.

Simulation is essential in learning high-risk and low-frequency or high-stakes situations. The simulation environment, if following the International Nursing Association for Clinical Simulation and Learning (INACSL) standards for best practice simulation [4], can effectively help learners develop a sense of salience and situated knowledge used to develop their nursing practice to work toward competency. Additionally, simulation integrates the five aspects of effective teaching in higher education articulated by Dr. Joshua Eyler [5]: curiosity, sociality, emotion, authenticity, and failure. These five aspects are essential in developing teaching and learning activities to engage learners and to build curricula that are maximally effective in achieving desired learning objectives and competence.

In creating either a simulation curriculum or individual simulation activities, faculty need to plan for evaluation of the efficacy of teaching and learning, and planning for evaluation is as important as planning the actual simulation scenarios. Understanding evaluation frameworks and theories is essential for simulation faculty to understand learning styles, clinical performance, and competence. Therefore, this chapter aims to review three theories and frameworks focused on learning and learning evaluation for faculty to adopt when creating simulation activities and assessing learner performance and competence.

VARK: Visual, Aural, Read/Write, Kinesthetic

Simulation is essential to develop a practice in a safe environment. Traditional teaching pedagogies have focused on teaching theories and the application of those theories in practice. Conversely, simulation helps learners develop a sense of salience and asks learners to engage in situations with an interpretive, dialogical use of theory in practice. This change from a purely cognitive application of theory to a dialogical use of theory in practice may be easier for some learners than others depending on learning styles.

We know learners learn best when their preferences for receiving information and engaging in curriculum topics match the teaching activities. Understanding learning styles and metacognition is helpful to faculty in planning simulation events because all learners receive and process information differently. A comprehensive learning style assessment could include aspects such as what time of day someone best learns, whether the person learns best by themselves or in a group, or whether ambient noise or silence help learning. One additional aspect of metacognition and understanding learning styles focuses on the modal preferences of receiving, perceiving, and conveying information a person has. One popular model to assess this aspect of learning style is the VARK model. VARK is an acronym for **v**isual, **a**ural, **r**ead/write, and **k**inesthetic and was created by Fleming and Mills [6].

G. K. Chan (✉)
University of California, San Francisco, CA, USA
e-mail: Garrett.Chan@ucsf.edu

J. M. Kutzin et al. (eds.), *Comprehensive Healthcare Simulation: Nursing*, Comprehensive Healthcare Simulation,
https://doi.org/10.1007/978-3-031-31090-4_25

Visual learners prefer using graphic ways to receive information and communicate. These learners respond well to and convey information through charts, graphs, diagrams, outlines, or process maps. Information is understood and communicated in a symbolic form. Aural, or auditory, learners prefer listening to information. They learn best from lectures, discussions, and tutorials. Aural learners prefer to engage in conversation to learn and communicate. Read/write learners prefer information printed as words or text and learn through the printed words of others. These learners prefer reading books, lists, or diaries. Kinesthetic learners, estimated to be the largest type of learner, learn best through experience and practice by utilizing multiple senses of sight, touch, hearing, smell, and taste. Kinesthetic learners prefer concrete experiences such as case studies, simulations, or problem-solving through real-life examples. It is common to have multiple modal preferences. These multi-modal learners can have two, three, or all four modal preferences and likely will engage more with the topics and teaching if the pedagogies use multiple modalities.

Faculty may want to consider two things if a learner needs help during simulation scenarios or with simulation in the curriculum. First, how are the faculty preparing or briefing students before the simulation scenario? Faculty can assess the modal preferences of learners through an online assessment tool found at https://vark-learn.com/. By assessing the modal preferences, faculty can create briefing materials to help situate the learner for the simulation scenario.

Second, faculty should ensure that all modal preferences are included in the facilitation and debriefing of the scenarios. Simulation faculty often rely heavily on an interactive discussion in the debriefing sessions. Adding summative diagrams, outlines, or process maps in the debriefing can help visual learners. Articles or websites can also be given as reference documents for read/write learners. While these adjunct teaching materials are helpful, faculty should reinforce to the learners that nursing is not solely theoretical but is thinking-in-action and engagement with patients, families, communities, and interprofessional colleagues. So, the immersive simulation experience needs to encourage solely visual, aural, and read/write learners to become more kinesthetic in their learning.

Honey & Mumford Learning Styles Questionnaire

Peter Honey and Alan Mumford [7] identified four distinct styles of preferences people use while learning: activists, theorists, pragmatists, and reflectors. They created the Learning Styles Questionnaire, an 80-item questionnaire designed to assess which learning style is dominant in a learner. An online version of the LSQ can be found at www.mint-hr.com/mumford.html. Honey and Mumford suggest that most learners follow one or two of these styles.

Activists learn by doing. They learn best when involved in new experiences, problems, and opportunities; thrown into situations where they need to solve problems, engage in role-playing exercises; and lead a group. They are disengaged from learning when they have to listen to lectures, read long explanations, work independently, analyze or interpret lots of data, or follow precise instructions.

Theorists learn by understanding the theory behind the actions. They need concepts, models, and facts in order to learn. They focus on analysis and synthesis to create a theory, and they sometimes feel uncomfortable with subjective judgments. Theorists learn best when the activity is supported by ideas and concepts that form a model or theory, are in a structured situation with a clear purpose, have the chance to question and investigate the situation, and need to understand the complex situation. Theorists do not learn in situations where emotions and feelings are emphasized, activities are unstructured and ambiguous, and they are asked to act without knowing the principles or concepts involved in the situation.

Pragmatists prefer to try putting learning into practice in the real world by looking for new ideas that can be applied to the problem. They experiment with new ideas and theories to check whether they work. They learn best by thinking about how to apply learning in reality through case studies, problem-solving, and discussions. They learn least when there is no apparent practical benefit, there are no clear guidelines or theories to solve an issue, or the issue is completely a cognitive, theoretical problem.

Reflectors learn by observing and thinking about what happened. They prefer to gather data and consider all the possible perspectives and implications before considering an opinion. They spend time listening and observing and tend to be cautious and thoughtful. Often, they prefer to stand back and watch from the periphery. Reflectors learn best through paired discussions, self-analysis questionnaires, taking time out for reflection, observing activities, seeking feedback from others, and are given time to think and investigate before commenting or acting. Reflectors learn least when forced to lead a group, do things without preparation, or rush into action.

Similar to the VARK model, simulation faculty can use the Honey and Mumford framework to evaluate the learners' style of learning and engagement in the simulation. By understanding the learning style, faculty can help learners process their inherent learning styles and find ways to engage all learning styles in the simulation experience to develop their nursing practice. For example, by understanding how each learning style learns best and the detractors to learning, simulation faculty can ensure briefing, simulation scenarios, and debriefing support learning and diminish detractors to learning.

Kirkpatrick Model of Training Evaluation

Fundamental in teaching and learning in graduate academic environments is the development of skill acquisition, clinical reasoning and decision-making, and embodiment and formation as a clinician, educator, leader, administrator, and scientist. Simulation programs must evaluate the success of the education and training in the curriculum. One training and education evaluation model is the Kirkpatrick Model of Training Evaluation [8]. This model has been modified since the 1950s, and the newest version, the New World Kirkpatrick Model, has four levels: (1) reaction, (2) learning, (3) behavior, and (4) results.

Level 1, reaction, focuses on the degree to which participants find the training favorable, engaging, and relevant to their learning. Learners should feel engaged, find value, and perceive the relevance of what they learned and apply it to their practice as a first step in understanding teaching effectiveness. It is important to measure reactions because it helps the faculty understand how well the learners received the education, and it can help improve the educational experiences for future learners, including identifying important areas or topics missing from the simulation experience. Interviews, surveys, and Likert scale reaction questions in the domains of engagement, value, and relevance can assess the reaction to the simulation scenarios and curriculum.

Level 2, learning, assesses the degree to which learners acquire the intended knowledge, skills, attitudes, confidence, and commitment based on the educational event. The learning objectives of the simulation scenario will be clearly articulated in the simulation design, outcomes, and objectives. Measuring or evaluating all of the dimensions of Level 2—knowledge, skills, attitudes, confidence, and commitment—are essential in understanding the efficacy of simulation teaching. In a simulation, it is easy to understand if knowledge and skills are being applied in the simulation. In debriefing, understanding the attitudes, confidence, and commitment can be elucidated in the discussion. According to the INACSL standards of best practices, sensitive debriefing is essential in providing a psychologically safe environment to assess Level 2 dimensions.

Level 3, behavior, is the degree to which the participants apply what they learned during the educational event in the clinical setting or their job. Behavior change can only happen if the learner has had favorable Level 1 and 2 experiences. Behavior change can only happen if the environment supports the behavior through supportive work environments, interpersonal relationships, structures, and processes. The link between simulation scenarios and precepted clinical practice experiences should be in alignment and reinforce behavior change through positive reinforcement. Preceptor evaluations, observations in simulation scenarios, 360-degree feedback, and self-reported behavior changes are examples of measuring Level 3.

Level 4, results, is the degree to which targeted outcomes occur due to the education, support, and accountability to the education and behavior change. Level 4 evaluation looks at macro-level outcome metrics that reflect the efficacy of the education and training and represents the impact on the practice, business, employee satisfaction, and return on investment. A practice and return on investment metric example could be the incidence of surgical site infections after a surgical simulation and the impact on payor reimbursement due to complications. These metrics may be difficult to measure in graduate education; however, Level 4 outcome metrics are essential in ensuring high-quality and safe patient care sustained over time.

Graduate programs should incorporate at least Levels 1, 2, and 3 in their assessment and evaluation of the simulation scenarios and curricula. Getting real-time feedback can improve the simulation programs in the spirit of continuous process improvement.

Conclusion

Simulation scenarios and curricula play an important role in graduate nursing education. It helps in the formation of learners to practice at the graduate level. Not all learners learn in the same way. Some are engaged, kinesthetic, and activists. Others are read/write and reflectors. Simulation faculty should be aware of the different types of preferred modes of learning and learning styles to ensure that the simulation experience can support all types of learners. Additionally, assessing and evaluating the simulation program and curriculum from a Kirkpatrick Model [8] of Training is essential for continuous process improvement.

References

1. Benner P, Sutphen M, Leonard V, Day L. Educating nurses. In: A call for radical transformation. San Francisco: Jossey-Bass; 2010.
2. Lucey CR. Achieving competence-based, time-variable health professions education. In: Proceedings of a conference sponsored by Josiah Macy Jr. Foundation. New York, NY: Josiah Macy Jr. Foundation; 2017.
3. American Association of Colleges of Nursing. The essentials: core competencies for professional nursing education. American Association of Colleges of Nursing; 2021. April 6; [cited 2021 May 11]. Available from: https://www.aacnnursing.org/Portals/42/AcademicNursing/pdf/Essentials-2021.pdf

4. International Nursing Association for Clinical Simulation and Learning. INACSL standards of best practice: Simulation^{SM}. 2021; [cited 2021 May 11]. Available from: https://www.inacsl.org/inacsl-standards-of-best-practice-simulation/.
5. Eyler J. How humans learn. In: The science and stories behind effective college teaching. Morgantown: West Virginia University Press; 2018.
6. Fleming ND, Mills C. Not another inventory, rather a catalyst for reflection. To Improve Academy. 1992;11:137–55.
7. Honey P, Mumford A. The manual of learning styles. London: Peter Honey Associates; 1982.
8. Kirkpatrick JD, Kirkpatrick WK. Kirkpatrick's four levels of training evaluation. Alexandria, VA: Association for Talent Development; 2016.

Simulation for Nursing Leadership Development

26

K. T. Waxman and Christine Delucas

The greatest leader is not necessarily the one who does the greatest things. He/she is the one that gets the people to do the greatest things.—Ronald Reagan

Introduction

Simulation is an effective tool in preparing nurses for leadership positions and for enhancing current leaders' knowledge and competencies. Many graduate programs have integrated simulation into leadership and organizational change courses. As leaders, we have used role play in multiple scenarios over time. Given that there is a nursing shortage, in leadership positions in particular, simulation can be used for succession planning and professional development. [1] We all know those nurses who were promoted into leadership and management positions because they were great clinical nurses but had little or no skills in leadership. Over the years, we have validated that simulation can make a difference in learning and application to practice. Simulation has been more clearly defined, and we can use the tools and skills we have acquired to apply to preparing nurses for leadership positions, hiring, and returning to work.

It is often thought that simulation only occurs in a specifically designed center and in person. The proliferation of online leadership educational programs, and subsequently the pandemic of 2020, provides a challenge to simulation. The synchronous virtual environment provides a safe environment for students to experience and develop leadership skills.

High-fidelity simulation occurs primarily in three areas: physical, functional, and psychological. Leadership simulations often rely more heavily on psychological fidelity, though more challenging to achieve than it is cognitive in nature [2]. However, leadership simulations are easily completed in areas outside of a center and may not require expensive equipment, provided the environment allows for participation and observation followed by debriefing. Offices and conference rooms, in person or virtual, all offer appropriate simulation experiences.

This chapter will review key points in creating simulation scenarios for leadership development, and examples will be shared.

K. T. Waxman (✉)
University of California, San Francisco, UCSF School of Nursing, San Francisco, CA, USA
e-mail: KT.Waxman@ucsf.edu

C. Delucas
College of Nursing, University of New Mexico, Albuquerque, NM, USA

Context

Simulation is not all manikin based. There are multiple types of simulation: role play; virtual reality; computer-based learning; standardized participants; task trainers; and manikin-based simulation. For leadership development, you may use a combination of these types, depending on your learning objectives. For example, a leadership scenario could occur in a simulated patient room with a manikin with the focus on the charge nurse or nurse manager needing to make an important decision. The scenario may occur in a board room setting, around a table, with the learner presenting a budget to the C-suite executives.

When creating a scenario, consider developing your learning objectives based on the American Organization for Nursing Leadership's nurse executive or nurse manager competencies, the National League for Nursing, the American Nurses Credentialing Center, or other reputable nursing leadership organization. It is also recommended that the objectives follow the International Nursing Association for Clinical Simulation and Learning's (INACSL) Healthcare Standards of Best Practice: Simulation Outcomes and Objectives [3].

Examples of objectives could include:

- Demonstrate effective communication skills
- Demonstrate situational leadership techniques

J. M. Kutzin et al. (eds.), *Comprehensive Healthcare Simulation: Nursing*, Comprehensive Healthcare Simulation,
https://doi.org/10.1007/978-3-031-31090-4_26

- Utilize leadership strategies in verbal and nonverbal communication
- Provide a presentation to your superior or another group
- Articulate the communication process in response to a complaint
- Analyze the interprofessional dynamics of the group

Case Studies to Consider Using for Leadership Development

Case 1

A large hospital system requires that each hospital within its system have a patient satisfaction score of 90 or above on the HCAPHS. The system as a whole has an average of 77.5 among all its hospitals. One of the key elements in the patient experience is the nursing handoff at the end of each shift, which includes the patient. Compliance with the nursing handoff is low in certain hospitals due to staff perceived barriers and need for management engagement.

The manager (*learner*) of a Medical/Surgical floor has a scheduled meeting with the three Assistant Nurse Managers who oversee the eight-hour shifts to discuss the review of the Patient Experience Scores for the last three months for the unit. The identified area of concern is the need for compliance with the nursing handoff being completed consistently at the change of each shift.

Case 2

This scenario presents the Nurse Manager (*learner*) with a situation in which a senior director/physician is refusing to work with staff. The director/physician complains to the manager that his requests/orders are not fulfilled in a timely manner or not at all.

He/she verbalized that yesterday he requested that a patient be ready for discharge upon his arrival this morning, only to find out this had not occurred, and the patient was transferred to a step-down unit in the middle of the night.

Alternate case for inter-professional: Director requested that specific supplies be ordered for.

today and they are not here.

A staff RN/another employee is standing nearby and overhears the entire conversation.

Case 3

You are the Chief Nursing Officer (CNO) (*Learner*) of a 268-bed acute care hospital. At your last Executive Leadership meeting, your Chief Financial Officer said, "I'm concerned. Our margin is dwindling. If we continue at this rate, we'll need to make cuts, so I recommend an across-the-board budget cut of 15%. We will gain a significant amount to the bottom line as nursing is the largest department." He will be taking this recommendation to the Board of Trustees at their next meeting. The Chief Executive Officer asked you to respond with an executive summary to the board and for you to be prepared to address any questions from the board.

Case 4

You are the Vice President (Learner) for a large provider practice that functions in collaboration with a multi-facility health care system. The physician practice has opened six school-based clinics, each with approximately 500 students and their families. The clinics are open Monday through Friday, days and evenings. Reimbursement is largely Medicaid or self-pay. You have determined that the practice group needs more infrastructure to maintain the clinics. The president of the practice group has asked you to create an executive summary for the hospital board requesting that they assume responsibility for the clinics.

Case 5

A nurse manager (Learner) presents an idea to enhance patient care or decrease costs to his/her Director. The Director likes the idea and asks the nurse manager to create a PowerPoint presentation and present it to senior leadership at their bi-weekly meeting, which occurs next week. The nurse manager complies, and the scenario unfolds to show the learner at the meeting presenting their idea with identification of the problem, the solution, and the return on investment.

Pre-briefing and Debriefing Leadership Scenarios

Pre-briefing

Pre-briefing in leadership development is as important as in the clinical environment. Pre-briefing is defined as [4, p. 37] "an information or orientation session held prior to the start of a simulation activity in which instructions or preparatory information is given to the participants. The purpose of the pre-briefing is to set the stage for a scenario and assist participants in achieving scenario objectives." The pre-briefing should include assigned readings, a review of the case, and objectives. The learner should only enter a scenario if they are pre-briefed.

Debriefing

Debriefing a leadership scenario is critical to facilitate self-reflection and provide feedback. Include all participants in the debriefing and encourage them to provide feedback to the learner in a safe, confidential environment. The debriefing should be approximately twice as long as the scenario itself

Table 26.1 Scenario examples

Communication during a management meeting	Coaching staff nurses
Addressing lateral violence in the workplace	Showing empathy
Difficult conversations with a direct report	Witnessed HIPAA violation and consequences for staff
Listening	NP/RN/MD communications
Integrity	Leading a meeting
Cultural sensitivity	Teamwork and collaboration

and end with how the learner will apply what they have learned to the practice setting. Skilled debriefers are critical, and it is recommended that anyone conducting a debriefing should have attended a course on debriefing either online or in person and that they are open to feedback on their debriefing skills.

Active observers in the simulation can and are encouraged to participate in the debriefing. Often, in leadership scenarios, there is only one learner, and the remainder of the group are actors, so it is important for others to be involved in providing feedback. To keep the observers engaged, consider giving them an assignment such as observing communication or body language, or professionalism (Table 26.1).

Summary

Simulation is an effective tool in leadership development. Using the evidence-based tools already established by the simulation community and in this book, faculty and nurse leaders can utilize these frameworks to prepare students and staff for leadership positions. Ongoing leadership development is important when training emerging leaders, as many learn on the job and can become intimidated by different scenarios that may occur during their work. Increasing confidence and competence can be established through ongoing, evidence-based simulations. Simulation is a great way to allow them to practice and gain confidence in these new roles.

References

1. Waxman KT, Delucas C. Using simulation for succession planning and leadership development. Nurse Leader. 2014;12(5):24–8. https://doi.org/10.1016/j.mnl.2014.07.009.
2. Dow AW, Salas E, Mazmanian PE. Improving quality in systems of care: solving complicated challenges with simulation-based continuing professional development. J Contin Educ Heal Prof. 2012;32(4):230–5. https://doi.org/10.1002/chp.21150.
3. International Nursing Association for Clinical Simulation and Learning Standards Committee. INACSL standards of best practice: simulation outcomes and objectives. Clin Simul Nurs. 2016;12:S13–5. https://doi.org/10.1016/j.ecns.2016.09.005.
4. Lioce L, Loprieto J, Chang TP, Robertson JM, Anderson M, Diaz DA, Spain AE, editors. Healthcare simulation dictionary. 2nd ed. Rockville (MD): Agency for Healthcare Research and Quality; 2020. 75 p. Publication No. 20–0019. https://doi.org/10.23970/simulationv2.

Part IV

Simulation for Continuing Professional Development

Simulation Modalities for Nursing Professional Development

27

Susan Doolittle and Virginia Riggall

Background

Simulation, in its many forms, is not a new phenomenon in professional healthcare education. Evidence shows that rudimentary task trainers were in use in the mid-eighteenth century to train midwives how to assist women in giving birth [1]. High-fidelity human simulators were first developed in the 1960s in academic settings. However, they did not become commonly used until the technology advanced enough to allow the production of lower-cost, easier-to-use manikins [2]. Standardized patients were first introduced into medical school curricula in the 1960s and are now commonly used to educate healthcare professionals in academic settings [3].

Although the use of simulation in healthcare education began in academia, the changing environment of healthcare has driven healthcare organizations to adopt simulation as one strategy to prepare healthcare professionals to adapt to changing demands. Increasing complexity in the healthcare system, evolving regulatory and accreditation requirements, increasing focus on improving patient safety, changing healthcare reimbursement practices by third-party payers, public reporting of healthcare outcomes, and increasing demands by patients for care to be provided in a caring and empathic manner have all led some healthcare organizations to the use of simulation as one means for preparing healthcare workers to manage the demands of their professions.

It is difficult to ascertain to what extent healthcare organizations use simulation to meet their staff's continued professional development needs. Healthcare organizations vary widely in size, structure, resources, and affiliations with academic institutions. Diversity in patient populations served and the types of care provided at an institution will also affect if and how institutions use simulation to meet their needs. A 2018 survey of acute care hospitals' use of simulation in the United States revealed that among the survey participants, task trainers were used by 91%, low-fidelity simulators were used by 90%, high-fidelity simulators were used by 86%, standardized patients were used by 59%, and computer-based simulation was used by 48%. Simulation was mainly used for education but also used to a lesser extent for interprofessional education, system testing, and patient/family education. Identified barriers to using simulation in acute care hospitals include cost, lack of space, lack of supplies, lack of equipment, lack of leadership support, and staff being too busy to participate. A 3% response rate severely limits the findings from this survey [4].

The future of simulation for professional development will likely be shaped by research studying the effects of simulation on patient outcomes, learning outcomes, and cost-effectiveness. The simulation will continue to evolve as more common practices in academia become more commonplace in medical centers, such as expanding the use of standardized patients for training with frontline staff to develop and maintain the interpersonal skills required when working with patients. One area of simulation that is beginning to get more traction is the use of extended reality technologies that include virtual reality, augmented reality, and mixed reality to provide a means for staff to participate in simulation exercises for professional development.

Best Practices

Successful simulation programs require more than fancy equipment and state-of-the-art simulation labs. High-tech equipment and simulation labs may not be required at all. A successful program clearly understands what outcome is to

S. Doolittle (✉)
Kaiser Permanente Santa Rosa Medical Center, Santa Rosa, CA, USA
e-mail: susan.j.doolittle@kp.org

V. Riggall
Kaiser Permanente, Risk & Patient Safety Northern California Region, Santa Rosa, CA, USA
e-mail: virginia.k.riggall@kp.org

J. M. Kutzin et al. (eds.), *Comprehensive Healthcare Simulation: Nursing*, Comprehensive Healthcare Simulation,
https://doi.org/10.1007/978-3-031-31090-4_27

be achieved for the healthcare organization and what resources are available to achieve the desired outcome. For this reason, staff development personnel must clearly understand each simulation modality so that simulation programs can acquire the resources needed so that the best modality can be chosen for the learners to achieve the learning objectives. Simulation modalities are not created equal. Each modality has advantages and disadvantages that need to be considered when determining how to structure a simulation exercise or how to use finite resources when developing a simulation program to meet the organization's needs.

Task Trainers

There is an incredible array of task trainers for simulation educators to consider when determining what is needed for a simulation program. Task trainers come in all shapes and sizes. They range from simple to complex. Some are inexpensive (costing a few dollars), and some are considerably more expensive, costing several thousand dollars. Some task trainers can be constructed by an educator using supplies readily available at the local grocery or hardware store, and some are available only through companies specializing in simulation equipment. Some task trainers are so simple that they can be operated without instruction; other more complex models may require many hours of specialized training to operate safely.

Task trainers are generally less expensive than full-body simulators, and they are usually smaller and easier to store than full manikins. They are used primarily in developing or maintaining psychomotor skills through deliberate practice of the specific steps of a procedure. Task trainers offer the advantage of allowing learners to practice these skills in a low-risk environment on a relatively inexpensive piece of equipment instead of on a very expensive simulator or with patients or colleagues, as was commonplace in the past in nursing education. The primary limitation of task trainers is that they often serve only one purpose and may be less useful in more complex simulations with objectives that focus on clinical judgment, interactions with a patient or family, or teamwork.

Simulation Manikins

Simulation manikins vary greatly in size, purpose, cost, ease of use, and ability to simulate the physiology of human responses to conditions commonly encountered in healthcare. Simulation manikins can range from low-fidelity plastic body forms that are completely static to high-tech simulators that are controlled by computers and can simulate a variety of physiological states and respond to various actions taken by the simulation participants. Simulation manikins are ideal when the objectives require the learners to consider a broad range of physiological responses in a healthcare situation. When considering the differences between a task trainer and a manikin, the educator will decide which equipment best suits the scenario objectives. For example, in a scenario about cardiac resuscitation, a task trainer may be helpful for participants to learn how to effectively provide chest compressions and artificial ventilation. A high-fidelity manikin can allow learners to do compressions and ventilation, interpret the cardiac rhythm, defibrillate, intubate, inject medications, evaluate the patient's response to them, feel pulses, and check pupil responses, among other activities. If the objectives for the simulation are about the basic life support skills of chest compressions and artificial respiration, a CPR task trainer may be all that is needed. If the objectives include aspects of resuscitation care beyond that, a high-fidelity manikin is better.

Simulation manikins offer many advantages for the educator to consider when planning an educational activity, but some limitations must be considered. Simulation manikins can simulate many human physiological states, but there are some conditions that manikins cannot recreate effectively. For example, many manikins' limbs cannot be articulated in a manner that resembles normal human flexibility. Also, many manikins can demonstrate acrocyanosis by having a blue light shine in the manikin's mouth. However, they cannot create other skin hues that are part of the human experience, such as mottling or pallor. In addition, manikins cannot create authentic-appearing grand mal seizures.

High-fidelity simulators take time to set up, program, and take down, and this investment of educator time may not be feasible for every program. Simulation manikins may be programmed for certain pre-recorded sounds or phrases but require special equipment for an educator to be 'the voice of the patient' in real-time. Having an educator provide the voice for the manikin may lower the fidelity of the simulation if the scenario is being conducted in situ and the participants can hear or see the person who is providing the voice. Simulation objectives focusing primarily on communication, caring, empathy, and other interpersonal skills will be better achieved by having learners interact with a live human instead of a manikin.

Some simulation manikins have capabilities that are not needed to achieve the learning objectives for a given scenario. Some novice educators may be enticed to use those features when they are unnecessary because they are fun and interesting but may distract learners from the scenario's objectives. An example of this phenomenon is some novice educators wanting to include unneeded vomiting sounds or pupil reactions when those things are not necessary for the learners to achieve the scenario objectives. Lastly, simulators are complex, computer-run machines. They can be prone to unexpected hardware problems and software glitches that can disrupt the learning flow if the educator needs to troubleshoot a problem in the middle of a program.

The variety of available simulators on the market makes it imperative that those charged with purchasing simulators do so in a manner that demonstrates sound clinical, educational, and business decisions for their organization [5].

Standardized Patients

Standardized patients (SPs) are people trained to play patients or family members in simulations, evaluate aspects of the participant's performance and provide feedback to learners. The term "simulated patients" is also sometimes used.

Standardized patients are most commonly used in undergraduate medical education for training and evaluating medical students. Some advanced practice nursing programs also use standardized patients to prepare their students for work in the healthcare industry. Use of standardized patients is less commonly used in staff development for nurses in the service sector. The term "standardized patient" is often used broadly in simulation literature, usually to describe simulations where the learners are not using a simulation manikin but are interacting with a live human. Whether or not it is important for people playing the part of patients in simulations to be standardized depends on the purpose of the simulation. For simulations run as high-stakes exams where learners are evaluated to determine if they are competent to practice or advance in their education, standardization of the humans playing the patient is extremely important so that all participants have the same opportunity to demonstrate their abilities. However, some degree of standardization is important, even if the simulations are not high-stakes exams. Simulations done to provide training or deliberate practice need some degree of standardization so all participants have the same opportunity to achieve the scenario's objectives.

Standardized patients may be professionals who are hired to perform this role, volunteers from the community, hospital staff who are assigned to help with education, or participants in a course whom the course facilitator assigns to act as the patient or family member with little or no direction regarding how to accomplish the assignment.

Standardized patients, to be effective, at a minimum, need to be trained on the course's learning objectives, the expectations of the SP, the details of the current problem, relevant past medical and social history, how to simulate specific signs or symptoms to be displayed during the scenario, how to answer questions that would be commonly asked of the patient in the scenario, and how to simulate the emotional condition of the patient. To provide effective feedback, SPs need to be trained on the parameters of appropriate feedback [6]. Standardized patients must also be given directives about helping participants struggling during the simulation. If help is to be offered, it needs to be communicated to the person playing the patient before the simulation on how that help should be given. Standardized patients also need to know how to answer questions that come up that were not specifically covered in the training.

For nurse educators, it is often necessary to limit the number of participants in a simulation so all participants can participate. This reality often requires that educators frequently run the same simulation many times. If the simulations are using standardized patients, many SPs may be needed to cover multiple sessions. If this is the case, all the SPs must be trained together to understand the purpose of the simulations, the learning objectives, the SP's role in the scenario, and training directives about the expectations for their performance. If the SPs are to give feedback to the learners during the debriefing, SPs must be trained on techniques to give feedback to learners so that psychological safety for learners is maintained. SPs should also be given specific criteria against which to evaluate learners' performance, and all SPs should have a common understanding of the evaluation criteria. Robust training before the simulation is essential for the success of simulation using standardized patients. It may be tempting for the busy educator to cut corners on this preparation, but poorly prepared standardized patients who unexpectedly adlib can lead learners down a path that is not conducive to meeting the learning objectives. Standardized patients who are not properly trained to evaluate learners or give feedback may cause psychological harm to participants and derail the learners' ability to reflect on the experience and learn from the debriefing.

Standardized patients offer simulation educators advantages over manikins in simulation training. Standardized patients are human beings, and it is easier for some simulation participants to *suspend disbelief* and believe they are in a *real* patient care situation than when they are working with a manikin that is not human. Standardized patients are superior for simulations that focus on interpersonal skills that clinicians use with patients and families. They are also superior, with the proper training, for simulating certain types of patient conditions that require physical movement that simulators cannot authentically replicate. Such movements may include limb movement for the assessment of stroke symptoms, complex behaviors seen in patients suffering from the agitation associated with delirium, or grand mal seizures seen in patients suffering from eclampsia. Standardized patients can also be used to augment manikin-based scenarios to serve as loved ones for the patient, which allows learners the opportunity to practice the skills needed to communicate with family members and manage their behavior in healthcare situations. During debriefing, standardized patients can share the patient's perspectives with learners about how care was perceived.

Standardized patients are not the appropriate modality for every simulation. Simulations that require participants to detect abnormal assessments, such as wheezing during a lung assessment, a specific cardiac rhythm on a monitor, specific pupillary response during a neuro exam, or very weak or bounding pulses, will require the use of a simulation manikin because standardized patients cannot alter their physiology on demand. Standardized patients are human and can be harmed by certain interventions the participants perform. Interventions such as defibrillation, intubation, procedures that break the skin, or painful interventions should be performed on a manikin or task trainer and not a standardized patient.

With the proper training, standardized patients can be used to evaluate certain aspects of physical assessment, such as whether a lung exam is performed according to established criteria. They can also evaluate if the learner asked the appropriate questions during the interaction based on a checklist developed by the scenario author. They cannot, however, evaluate the clinician's clinical judgment.

Not every standardized patient is right for every simulation scenario. Human characteristics like age, gender, size, and appearance all impact the learner's ability to suspend disbelief and engage in the scenario to meet the learning objectives. For very specialized scenarios with objectives that address specific patient populations, it may be difficult to find a standardized patient with the desired characteristics. Suppose the simulation is repeated in multiple training sessions and will require more than one standardized patient. In that case, care must be taken to prepare all the standardized patients to the same criteria so there is standardization across multiple sessions.

It is necessary to differentiate standardized patients from that "embedded simulation persons," previously known as "confederates." Embedded simulation persons are people who play a healthcare team member in a scenario, but they are not part of the target audience for the simulation. Embedded simulation persons may be used with either manikin-based or standardized patient simulations. In continuing nursing education, a common example of an embedded simulated person is using an interested physician to serve as the physician in a nursing scenario when the objectives require the nurse to report a patient's changing condition to the physician. In this example, the physician will receive the report, request additional information as needed, and give orders as indicated. Unlike a standardized patient, the embedded simulated person usually does not have extensive training before the simulation but should have a clear understanding of the scenario objectives, the level of training of the scenario participants, and knowledge of the roles of the simulation participants on the health care team [7].

Extended Reality

Extended reality is the newest frontier in healthcare simulation education. Extended reality is an umbrella term used to describe the various forms of immersive technologies that may be employed in a simulation experience, such as virtual reality (VR), augmented reality (AR), and mixed reality (MR). These technologies differ in the degree of immersive experience for the learner during a simulation. Virtual reality allows learners to only see digital images, whereas augmented reality allows participants to see their physical environment with digital images added. Mixed reality describes blending the student's physical and digital worlds using various devices [8]. Studies have shown that undergraduate nursing students who participated in virtual simulation achieved the desired learning outcomes [9]. However, it is unknown if virtual simulation for continued professional development will demonstrate the same results.

The advantages of extended reality simulation include the ability to have a simulation that allows any number of participants to participate from multiple locations. This simulation training allows participants to participate in training in clinical areas, such as operating rooms, that are challenging to use for other types of simulation. Because the training environment is computer-generated, it does not require a dedicated training space for the training to occur, and learners can participate in the scenario at any time that is convenient for them. Because the virtual simulation patient is computer-generated, that patient can display complex and rare symptoms that would not be possible to simulate with a manikin or a standardized patient. Learners may repeat scenarios as often as needed to achieve the learning objectives.

While extended reality simulation allows for learner flexibility in when they participate and eliminates the need for dedicated training space, those advantages come at a price. Expenses associated with extended reality include the purchase and maintenance of headsets and licensing fees for using the computer platform to run the scenarios. Expenses are associated with training simulation educators to write and program scenarios or contracting with a vendor to create scenarios. Once scenarios are written, there is the ongoing expense of adding new scenarios or updating old ones as healthcare practices change. The other expense, as with all forms of technology, is to replace or update obsolete technology. Another disadvantage is that some learners may become nauseated or claustrophobic while using extended reality headsets [10].

Sample Curriculum

When one thinks of simulation, what comes to mind is often a team exercise involving healthcare clinicians managing a patient whose condition is deteriorating or experiencing a specific event, such as the birth of a child or an operative procedure. Simulation can be used much more broadly than that. Subsequent chapters will detail the use of simulation in more traditional ways in various clinical settings. The following is an example of a simulation program that was developed to deal with the problem of injuries sustained by healthcare workers while assisting patients with mobilization. It was chosen to share in this chapter to illustrate the use of simulation for issues other than what is traditionally addressed with simulation.

Workplace injuries are a significant concern to any healthcare organization. Injured employees create a financial burden for the organization with the cost of replacing injured employees who cannot work, paying injured employees for time off to recover, and providing treatment for the injuries. There is also a human cost for the injured employee who experiences the pain of the injury and the possible long-term consequences the injury may have on the employee's ability to return to work in his or her chosen career. One medical center implemented a robust Workplace Safety Program to manage the risks of injury associated with patient care. The Workplace Safety Program staff are responsible for having the correct patient mobility equipment available on patient care units, training staff on workplace safety practices and use of the patient mobility equipment, analyzing all workplace injuries to determine their root cause, and developing mitigation plans to minimize risks. Analysis of workplace injuries to nursing staff that occurred during patient mobility revealed that although injured workers knew at the time there was a safety risk in their situation, they chose to act in a manner that was not congruent with safety best practices. Some of the reasons for this included pressure from patients and their families for immediate assistance without waiting for help, a sense that safe practices take too long, the staff being too busy to wait for help or equipment to arrive at the bedside, believing that delaying care to assure safety would be detrimental to the patient experience, and mistakenly believing that they would not get injured if they did not follow all the recommended safety practices.

Traditional training methods (online computer modules about safe mobilization techniques and in-person demonstrations of the use of patient mobility equipment) are not designed to address the types of issues that contributed to the injuries that employees experienced. The simulation was identified as an appropriate methodology to address the training and systems issues that appeared to negatively impact workplace safety. Simulation methodology places the learner in a realistic environment. It requires the learners to remember correct safety practices and perform them in real-time in the patient care setting. This allows for not only the training of participants but also system analysis to determine if system issues are contributing to the workplace injury problem.

It was anticipated that the use of standardized patients in the safe patient mobility training would be superior to using a manikin because of the need for a "patient" that could actively participate in a mobility exercise that required the patient to stand, evaluate the participants' communication with the patient during the exercise, and provide feedback to participants about the patient's perception of the care provided during mobilization.

The learning objectives for the patient mobility simulations were as follows: After the training, the participating teams will be able to:

1. Demonstrate caring behaviors and communication with the patient in a patient mobility simulation.
2. Demonstrate safe patient mobility practices in a patient mobility simulation.
3. Demonstrate effective teamwork and team communication during a patient mobility simulation.
4. Discuss systems issues that affect their ability to mobilize patients safely.

The training plan for this simulation program was developed after a needs assessment was conducted with the identified stakeholders, which included the Workplace Safety Leader, the director of Adult Services, the manager of the medical/surgical unit with the highest injury rate, the Patient Mobility manager, and the director of Nursing Education. The focus of the training was to provide an opportunity for nursing teams to practice patient mobility in a scenario with a standardized patient. The scenario was designed to address the root causes of injuries that occurred with patient mobility and to allow the participants to use infrequently used patient mobility equipment in a low-risk, realistic environment. The use of an SP allowed participants to practice communication and caring skills in caring for patients and receive feedback about the patient's perception of the experience.

Eight training sessions were held in 4 weeks. The training was 2 hours in length and included two scenarios. Participants included RNs, patient care technicians (PCTs), and assistant nurse managers in the designated medical/surgical unit with the highest injury rate. Up to 10 participants could be accommodated in each training session.

Large groups (>6 learners) were divided in half, with one group participating in each scenario. Smaller groups participated in both scenarios. All learners participated in the debriefing session after both scenarios.

The training occurred in a closed patient care unit in a semi-private room. The room had one bay for patient care, and the other bay for video-recording equipment. All scenarios were recorded, and the videos were reviewed during the debriefing. Course facilitators were not present in the training room; only the operator of the video equipment was in the room during the scenarios. The video operator was unknown to the participants and did not participate in any way during the scenarios. It is important to note that the decision was made not to have observers in the training room as this affects the participants' behavior during the simulation. The lack of observers and the fact that the participants did not know the SP added greatly to the environmental and psychological fidelity of the training (the degree to which the simulation looked and felt real). This degree of fidelity was vital in achieving the goals of the program.

Participants received a briefing from the Simulation Project manager before participating in the scenario. Various types of patient mobility equipment were present on the unit, and participants were instructed to mobilize the patient according to their professional judgment and facility guidelines for patient mobility. Participants were briefed about the scenario's objectives and reassured that the goal of the simulation was patient mobility and not the identification of possible clinical deterioration of the patient. The briefing also included a brief review of the steps of safe patient mobility based on their previous training using traditional methods.

Participants who were not active in the scenario (either because they were participating in the other scenario or because they had not yet been called into the room to help) were in the nursing station just outside the training room.

Once the scenario was completed, all participants were invited into the training room to debrief and watch the video of the scenario. During the debriefing, participants were asked to analyze the scenario and articulate positive and negative aspects of how the scenario unfolded. Participants were asked to identify anything they would do differently if they could repeat the scenario. Participants were also asked to identify any systems issues that enhanced or diminished their ability to practice safe patient mobilization. The participants watched the video to identify examples of safe practices and practices that were unsafe that occurred during the simulations. The SP from the scenario was present for the debriefing and gave feedback to the participants based on a standardized checklist regarding the patient experience. Participants were invited to ask for feedback from the SP. Participants were also asked to reflect on the experience and identify specifics about how they planned to implement practice changes based on this training. Notes from the debriefing session were captured on a chart pad for later analysis.

Scenario #1 is about an older woman of size who is admitted for heart failure. The cardiologist is adjusting her medications. She had a past medical history of a stroke four years ago and has minimal left-sided weakness. She lives alone and is independent with ADLs. On admission to the hospital yesterday, she was determined not to be a fall risk, and she has been up and ambulating in her room independently. Her Schmidt score was one based on her slight weakness after her stroke. Other information the SP had but was not shared with participants unless they asked was that she has a grown son who is very concerned about her living alone. She is terrified that he will "put her in a home" if she can't care for herself. She is adamant that she must be able to get to the bathroom because if she can't, her son might "put her away somewhere."

This morning, she received a dose of a diuretic and now needs to urinate urgently. Upon standing at the bedside, she becomes slightly dizzy and needs to sit back down. Her vital signs are at baseline. She can bear weight but feels unsteady on her feet. The scenario progresses until the patient gets to the bathroom and returns to the bed. If participants insisted that she try the bedpan or bedside commode, the SP responded, "I can't go using this. I need to use the toilet."

Scenario #2 is about a 30-year-old quadriplegic patient admitted two days ago for pneumonia. The patient's pneumonia is resolving, and the patient expects to be discharged the next morning. The patient has slid down in bed and is now experiencing shortness of breath. The patient's vital signs are at baseline, and the skin color is normal. The patient is lying on a Hovermat. The scenario begins with the participants entering the room, and the patient complains of shortness of breath. The scenario progresses until the patient is repositioned in the bed.

After the simulations, participants completed a four question post-simulation survey that focused on their perceptions of their ability to deal with patient pressure to act immediately in an unsafe manner and their perceptions of their skills in caring communication that maintain the nurse-patient relationship when a delay in care is necessary to maintain safety.

The data gathered from this training came from several sources: the injury rate on the unit where the training occurred, the information shared during the debriefing sessions after each scenario, observations of the course facilitators during the video review, and the post-simulation questionnaire. The results of the analysis of this data are described below.

In general, the participants used safe practices during the patient mobilization simulations. Excellent teamwork and team communication were consistently demonstrated in all scenarios. Teams also consistently demonstrated consideration and discussion of alternatives before deciding on a mobility plan for the patient. Appropriate patient mobility equipment was used in each scenario.

Some safety practices were not consistently used by all the teams and in all scenarios. Some teams did not ask the patients how they could assist during the mobilization process and did not include them in developing the mobilization plan. Some groups of learners did not adequately explain the mobility equipment to the patient, resulting in the patient feeling fearful of the mobilization process. The use of safe patient mobility resources posted in the patient care room was not consistently used by all teams, resulting in consideration of a piece of equipment with a weight limit that made it unacceptable for use with a patient of size.

There were also a few actions that were not congruent with safe practices that occurred during simulations. These were all discussed during the debriefing sessions and while watching the video.

Training participants showed consistent interest and motivation to protect the patient's comfort and dignity. Learners in all groups asked the SP during the debriefing how their actions and words were perceived and asked for recommendations for improvement if warranted. The SP shared specific, observable behaviors (such as when touched, social conversation, or specific instructions) that either enhanced or detracted from a positive patient experience during the scenario.

Mobility Equipment

As with many in situ simulation training exercises, this program revealed system issues that had not yet been identified that are detrimental to safe patient mobility and workplace safety. For example, the piece of equipment that the Patient Mobility manager had identified as the most appropriate equipment for use in the first scenario was avoided by all the participants. The staff shared in the debriefing that this piece of equipment is too large to maneuver easily in a semi-private or cluttered room, is difficult to use because it has many steps to secure the sling correctly, requires more than one person to use, and a second person is often not immediately available, the slings have special cleaning requirements, and the staff struggles to use the process in place for cleaning, and the equipment is not used frequently enough for the staff to feel comfortable using it and they are concerned about the patient's perception of them if they appear to "not know what they are doing."

The course facilitator made several pieces of patient mobility equipment available immediately outside the training room for use during the simulation. The only available equipment was those available on the unit where the participants worked. In the first scenario, when the participant went to survey the available equipment, she stated she wouldn't use any available equipment. She saw a different piece of mobility equipment that was being stored for another unit. She went and got that equipment and used it in the scenario without incident. During the debriefing, the participants all agreed that the equipment that had been used was far superior to the other options. They questioned why that piece of equipment was not available on their unit. Several months before the simulation, the Patient Mobility manager put that piece of equipment on the participants' unit and requested that the staff try it out and provide feedback. The Patient Mobility manager received no feedback in 6 months, so the equipment was removed. The participants in the simulation stated they did not know they were being asked to evaluate the equipment and provide feedback. The participants did, however, provide feedback during the debriefing that the equipment worked well and that they felt they would use consistently on their unit. This information was shared with the Nurse Manager on the unit, and the equipment was ordered and available to use on that unit within a month.

Bedside Staff Competing Mandates

During debriefing sessions, the learners in this program revealed that it is difficult to continually juggle all the competing priorities regarding patient care. The participants acknowledged that the mandates are all intended to improve patient care, but staff found it difficult to meet those standards and take time to maintain their safety while providing care. There was concern that taking appropriate steps to maintain their safety would be detrimental to providing an optimal patient experience, timely medication administration, same-time documentation, and completing all their work while not incurring overtime. Some staff stated that maintaining their safety often fell to the bottom of the list of priorities.

The Use of SPs for Patient Mobility Training

Participants in this simulation program stated that training with this methodology with standardized patients was more effective than traditional methods of patient mobility training. The added element of the "real person" who could give feedback from the patient's perspective was a valuable element of the training. The participants also observed that providing the training in a patient room was an element that made the training more realistic and provided a better learning experience than more traditional methods.

Results

The injury rate improved significantly after this simulation program was completed. The results from the post-simulation questionnaire demonstrated a statistically significant improvement in the staff's self-perceived skill in managing a patient care situation where delays in care were needed to maintain safety and their confidence in maintaining their relationship with the patient who experienced delays in care related to using recommended safety practices.

Based on the initial success of this program, simulation has frequently been included in the training plans for safe patient mobility across the medical center. Aspects of patient mobility that have been deemed problematic, such as consistent use of patient mobility assessments and care for managing patients who display impulsive behavior during mobilization, have been addressed with simulation.

Integrating Simulation into Existing Education

Simulation can be used as an adjunct to the traditional education used for years. When an educator assesses that a problem is appropriate to be addressed with staff training, but the educator is concerned that traditional training methods will not result in the desired change of practice, the educator should consider whether simulation would serve as a useful tool to augment the traditional training.

In one medical center, the care of patients experiencing alcohol withdrawal was identified as problematic. Several changes were planned to address the identified issues. These issues included how physicians order treatment for these patients, how nurses assess this patient population, how nurses communicate patient condition to hospitalist physicians, which medications were used to manage the patient's symptoms and behavior, and the risk of injury to staff when caring for patients who demonstrate combative behavior when experiencing withdrawal.

The standardized physician orders were being updated to reflect updates in the practice guidelines for alcohol withdrawal patients, including nursing assessment parameters and medication administration. The assessment tool for alcohol withdrawal in the electronic medical record was changed to a more robust tool. Analysis of care of patients who experienced sub-optimal outcomes revealed that communication between bedside nurses and hospitalist physicians was not always clear, and the care team was not consistently working with a shared mental model about the status of these patients. The updated treatment protocol included medications that had not been used with this patient population before, and their administration route was unfamiliar to many nurses caring for these patients. To address the workplace injury risks for the staff caring for these patients, caregivers needed training in techniques to maintain their safety during interactions with these patients.

Historically, nurses would have been trained on the new expectations through some combination of online computer modules, videos of new order sets in the electronic medical record, discussions during staff meetings, in-person lectures, and coaching from nurse educators and nurse leaders on the unit. In addition to the usual training, simulation was deemed to be a useful adjunct to the traditional training so the nurses would have the opportunity to practice using the new order sets, the new assessment tool, focused communication with a physician regarding patient condition, administration of the new medications, and communication with the patient and family in a single training opportunity.

Once the decision was made to incorporate simulation into the training to prepare the nursing staff for the changes in the care for these patients, choosing the most appropriate simulation modality for the learning objectives was necessary. The learning objectives for this program are listed. After this program, the participants will be able to:

1. Demonstrate the use of the new physician order sets.
   (a) For this objective, either a standardized patient or simulation manikin would be an appropriate modality for this simulation.
2. Demonstrate correct use of the new assessment tool.
   (a) For this objective, a standardized patient with robust training on the simulation of advancing alcohol withdrawal symptoms, including agitated behavior and specific vocalizations, was deemed superior to using a manikin.
3. Demonstrate the use of SBAR (Situation-Background-Assessment-Recommendation) communication when reporting a change in patient condition to the hospitalist physician.
   (a) For this objective, interaction with a human trained to simulate agitation symptoms was deemed superior to using a manikin for the nurses to practice developing a concise report for a physician that accurately describes the patient's behavior that occurred during the simulation.
4. Demonstrate appropriate application and labeling of transdermal medications to treat alcohol withdrawal symptoms.
   (a) For this objective, a standardized patient or a manikin could reasonably be used for nurses to practice applying and labeling mock transdermal medication patches.
5. Demonstrate caring behaviors while maintaining safety when interacting with a patient experiencing alcohol withdrawal.
   (a) For this objective, the standardized patient is the superior modality for achieving this objective because the standardized patient can provide feedback to participants about the SPs' perception of their care.

After considering the objectives of this program, it was clear that standardized patient simulation was the appropriate modality for the learners to achieve the learning objectives.

A simulation scenario in 3 parts was developed to allow nurses to practice using the three different order sets that would be implemented for this patient population. The three order sets included a set intended for use for patients at risk for developing alcohol withdrawal during their hospital stay, a set for those experiencing mild withdrawal symptoms, and a set for those whose withdrawal symptoms are worsening. The simulation included having participants assess the patient using the new assessment tool, review the appropriate order set based on the assessment, implement appropriate interventions based on the patient assessment, notify the physician of a change in the patient's condition, apply and label mock transdermal medication patches per order, and interact safely with the patient and/or family member in a way that demonstrated caring while maintaining personal safety.

Two standardized patients were used in the scenario. One SP played the patient, and the other was the spouse. Each SP was trained on the purpose of the training, the physiology of alcohol withdrawal, the behavior and speech patterns associated with varying degrees of agitation in withdrawing patients, and common behavior exhibited by close family members who live with patients who suffer from alcohol use disorders.

Before participating in the simulation, learners were assigned online computer modules and instructional videos as an introduction to the changing aspects of care.

Six learners participated in each simulation. The participants included bedside registered nurses, patient care technicians, and nurse leaders on the medical/surgical units. Teams of 2 learners participated in each of the three sections of the simulation. Debriefing occurred after each of the three sections of the scenario. The participants who were not participating could watch the simulation and participated in all debriefings for all three sections of the scenario.

A pre-survey was administered to participants immediately before and after the simulation to assess the participant's perception of the training. The incidence of workplace injuries related to the care of these patients was assessed before and after the training, as well as reports to the Quality department regarding problems associated with the care of these patients. After the training, it was determined that when the patient's agitation was managed appropriately using the new tools, injuries declined, and fewer problems were reported. Participants found the training to be useful.

Challenges and Solutions

Every simulation modality has its challenges. Sometimes when considering which simulation modalities are available to use for a given program, it boils down to which modality presents the fewest challenges or the challenges that are the easiest to overcome. Challenges associated with simulation modalities fall into several common categories: educator time required, space required, equipment/supplies required, and technical expertise required by the facilitator.

Time

All simulation modalities require preparation time. How much time is required to prepare depends on the modality and the complexity of the scenario. Simulators and task trainers must be set up at the training location, assembled if necessary, and necessary equipment and supplies to run the simulation must be acquired and moved to the training site. Simulation computers needed to run manikins or display vital signs for standardized patients take time to set up before the training. Standardized patients need to be trained on how to perform their role, the criteria by which they will be evaluating learners, and feedback techniques if required for the simulation. Educators will also need to consider acquiring any supplies needed for the standardized patients, such as nasal cannulas for each SP who is playing the patient or orthopedic boots in all the sizes needed for SPs in a scenario with an orthopedic patient. Virtual reality will require educators to develop scenarios and program them into the software or consult with the virtual reality company programmers about elements needed in scenarios for each scenario. Educators must be able to accurately predict how much time preparing for a simulation will take based on the modality to be used. Ideally, educators should document the time required for set-up before and take-down after a simulation as a key component to determining the cost of running a simulation and the potential return on investment for the organization. Demonstrating return on investment for simulation programs provides needed evidence to healthcare organization leaders when simulation programs request additional resources.

Space

Space to conduct simulation training is an ongoing challenge for many healthcare organizations. In situ simulation with manikins or standardized patients has the advantage of better environmental fidelity, but the reality of fluctuating hospital census makes in situ training impossible at times. Simulation labs or spaces dedicated to simulation training are not subject to changing patient census. However, they may have scheduling challenges related to sharing space with others in the facility who also need to do training. Simulation spaces often lack enough storage space, electrical outlets, and patient care equipment and supplies to efficient run simulations. The challenge of finding adequate space to run simulations in a dynamic environment will require the educator to partner with hospital leadership to determine if the simulations are a priority for the organization and collaborate with them to find a workable solution. Even with the best-laid plans, it is always a good idea to have a contingency plan for the day of the training in case unforeseen events make last-minute location changes necessary. For organizations with very limited space, extended reality simulation training, which can allow participants to participate from any location, may be a viable solution.

Technical Expertise

Technical expertise for each simulation modality the educator will use will take time to develop and maintain. Using simulation manikins and some task trainers requires the educator to develop and maintain expertise in the programming and troubleshooting of computer equipment and manikins. The simulation educator also needs to plan for the activities needed to maintain the integrity of the equipment, such as computer updates and regular manikin cleaning. The standardized patient simulation requires the educator to effectively train and evaluate the standardized patients and create the documents the SP will need to use, such as training directives and learner evaluation checklists. Many resources are available for interested educators to increase their expertise in various simulation modalities. Simulation professional organizations have various resources available to people interested in learning about various modalities. The Society for Simulation in Healthcare and the Association of Standardized Patient Educators are two well-known organizations. Vendors who sell simulation equipment often have educational services available for a fee or sponsor conferences to help those new to their equipment learn to use it effectively.

Availability of Resources

Every simulation educator has a wish list of things or people that would benefit their simulation program. Most simulation programs, however, have finite resources allocated. This reality makes it necessary for those developing or growing their simulation programs to prioritize what they need based on the goals they are trying to achieve and then pursue the most feasible way to proceed.

Making more simulation modalities available for use will increase the possibility that the educator can use simulation to meet the organization's goals. Several avenues may be pursued to try to acquire resources to increase the availability of simulation modalities.

First, make a business case to the organization's leadership about how simulation can be used for more than just mock codes or other emergencies. Research how other organizations have used simulation to meet their needs. Consider how much the addition of any new simulation modality may cost. Adding equipment involves not only the purchase price but the cost of ongoing maintenance, the cost of training educators to use the equipment, the cost of consumables, and the cost of potential upgrades to infrastructure (such as Wifi capability, availability of electrical outlets, secure storage space) that may be required. Compare the costs with the potential return on investment to see if the organization can find funds for the request.

If funding within the organization is not an option, investigate possible partnerships with outside organizations that have the needed resources. Academic institutions that educate healthcare professionals may already have the resources that a healthcare organization wants to use. Develop relationships with leaders of those academic institutions to determine if a mutually beneficial relationship can be pursued.

Another potential source of funding from outside the healthcare organization is grant funding that may be available from various entities that wish to support the ongoing development of healthcare professionals. Networking with other educators interested in simulation may lead to information about specific organizations that offer funding for simulation projects.

Interface with Regulatory Bodies

Organizations that accredit healthcare organizations or credential healthcare professionals exist to assure that healthcare consumers are protected from organizations or clinicians who are suboptimal and may harm them. These regulatory agencies do not have rules about which simulation modalities are acceptable to use to train healthcare professionals to provide care that meets the needs of their patients. It is incumbent upon the simulation educator to choose the modality that is most likely to provide the best opportunity for the simulation participants to meet the course's learning objectives.

The needs of healthcare consumers, and the clinicians who care for them, are broad and complex. Ideally, the simulation educator has various simulation modalities available to meet these diverse needs.

References

1. Meyer HS, Eldredge JD, Hogan R. History: The king's midwife: a history and mystery of Madame du Coudray. JAMA. 1998;280(24):2131–2. Available from http://jamanetwork.com/journals/jama/fullarticle/1839275. https://doi.org/10.1001/jama.280.24.2131-JBK123-7-1.
2. Bradley P. The history of simulation in medical education and possible future directions. Med Educ. 2006;40:254–62.

3. May W, Park JH, Lee JP. A ten-year review of the literature on the use of standardized patients in teaching and learning: 1996–2005. Med Teach. 2009;31:487–92.
4. Harper MG, Gilbert GE, Gilbert M, Markey L, Anderson K. Simulation use in acute care hospitals in the United States. J Nurses Prof Dev. 2018;34(5):242–9.
5. Sloane FL, Lampotang S. Mannequins: terminology, selection and usage. In: Palaganas JC, Maxworthy JC, Epps CA, Mancini ME, editors. Defining excellence in simulation programs. 1st ed. Philadelphia: Wolters Kluwer; 2015. p. 573–617.
6. Lowens T, Gliva-McConvey G. Standardized patients. In: Palaganas JC, Maxworthy JC, Epps CA, Mancini ME, editors. Defining excellence in simulation programs. 1st ed. Philadelphia: Wolters Kluwer; 2015. p. 618–51.
7. Sanko JS, Shekhter I. Using embedded simulated persons (aka "confederates"). In: Palaganas JC, Maxworthy JC, Epps CA, Mancini ME, editors. Defining excellence in simulation programs. 1st ed. Philadelphia: Wolters Kluwer; 2015. p. 652–85.
8. Foronda CL, Fernandez-Burgos M, Nadeau C, Kelley CN, Henry MN. Virtual simulation in nursing education: a systematic review spanning 1996–2018. Simul Healthc. 2020;15(1):46–54.
9. Andrews C, Southworth MK, Silva JNA. Extended reality in medical practice. Curr Treat Opt Cardiovasc Med. 2019;21(4):18. https://doi.org/10.1007/s11936-019-0722-7.
10. Chang E, Kim HT, Yoo B. Virtual reality sickness: a review of causes and measurements. Int J Hum Comput Interact. 2020;36(17):1658–82.

Writing Clinical Simulations for Continued Professional Development

28

Virginia Riggall and Susan Doolittle

Background

Historically the concept of professional development for nurses began with Florence Nightingale. When she returned from the Crimea War, she worked to promote education for all nurses as an essential component of all healthcare systems. Nightingale advocated for nurses to continue learning throughout their professional life by urging them to remain current and competent in their nursing practice [1]. It would take 70 years until the concept of professional development for employed nurses was formally introduced at the National League for Nursing Education Conference [2]. After World War II, there was a shift in the delivery of healthcare from clients' homes to hospitals [3]. With a growing need to prepare nurses for careers in the acute environment, retraining in the form of "in-service education" became necessary. The nurse educator role was created in many hospitals to provide this training. However, it was not until 1954 that the American Nurses Association (ANA) started to discuss the scope and standards to guide professional development for nurses [2]. In 1975, the ANA published the first guidelines for staff development. It clarified the term "in-service education" as "education and training delivered in the practice setting to facilitate an individual's ability to function within a given agency" [4]. It would take until 1990 for the ANA Council on Continuing Education and Staff Development to publish the first Standards for Nursing Staff Development [2]. With the slow process of developing guidelines and standards for educating professional nurses, it would take many years for the use of simulation to be utilized in advancing the training of the profession of nurses.

The first introduction of simulation-based concepts occurred with task trainers to teach psychomotor skills during orientation or annual competencies [5]. As educators became more comfortable teaching with task trainers, they added patient teaching and narrating care to the skill as part of the competency. As nurses became more confident in their ability to perform skills, they increased their competence level with many procedures and became focused on performing tasks. During this evolution in professional nursing education, it was noted that as the skill levels around performing tasks increased due to practice, critical thinking skills in nurses declined [5]. Team training needed to be clearly defined, and many hospitals felt it was better to have the professions train separately.

In 1999, the state of healthcare safety was defined in the Institute of Medicine (IOM) *To Err is Human* report, which highlighted the need to increase patient safety and the quality of care delivered [6]. In response to the IOM report, healthcare team members and physicians started to explore simulation for team training to reduce obstetric emergencies and critical events in intensive care units. In 2002, The Joint Commission published the first National Patient Safety Goals to provide accredited organizations with suggestions on addressing patient safety concerns [7]. The Patient Safety Advisory Group works with The Joint Commission annually to identify events that could harm patients and recommends specific education and training to address potential risks. From 2004 until 2014, The Joint Commission identified ineffective communication as one of the top three root causes of all sentinel events reported. Every year since 2010, The Joint Commission has recommended team training to improve communication between team members [8]. In 2019, The Joint Commission provided clear guidance on the specific education and team training requirements for healthcare teams to reduce the incidence of Postpartum Hemorrhage

V. Riggall (✉)
The Permanente Medical Group, Risk & Patient Safety Northern California Region, Oakland, CA, USA
e-mail: virginia.k.riggall@kp.org

S. Doolittle
Kaiser Permanente Santa Rosa Medical Center, Santa Rosa, CA, USA

J. M. Kutzin et al. (eds.), *Comprehensive Healthcare Simulation: Nursing*, Comprehensive Healthcare Simulation,
https://doi.org/10.1007/978-3-031-31090-4_28

and Maternal Hypertension as part of their accreditation process for healthcare systems [9].

Development

Many hospital programs, due to limited resources, had focused their simulation-based education around acute and critical patient events that occur in the hospital. Nursing teams had focused on improving competency skills and using simulation scenarios for training on code blue practices for patients suffering from either cardiac or respiratory arrest [5]. In recent years, the focus has shifted from managing critical events only to training around early recognition of sudden changes in a patient and trying to prevent a critical event from either occurring or advancing. In addition to team communication skills being emphasized in scenarios, there is a current trend to add concepts around providing exceptional patient care experiences to each scenario.

As the business of healthcare continues to change and evolve, so does the need for expanded use of simulation-based education to prepare nurses for the ever-changing environment. From 1995 to 2005, many elective patient procedures transitioned from the hospital into ambulatory care centers and doctors' offices due to diminishing healthcare reimbursement dollars and growing procedure demand [10]. When procedures first moved from the hospitals to the clinics, staff education was focused on the competencies and skills to assist with the procedures. As more adverse and unexpected patient events occurred, training all the staff on what to do in an emergency became necessary. This training has traditionally taken place once a year and utilized a group lecture format to educate the staff and physicians [10]. Many clinical sites utilize more medical assistants and licensed practical nurses to assist physicians with procedures and have very few registered nurses. Offices and clinics also have limited patient monitoring equipment compared to the hospital setting. When an adverse patient event occurs, many offices and clinics may have the basic emergency equipment available. However, the staff may not have the knowledge or experience to use the equipment during an emergency. Simulation-based education is an excellent method to identify potential risks due to the office's limited supplies and emergency equipment. It is also an excellent training tool for communicating the scope of practice for licensed and unlicensed clinical staff and providing physicians with the knowledge of the resources available in the office setting.

As these new areas of education arise for simulation-based education, it is important to start with identifying the current mandatory educational requirements for the hospital, department, or clinic before creating a new scenario. One efficient method for identifying training gaps is to utilize a crosswalk grid to match what training or educational programs are currently available and where the training opportunities exist. The next step is reviewing quality data for areas of performance improvement around patient safety. This review should also include incident reports, sentinel events, and near-miss reports to provide a clear picture of the current state of safety within the organization or department. Once this data has been collected, a review to examine all sources of information should be done to identify common themes, correlations, or gaps in training. While this assessment can take time, it is imperative to clearly understand the current state before approaching leadership with a plan to develop a new or revise a current training program that includes simulation.

Identifying the different stakeholder groups as part of the needs assessment will be beneficial in identifying how to address each of the areas of need. Viewing the assessment data and plan from the perspective of the organization's stakeholders will effectively align the plan with each stakeholder's goal or objective. For example, if one of the stakeholders is a unit manager, looking at the training plan through the lens of the unit manager will provide the educator with information on how to gain the unit manager's buy-in for the plan. Stakeholders who manage the resources needed for the program will have different goals and objectives compared to the stakeholders who will be receiving the education. Therefore, understanding the different stakeholders and how the development of a new program can benefit their goals is a key program development step. For example, talking to the C-suite executive about funding for a program will be a different conversation than a discussion with a department manager or lead physician on the resource of staff and physician time. Developing the training needs assessment will provide valuable information for both types of stakeholders, but the presentation of the information will look different for each stakeholder. For example, when an educator meets with the perioperative nursing director and the chief of surgery to discuss implementing interprofessional simulation-based training in the department, the leaders will look at how this training will impact the operating room and the team's schedule. Suggesting using one of the already scheduled education times on a morning when the operating room starts later with cases as an option for a simulation provides the leaders with a plan of how to incorporate the training into an existing resource. Many leaders support simulation-based education because of its benefits, such as improved learning retention.

In addition to assessing the current need for simulation, assessment of the learner's skill level and how they prefer to learn is equally important as the content. Viewing the learners as stakeholders in the simulation program is an imperative step in planning. As a stakeholder, their buy-in is important for engagement during the training. Utilizing the Adult Learning Theory, as defined by Knowles, as a framework for developing a program takes into consideration the learner's prior experience and education [11]. Allowing the learner to lead the learning utilizes their internal motivation as adult learners to solve problems and increases the likelihood they will change their behavior. Nurses have busy schedules and must see how training or new education will benefit them. One way to engage nurses is to start every scenario with how the training will address an identified problem or a change in their work that will impact them. Sharing the scenario objectives with the learners prior to running a simulation is one way of being transparent about why the training is needed [10].

Maintaining the learner's interest in the training also requires creating a psychologically safe environment for learners to explore and engage in a dialogue about the scenario. Educators may not know what prior experiences the learners bring to the education. Building trust with the learners through collaboratively developing and planning a scenario will provide the educator rich insights into prior experiences. Engaging in conversations with the learners interested in being involved will provide the educator with valuable knowledge about the nurses' perspective of their past training and lived experiences in the clinical environment. These perspectives can help the educator set the stage for learning in a psychologically safe environment. Staff discussions will inform the educator of any sensitivities around past significant patient events that may trigger second-victim symptoms. These symptoms may include emotional or physical distress, including guilt, anger, fear, and doubt. Caution should always be used when creating a scenario or training around a significant patient event the learners may have lived through. An example of a training that did not take the possibility of staff suffering from a second victim occurred when an obstetric department used a simulation scenario to address a state reportable death of an infant during delivery. The scenario contained many of the original patient event's details, and the staff felt blamed for the event during the training. While retraining physicians and staff may have been a regulatory requirement for the department, emotional support for the staff should have occurred before the simulation to prepare the physicians and staff for training. Additionally, the scenario should have been written around the systems issues and should not have included the details of the specific patient that died.

Current State

The current state of utilizing simulation-based education programs for professional nursing development depends greatly on how the organization views staff training and education delivery. Historically, it has been difficult for nursing to correlate between implementing an educational program to address risk and showing the program's benefit through cost savings or a harm reduction. In recent years, many clinical nurse specialists, and nurse educators, have used a program evaluation framework when planning a simulation-based curriculum. Evaluation methods and specific outcomes are outlined in the program during the development phase, such as reducing central line infections in an intensive care unit by following the proper care and maintenance procedures for central lines. Additionally, nurse managers are working with educators to forecast the cost of wages and salaries in their budgets to account for the financial cost of training. These proactive methods help to support current programs and can be used to calculate return on investment or reduction in harm for specific training. In the past, the cost of a program may not have included the wages to backfill positions while nurses attended scheduled training.

Funding for simulation equipment and lab space remains challenging in the healthcare environment, with limited grants available to augment the equipment replacement cost. The budget for simulation equipment is often in the same budget that pays for hospital equipment for patient care. This has created challenges for developing and sustaining simulation programs for professional nursing education. Creative educators focus scenario development on the objectives and utilize low-fidelity manikins and task trainers as a solution to continue simulations. *In-situ* simulations that utilize low-fidelity manikins provide the simulation educator with equipment that is less expensive to purchase and easier to use. With limited space and time to run *in-situ* simulations, the equipment must be easy to move, set up, and take down. The technology must be user-friendly and easy to connect to the manikin. Utilizing a lower fidelity simulator in an *in-situ* simulation increases physical fidelity because it occurs in the clinical environment where the nurses work. *In-situ* requires nurse educators to create a schedule early in the year utilizing optimal times for training on the unit. For example, the perioperative department could schedule their monthly simulation training on one of the days that surgeries are started an hour later to accommodate the department meetings and education. Educators should plan simulations on patient care units when the census is low. Successful *in-situ* simulations require leadership support to help coordinate the resources, including space, that are needed for the training.

Future State

Simulation has been utilized for training frontline nurses in clinical scenarios. It has yet to be fully utilized to train nurse leaders and executives on advanced leadership and management skills. Many nurses complete a business degree to provide them with the skills to manage staff and departments. While these educational programs provide nurses with business theories and case studies to prepare for the complex business environment, the programs may not allow nurses to experiment with these concepts in a simulated environment. Adding scenarios around the topics of supply and demand using the cost of supplies and staffing hours to match patient care hours is one type of leadership scenario that would allow nurse leaders to practice the financial and management skills required in today's healthcare environments.

Simulation is a tool that is under-utilized in developing professional nurse leaders and preparing entry-level assistant nurse managers on the tools to maintain the operations side of a patient care unit effectively. Nurses are often chosen for entry-level leadership positions because they have exceptional clinical skills. Many hospitals train entry-level leaders by offering real-time learning from day-to-day experiences. On-the-job training often offers little support for entry-level managers, and they tend to leave their roles due to a lack of confidence and stress.

Simulation is a tool that can provide leaders with the skills to handle difficult conversations with employees or how to prepare a budget for the department. The business of healthcare is a very complex system of different processes that include scheduling staff, ordering supplies, and developing new workflows for the unit. Adding leadership scenarios to a nursing leadership development program that includes mentoring would be an excellent way to prepare future nurse leaders with the confidence and skills before they accept a role as a leader.

Best Practices

When defining what makes a hospital-based simulation scenario successful for developing nurses professionally, several common characteristics have been identified through the author's experience. When approached to create a new scenario, the first step should be conducting a needs assessment focused on the current situation requiring a scenario. A general assessment should include reviewing the current educational programs provided to the unit nursing staff. Surveying the resources that are available for the training, such as time allotted for staff education and leadership resources for education, should be included in the assessment. Identifying the common educational themes from the current and past education will provide the simulation educator with knowledge of how the nurses have been educated in the past and may provide an opportunity to integrate past education into the scenario. Scaffolding the learning is one way for the educator to build trust with the participants by building on their current knowledge and extending past learnings. It also reduces the common staff complaint of education overload or "one more thing" to learn. One key step the author always includes in their needs assessment is a site visit to talk with staff about the unit and to walk through the area where the learners work. This gives the author a lens into the learning environment and a view into the audience for which they are creating a scenario.

Once the general assessment is completed, a focused assessment should be done to clarify the purpose of the scenario further. Often simulation educators are asked to create a scenario to meet a regulatory requirement, such as The Joint Commission's 2021 accreditation requirement for healthcare team training to reduce the incidence of patient harm when a woman is having a Postpartum Hemorrhage or suffering from Maternal Hypertension. Defining the scenario's purpose will help identify the educator's next assessment steps. Suppose the purpose is to meet a new regulatory requirement. In that case, it will be important to understand what the governing body or hospital leadership defines as the criteria for meeting the new regulation. Reviewing pertinent data around an adverse or unexpected event would be part of the focused assessment before creating a training scenario that identifies latent patient safety issues or system issues. Lastly, if the purpose of the scenario is to test a new process or orient physicians and staff to a new work environment, delineating the key aspects of the new process or environment should be completed during the assessment. This would include listing the resources needed for the scenario and an evidenced-based literature review and guidelines about the new process. During the assessment, the simulation education should identify any new specialty equipment that should be incorporated into the scenario. This gives the scenario's creator the most up-to-date information and knowledge about the new equipment. Gaining this information during the assessment phase will provide the simulation educator with accurate information and an understanding of the relevance of the new piece of equipment within the context of the department. This step will show the leaders and learners that simulation educators highly regard their knowledge.

After compiling the information from the needs assessment, the simulation educator should meet with the stakeholders to confirm the assessment findings. This step will create a shared mental model between the scenario's creator and the stakeholders. During the planning and creation phase, regular meetings are scheduled with the stakeholders to help define the goal and three to five objectives for the scenario. Subject matter experts should be included in the planning process to check the clinical accuracy of the scenario. Including the leaders and stakeholders in the development process will foster a collaborative relationship between the simulation educators and the stakeholders that will build buy-in for promoting the current training and future uses of simulation-based education.

Selecting the level of evaluation for each scenario should be included in the development of the scenario. For example, if the scenario's goal is to educate the learners on a new process, then one of the objectives should be written as a knowledge-based objective with an outcome that can be measured. The evaluation could be a knowledge pre- and post-test or an observation of the behaviors during the scenario. Understanding the outcome the stakeholders are hoping to achieve because of the simulation will help the simulation educator choose the appropriate level of evaluation. The information obtained from communications with leaders will help to inform the simulation program leaders and educators on what is important to measure for outcomes. This knowledge will aid in the development of valid and reliable evaluation methods to show the value of simulation for the organization.

One effective method of creating an evaluation tool for a new scenario is tying the objectives to an existing performance improvement project. This is an effective way to test a new workflow or to observe how a new process has been incorporated into a common clinical scenario. A checklist of the key behaviors or the new workflow could be developed as an observation tool for the simulation scenario. See the example of the Critical Behaviors Checklist for the Local Anesthetic System Toxicity Syndrome Scenario. Data collected during the scenario could be presented to show how the simulation either tested a new workflow or was used to observe how the new workflow fit with other existing processes. The data could also inform educators about gaps in knowledge that must be addressed. Sharing this information through presentations to key stakeholders continues to show the value of simulation and the need for future financial support to continue to utilize simulation-based education.

Other best practices that the author has experienced include having certified dedicated educators to develop the scenarios and a simulation operations specialist to run the scenarios. This best practice ensures that the scenarios are created and delivered standardized, utilizing evidence-based protocols and guidelines. Engaging the frontline staff as subject matter experts during the scenario development will gain their buy-in and help set expectations for the frontline staff. Applying and receiving continuing education units for a scenario will help nurses meet certification requirements for professional certifications.

Lastly, developing a method to document each scenario's key creation and implementation learnings will provide the simulation educator with a rich amount of data for future scenarios. The documentation process should include the following information: the reasons why the scenario was created, the results of the needs assessment, source references used to create the scenario, and how the evaluation methods were determined. In addition to the resources used to create the scenario, capturing any best practices learned while running the scenario is also best. Notes should be captured on the appropriate target audience for the scenario. It should also be noted in the scenario development form if the scenario could be part of an unfolding case. Finally, any notes from the educator on any recommended changes to the scenario or technology should be included. These notes should be developed with the simulation operations specialist and the educator. Suggested tips or guidance about running the scenario should be captured in a best practices tip sheet and shared with other educators and simulation operations specialists to ensure standardized delivery of every scenario.

Sample Curriculum

While the benefits of utilizing simulation for team training and improving communication have been well documented, it remains challenging for many hospitals to implement. Team training creates an opportunity to build relationships between different roles by providing them a venue to work and talk in a safe environment. Planning to train a team comprised of different professional roles takes extra planning to develop relevant scenarios for all team members. Engaging subject matter experts during the creation of the scenarios is a key step to ensure the content of the scenario is relevant. It will provide a valuable educational opportunity for every member of the team.

In many departments within a hospital setting, the team members are fluid and continually changing throughout the shift, as well as changing from day to day. When team members transition in and out of multiple teams during a shift, there is little opportunity for a team to form, let alone develop a trusting culture. This constant fluctuation of team members can create chaos within any department, especially during an adverse patient event. Departments that utilize different professional roles with different scopes of practice add layers of confusion when there is no clear delineation of role responsibility. Often, this confusion leads to conflict when an adverse event occurs with a patient, and stress levels increase. One department that this scenario is common is the radiology department within a hospital where adverse events are rare. In the radiology department, the physicians have many roles throughout their shift, including nurses, radiology technicians, ultrasound technicians, patient care technicians, MRI technicians, and CAT Scan technologists. When an adverse event occurs with a patient, the physician may expect the technician performing the test to be able to assess the patient's condition by taking blood pressure. If the technician has yet to be trained in this skill, they will have to call for a nurse or patient care technician to take the patient's blood pressure. This delay in care can heighten the stress of the situation, especially if the patient's condition declines.

A simulation program for a large radiology department in a 500-bed urban hospital was developed to address the team training requirements for the care of a patient suffering from an adverse reaction to contrast media. The training was based on The Joint Commission National Patient Safety goals developed due to sentinel event reporting around patient and staff safety when utilizing contrast media. In addition, the American College of Radiology and the American Society of Radiologic Technologists established best practice standards to improve patient safety and reduce the risk of liability due to adverse reactions to administering contrast media.

The simulation program was developed to complement the department learning module, which included didactic information about the different types of contrast media used in the different imaging modalities and the possible adverse side effects that patients could suffer. This learning module was the first part of a new competency the department had created. The second part of the training included team training utilizing an interprofessional simulation to practice the skills described in the learning module. The staff included in the simulation training were from the following diagnostic imaging departments: X-ray, Ultrasound, Cat Scan, and Magnetic Resonance Imaging.

The radiology department was managed by a nurse and leaders from the four diagnostic imaging departments. In addition to the various professional roles that supported the outlined imaging services offered by the hospital, the department also served as a medical residency site for radiologists and had 12 residents rotating to the different services within the department each week. This further diminished the ability of the team to form and gain trust among its members.

The role of the nurses in the department included working in all four imaging modalities. Nurses prepared the patients for their diagnostic images and performed specific tasks, such as administering contrast dye. This required the nurses to rotate in and out of the different rooms assisting with medication administration and completing a quick assessment before moving on to the next patient. The nurses and physicians were the only roles that rotated to all four diagnostic modalities throughout the day. The different technicians worked in the specific diagnostic imaging rooms in the department that matched their specific modality. This geographic arrangement divided the department by segregating each specialty into a defined set of imaging rooms, creating a communication barrier between the departments.

With the nurses working in all four areas within the department, the nurse manager thought it would benefit the department and the patients if the nurses took on more of a leadership role in supporting the physicians in all four departments. The manager's goal was to fully utilize the nurse's professional role and to grow the nurses' leadership skills within the department.

With the nurse's role needing to be more cohesive due to the constant rotating in and out of the different imaging rooms within the four areas of the department, the nurses felt overworked and not supported by the other team members. When the manager communicated her desire to have the nurses play more of a leadership role within the department, the nurses stated they were already heavily taxed with their current tasks. This discussion further divided the professional staff and caused more resistance for the nurses. The nurse manager hoped that by utilizing simulation to train as a team, the different professions would come together and support one another as one team for the patient's benefit.

Planning for the simulation program started with the simulation educator meeting with all the leaders of the radiology department to plan the scenarios. It was decided that the teams would attend two simulations. A schedule was developed for the training, and each leader scheduled the members of their teams. In addition to scheduling the staff, the leaders decided that one leader from the group would be present for all the simulations to welcome the teams and introduce the simulation team. This unified approach provided the different teams with an example that the leaders shared a common goal for patient safety.

Each scenario included a radiologist, a radiology medical resident, a nurse, a unit assistant, and one technician from the four imaging departments. It was decided to utilize *in-situ* simulations to capture a higher level of physical fidelity for the learners. The training was scheduled to take place in imaging rooms in all four imaging modalities to orient the staff to the different supplies and emergency equipment available in each room.

It was determined that four contrast media adverse reaction scenarios would be created for the program and developed with the help of subject matter experts from the radiology department. The significance of developing the four distinct scenarios was related to the four different types of adverse reactions that can occur. The four scenarios included the following adverse reactions: Hypotension with tachycardia from anaphylaxis; hypotension with bradycardia; laryngeal edema with inspiratory stridor; and bronchospasm with expiratory wheezes. Each type of reaction requires different management. The learning objectives for the four scenarios were as follows: After the training, the participating teams will be able to:

1. Identify the specific contrast dye adverse reaction the patient was having.
2. Demonstrate the appropriate interventions for the patient in a timely manner.
3. Utilize effective patient-centered communication with the patient.
4. Demonstrate effective teamwork and team communication during the simulation.

An observation tool was created for each scenario with the appropriate interventions and team actions for each type of adverse reaction (see example). During the running of each scenario, the radiology department leader would observe the teams and document team behaviors on the tool. This data gave the leadership team an effective method of assessing the need for further education or identifying system issues during each scenario. A shared mental model was created when the leadership team worked together to develop the observation tools. Involving the leaders in the development of the program not only showed them the value of the training but also significantly increased their passion and dedication to the training.

The training plan consisted of each participant attending two simulation scenarios: one scenario in which the patient had an adverse reaction involving cardiac symptoms; and a second scenario involving a respiratory adverse reaction to contrast media. The leadership team decided to develop two phases of training with the patient's symptoms in the second scenario, increasing in complexity. The goal was to use the easier introductory scenario as an orientation to the simulation training. Building trust was key in promoting psychological safety during the training and a healthy work environment.

A simulation manikin was utilized for all four scenarios and was positioned on the imaging table at the start of each scenario. The simulation operations specialist was located out of the view of the team at the start of each scenario but close enough to the technician's control room that they could see the scenario. Once the technician left the control room, the simulation operations specialist relocated into this space to run the rest of the scenario. This provided the simulation operations technician with a clear visualization of the patient and the team during the scenario. Using a headset and a small microphone attached to the manikin; the simulation operations technician provided verbal responses to the team. They also were able to change the vital signs for the manikin utilizing a small handheld computer tablet. Having just the manikin, headset, and small computer tablet allowed for easy transfer of the equipment from room to room during days when multiple simulations were being run. For the scenarios, an intravenous line and a drainage bag were placed on the manikin's arm.

Moulage was used during the respiratory cases to create a dusky appearance on the manikin's face. This was created by using children's water-based blue and grey paints thinned with water and a make-up sponge to lightly apply to the face of the manikin. Thinned water-based red paint and a make-up sponge were used to create hives on the patient's trunk as part of one of the scenarios. The paint had been tested on an old manikin's skin before placing paint on the manikin, to test whether it would stain the skin. Mild soap and water easily removed the paint after each simulation session ended. For pertinent patient symptoms that could not be created on the simulator, white slap bracelets were utilized with labels describing the specific symptoms. For example, bracelets were placed on the extremities of the manikin with the key diagnostic symptoms, such as cool, clammy extremities, for the participants to find during the assessment of the patient.

Training supplies were labeled "For Simulation Education Only" and placed in each room. Simulated medications were created and placed in a new locked box to store emergency medications in each room. Staff in-services on the medication locked box were completed before the simulation program began. Each diagnostic testing room also had a blue code button that, when pushed, solicited help from the entire hospital. This process created chaos and confusion in the department. Care for the patient would be delayed while the department nurses waited for the critical care nurses to arrive. This resulted in a deterioration of the radiology nurses' critical thinking and code skills. To reduce the chaos in the department, a new workflow had been developed six months earlier to communicate when assistance is needed within the department. This workflow utilized the department paging system to page overhead "Doctor Stop to the specific radiology room." This new workflow was challenging because of the department's size, and many of the residents needed to learn the room numbers. This workflow would be built into the scenario to reinforce the existing procedure.

Briefing the participants started with reading the Basic Assumption, which is "We believe everyone participating in simulation is intelligent, capable, cares about doing their best, and wants to improve" [12]. In addition, the following guiding principles were shared with the teams: We ask you to keep what happens in the simulation confidential; suspend disbelief; treat each other and the patient with dignity and respect; critically reflect on the experience; and be curious!" [12]. The briefing continued orienting the participants to the equipment, resources, and medications available during the scenario. Additionally, the team was oriented to the specific functions of the manikin and how they could receive additional information, such as vital signs, if necessary. Finally, the team was briefed on utilizing the paging system for "Doctor Stop" if they needed a physician to care for the patient. They were informed to state "Doctor Stop Drill to room number" during the simulations. On the day simulations were scheduled, the leaders would announce in the morning huddle that "Doctor Stop Drill to room number" would be used for the simulation training that day. The scheduled staff was reminded of their training session information in the huddle. Patients in the waiting room and other imaging rooms were notified that training would take place in the department and would not impact their test. This helped alleviate miscommunications and provided patients with an explanation of sounds that may have been alarming.

Two introductory scenarios were created for the first round of training. Staff was randomly assigned to one of the two scenarios. Each of the introductory scenarios began with a technologist receiving report that the patient was positioned for a diagnostic imaging test and the nurse had completed the administration of the 100 ml contrast media. For each session, the patient's diagnostic test was changed to match the specific diagnostic imaging setting as the training rotated throughout the four different areas within the department. In scenario one, the patient was a 38-year-old woman who had just received contrast media for her MRI. As usual, the nurse would be called to see another patient as the test started. The patient starts to verbalize that she feels terrible and cannot describe the symptoms to the technician. The imaging technician would need to stop the procedure and check on the patient. As the patient declined, the goal for the technician was to call for help utilizing the workflow of paging "Doctor Stop Drill to room" overhead. In this scenario, the patient becomes bradycardic with hypotension. The patient improves if the team completes the critical actions for this scenario, which include placing the patient on the defibrillator to monitor the vital signs and cardiac rhythm, administering oxygen through a non-rebreather mask, elevating the patient's legs to 60°, starting a normal saline bolus, and calling "Doctor Stop Drill to room."

In the second introductory scenario, the patient is a 36-year-old woman who has received contrast media before her MRI. She starts to complain that she is feeling short of breath and states she has never had an MRI before. Her blood pressure and heart rate remain stable in this scenario. As she continues to complain, her speech becomes labored. Again, the technician should page overhead to alert the team that they are needed in the room. The patient will improve if the resident orders the appropriate interventions after listening to the patient's lungs to assess for expiratory wheezing and rales. The team would be expected to place the patient on the defibrillator to monitor vital signs, administer a beta-agonist inhaler with 8–12 L of oxygen through a non-rebreather mask, and call "Doctor Stop Drill to room."

As teams completed the first round of training, a second scenario was planned for each participant. If the participant had attended the cardiac scenario in the first round of training, they were assigned to the advanced respiratory scenario in the second training. And participants who had participated in the introductory respiratory scenario in the first round were assigned to the advanced cardiac scenario. These two scenarios started with a simulated nurse actor calling a resident to come to see a patient who was exhibiting deteriorating symptoms. If the resident asked for help, the nurse would page "Doctor Stop Drill to room" overhead to alert the training team that help was needed in the simulation. The patients deteriorated very quickly in the advanced scenarios, which added additional stress to the team to respond immediately. If the appropriate interventions were not identified and completed, the patient would undergo a cardiac or respiratory arrest.

Each scenario was designed to show one of the four possible adverse reactions that could occur and the correct treatment algorithms to treat the symptoms. If the wrong adverse reaction was diagnosed and the wrong treatment was prescribed, the patient would deteriorate. The teams had been given knowledge about contrast media reactions in a department presentation and by completing a learning module before attending the simulations. The simulations built on this knowledge and allowed the teams to practice using the new processes for emergency medications and to reinforce communicating for additional help by using the paging system.

During the debriefing, the teams expressed their appreciation for the opportunity to participate in the simulations. It was very helpful for them to learn about the different areas in the department. It was most helpful for the technicians unfamiliar with where supplies and emergency equipment were stored in the different imaging rooms. Many technologists stated they would like to learn how to set up the defibrillator and other monitoring equipment to help care for the patient. The teams expressed an interest in having continued practice with running codes and learning more about each other's areas of expertise. The residents were grateful to learn about the different professionals who worked in the department, their roles, and their scope of practice. They were also grateful to learn that each team wore a different color uniform to help distinguish the different roles. In each scenario, the team saw the nurses as the informal leader in the room. The nurses were surprised to hear the other team members' perception of them as the leader in the room. Several of the nurses stated they would be willing to help teach the other team members how to set up the emergency equipment. Several of the nurses asked to become American Heart Association Basic Life Support instructors to help run the skill training in the department. At the beginning of the project, the leadership team and the nurses expressed their doubts about changing the behaviors in the unit. Fortunately for the staff and the patients, the program helped to shape a new culture within the department while promoting the professional image of the nurses. The leadership team expressed their gratitude for the experience that brought their teams together and transformed the way they delivered care to patients.

Integrating Simulation into Existing Education

As mentioned in best practices, simulation program leaders that meet with stakeholders regularly to plan curricula can provide department leaders with ideas and plans to integrate simulation into existing skills sessions. Engaging simulation educators as soon as new training requirements are defined will provide the department leaders with resources to share the burden of adding additional training. Developing or adding new training to an existing simulation scenario or program will expand the current library of available scenarios and meet the new training needs of the department.

Many healthcare organizations are creating nurse residency programs to support new nurses transitioning from academia to the practice environment. Simulation is an educational modality that new nurses have experienced, and they welcome the opportunity to continue to practice skills during interprofessional simulations or with experienced nurses. Care experience and implicit bias are two topics that are being added into clinical scenarios for new graduate nurses to shift the culture in hospitals,

Incorporating experienced nurses into the residency program simulations creates a mentoring environment that benefits both the new and experienced nurses. Studies have shown that new nurses who complete a residency program transition from advanced beginners to competent professionals with improved critical thinking skills [13]. Developing a mentoring relationship with an experienced nurse promotes role development and socialization for the new nurse. Simulation provides a psychologically safe environment for the new nurse to explore their professional role and develop relationships with experienced nurses.

Challenges and Solutions

The nursing profession continues to be challenged with defining the minimum requirements for nurse educators and how nurses should be educated in the practice environment. Nurse educators traditionally train large groups of clinical staff with limited resources. In addition to providing education to clinical staff, many nurse educators are taxed with training interprofessional groups with no additional help from the other roles. Physicians and residency programs often expect nurse educators to run simulation programs for medical education and the nursing education they provide. These additional responsibilities can deter simulation educators from continuing in their roles because they need support. Hiring a simulation operations specialist to help set up and run a simulation can provide the much-needed support to meet the demands of competing groups. By providing a trained simulation operations specialist to utilize their expertise to run simulations, the simulation educator's expertise can be utilized more effectively to create and develop curricula.

Incorporating simulation into professional nursing development programs has traditionally been received very positively by nurses. Challenges are often created over scheduling time for education and dedicating space to run the simulations. One solution to this challenge is working with leaders early in the year to plan for the training. Developing a program plan with scheduled dates for training will help the schedulers in the department coordinate each nurse's schedule to include time for the training. Additionally, incorporating several skills stations for nursing competencies to be included in the training will efficiently meet competing priorities with scheduling.

Other challenges include obtaining leadership buy-in for using simulation as a teaching method. One solution to this challenge is scheduling the first simulation with the department leaders. Experiencing the power of a simulation as a teaching method is enough to convert leaders to support the program. Simulation educators must be flexible and willing to partner with other departments to help meet the increasing training demands required for staff. Reviewing the objectives of each new required training will provide an experienced simulation educator with the details to determine if the simulation is the best modality to use for the training. When a simulation-based program does not seem to be the best fit for the training, being honest with leaders and providing them with an explanation will develop further trust between the simulation educator and nursing leaders.

Interface with Regulatory Bodies

Simulation and team training is recommended by The Joint Commission to reduce the harm that is caused by poor communication among teams. In 2019, The Joint Commission approved a new standard for perinatal safety requiring drills to identify systems issues that may impact the care of women suffering from a postpartum hemorrhage or severe hypertension or preeclampsia [9]. During site visits starting in 2021, the Joint Commission will be looking for evidence that obstetric units and emergency departments conduct these trainings.

Healthcare organizations applying or re-certifying for the American Nurses Credentialing Center Magnet Recognition Program® can document stories about how simulation-based education was used to promote the Forces of Magnetism. Magnet® Recognition Program is a certification that recognizes healthcare organizations that align their strategic goals around elevating patient outcomes through creating and sustaining a culture of excellence [14]. The new Magnet model has configured the 14 Forces of Magnetism into five model components to help organizations streamline the required documentation. Under the Structural Empowerment component, simulation-based education can be shown as a method of developing professional nurses and improving the image of nursing within an organization. A story about how simulation benefited nursing in an academic-practice partnership that was developed to socialize new nurses to the profession before transitioning to the practice environment would exemplify the Professional Development of Nursing. It would provide evidence of Nurses as Teachers (Force #13). The example curriculum that was provided for the radiology department would also be an excellent story to document Nurses as Teachers under the Exemplary Professional Practice [14].

Sharing a story about how a bedside nurse worked with a nurse researcher to develop a program to improve a clinical outcome through simulation training would be an excellent story to be shared during a Magnet site visit. The nurse could describe the evidence-based steps she learned and implemented in a simulation-based program to improve patient safety. This story would be evidence of Quality Improvement (Force #7) [14]. Incorporating evaluation methods into every simulation program provides nursing with a rich amount of data that could be used to document how the organization met the New Knowledge, Innovation, and Improvements component. Data showing a reduction in nurse turnover rate due to the implementation of a residency program that provided a safe learning environment for experienced nurses to mentor new nurses would support the Global Issues in Nursing and Healthcare category, as well as Professional Development (Force #14) under Structural Empowerment and Nurses as Teachers (Force #1) under Exemplary Professional Practice.

Developing a middle manager nursing leadership simulation program to support the development of new nursing leaders would show evidence that the organization is investing in the future of professional nursing. Utilizing an innovative program to provide education and simulations around current and future challenges for leaders would show evidence of Transformational Leadership.

In addition to using simulation-based education for regulatory requirements and Magnet® recognition, organizations can utilize simulations to address required training associated with sentinel events. Simulation educators can provide support in developing specific training to address action plans after an adverse event occurs. Working with the risk and quality departments to meet a deadline for training can be supported through existing or new scenarios developed to provide support for the departments or teams. Utilizing a simulation educator during training to address a sentinel event provides a neutral person to work with the teams around a potentially emotionally charged situation. Simulation educators are trained to guide the learning to meet the learner's needs non-judgmentally.

Summary

Simulation-based education provides many professional development opportunities for nurses throughout their career path. Nursing skills and knowledge can be enhanced by utilizing simulation-based education to expand the nurse's role to improve clinical practices and patient experiences. Simulation is an innovative tool that professional nurses can utilize to develop solutions that improve access to care, improve the quality-of-care patients receive, and reduce the cost of healthcare. Leveraging simulation to meet the evolving needs of healthcare organizations elevates the value of the professional nurses' contribution to reforming healthcare.

References

1. Selanders LC, Crane P. The voice of Florence Nightingale on advocacy. Online J Issues Nursing. 2012;17(1):F1. Available from https://ojin.nursingworld.org/MainMenuCategories/ANAMarketplace/ANAPeriodicals/OJIN/TableofContents/Vol-17-2012/No1-Jan-2012/Florence-Nightingale-on-Advocacy.html
2. Maloney P, Woolford L. Ninety years and counting: the past, present, and future of the nursing professional development specialist. J Nurses Prof Dev. 2019;34(2):56–65.
3. Miller MA. Trends of in-service education. In: Cowan MC, editor. The yearbook of modern nursing. G. P. Putnam Sons: New York, NY; 1956.
4. American Nurses Association. Scope and standards of practice for nursing professional development. Washington, DC: Author; 2000.
5. Nehring WM. Nursing simulations: a review of the past 40 years. Simul Gaming. 2009;40(4):528–52.
6. Kohn LT, Corrigan J, Donaldson MS. To err is human: building a safer health system. Washington, DC: National Academy Press; 2000.
7. The Joint Commission. The Joint Commission: over a century of quality and safety. 2020. Available from: https://www.jointcommission.org/-/media/tjc/documents/about-us/tjc-history-timeline-through-2019-pdf.pdf.
8. The Joint Commission. Joint Commission Online. 2015. Available from: https://www.jointcommission.org/-/media/deprecated-unorganized/imported-assets/tjc/system-folders/joint-commission-online/jconline_april_29_15pdf.pdf?db=web&hash=DEFFBC416 23A360F1C1428A5E9602773.
9. The Joint Commission. New standards for perinatal safety. 2019. Available from: https://www.jointcommission.org/standards/prepublication-standards/new-standards-for-perinatal-safety/?_ga=2.45266662.319791927.1604866353-2070799425.1604866353.
10. Uman RD, Punwani N, Shapiro FE. Office-based surgical and medical procedures: educational gaps. Ochsner J. 2012;12(4):383–8.
11. Clapper TC. Beyond Knowles: what those conducting simulations need to know about adult learning theory. Clin Simul Nursing. 2010;6:e7–e14.
12. Center for Medical Simulation. The basic assumption. Harvard Medical Simulation. 2004–2019. Available from www.harvard-medsim.org.
13. Letourneau RM, Fater KH. Nurse residency programs: an integrative review of the literature. Nursing Educ Perspect. 2015;36(2):96–101.
14. American Nurses Credentialing Center. ANCC Magnet Recognition Program®. 2020. Available from https://www.nursingworld.org/organizational-programs/magnet/.

Simulation for New Hire/Pre-Hire Orientation

29

Karen Josey and Carrie Brandon

Background

Developing a standardized curriculum that includes simulation for both experienced and New Graduate Nurse Orientation allows for consistent assessment and the measurement of opportunities and strengths. During an onboarding curriculum, there is a focus on remediating staff that don't adhere to critical actions or make errors in knowledge, judgement, or skill thereby improving the quality and safety of patient care. Simulation allows for the creation of standardized experiences so that learners progression can be fairly assessed as well as ensuring that important clinical conditions are experienced, thereby supporting the new graduate and.

Best Practices

Banner Health, a large not-for-profit healthcare organization, has 29 hospitals including three academic medical centers in 6 western states and over 55,000 employees. Banner Health offers a simulation based, standardized, centralized basic skills assessment and remediation model for nurse onboarding, originally developed and implemented in 2009. Basic skills checklists are created using critical actions and common errors that had been identified through patient safety reports. Learners are assessed using these checklists and an individualized report is generated for the learner and faculty. This system-wide standardized process decreases variation in onboarding with the goal of assisting and preparing the new employee for success in their journey within the organization.

Supplementary Information The online version contains supplementary material available at https://doi.org/10.1007/978-3-031-31090-4_29.

K. Josey (✉)
HCA Healthcare, Nashville, TN, USA
e-mail: karen.josey@hcahealthcare.com

C. Brandon
HCA Healthcare, Nashville, TN, USA

Banner Healthcare, Loveland, CO, USA

The onboarding program requires nurses that are employed in a simulation specialist/educator role where they develop curriculums, program manikins, run simulations, as well as assess learners, collect data, and debrief scenarios. Initially Banner simulation employed both educator and simulation specialist positions, but found it was more efficient to combine the roles because of the overlap in responsibilities. Through combining the educator and simulation specialist role, funding was available to hire a data analyst. This role has been critical in developing reports and assessing data to demonstrate the value of a simulation activity. The data analyst also runs reports on the learner evaluations completed by the assessors (simulation specialists) and provides feedback on the inter-rater reliability of the assessors evaluating simulation skills and scenarios. This is important to assure learners are evaluated consistently and that the needed remediation occurs.

The simulation curriculum has morphed throughout the years based on feedback from Risk Management, Quality, Patient Safety, and Infection Prevention personnel as well as hospital-wide initiatives and practice gaps. Some examples of how simulation curriculum as evolved:

- Basic skills that were part of the standard education during onboarding for any single facility at Banner were incorporated into the onboarding Simulation Skills starting in 2009.
- New Grad *a day in the life* scenarios were added to facilitate assimilation into practice. These scenarios mimicked a six-hour day of caring for two patients in a simulated patient care environment.
- Content for New Grad scenarios was based on:
  - Med-Surg based competencies.
    Because specialty specific scenarios didn't work as new grads were novice and needed more experience in basic nursing care
  - Common diagnosis-related groups (DRGs) of admitted patients
  - Organization initiatives and feedback from Patient Safety, Quality, Infection Prevention, and Risk Management departments

J. M. Kutzin et al. (eds.), *Comprehensive Healthcare Simulation: Nursing*, Comprehensive Healthcare Simulation,
https://doi.org/10.1007/978-3-031-31090-4_29

- National Safety Goals, Sepsis, Surgical Site Infections, Hospital Acquired Conditions (HAC), Organizational Initiatives, Never Events
- High alert medications such as heparin and insulin
- Medication administration issues using automated medication dispensing system reports from the Pyxis (medication dispensing machine)
- Incorporating the electronic medical record using the training environment and simulated patient scenarios

A metric tool (Table 29.1) was created to capture quality measures and provide a guide for choosing priorities that were important to Banner. The tool has changed throughout the years and has included Banner Strategic Initiatives, AANC Magnet

Table 29.1 Partial snapshot of quality measures tool used in building simulation curriculum

Banner Health Simulation Education Quality Measurements Tool

Submission Date:	Scenario Name:	Target Audience:
March 2019	Pneumonia/Sepsis – P.O.	Novice RNs

2019 Banner Health Strategic Initiatives

Quality Measures listed below are addressed in the Simulation Education Document

Sepsis

Notify provider when SAFE alert fires
Provider to determine if confirmed or suspected infection- If yes initiate Sepsis 3-hour bundle
- Initial lactic acid
- Blood cultures before antibiotics
- Start Broad spectrum IV antibiotics
- Fluids @ 30ml/kg IF initial lactic acid >4, hypotension or septic shock
- Repeat lactic acid IF initial lactic acid >2.0 to reassess tissue perfusion
- Provider reassessment of tissue perfusion status after initial fluid bolus

Healthcare Acquired Pneumonia

- Assess for risk of aspiration every shift
- Document in the Neuro section of the adult assessment
- Caution all patients to eat and drink sitting up to avoid aspiration

If assessment reveals risk for aspiration:
- Obtain order for Speech Therapy Swallow Evaluation
- Keep HOB up to 30-45 degrees unless contraindicated
- Provide oral hygiene BID (1 x shift)
- 1:1 Supervision at meals
- Keep suction at bedside

Implement risk of aspiration IPOC
Documentation – ARA (1 x shift), Oral care (1 x shift), HOB up (1 x shift), IS 8 times/day (4 x shift)

Surgical Site Infections

Inpatient/OBS patients:
- CHG full body skin bath preoperatively
- Nasal decolonization for total hip/knee patients only
- Removal of hair only if necessary
- Pre-and post-operative glucose monitoring on ALL surgical patient to maintain BG 110-180
  - POCT </=70 mg/dL, notify provider, initiate hypoglycemia protocol
  - POCT >/=150 mg/dL, notify provider, initiate the subQ low resistance insulin sliding scale
- Antimicrobial prophylaxis prior to skin incision
- Normothermia (temp ≥ 36 C) during the perioperative phase
- Intraoperative application of alcohol-based antiseptic agent
- Oxygen therapy initiated in PACU for patients receiving general anesthesia if <94%
- Keep sterile dressing intact for 48 hours postop (cardia and C-section dressing 24°
- Appropriate post-op dressing (silver for colon/hip/knee up to 7 day per manufacturer instructions
- Patient education – provide BH Surgical Incision Care and Pre-venting Surgical Site Infections at d/c

Model Components and Forces, National Patient Safety Goals, ARHQ, IHI Protective Five Million Lives from Harm Campaign, CMS Hospital Acquired Conditions "Never Events", Standards and Initiatives from the Agency for Healthcare Research and Quality (AHRQ) and the Center for Disease Control and Prevention (CDC) . Banner Annual Initiatives that focus on Quality and Patient Safety included National Database of Nursing Quality Indicators (NDNQI) and Joint Commission components. Hospital acquired infections and adverse drug events are examples of what Banner focused on and the simulation team supported in the curricula. Depending on the safety focus for any given year, it was easy to add different quality metrics to skills or scenarios such as sepsis, healthcare acquired pneumonia, and surgical site infections. This tool allowed Banner Simulation to capture and illustrate how learners were performing in these important quality-based metrics [1, 2].

Sample Curriculum #1: New Hire RN Skills and Scenarios

New hire nurses must attend a skills assessment in the Simulation Center as part of the onboarding process. The purpose of the skills assessment is to establish the learner's baseline performance data on basic clinical skills, which will drive an individualized orientation program. Although not every skill applies to every specialty area, there are critical elements that are transferable to all areas such as sterility in the skills of foley insertion and central line dressing change that translate across departments. Should a participant miss a step during the assessment, they are immediately remediated at the skill station. Each objective on the checklists is cross-referenced and aligned with current procedures and guidelines of nursing care as well as Banner Policies and Procedures. Periodically, the skills assessed are reviewed and cross-walked with different teams such as Risk Management, Patient Safety, and Quality and the simulation remediation data to determine if changes are needed. The individualized report consists of the data collected from the individualized performance at each skill station. An overall percentage of the first attempt to complete the skill (without prompting or instruction) indicates the employee's performance given the knowledge and experience on that day.

The preceptor, manager, and educator review the report to become familiar with the learner's strengths and opportunities for improvement and share it with the employee to create an individualized orientation. The report is then filed in the employee's record. The Simulation Specialist may contact the educator or manager if there are significant concerns regarding a new hire's knowledge, skills, or attitude.

Standard onboarding skill curriculum may include basic skills and scenarios such as:

- Peripheral IV insertion
- Foley insertion
- Central line dressing changes
- Mock codes/COVID Codes
- PPE
- Culture of Safety
- Sepsis Escape Room

Registered Nurse New Hire Data

Attendance data is significant for addressing resources needed for each type of learner and for reviewing the impact on simulation operations. Attendance data can be a part of showing program value. Banner Health hired over 4800 new nurses in 2020, making the topics covered in onboarding extremely important. The specific type of learner, new grad, experienced nurse, change of specialty, etc. helps to define the content covered in the simulation experiences. For example, new grads may not be familiar with giving blood, so a blood administration simulation would be a brand new learning event important for the new hire to experience. Data

Table 29.2 Blood administration simulation

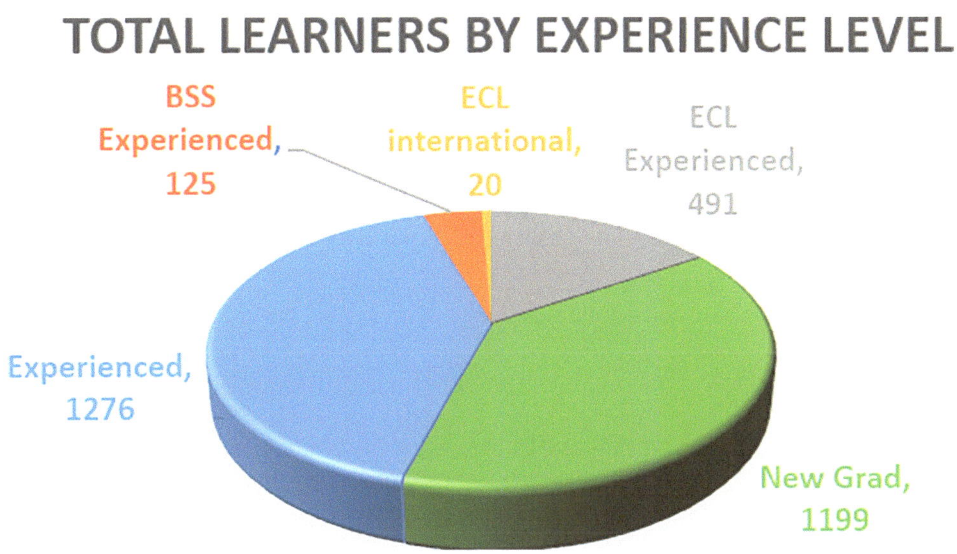

showing learners by experience level from 2020 is displayed in Table 29.2. Learner type includes nurses that are New Grads, Experienced Nurses, Banner Staffing Experienced (BSE), External Contract Labor (ECL) International, and External Contract Labor.

The Escape Room scenarios used a Room of Errors (ROE) model that was a new addition to the curriculum started later in Q4 so the total participants are lower than Total Learners.

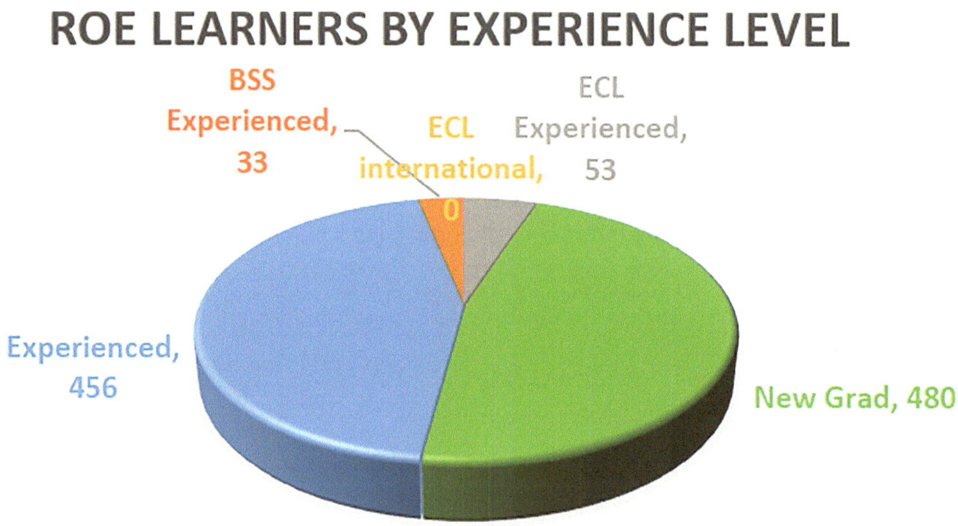

Specific risk management, quality, or safety issues are incorporated into the onboarding training once identified. For example, issues maintaining sterility across skills was commonly identified by the assessors. Because of this, donning and doffing PPE was added to the curriculum. Adding donning and doffing PPE helped learners to experience the importance of keeping themselves safe. Data consistently showed that experienced nurses also had gaps in basic skills and needed some components such as sepsis care skills that were in the New Grad scenarios. Based on this data, the Banner Simulation Team adjusted the curriculum and added a Sepsis Escape Room and Culture of Safety scenarios to the onboarding skills for both the Experienced and New Grad groups.

RN New Hire Simulation Course Data Includes Data from Clinical Events

Errors occur throughout healthcare. Nursing errors in particular may occur when programming an IV Pump, placing a peripheral IV, donning or doffing PPE, maintaining a Central Venous Catheter (CVC), or placing a urinary catheter. These skills are broken down into critical components to identify where the error may occur. If a learner makes an error when preforming a skill, remediation occurs immediately. However, the data demonstrating that an error was made is collected to that the performance data demonstrates the learning need. If the majority of learners are able to complete the skills and scenarios with little to no remediation necessary, then the skill may be removed from the curriculum. However, if many learners continue to demonstrate a need for remediation, then the skill or scenario is continued and periodically reviewed for improvement to better meet learning needs. Examples of critical components during which an error may occur are:

Blood administration errors:

- Forgetting to check if the consent is signed
- Missed Blood Bank ID verification or does not know what that is.
- Missed checking transfusion record against blood product: demonstrate verifying unit #, blood product type, unit ABO/Rh type, patient ABO/Rh type compatibility, expiration date with two licensed personnel. Often missed checking one of these four categories and usually gets two out of four but not all four.

Equipment (IV Pump) errors:

- Does not know what information to enter in the pump. Enters patients name or does not enter anything at all.
- Does not enter the correct rate to match the order given
- Does not choose Guardrail IV fluid option and program under Basic infusion
- Does not extend hanger full 9.5 in. or forgets to open roller clamp when hanging secondary IV
- Often misses and it does not match medication order given and usually runs the IV twice as fast when programing secondary drug-rate
- Often misses the correct dose for the IV bolus
- Incorrectly programs or does not read protocol correctly
- Set up the infusion with the blood and NS clamps open at same time so fluids mix

Procedures:

Central Venous Catheter or CVC errors:

- Does not put mask on self or patient
- Does not perform hand hygiene after removing gloves.
- Does not perform full 30 s friction scrub of dressing change site
- Forgets to label or doesn't include insertion and dressing change information
- Often contaminates caps/line and does not use alcohol to disinfect cap
- Breaks sterility mostly during cap change

Urinary catheter insertion errors:

- Does not use castile wipes or know why they are used
- Does not use fenestrated drape
- Does not insert catheter far enough before inflating
- Does not know how to use the stat-lock because they have not used prior
- Often breaks sterility during insertion process as sterile glove touches the patient's skin while inserting or they use the dirty hand to reach back in sterile kit

Workplace Safety (Personal Protective Equipment or PPE) concerns:

- Forgets to wash hands after removal of PPE
- Puts gown on but ties it in the front
- Contaminates self

Skills requiring significant remediation are listed in Table 29.3.

Table 29.3 2020 Compiled skill data breakdown and remediation data

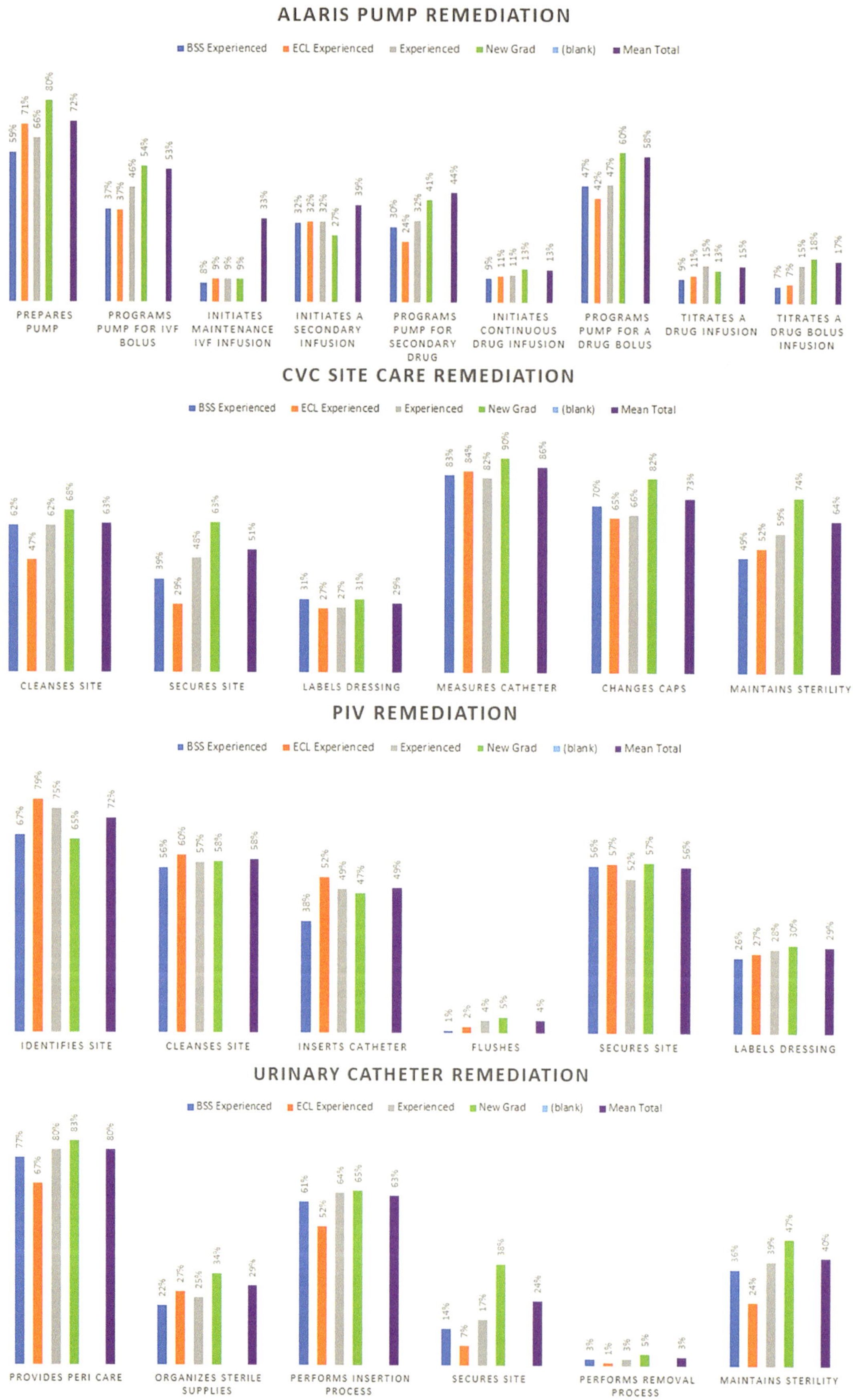

Sample Curriculum #2: "A Day in the Life" New Grad Scenarios

New Grads have an additional experience in simulation onboarding that includes a 6-hour *Day in the Life* scenario. During this onboarding simulation, newly hired graduate nurses are assigned to care for two typical medical surgical patients simultaneously at a Banner Simulation Center. During the 6-hour day, the learners care for patients as they would in a normal day. They get report, give report, complete assessments, take vital signs, prioritize patient care, give medications, communicate using SBAR format, and chart using a live training environment that gives alerts as would occur in the normal the Electronic Medical Record (EMR). Originally the program was a 3-day event of caring for the same patients with different needs as well as a new patient assignment. Scenarios were programed and timed to not overwhelm the learner by having too many events occur at the same time. These scenarios decreased to two days and then one day of scenarios over the years due to increased hiring and onboarding.

Each session includes a pre-brief, scenarios, and a facilitated debrief (Appendix 1).

New Grad Scenarios include a mixture of clinical experiences:

- Basic assessment on two patients
- Prioritization of care
- Electronic Medical Record documentation
- Communication using SBAR format including during handoffs
- Medication Administration
- Alaris pump IV management and administration (Guardrails/titration/fluid bolus)
- Heparin calculation based on labs
- Implementing order sets
- Fall Risk assessment
- Change in condition situations
- Assessment of oxygen needs
- Signs and Symptoms of deterioration
- Sepsis evaluation
- Respiratory distress management
- Asthma management
- BLS Code management
- Utilization of resources
- Fluid therapy/bolus management
- Pain management/documentation on MAR
- Contact precautions
- Smoking cessation/education
- Blood transfusion education S/S reaction
- Diabetes management:
  - Hypoglycemia
  - Insulin calculations
  - S/S diabetic ketoacidosis
- Patient education
- Wound care
- Pain Management
- Hospital Acquired Pneumonia Protocol
- Abnormal lab identification and management
- Ordering labs
- Blood Transfusion
- General post op care
- Dressing changes
- Addressing diversity, attending to emotional needs and patient education

Communication using SBAR format including a readback and verify is assessed during the simulation. SBAR is broken down into sections and each section, Situation, Background, Assessment, Recommendation, are measured separately. The learner is expected to use SBAR throughout the 6-hour day by communicating with physicians and other care staff.

The 6-hour day of caring for two patients is followed by a two hour debrief which allows the participants time to self-reflect, learn from each other, process what they learned, and conclude with takeaways to improve their patient care and practice.

The facilitators complete an assessment checklist based on critical actions and errors (Appendix 2) while observing the participants, which is used to guide remediation and generate an individualized report. Each section lists the objectives, overall percent completed, and a breakdown of missed steps.

The Simulation Specialist may contact the educator or manager if there are significant concerns.

New Grad scenario patient care behaviors are categorized into the following Domains:

- Patient Assessment
- Communication with patient
- Critical Thinking
- Documentation
- Impact on Patient Experience [3]
- Medication Administration
- Patient Education
- Patient Safety
- Skills

Timely Interventions

New Grad Scenario Domain and SBAR Data ($n = 221$)

The preceptor, manager, and educator should review data in the individualized report to become familiar with the learner's strengths and opportunities, share it with the employee to create an individualized orientation, then file the report in the employee's record. The charts and tables included in the report summarize the participant's simulation experience broken out by the different domains in the scenarios.

The Measured Domains compiled from the New Grad Onboarding Scenarios are results from the work of the learners caring for two patients for 6 hours. Assessment components including initial, ongoing, and specific additional assessments are grouped into the Assessment Domain. Communication opportunities such as communicating with the patient, a peer, or a physician are grouped into the Communication Domain. Timely interventions may include addressing the patient's pain appropriately. Many of the care objectives crossed over into more than one domain. There was a limit of three domains that were prioritized for each objective.

The SBAR compiled data from the New Grad Onboarding Scenarios reflect each time the learner had the opportunity to use SBAR and breaks it down into how they performed in each component.

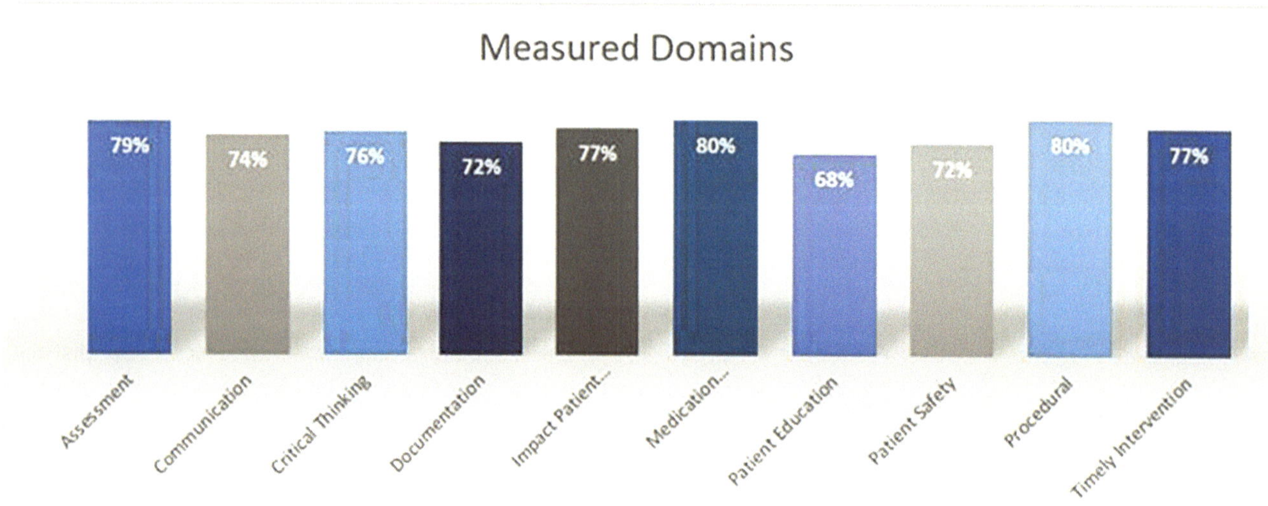

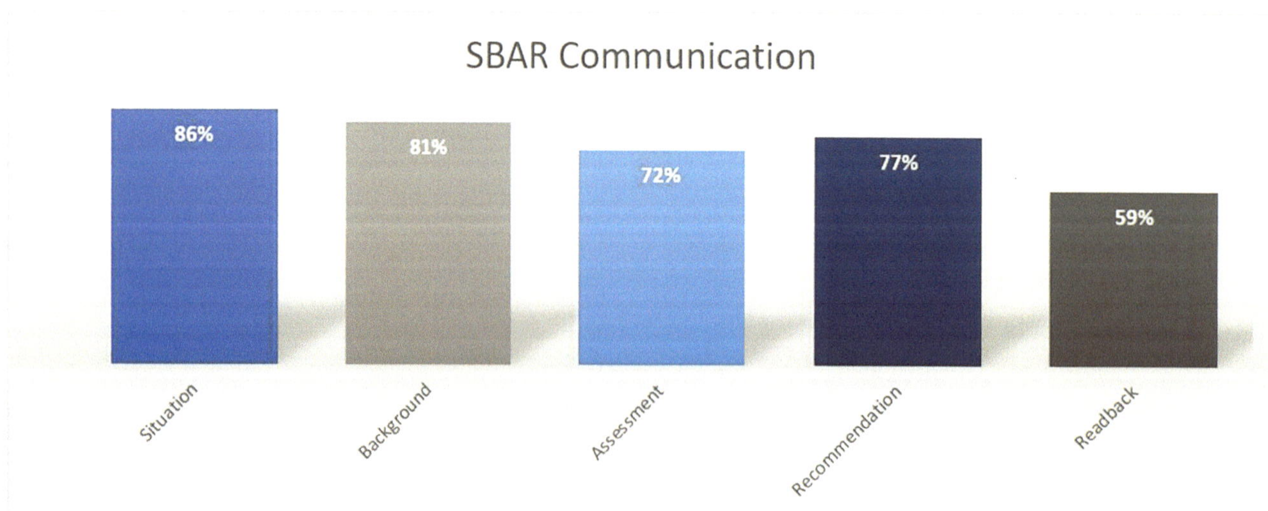

Integrating Simulation into Existing Education

Expanding the onboarding curriculum into the in-situ setting was an easy task because the simulation was already developed and piloted during onboarding with large numbers of learners. Additionally, there is value in using some of the onboarding skills and scenarios in-situ in addressing areas of improvement, such as catheter associated urinary tract infection (CAUTI) and central line bloodstream infection (CLABSI), especially as those simulations already existed. Adding new curriculum into the existing program was easier to accomplish because the basics of the program had already been developed and learners were already scheduled to attend. Prioritizing simulation events, fitting an event in that takes a different amount of time than the one it replaced, space, and equipment needed, and the ratio of simulation staff needed to deliver the simulation were the main issues to be solved.

New Groups of Learners

Reviewing and updating simulation program components is ongoing and vital in delivering the most valuable experience and identifying what is most important to the organization and impactful for patient safety. Integrating new types of learners into the existing programs included developing a program for nurses trained internationally.

International nurses have historically been great additions to Banner Health teams because of the potential for long-term retention. International nurses that came from countries that do not have the same technology or scope of practice participated in the New Grad scenarios to allow for a more comprehensive individual assessment and orientation to help them be successful in their nursing journey.

A simulation assessment was developed based on gaps observed during the International RN scenarios. This allowed educators to expedite early in the onboarding process any additional education needed such as EMR and IV pump training if needed. As with New Grads, the International nurses, and the direct report leader, usually the unit Sr. Manager, were included in the data collection process to assist in developing onboarding specific to their needs. Listed below are needs identified:

General Needs

- Unfamiliarity with the medications. Many countries go by Generic names only.
- Assessment capabilities vary. In some countries, nurses do not do assessments as the providers are responsible for assessments.

Language/Communication Needs

- Unfamiliarity with a term, acronym, medication name, or surgical procedure. Examples include:
- Situation-Background-Assessment-Recommendation (SBAR) Communication Tool
- Sepsis And perFusion Evaluation (S.A.F.E.) alert which expands the scope of the Sepsis alert
- Early Warning System (EWS) evidence-based scoring tool that looks at 5 vital signs metrics and calculates score to identify at risk patients for deterioration.
- Open Reduction Internal Fixation (ORIF)
- Discontinuing (DC)
- The term "full code"

Electronic Needs

- Had never used computer documentation.
- Had never used medication barcode scanner.

Rapid Onboarding to Meet Crisis Staffing Needs

Expedited onboarding was developed to facilitate staff getting onto units quicker to assist with crisis staffing needs. This involved large volumes of crisis staffing including External Travelers nurses and new hire experienced core nurses being onboarded quickly. When COVID surges called for rapid onboarding of the External Travelers to get them on units quickly to care for patients, the simulation team took the normal onboarding process and condensed it into a two-hour block and the Clinical Education team condensed the EMR training and Nursing onboarding to allow travelers to orient to the unit on Day 2 and take care of patients by Day 2 and 3.

A Program called *Core Experienced RN Onboarding Compression* was also developed to meet the increased, immediate need for nurses on units during the COVID pandemic. The *New Hire Experienced RN* simulation was moved to week 1 from week 2. The changes to the program consisted of condensing Simulation RN Onboarding and temporarily removing the Sepsis Escape Room and adding the regulatory components of Point of Care testing and restraints to the simulation skills program. This facilitated the Experienced RNs getting on the units to help with patient care by the end of the first week of hire.

Errors in practice that were identified during simulation helped identify Skill Labs that would be offered in situ or at the Simulation Center. In addition, specific skills such as Chest Tubes, Trach Care, $ETCO_2$ are often requested. The most frequently requested scenario is Mock Codes. Mock Codes are included at onboarding as it is a high-risk, low-frequency event for most healthcare professionals. The onboarding Mock Code is BLS based focused on primary ABCD skills and roles in a Code. In 2012, the Simulation Team led the development of a standardized in-situ system Mock Code process to capture the learner outcomes. An electronic assessment form was developed that incorporated the main components in a Code and the timing of each response [4] (Appendix 3). This electronic form produced immediate debriefing feedback and data that facilitated a timely in-situ debriefing The in-situ Mock Code was developed to be a quick simulation; 5 min for the Code and a quick debriefing to help identify critical remediation needs of each group (Appendix 4). [4] Mock Codes are included in all in-situ facility simulation events.

Most recently, Mock Codes (Appendix 5) were developed to include COVID precautions needed to keep healthcare workers safe and to include the changes in how many healthcare team members could be in a room for a COVID code, roles and what equipment could be brought into a room.

One of the major changes to the Code process was that the participant had to assure their safety first. Instead of running right into the room to assess the situation, if the patient had COVID, they had to first assure their own personal safety and don personal protective equipment (PPE). To not use scarce and precious resources, the participants would tell the simulation staff how to don PPE instead of them using the resources. This allowed participants the opportunity to experience the time it would take to complete this important step and feel the anxiety of being delayed in entering room to care for patient. They experienced roles differently as only minimal staff could enter the room and the Code cart stayed outside the room. Debriefing discussion was rich in the barriers experienced during the mock. Masks and closed doors, even if there were windows, hindered communication between those in the room and those outside of the room. Staff weren't sure where to put the defibrillator which was usually on the Code cart and now not taken into the room. Medication and other supplies had to be handed off from outside the room to someone inside the room without touching each other. This all caused a major change in workflow and normal procedures in caring for deteriorating or coding patients.

The Culture of Safety simulations were offered insitu to existing facilities and included in a new facility pre-opening education. These simulations addressed both team building and communication. Teams that had worked together could refine their communication skills with each other while the simulations gave newer teams the opportunity to develop relationships and skill sets. Debriefing was critical for identifying take-aways and supporting each other by identifying the importance of situational responses for the Culture of Safety and the importance of a team in escaping the Escape Room. During debriefing participants transferred learning to other events in their work environment where it would be valuable.

Sample Curriculum #3: Sepsis Escape Room

Sepsis prevention and early recognition and treatment is a Banner Health Strategic Initiative. Sepsis contributes to increased patient mortality, length of stay (LOS), and readmission rates [5, 6]. Time is critical in diagnosing and treating sepsis. An Escape room was a perfect fit for simulation where a team participates in an interactive engaging event with puzzles to be solved within time constraints to be able to "escape the room". Curriculum addressed in the simulation includes:

- Identifying the signs and symptoms of sepsis
- Identifying Early Warning Signs of Sepsis and perfusion Evaluation (SAFE alert) clues
- Reviewing Systemic Inflammatory Response Syndrome (SIRS criteria)
- Demonstrating effective communication using SBAR
- Initiating sepsis bundle in the correct order
- Working effectively as a team.

An Escape Room is an active learning strategy that incorporates different learning styles and facilitates critical thinking, teamwork, and communication [7, 8]. Banner Simulation uses a modified, facilitator-guided 3 A's debriefing model in which open-ended questions are asked to encourage the learner to self-reflect on their experience and discuss opportunities for improvement [9–14]. The Escape Room required a more advanced level of facilitation and ability to take the competitive game and link the experience to caring for a patient with sepsis. Feedback from learners has been that the Escape Room is a meaningful exercise and even though they know about the Sepsis Protocol, this learning event has made an impact on remembering what to do when a patient is septic.

The Escape Room Simulation Specialist Learner Assessment Form (Appendix 6) is used to assess if the learning event objectives were met. This document assists the facilitator during debriefing and allows the learner to self-reflect and discuss why they responded the way they did and takeaways that would impact their clinical response. The learner report generated for the preceptor educator, and leader, describes the simulation event, objectives, and details of how the group performed in completing the Sepsis Bundle components.

The Sepsis Escape Room 2020 Q4 Learner Outcome data graph shows data from 52 groups that had an average of 5 learners per group. This data reflects the percentage of successful completion of each objective. For example, only 17% worked effectively as a team to escape the room and 60% were able to initiate the sepsis bundle in the correct order.

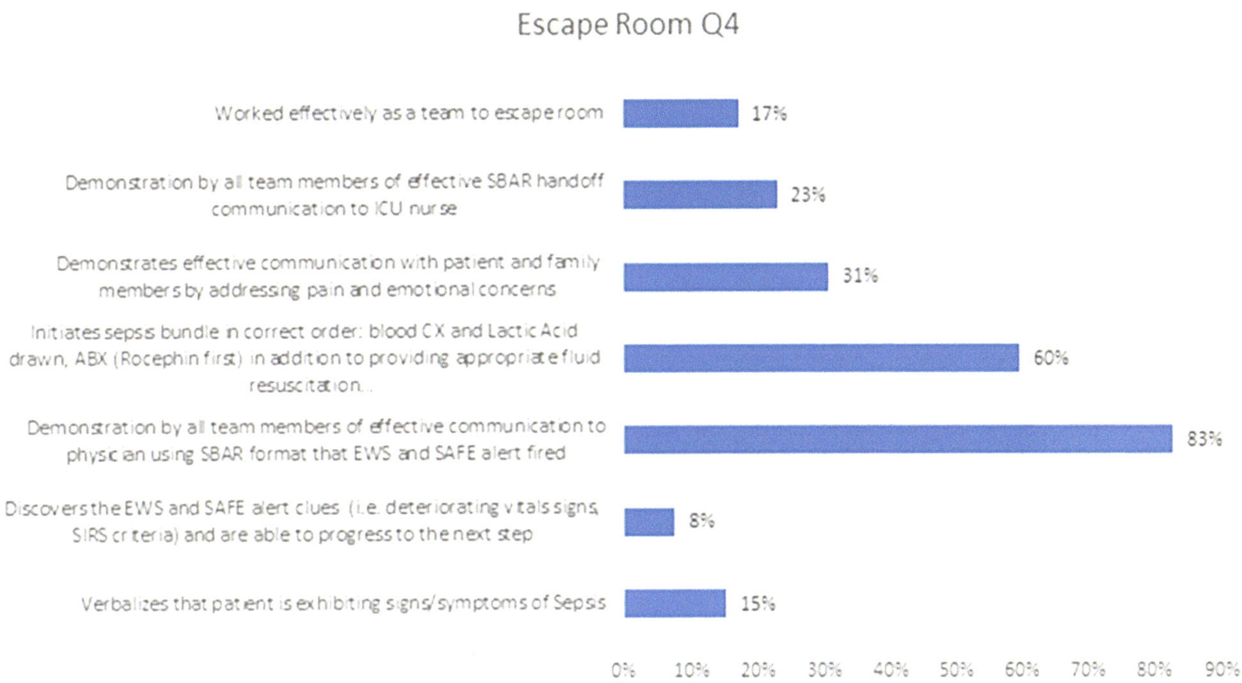

Curriculum #4: Culture of Safety

The Banner Culture of Safety simulation addresses situational safety responses such as asking for help, speaking up, clarification, calling a halt, escalation, and going up the chain of command. This simulation was prioritized to allow participants to practice situational responses and then debrief with the goal of improving competence and confidence in the real environment. Simulation is an intervention that is supported in Patient Safety Strategies in *The Safety Playbook* [14]. It isn't easy questioning another healthcare worker by asking for clarity from the bedside nurse if the pump rate reflects the correct dose for a heparin drip that is running on their patient. An example of this difficulty was exemplified in a Banner Culture of Safety simulation debriefing when learner feedback was given that "You have to have courage" in using the situational responses. Feedback from learners in this simulation also described hierarchy as a barrier to addressing safety concerns; learners admitted they didn't feel comfortable going to a leader and providing feedback.

Speaking up to address a patient safety concern is paramount in-patient safety. There are barriers that prevent people from addressing safety issues [15] and leadership support is crucial. Hierarchy can play a role in barriers to reporting events even when leaders are supportive. 'Speaking up' is one of the critical behaviors of patient safety that both provider and patient can improve [16]. Simulations that include interprofessional members and teamwork are more reflective of the complex real environment and is a great venue to incorporate and practice Culture of Safety situational responses, especially 'speaking up'. In situ simulations capture multiple events happening at the same time which includes interruptions and interactions and can offer a great opportunity for the team to work through and use important and pertinent situational responses. Communication and collaboration are vital behaviors for ensuring patient safety especially in "transitions in care and handoffs" [17].

Barnsteiner [18] shared a table outlining simulation activities that promote the Culture of Safety that includes a clinical room with hazards and errors.

Simulation Activities for Culture of Safety from Teaching the Culture of Safety [18]

Banner Simulation used "Room of Errors" format to address patient safety issues and connect them to Culture of Safety actions. The learners go into a patient's room and identify safety issues and what their response for handling the situation would be for each error. The Culture of Safety simulation was designed with the result of preparing learners with the knowledge and confidence needed to apply these principles in their workday to have a positive impact on patient safety.

Self-reflection and debriefing are focused on barriers to communication and how to navigate feeling safe, confident, and empowered to act on a patient safety issue and on being proactive and predictive. Improving situational awareness and exploring ways to accomplish this is covered in debriefing as well.

Situational responses to the errors in the Culture of Safety simulation include six responses for the learner to choose from. These responses include error wasn't identified, calling a halt, further discussion on choice of action was warranted, error identified but no action selected, speaking up/clarification issues, and escalation/chain of command issues.

The Culture of Safety Pie Graphs data illustrates the situational response (Appendix 7).

The top 3 common responses were the error wasn't identified, speaking up/clarification, and calling a halt. The least common responses were asking for help, escalation/Chain of Command, and error identified with no action selected. In debriefing sessions learners discuss the common responses and take-aways such as being more situationally aware and open to feedback.

Note: Calling a Halt is the correct answer for the Blood and Heparin errors due to their severity. If the learner doesn't choose Calling a Halt then it is discussed in debriefing and the graph data captures the error as *Further discussion on choice of action*.

Challenges and Solutions

One of the biggest challenges in running a simulation program is having adequately trained simulation team staff. Many times, staff have experience in education but rarely do new applicants have simulation experience. Staff training is extensive and time consuming. Onboarding skills and scenarios usually take 6 months to a year for a new simulation staff member to become fully independent. Staff progressively start by observing and then independently running one skill station at a time. Running a 6-hour simulation session and debriefing take considerably more time to learn and competence than shorter scenarios. In addition, debriefing takes time to gain competence in. Typical debriefings last 30 minutes to 1 hour but debriefing a 6-hour long scenario is much more complicated. Other simulation events, besides onboarding, that occur may take over a year to incorporate into the competency of the simulation specialist. The time it takes to onboard can impact the program's ability to deliver impactful curriculum for patient safety.

As a simulation program grows and transforms, the number of simulation positions needed can change. The number of new hire RNs being onboarded is fluid and changes from week to week and month to month. Historically, some of this is cyclative, with higher needs for nursing staff during the winter months in the Arizona Banner Health Region. This is when our facilities are more likely to be full of patients and have a higher need for nurses. For example, External Traveler RN onboarding can double and triple the normal weekly numbers of participants in the first few weeks in January. The solution, as in COVID high onboarding, is to modify the simulation program. Focusing on the critical actions and knowing common errors helps assure the important components are addressed.

Simulation staff assessment and remediation reliability are critical and takes ongoing assessment of staff. This is important as the data is critical in identifying the opportunities and strengths of the learner and to get help if needed to be successful. Inter-rater reliability of the simulation staff is assessed using their assessments of learners and comparing to norms. Data points are reviewed, and staff review for understanding and consistency in ratings.

Student to learner ratio varies with each simulation event. New Grad scenarios have a 1:2 simulation specialist to learner ratio. This is a high resource simulation that is greatly influenced by the number of new grads hired any given week. Simulation skills have a 1:4-5 simulation specialist to learner ratio.

It is recognized that it is harder to get learners back to training/simulation after they are off orientation, as they are caring for patients. Therefore, when onboarding numbers have been high, the solution has been to prioritize skills for the experienced and new graduate nurses and delay new graduate scenarios. The reason being that new graduates have a longer onboarding period and there is a high probability that they can be scheduled for their scenarios while they were still being onboarded without eliminating the skills assessments for the experienced nurses.

A significant challenge is ensuring that the learners all move through the day at a roughly equal pace. However, the most updated Banner Simulation RN New Hire Onboarding Day consists of skills and scenarios that take different amounts of time to complete. When there is variation in the time it takes to do a skill or scenario, the flow of the learners going through the events must rehearsed and modified to be successful.

A Preceptor Checklist (Appendix 8) was developed to use at the bedside to address most missed steps observed in simulation onboarding skills. Consistent errors in basic skills resulted in the development of this checklist that could be used at the bedside and tracked with a QR Code. The purpose of the checklist is to ensure follow through at the bedside on the most missed steps that are seen in simulation skills. The list gives the preceptor a focused guide and allows for remediation at the point of care. It also can provide data on continued errors. This process at Banner has been delayed due COVID priorities.

Summary

Use of simulation for pre-hire and new hire orientation provides the opportunity to develop standardized processes focused on organizational needs and curriculum that is impactful for patient safety. Simulation onboarding orientation curriculum can cover a variety of important clinical and behavioral aspects to help the new hire be successful in the clinical setting. Metrics are key in assessment, remediation, and learning outcomes as well as showing the value of the simulation program.

Appendix 1 Pre-brief and Orientation to New Grad Scenario Simulation Tool

Simulation Scenario Orientation

Welcome to SIM:

- No tricks, No strange diagnoses
- Independent functioning with resources

Objective of Simulation:

- Safe patient care
- Begin to develop patient time management, prioritization skills, etc.

Professionalism:

- Best practice: 4 critical behaviors
- Allow others their discovery moments. Be mindful of voice volume & save your "discoveries" for debriefing

Agenda:

- Clock out: lunch (12pm-1pm) and end of day
- Debriefing (Most important component of simulation) at 2:30pm (safe zone to review, reflect, & clarify)

Latex allergy/sensitivity:

- Ask learners. Use non-latex gloves

Linen Cart

- If bed linens become wet please change them out

Supply Room (Clean Utility)

Pyxis (med Room):

- Pills are beads. Do NOT open med package. DO NOT throw away Pills/syringes. ALL MEDS (even torn or damaged) need to be returned to buggies/bins. Patches attach to velcro - Do not write with marker on patch. IV/PB location (ED)
- Advise learners of login and password, explain override functionality.
- All IV fluids are refilled. Spike ↓
- All IV and SQ medications in syringes are filled with air.
- No meds in manikins mouth, simulate IM and SQ's
- Do accurate narcotic count. Inform facilitator of any discrepancies made ASAP
- If you are having problems with sign in with Pyxis, DO NOT continue to put a wrong password in. Please ask for help or the Pyxis will lock you out. Check to ensure CapsLOCK is not on.
- If Pharmacy is working around the Pyxis and you need meds, please ask them if you could grab the meds you need
- Medication scanners are on WOW's. Use BCMA at Sim center.

Code Cart:

- Live energy. Stocked w/ meds

Patient Room:

- Beds work, O2 and suction work, Alaris IV pumps work
- Blue basket for used pills, syringes
- Baby buggy for used supplies
- ELO monitor (if in ICU)
- Use whiteboard
- BS drawers for facilitators only

Manikin:

- Inspect manikin: simulated spontaneous respirations, pulses, lungs sounds, heart tones, bowel sounds, explain vocals (driver and manikin voices may interchange). defib/hands free pads over metal posts
- Fluids on one side/pulses on other
- Name bands
- How to take VS (Learner takes 1st set VS manually –then can delegate other VS). Temp and O2 sat cards on pts chest are current
- Do NOT start or discontinue any IVs in manikin. Use IV arm
- IVs covered by stockinette are not in use. Functional IV w/drainage bag
- Ask for help to turn manikin
- Ask us for anything you cannot assess… (e.g. grips, pushes, pulls). Do not assume

IV Arm:

- Use for any restarts or new IVs needed in your manikin. Supplies in drawers

Signage/Krames education:

- Pt education, arm bands, room signs, blank consents

Patient Board:

- NAME ALERT…Patient name, learner name, facilitator

Documentation:

- (Done with assigned facilitator in groups of 2) Choose a WOW, TrainB Power Chart>User Name = SIMRN# > password = training > It opens to Care Compass > Assign relationship
- Physician: Physician, X (Ph, X)
- Other RN (handoff, witness): SIMRN, SIMRN30
- We expect charting in EMR (VS, assessments, med administration, handoff and notification, procedures, etc.)
- Labs, Radiology, H&Ps, Progress Notes, Op Notes are all in Cerner (Results Review and Clinical Notes)
- If you can't find where to chart or don't know how to chart something, ask

Miscellaneous:

- Hand gel only (no running water)
- Facilitator is your CNA, experienced nurse, HUC, doctor, R.T., etc.
- Need 2nd nurse med verification? Ask facilitator only
- If we are busy with other learner, don't wait (do other tasks until we are available)
- Plug in WOW's whenever possible
- Please empty pockets of alcohol wipes, NS syringes, etc into basins before debriefing

11/14/19

Appendix 2 Critical Actions and Errors-Based Learner Assessment Checklist

Banner
Simulation System

New Hire Skills Assessment

CVC Site Care

Onboarding Skills Station

Participant Name: 0 Lawson#: 0 Date: 1/0/1900

Experience: 0

Instructor:

CVC Site Care

	Steps	✓ = done; X = not done
Perform Critical Behaviors: confirm order, verify pt with 2 identifiers, explain procedure, & hand hygiene		
1	Removes dressing: demonstrate applying face mask to self and patient, apply gloves, removing old dressing and Biopatch, removing gloves, and performing hand hygiene.	✓
2	Cleanses site: demonstrate cleansing site and catheter with 2% chlorhexidine for 30 second friction scrub.	✓
3	Secures site: demonstrate applying Biopatch, skin prep, stabilization device (if applicable) and transparent dressing.	✓
4	Labels dressing: demonstrate labeling with date and time of dressing change and initials.	✓
5	Measures catheter: demonstrate measuring external length of PICC.	✓
6	Changes caps: demonstrate changing needleless connectors, cleansing hub with alcohol, and placing, without contaminating caps/line.	✓
7	Maintains sterility: demonstrate performing all steps without breaking sterile technique.	✓

Appendix 3 Mock Code Electronic Checklist to Capture Learning Performance [1]

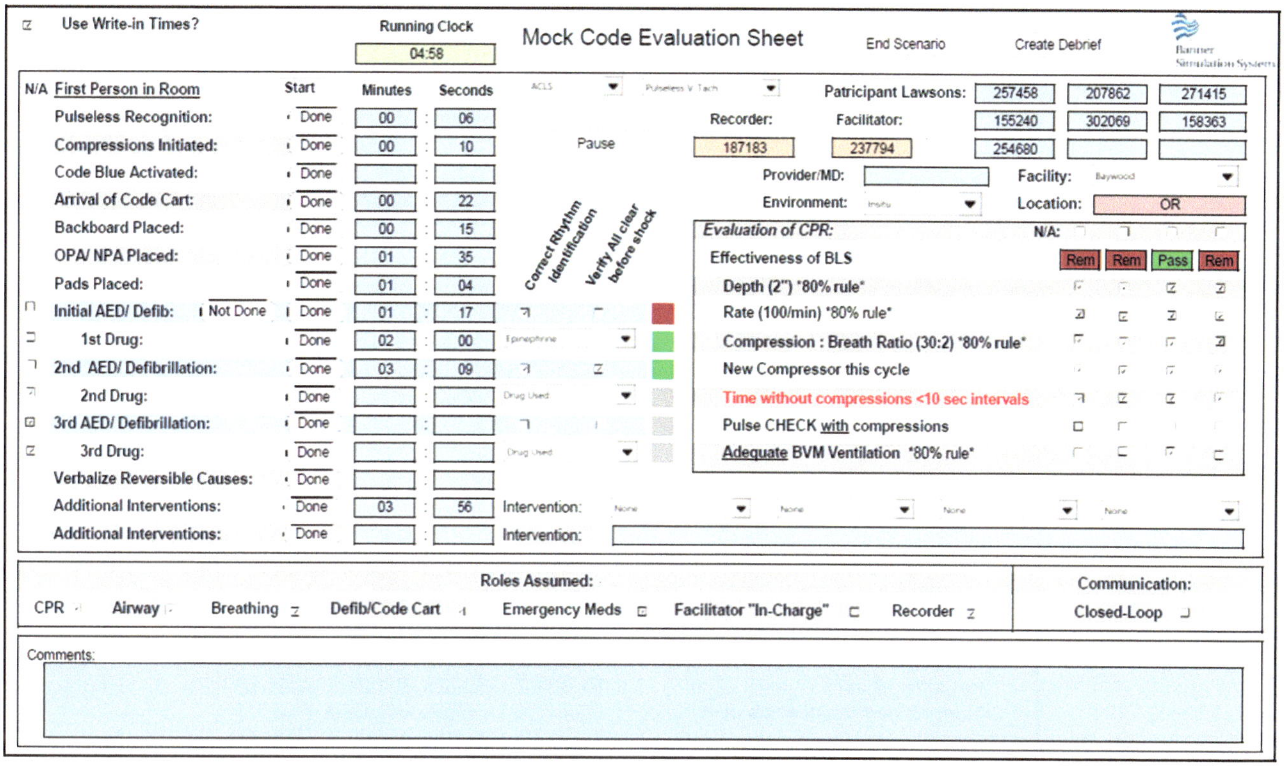
Use Write-in Times?

Running Clock 04:58

Mock Code Evaluation Sheet

End Scenario Create Debrief

Banner Simulation System

N/A First Person in Room	Start	Minutes	Seconds
Pulseless Recognition:	Done	00	06
Compressions Initiated:	Done	00	10
Code Blue Activated:	Done		
Arrival of Code Cart:	Done	00	22
Backboard Placed:	Done	00	15
OPA/ NPA Placed:	Done	01	35
Pads Placed:	Done	01	04
Initial AED/ Defib: Not Done	Done	01	17
1st Drug:	Done	02	00
2nd AED/ Defibrillation:	Done	03	09
2nd Drug:	Done		
3rd AED/ Defibrillation:	Done		
3rd Drug:	Done		
Verbalize Reversible Causes:	Done		
Additional Interventions:	Done	03	56
Additional Interventions:	Done		

ACLS Pulseless V. Tach

Pause

Correct Rhythm Identification

Verify All clear before shock

Epinephrine

Drug Used

Intervention: None None None None

Intervention:

Patricipant Lawsons: 257458 207862 271415

Recorder: 187183

Facilitator: 237794

155240 302069 158363

254680

Provider/MD:

Facility: Baywood

Environment: Insitu

Location: OR

Evaluation of CPR: N/A:				
Effectiveness of BLS	Rem	Rem	Pass	Rem
Depth (2") *80% rule*				
Rate (100/min) *80% rule*				
Compression : Breath Ratio (30:2) *80% rule*				
New Compressor this cycle				
Time without compressions <10 sec intervals				
Pulse CHECK with compressions				
Adequate BVM Ventilation *80% rule*				

Roles Assumed:

CPR Airway Breathing Defib/Code Cart Emergency Meds Facilitator "In-Charge" Recorder

Communication:

Closed-Loop

Comments:

Appendix 4 Mock Code Electronic Checklist Debriefing form Automatically Generated from Learning Performance [1]

Pulseless V-Tach Mock Code Debriefing Sheet

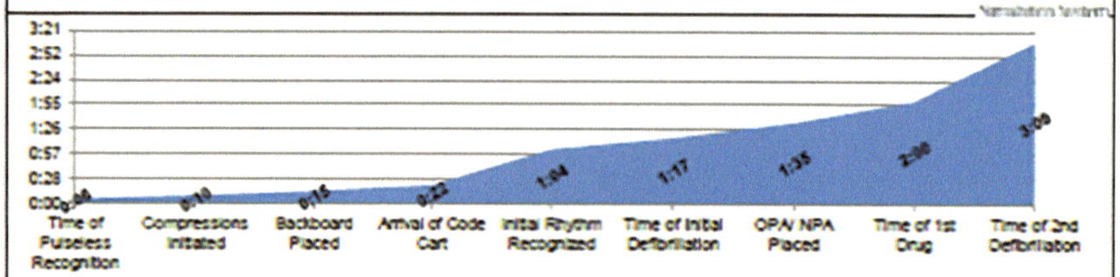

Intervention Timeline	Time from start	Time Success Criteria Met or Missed?
Time of Pulseless Recognition	00:06	Completed Successfully
Compressions Initiated	00:10	Completed Successfully
Backboard Placed	00:15	Completed Successfully
Arrival of Code Cart	00:22	Completed Successfully
Initial Rhythm Recognized	01:04	Completed Successfully
Time of Initial Defibrillation	01:17	Completed Successfully
OPA/ NPA Placed	01:35	Not performed
Time of 1st Drug	02:00	Completed Successfully
Time of 2nd Defibrillation	03:09	Completed Successfully

Team Roles Filled:

Defib/Code Cart	Breathing	CPR	Facilitator "In Charge"
Emergency Meds	Recorder	Airway	Closed-Loop Communication

CPR by Cycle

Effective Compressions	Cycle One	Cycle Two	Cycle Three	Cycle Four
Depth (2") "80% rule"				
Rate (100/min) "80% rule"				
Compression : Breath Ratio (30:2) "80% rule"				
New Compressor this cycle				
Time without compressions <10 sec intervals				
Pulse CHECK with compressions				
Adequate BVM Ventilation "80% rule"				

Critical Errors:

On the first Defib did not properly execute an all clear before shocking

Debriefing Notes:

Remediation Methods used:

Commonly remediated items:

Compression Depth	☐	OPA Insertion	☐	AED/Defib equipment usage	☐
Compression Technique	☐	BVM technique	☐	Hands free pads	☐
Hand position	☐	2 people on airway	☐	Connection problems	☐
30:2 Ratio	☐	"E" or "C" technique	☐	Pads versus 3-5 lead	☐
Counting aloud	☐	Each breath over 1 second	☐	ALS algorithm	☑
2 full minutes on chest	☐	Just enough to make chest rise	☐		
Off chest time < than 10 sec	☐	Correct Backboard usage	☐		
Pulse check with compressions	☑				

SUBMIT TO SHAREPOINT

What went well?

Everyone knew role, Good compression rate and depth, quick to first defib

What could be improved?

Safe defib, fully release with each compression, pulse check with compression, ALS Algorythm

Feedback Mannequin Information: (Only for use when a feedback mannequin has been utilized)

Ventilations:		Compressions:	
Average Volume		Average Depth	
Average number per minute		Average number per minute	
Minute Volume		Average compression rate	
Total Number		Total number	
Number Correct		Number Correct	
Percent Correct		Percent Correct	
Too Much		Too Deep	
Too Little		Too Shallow	
Too Fast		Wrong hand position	
Compr: Vent Ratio	:	Hand Position too low	
		Incomplete release	

Appendix 5 COVID Mock Code Outline

Covid Codes (30 minutes total)

Pre-brief:

- **BLS, covid code**
- **Code cart:** Plugged in - Zoll defibrillator with AED/ACLS mode – pads with velcro – Live energy - Ambu bag - recorder board
- **Manikin/room:** Bed works, O2 works, Manikin has velcro front and back for pads
- **PPE:** 1 person (to limit supply use) needs to do hand hygiene, don PPE gown (use pt. gown), gloves, simulate applying mask and shield before any staff can enter room; other staff wear gloves

Debrief:

- **Teamwork:**
  Assign Roles: Identify team members inside and outside room. Goal to minimize number of staff in room
  Communication: closed loop, Vocera, room phone, cell phone on speaker, Care aware phones, Ascom phone, disaster walkie talkies
- **Covid code:**
  - Room door remains closed during code.
  - Outside staff do not cross threshold.
  - Code cart stays outside room with defibrillator brought inside rm.
  - Meds prepared by outside nurse, labeled, placed in basin and handed to nurse inside room at doorway without touching each other's hands (outside nurse touches only outside of basin- inside contaminated).
  - Check with facility regarding supplies/meds used in code; dispose of properly.
  - During intubation; follow Banner Covid-19 intubation workflow
- **Remediate only to missed steps per AHA. Circle any missed steps below:**

Initial: Scene safe (PPE), check responsiveness, call code, check pulse (5-10 sec), begin compressions

Compressions: 100-120 min, 2-2.4 inches, recoil, 30:2 ratio (count out loud), backboard, change compressor Q 2 min, Check pulse with compressions, off chest <10 seconds

Airway/breathing: 2 people if able; *Airway* stands at HOB- *Breathing* at side of pt., Pillow out, C & E, OPA, Bag just to chest rise, O2 all the way up,

Defibrillation: Clear to analyze, then back on chest for charging; clear again and deliver safe (Eyes on pt. while shocking)

NOTE: Document "Covid code: Enhanced precautions used" on excel code sheet.
Return rhythm generator to office when done.

11/11/20

Appendix 6 Escape Room Simulation Specialist Learner Assessment Form

Escape Room is a challenging, creative opportunity for participants to recognize, identify and intervene for a deteriorating Septic patient. The participants work as an interactive team in a scenario-based game that is engaging and memorable. Team members will work to discover clues that lead them down several pathways to prioritize and implement the Sepsis bundle. Following the pathways and providing initiative driven care eventually leads them to escaping the room. The experience concludes in a reflective, objective driven debriefing session involving: EWS/SAFE alert, SIRS criteria, Cerner components, SBAR, and prioritization of interventions.

A copy of the team's Escape the Room performance will be attached to each learner's report for review and will include the team's participation as well as any relevant individual learner participation comments.

Station Goals:

1. Recognizes and notifies physician of Sepsis, SIRS criteria and patient deterioration that triggered EWS and SAFE alerts
2. Initiates all Sepsis Bundle Components in correct order.
3. Model professional behaviors of communication and effective teamwork with team members, patient and family

Escape Room		*X = Remediated*	*Comments*
1	Verbalizes that patient is exhibiting signs/symptoms of Sepsis		Instructor: Amy Simms
2	Discovers the EWS and SAFE alert clues (i.e. deteriorating vitals signs, SIRS criteria)		Mix of NG and Experienced
3	Demonstration by all team members of effective communication to physician using SBAR format that EWS and SAFE alert fired	X	Group escaped with 17 minutes remaining
4	Initiates sepsis bundle in correct order: blood CX and Lactic Acid drawn, ABX (Rocephin first) in addition to providing appropriate fluid resuscitation		
5	Demonstrates effective communication with patient and family members by addressing pain and emotional concerns		
6	Demonstration by all team members of effective SBAR handoff communication to ICU nurse		
7	Worked effectively as a team		
Learner Specific Comments:			

Appendix 7 Pie Graphs of Culture of Safety Situational Responses Illustrate Situational Responses

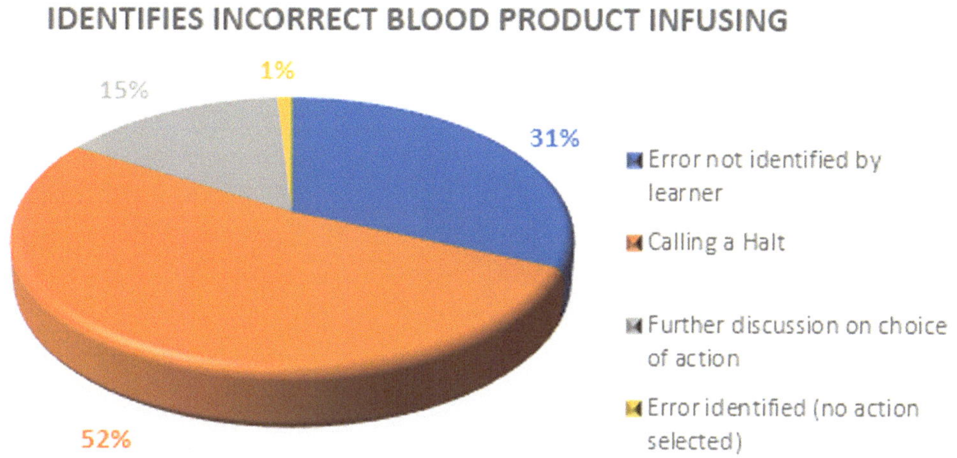

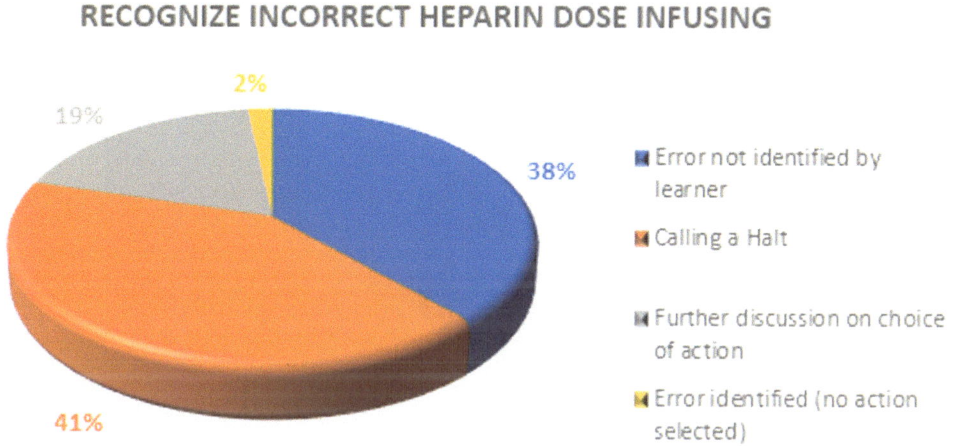

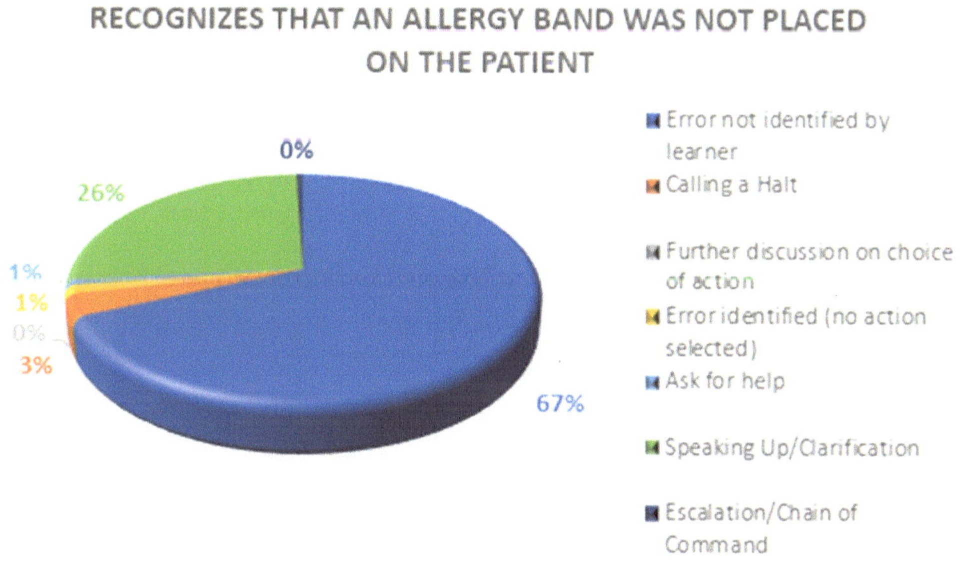

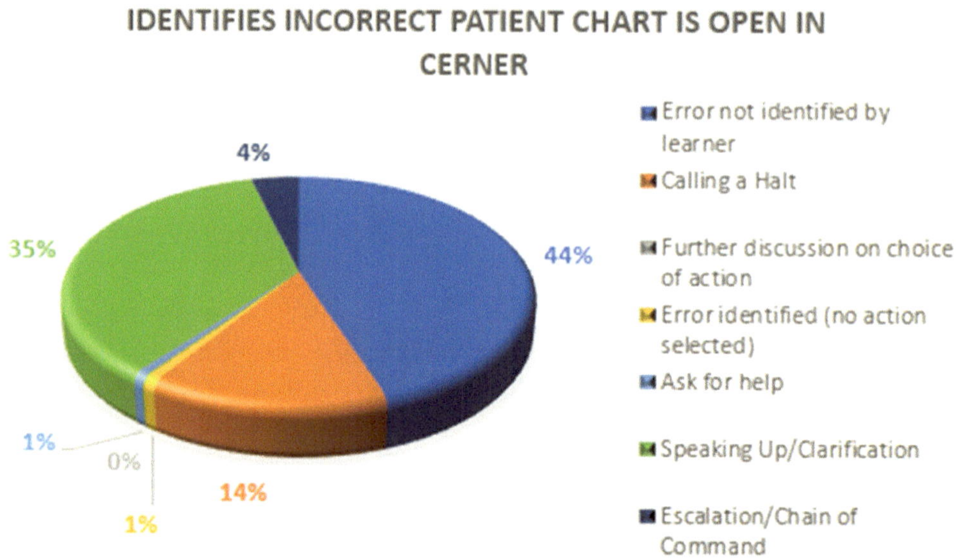
IDENTIFIES INCORRECT PATIENT CHART IS OPEN IN CERNER
4%
44%
35%
1%
0%
14%
1%
Error not identified by learner
Calling a Halt
Further discussion on choice of action
Error identified (no action selected)
Ask for help
Speaking Up/Clarification
Escalation/Chain of Command

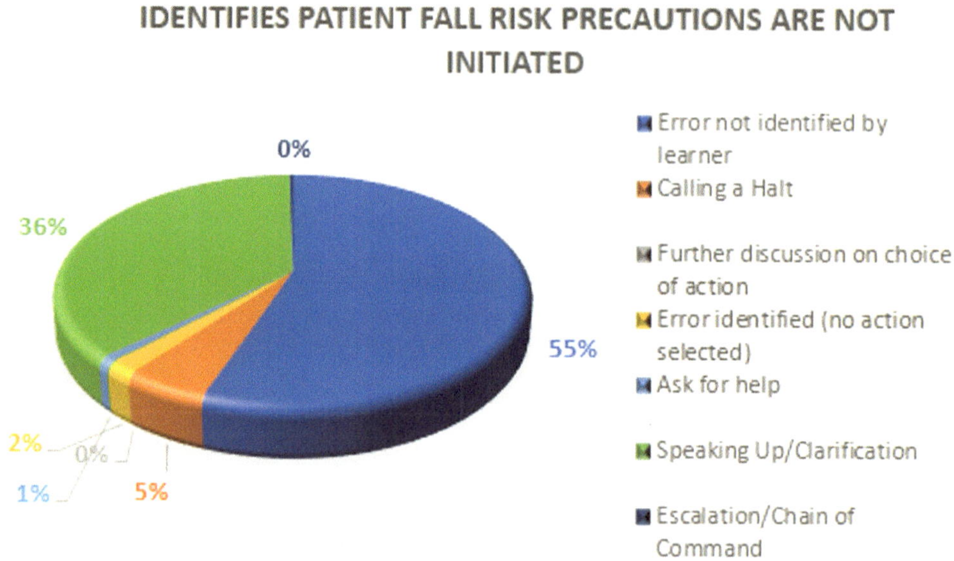
IDENTIFIES PATIENT FALL RISK PRECAUTIONS ARE NOT INITIATED
0%
36%
55%
2%
0%
1%
5%
Error not identified by learner
Calling a Halt
Further discussion on choice of action
Error identified (no action selected)
Ask for help
Speaking Up/Clarification
Escalation/Chain of Command

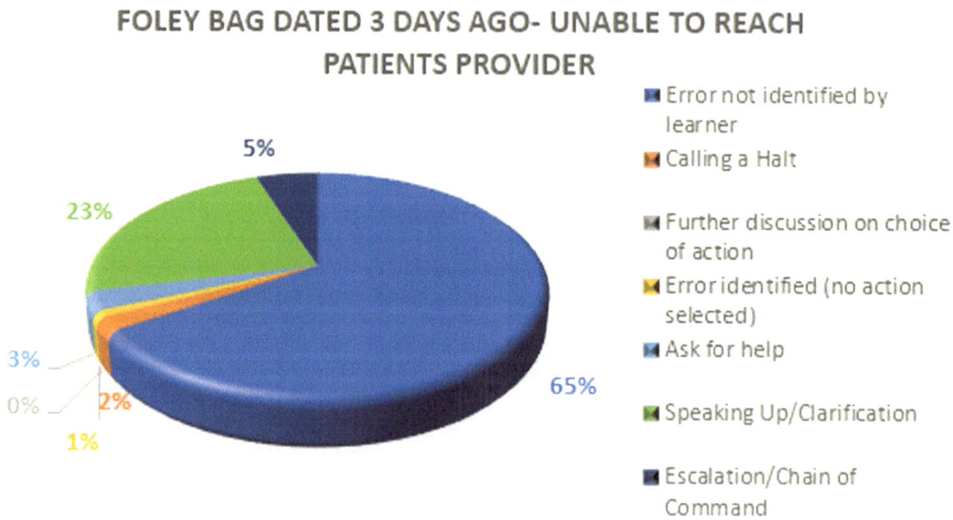
FOLEY BAG DATED 3 DAYS AGO- UNABLE TO REACH PATIENTS PROVIDER
5%
23%
3%
0%
2%
1%
65%
Error not identified by learner
Calling a Halt
Further discussion on choice of action
Error identified (no action selected)
Ask for help
Speaking Up/Clarification
Escalation/Chain of Command

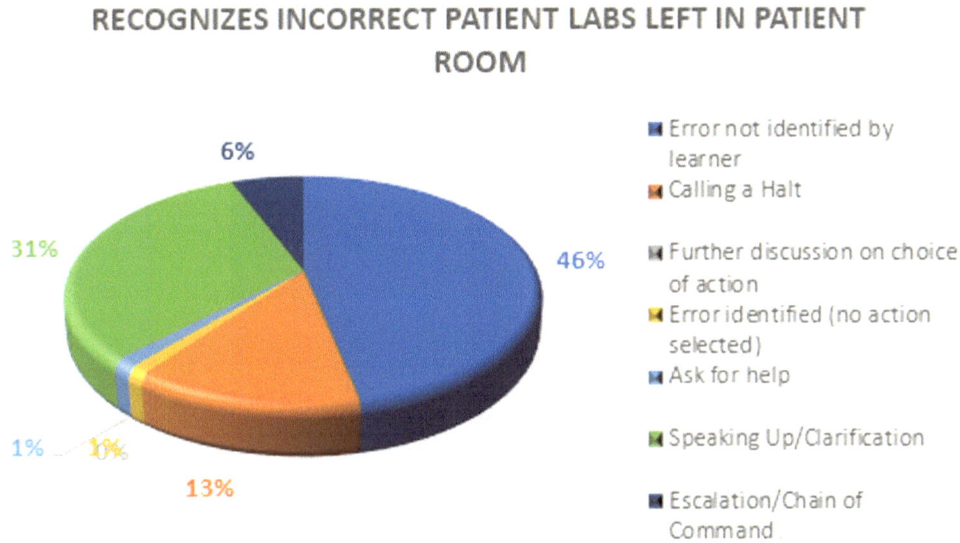
RECOGNIZES INCORRECT PATIENT LABS LEFT IN PATIENT ROOM
6%
31%
46%
1%
1%
0%
13%
Error not identified by learner
Calling a Halt
Further discussion on choice of action
Error identified (no action selected)
Ask for help
Speaking Up/Clarification
Escalation/Chain of Command

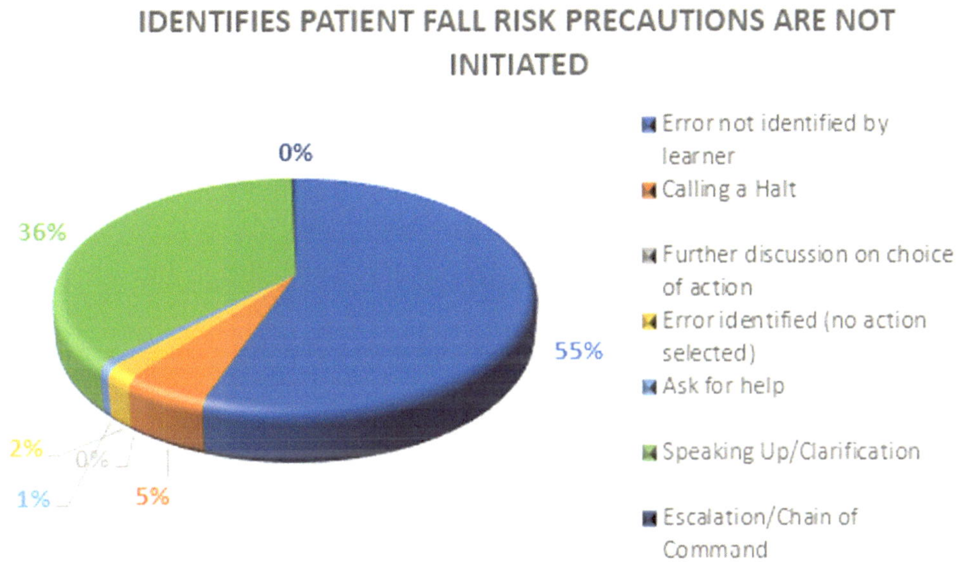
IDENTIFIES PATIENT FALL RISK PRECAUTIONS ARE NOT INITIATED
0%
36%
55%
2%
0%
1%
5%
Error not identified by learner
Calling a Halt
Further discussion on choice of action
Error identified (no action selected)
Ask for help
Speaking Up/Clarification
Escalation/Chain of Command

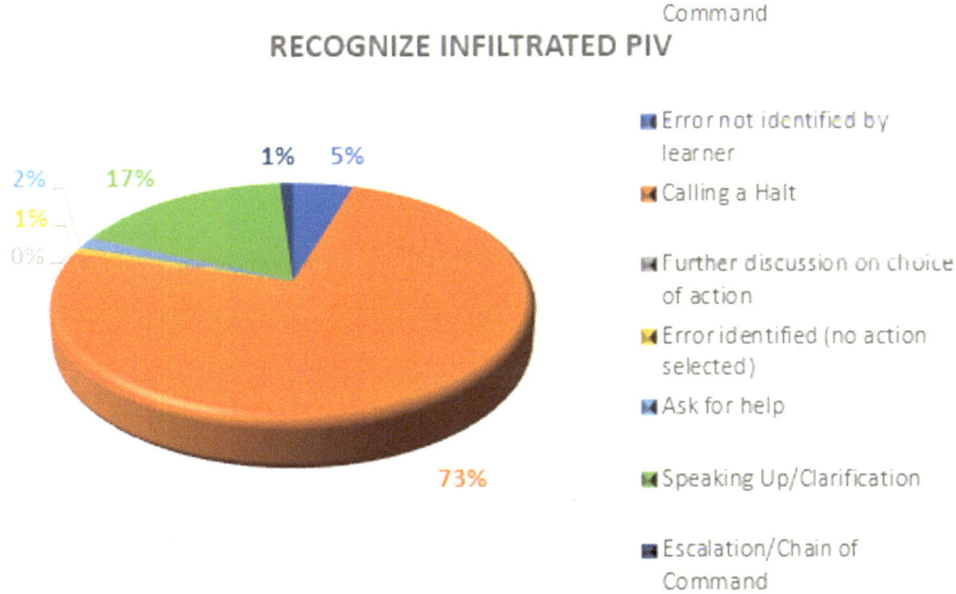
RECOGNIZE INFILTRATED PIV
1%
5%
2%
17%
1%
0%
73%
Error not identified by learner
Calling a Halt
Further discussion on choice of action
Error identified (no action selected)
Ask for help
Speaking Up/Clarification
Escalation/Chain of Command

Appendix 8 Preceptor Checklist

Preceptor Checklist for Most Missed Steps in Simulation

New Hire Name: ______________________ Exp RN ☐ New Grad RN ☐ Preceptor Name: ______________________
New Hire Lawson: __________ Hire date: __________ Facility: ________ Preceptor Lawson: __________

Directions for paper version: Below are the steps that nurses miss the most when performing each of these skills. Observe the new hire when they perform these skills. Note any breaches in technique that align with the bullet points below. Provide feedback as needed. If the new hire performs the skill flawlessly, check "MET." If the new hire has room for growth on the skills, check "NOT MET" and then refer them to policy/clinical skills. At end of orientation, scan to Stephanie.Latus@bannerhealth.com.
To access the electronic version: Scan the QR code either with your phone's camera or your scanning app. You will be taken to an electronic checklist. Complete the electronic checklist after each skill attempt.

	MET	NOT MET	POLICY/ CLINICAL SKILLS	QR CODE
Blood Administration	☐	☐	☐	
• Checks transfusion record – Possible errors include missing the patient ID, blood bank ID, unit number, or product number.	☐	☐	☐	
• Prepares tubing- Primed correctly with entire filter covered in normal saline.	☐	☐	☐	
• Employee specific (see report) ____________	☐	☐	☐	
CVC (central line dressing change)				
• Maintains sterility Common errors include breaking sterility w/cap change, donning gloves incorrectly	☐	☐	☐	
• Changes caps- Employee might forget to change caps with each dressing change, change them improperly, or fail to properly scrub end of catheter with alcohol before applying a new cap	☐	☐	☐	
• Measures catheter – Employee might forget or might not know how to measure external length	☐	☐	☐	
• Employee specific (see report) ____________	☐	☐	☐	
IV Insertion and Removal				
• Identifying site- The most common error involves leaving the tourniquet on while cleansing site and/or organizing supplies	☐	☐	☐	
• Cleanses site- The employee may incorrectly cleanse (should scrub with chlorhexadine for full 30 seconds, hashtag pattern, friction)	☐	☐	☐	
• Employee specific (see report) ____________	☐	☐	☐	
PPE (donning and doffing gloves, gown, and mask)				
• Doffing Doffing (removing) the mask is the step that most often results in contamination.	☐	☐	☐	
• Employee specific (see report) ____________	☐	☐	☐	
Urinary Catheter Insertion and Removal				
• Maintains sterility Possible errors include incorrectly organizing equipment (i.e., too far from patient), touching patient on insertion with sterile glove, or crossing sterile field.	☐	☐	☐	
• Provides Peri care Possible errors include incorrectly discarding castile wipes (i.e., they assume that soap and water pericare is sufficient and neglect to use castile wipes for 2nd round of pericare), or only one or two wipes are used rather than all three.	☐	☐	☐	
• Employee specific (see report) ____________	☐	☐	☐	
Alaris Pump				
• Prepares pump Errors include entering pt's MRN or last name instead of correctly entering patients FIN / ACCT number.	☐	☐	☐	
• Programs pump for drug bolus Errors include going outside of Guardrails or programming incorrect dose	☐	☐	☐	
• Programs pump for IV fluid bolus Errors include using basic infusion, not following orders or programming the bolus too fast	☐	☐	☐	
• Employee specific (see report) ____________	☐	☐	☐	

References

1. Health Care-Associated Infections. Office of disease prevention and health promotion; 2020 [cited 2021 April 1]. Available from: https://health.gov/our-work/health-care-quality/health-care-associated-infections.
2. Get Ahead of Sepsis. Centers for Disease Control and Prevention; U.S. Department of Health and Human Services [cited 2021 April 23] Available from; https://www.cdc.gov/sepsis/education/index.html.
3. What is patient experience? Agency for Healthcare Research and Quality, Rockville, MD; 2021 [cited 2021, April 10]. Available from: https://www.ahrq.gov/cahps/about-cahps/patient-experience/index.html.
4. Josey K, Smith ML, Kayani AS, Raschke RA, et al. Hospitals with more-active participation in conducting standardized in-situ mock codes have improved survival after in-hospital cardiopulmonary arrest. Resuscitation. 2018;133:47–52. https://doi.org/10.1016/j.resuscitation.2018.09.020.
5. Centers for Disease Control and Prevention. Sepsis. [cited 2021 Jan 8]. Available from: https://www.cdc.gov/sepsis/clinicaltools/index.html.
6. Society of Critical Care Medicine and the European Society of Intensive Care Medicine. Surviving Sepsis Campaign [cited Jan 8, 2021]. Available from: https://www.sccm.org/SurvivingSepsisCampaign/Guidelines/Adult-Patients.
7. Adams V, Burger S, Crawford K, et al. Can you escape? Creating an escape room to facilitate active learning. J Nurses Prof Dev. 2018;34(2):E1–5. https://doi.org/10.1097/NND.0000000000000433. [cited Aug 27, 2020]. Available from: https://journals.lww.com/jnsdonline/Fulltext/2018/03000/Can_You_Escape__Creating_an_Escape_Room_to.15.aspx'12
8. Laerdal. Simulation escape room workbook. [monograph on the Internet]. [cited Aug 27, 2020]. Available from: Simulation Escape Room Resources (laerdal.com).
9. Cantrel MA. The importance of debriefing in clinical simulations. Clin Simul Nursing. 2008;4(2):e19–23.
10. Fanning RM, Gaba DM. The role of debriefing in simulation-based learning. Simul Healthc. 2007;2(2):115–25.

11. Gladwell M. The tipping point how little things can make a big difference. Little Brown; 2000.
12. Jaye P, Thomas L, Reedy G. The Diamond: a structure for simulation debrief. Clin Teacher. 2015;12(3):171–5.
13. Lacroix D. Debriefing in simulation train the trainer, laerdal medical educational services, simulation user network. 2016.
14. Rudolf JW, Simon R, Dufresne RL, et al. There's no such thing as "Non-Judgemental" debriefing: a theory and method for debriefing with good judgement. Simul Healthc. 2006;1(1):49–55.
15. Byrnes J, Teman S. The safety playbook. Chicago, IL: Health Administration Press; 2018. p. 110.
16. Culture of safety: an overview. ECRI. [cited Aug 27, 2020]. Available from: https://www.ecri.org/components/HRC/Pages/RiskQual21.aspx?tab=1.
17. Nacioglu A. As a critical behavior to improve quality and patient safety in health care: speaking up! Safe Health. 2016;2:1–25. [cited 2021 Jan 8]. https://doi.org/10.1186/s40886-016-0021-x.
18. Barnsteiner J. Teaching the culture of safety. American Nurses Association; 2011. Available from: https://ojin.nursingworld.org/MainMenuCategories/ANAMarketplace/ANAPeriodicals/OJIN/TableofContents/Vol-16-2011/No3-Sept-2011/Teaching-and-Safety.html?css=print#Integrating

Simulation for Nursing Competencies

30

Cynthia Shum

> Tell me, and I will forget, show me, and I may remember; involve me, and I will understand.—*Confucius*

Background

Consumers of healthcare expect and deserve to have care delivered by competent nurses. Healthcare is a high-risk industry continuously evolving and becoming more complex daily. The advent of new technologies, treatments, and equipment demands a high level of knowledge, skills, and attitudes (KSAs) for nurses. Healthcare administrators are responsible for ensuring their staff are prepared at all times. Registered nurses practice under a professional license and have a defined scope of practice in their work areas.

The Nursing Scope and Standards of Practice describe the "who," "what," "where," "when," "why," and "how" of nursing practice [1]. Scope of practice describes the services that a qualified health professional is deemed competent to perform and permitted to undertake—in keeping with the terms of their professional license. There are numerous specialties in healthcare and an ever-increasing set of new skills that are being added to the scope of practice for nursing. Furthermore, as healthcare evolves, the nursing staff must be prepared to keep up. It is the responsibility of individual organizations to define what competencies the nursing staff need in order to conduct their specific jobs correctly and safely. Competency is a set of defined KSAs necessary to fulfill organizational and specific work area requirements and is considered a fundamental element in the provision of nursing care.

Competencies are driven by regulatory and organizational mandates and policies, which commence during orientation to a new job and continue throughout employment. Nursing competencies can be divided into three major groups—General (those that all nurses need to work in the particular organization), Work Area Specific (those that are needed for a particular area of work, e.g., Medical/Surgical), and Specialty Skills (e.g., Chemotherapy administration). Competency assessment is designed to ensure the best possible evidence-based care delivery, which ultimately impacts patient care outcomes [2]. Most competencies are written into hospital policies and have an annual frequency. The model of an "Annual Nursing Skills Fair" was a solution first embraced to tackle the immense task of competency verification and is still commonly used. There is no strong rationale for the annual frequency [3], and it was most likely chosen as it seemed reasonable and manageable. Traditional approaches to skills fairs utilize an open forum with multiple skills stations where didactic content is presented in lecture or poster form with a written assessment of knowledge and minimal return demonstration of skill [4]. Waterval et al. [5] add that many hospitals lack a structured, standardized method or model for evaluating clinical skills. A primary problem with the Annual Nursing Skills Fair is that the learning is mostly passive, with little relevance to the true breadth of the competency.

The apprenticeship model, an arrangement in which someone learns an art, trade, or job under someone at a mastery level, has been the long-favored continuing education model for most healthcare professionals. It is still commonly used, but it is more common now to see formal education departments in hospitals. The development of a formal nurse educator role was first introduced in the 1950s to keep up with the demands of managing the ever-increasing list of nursing skills. Over the years, hospitals have created unique positions for nurse educators whose primary role is to deliver education to the nursing staff and manage their competencies. Nurses regarded as experts in their fields were commonly chosen to fill these roles with little regard given to their skills in education. Today it is expected that healthcare organizations have educators who have specialized education and certifications in the field of healthcare education, and it is becoming commonplace to refer to them as Nursing Professional Development Specialists

Supplementary Information The online version contains supplementary material available at https://doi.org/10.1007/978-3-031-31090-4_30.

C. Shum (✉)
VA Palo Alto Health Care System, Palo Alto, CA, USA
e-mail: Cynthia.shum@va.gov

J. M. Kutzin et al. (eds.), *Comprehensive Healthcare Simulation: Nursing*, Comprehensive Healthcare Simulation,
https://doi.org/10.1007/978-3-031-31090-4_30

(NPDS). NPDSs have specialized knowledge and skills in various educational methods and are responsible for meeting annual and ongoing nursing competencies. NPDS also has its association, the Association for Nursing Professional Development [6], which oversees its scope and standards of practice [7].

Professional development, which includes nursing competencies, should be meaningful and meet the learner's needs. Traditional methods often need to catch up as they are aimed at knowledge. Over a decade ago, Kennedy et al. [8]conducted a literature review of over 2000 articles that looked at nursing orientation and teaching methods. In this study, they concluded that the traditional orientation is taught in a passive learning format that does not consider the adult learner and the need for interactive learning methods to meet the dynamics of the healthcare environment. Further, the articles all showed that little has changed in over 60 years of nursing orientation.

As healthcare has advanced, the list of nursing competencies has increased significantly. The Joint Commission [9] created standards for organizations to use when developing their competency process and included various assessment methods, including test taking, drills, and peer feedback. Although simulation is not directly stated, drills are simulated events.

Education and training should be designed utilizing methodologies that align with the specific competency and meet the level of complexity required. Simulation offers learners an immersive experience that can replicate real life but in a safe environment that can be controlled for optimal learning outcomes. Simulation allows learning to move beyond the knowledge level and move into being able to apply and analyze, which gets at critical thinking [10]. Furthermore, adding a debriefing session to the simulation activity allows learners to reflect on their practice and hopefully translate what they learned into practice [11].

Orientation is where nursing competencies are first introduced. A literature review demonstrated a need for more information specifically addressing hospital-based nursing competencies and even less that mentioned the use of simulation. Academia has embraced simulation, and in the United States, the National Council of State Boards of Nursing [12] provided strong evidence to support replacing traditional clinical hours with simulation. Moreover, during the last year, the pandemic has forced more people to consider using simulation to replace lost clinical hours. Conversely, hospitals have limited in-person teaching and simulation due to safety restrictions in place for COVID. These safety concerns have led to many creative solutions, and we are seeing industry leaders and simulation experts embrace alternate methods, such as virtual platforms and creative thinking, when it comes to immersive simulation.

Best Practices

With the rise in available simulation technology and the growing body of knowledge around simulation pedagogy, changes in how hospital-based nursing education is delivered started around 2010. Large hospital systems began embracing simulation methods. Hospitals purchased simulation equipment, some even built centers for training, and many provided training to their staff. Kaiser Permanente, Sutter Healthcare, and the Veterans Affairs Health Care System are a few large organizations leading the way. Lucile Packard Children's Hospital at Stanford Nursing Department transformed their traditional skills fairs to a simulation-based model in 2008 and called the program CHILD - Collaborative Healthcare Immersive Learning Dynamic [4]. They recognized that the traditional model lacked relevancy and that the time spent could be better allocated to offer an enhanced, immersive learning experience.

Further, they argued that the traditional model of skills fairs lacked evidence to support the translation of KSAs to the bedside or improved healthcare outcomes. The focus of CHILD was on quality rather than quantity. Short lectures followed by immersive scenarios reinforced the learning objectives.

Additionally, the group embedded several competencies in one scenario, making the learning experience interprofessional. The outcomes were positive, and the program remained cost neutral. Forward-thinking nurse leaders who were not afraid to challenge the status quo proved that nursing competencies could be managed in alternative ways. Some of the key benefits of this program were:

1. increased ability to train in a realistic environment
2. interprofessional teamwork
3. increased satisfaction with education.

The program has been so successful that CHILD continues today. As with every program, it is essential to train new staff to use simulation.

In 2009, the Orlando Regional Medical Center recognized a gap in their annual clinical competency review for nurses. It noted a lack of process and no standardized method or model for evaluation [5]. This group also recognized that the traditional skills fair and observation of daily work needed to translate into the outcomes they needed. This group concluded that multiple competencies could be incorporated into one simulated skill station. Scenarios were created that were front-loaded with independent pre-work. During the scenario, the nurse would have to interface with a patient case and perform multiple skills, much more representative of real clinical care. During the pilot, this new program showed cost savings, increased participant satisfaction, and decreased waiting time. This new model also incorporated interprofessional team training, an important goal of patient safety.

Transforming a traditional annual nursing competency model from a passive learning encounter into an active, experiential experience requires someone to take the first step to realize that things can be done differently. An important consideration is using the already available information and starting slowly with one area at a time.

Integrating into Existing Education

Donna Wright (2005) redefined nursing competencies and outlined six aspects of meaningful competencies. The first two aspects are of particular relevance, which dictate that Nursing Professional Development Specialists select the correct competencies and the right verification method. The Wright model emphasizes that competency is not simply a 'checklist' nor a task that only occurs annually Wright [2] (Fig. 30.1).

Verification methods are used to measure the KSAs of an individual for a specific competency [2]. This is the toughest part of the job for the NPDS, as numerous factors must be considered and weighed. The more complex a competency is, combined with the greater the associated risks related to that competency, will impact the verification methods chosen. Single verification methods should be discouraged, with a focus on developing a comprehensive competency process. All three domains of competency (technical, critical thinking, and interpersonal) must be verified, and more than one method is required. Competency verification methods include tests (pre and post), return demonstrations, observation, case studies, exemplars, peer reviews, self-assessments, participation in discussion groups, presentations, mock events (immersive simulated scenarios), and quality improvement monitors (observation of clinical work). Wright [2] suggests a minimum of two to three verification methods for any competency. Tests and observation of skills with checklists are the most common verification methods but only measure knowledge and technical ability in a controlled, non-stressful environment. It is well recognized that knowledge is often not the problem [13] but, rather, the system's complexity and the high stress of the job that challenges individuals to deploy their knowledge.

Verification methods, including simulations that match the level of complexity, should be favored. Furthermore, the NPDS should build their competency verification methods in a tiered process. A simple three-tier process could look like this: (1) review of knowledge with tests (pre-work), (2) skills practice, and (3) a simulated scenario, remembering that one scenario could have multiple competencies. Other verification forms could be added to enrich the learning experience. This type of tiered process would cover all three domains and have a higher translational impact on healthcare delivery and outcomes.

Below is Table 30.1 of competency verification methods as outlined by Donna Wright [2] in her 2005 book "*The Ultimate Guide to competency assessment in health care. Creative Health Care Management*," which has been adapted to include a description of how simulation-based learning (SBE) fits with this model (note—a few of the verification methods were removed as they do not have any application to simulation).

In reviewing existing educational plans for managing competency validation, the NPDS should look at replacing many passive educational methods with active learning experiences. The concept of a 'Flipped Classroom' reverses the order of education, with learners independently reviewing lecture information and then in-person time spent practicing and applying what they learned. Learning moves from a passive model to an active one and is also meaningful as the learner can be deliberate about what they need to practice. Education plans should have layers that build on each other, tiers—independent learning aimed at knowledge gaps or refreshers, skills/task training, immersive and/or team training. NPDS should consider the type of competency and then add appropriate layers of verification methods. Things to consider are the complexity of the skill or procedure, the frequency the skill or procedure might be performed, and the consequences if something goes wrong while performing the skill or procedure. A higher number of all these factors would lend itself to competency with multiple layers of SBE, including a fully immersive simulated scenario.

Educators must understand how learning happens. There are three domains: Affective, Cognitive, and Psychomotor [10]. The technical domain of skill is addressed in the Cognitive and Psychomotor while critical thinking and interpersonal fall in the Affective domain. Fully immersive simulation allows the educator to impact all three of these domains. Task training and skills assessment does not necessarily impact the affective domain. However, they are still in a higher order than traditional didactic presentations and tests of knowledge. Task training can be elevated to increase

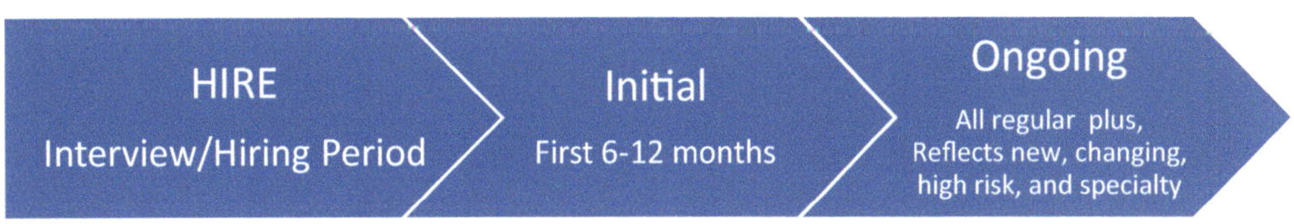

Fig. 30.1 Competency continuum—Adapted from Donna Wright

Table 30.1 Donna Wright verification methods—Adapted from Donna Wright

Verification method	Domain	Examples	Simulation methods
Tests/exams	Cognitive skills and knowledge (measure attainment of cognitive).	Written tests, quizzes, oral exams, surveys, calculation tests, crossword puzzle tests, and word games (some forms).	*Not a simulation method. If uncertain how to evaluate it, NPDS will often use a pre-posttest to augment a simulated event. This method only measures knowledge.
Return demonstrations	Technical skill (psychomotor).	Demonstrate a set of skills (techniques) to a skilled observer. (on a real patient). Observers must keep the environment safe-stop skill if unsafe or negative consequences for the patient, the public or employee.	Skills may be practiced on a task trainer during an education session. Just-in-time training: set up a training cart for staff to practice and perform a return demonstration. Ideal for skills that are not performed regularly and for skills that are new to staff (new graduate nurses, recently hired).
Case studies	Critical thinking skills.	Create case study questions that reflect the situation and capture the nature of the competency you are measuring. OR Identify questions that capture the nature of the competency and have employees use their real-life situations as the story. Then use the list of general questions to demonstrate their critical thinking skills in a real-life situation.	Case Studies are scenarios that allow the learner to immerse themselves into a situation and walk through their mental model. Case studies can be presented in a Tabletop scenario where different learners play out the various roles; learners can stay within their real role or take on a different one. This level of education is ideal as one of the tiers in a competency verification plan. For interprofessional teamwork, a tabletop scenario will allow multiple participants to plan and practice before moving into a fully immersive simulation. As a stand-alone exercise, this method can highlight critical thinking and gaps.
Exemplars	Critical thinking skills and interpersonal skills.	The story you tell or write yourself. Describe a situation you have experienced or may experience; describe a rationale you thought about and choices you made in a situation.	The equivalent in a simulation would be a reflection post a simulated event. The learner will either verbalize or write out their reflection. This is a powerful way for new nurses to reflect and identify their strengths and areas to improve.
Self-assessment	Some Critical thinking skills (especially those associated with values and beliefs). Best used to assess aspects of the Affective Domain of Learning.	Valuable in measuring competencies related to values, beliefs, myths, and assumptions that help/hinder us in achieving our desired outcomes (conscious and previously unconscious thoughts).	This is the Reflection piece in simulation. The person debriefing can direct or advocate for a discussion around any piece of the scenario to facilitate the learner's reflection.
Mock events/ surveys	Used to assess responses in daily work or practice (simulations of real-world situations).	Used in conjunction with an education event or stand alone as merely a verification of skill(s). *Mock Events reflect individual performance. Debriefing after the event is essential. Reflective learning-recognizing mistakes and identifying future actions are essential to ongoing learning and development.*	Mock events are simulated events. Mock events are usually fully immersive simulated events that should be a capstone for competency verification. They may be a single discipline, interdisciplinary or interprofessional. The simulated scenario may have multiple competencies embedded. Checklists combined with debriefing and reflections are used to evaluate the scenario outcomes for a learner.
Quality improvement monitors	Measure all three skill domains. *Critical Thinking, Technical, and Interpersonal.*	Any time a QI monitor r*eflects individual performance*, it automatically verifies competency. • Monitor outcomes and environment. • Compliance with policies and protocols.	This allows for evaluating the transitional outcomes of education.

Table 30.1 (continued)

Verification method	Domain	Examples	Simulation methods
Discussion/ reflection groups	Critical thinking skills (when linked to mock events, it may also measure technical and interpersonal skills).	This a valid way to look at critical thinking skills and promote group cohesiveness and mutual support. The purpose is to allow the group to share their thoughts and strategies on an issue and discuss the merits and consequences of each aspect.	This is Debriefing. The session should allow the learners to reflect on their actions through a facilitated discussion. There are opportunities for Reflection in Action—this is when the simulation facilitator will pause the scenario and have the learner reflect on the moment. This style corrects mistakes and gets the learner on the right path.

realism by adding additional factors. For example, the management of a central line on a task trainer can be more authentic if it is attached to a real person who is moving and talking. As a result of simulation, retention of knowledge and the experience of what could happen if an alternate choice was made are explored are superior education methods and translate into better outcomes [14].

Beyond retention of knowledge and psychomotor skills, nurses need to be able to think critically. Research shows that half the adult population never reaches formal operations, where you can think critically. Higher educational methods should be utilized for nursing competencies if positive outcomes are desired. Simulation-based education is consistent with the cognitive learning theory that the nurse only enters into practice with displaying sufficient knowledge and demonstrated competencies and ensuring that they analyze themselves during the simulated event and reflect on the results during the debriefing stage [15].

Challenges and Solutions

Transforming an education plan for managing nursing competencies from a traditional model into one that utilizes SBE requires deliberate planning that includes longitudinal goals and a sustainability strategy. A key piece of advice is to get started with SBE and start where you are. If you already are using simulation in your organization, leverage your existing resources; you may have some equipment or staff who are trained, or perhaps even space. Simulation is simply an alternative educational method. If the organization has people trained in simulation, the NPDS should partner with them. Together they can review the competency and replace passive learning or add simulation to the verification methods. A simulated patient care monitor can be added to a case study with a higher fidelity level. The learner has to view the monitor and interpret the information while working on the case study. For those organizations that do not have any existing simulations, there are simple ways to get started. Simulated patient care monitors are available for free download or nominal cost and are a great way to augment education.

For every challenge, there is a solution. One of the best solutions is to become educated on simulation pedagogy. A common misconception among educators and healthcare staff is that simulation is only the part with the manikin, the full simulated scenario. As we have noted, there are many types of simulation methods, and anything that gets the learning to be active is truly a simulation method. This is one of the biggest barriers; thinking it is more than it is.

Another barrier is the belief that simulation takes more time. We have reviewed the evidence that has proven this is **not** the case. The solution is to think about your competency verification plan differently. There is nothing that dictates you must show a test of knowledge, yet this is a common choice. Testing is a comfortable, well-known educational strategy our education system has instilled in us. In healthcare, we want our nurses to deliver care without any errors and to be able to reproduce this over time. Testing does not demand this and usually has a minimum passing score. How does 80% reflect competency? Conversely, simulation allows for practice in a realistic environment that can translate to positive outcomes [16].

Further challenges are the sheer number of nurses in any organization and the number of competencies that must be accounted for; this is on top of all the other ongoing education needs. Traditional models treat every competency as a stand-alone item and validate them separately. This is highly time-consuming and takes enormous effort to schedule. Conversely, immersive simulation scenarios will have multiple competencies that are mandatory for one nurse. Multiple nurses from the same area can participate, and the experience can further be enhanced by making it interprofessional. The scenario will outline the various competencies and criteria for meeting the requirements of each competency. This method demands a new way of thinking about competency validation. In a team scenario, as in real clinical practice, the clinical nurse demonstrates competency by managing the work needed while interfacing with other healthcare professionals. It is important to note that certain competencies with regulatory requirements may need individual assessment. In this case, a test of knowledge or return demonstration of skill could be added to the overall competency.

Other challenges are space, equipment, and staff for conducting the simulation. Once again, if you do not have a full simulation program, the goal is to start small and create your business case for building the program. Simulation can be done in any room and does not necessarily require the whole expensive setup of a simulation center. Even hospitals with dedicated simulation space, scheduling it when needed is often challenging. In this case, NPDS should consider the in-situ environment, which adds even more fidelity. However, with in-situ simulation, NPDS will have to manage the expectations of the nurses to ensure they stay focused on the ongoing clinical work.

Sample Curriculum with Sample Case

Nursing competencies should be managed in the same manner that you would an educational course. NPDS should consider the gamut of nursing competencies required in specific units and treat them as units rather than individual pieces. Patient care is complex, and building a comprehensive plan for competency management presents the nurse with a more realistic educational plan. Building competencies into a simulation scenario allows the nurse to reflect on the challenges and barriers to delivering care in a complex environment and translate lessons learned into the real clinical world.

A nursing competency should have a complete educational curriculum that includes the following items:

- The competency (ies)—define the scope of KSAs
- The competency verification plan
  - Detailed validations methods
    Simulation methods:
    - Task training
      - provide details of which trainers will be used with instructions on setting up
      - Checklist
    - Immersive simulation
      - Complete the scenario using a template—will identify the competencies
      - Debriefing guide
      - Resources required—staff, space, equipment
      - Assessment and evaluation tools for scenario

An example competency curriculum for pediatric nursing is attached in the Appendix. This curriculum outlines all the competencies a nurse in this area would need and defines the verification methods. There is a progressive plan which culminates with a fully immersive scenario. The pediatric respiratory scenario is designed to be interprofessional and to allow the nurse to manage multiple competencies. No checklists are associated with this scenario, but the competencies will be addressed in the debriefing. Checklists are helpful for skills that require a learner to follow a prescribed set of actions but are less desirable for reflecting on an immersive scenario. This approach to competency management moves away from the siloed approach of checking off individuals to a deliberate strategy that recognizes and emphasizes the importance of having nurses practice in realistic ways.

Conclusion

The nursing workforce constitutes the largest group in healthcare today. Healthcare organizations understand the importance of retaining competent and confident nurses who can adapt and meet the increasing demands of providing safe and effective care for complex patient populations [5]. High-performing organizations recognize the significance of professional development plans for new and incumbent nurses. The IOM's Report, *The Future of Nursing: Leading Change, Advancing Health*, highlights the importance of lifelong learning and the need for a process designed to promote areas of improvement for nurses, such as patient care and population health [17]. Nursing professional development is critical in ensuring quality care, career satisfaction, and a solid pipeline for tomorrow's leaders.

Additionally, nurses should plan for ongoing professional development and consider lifelong learning part of a healthy work environment [18]. Position changes to new areas are also common and to be expected, and this offers a new set of KSAs. Nurses must be competent, at a minimum, to deliver safe, evidence-based care. Therefore, organizations must prioritize professional development, from new graduates to seasoned veterans, across each nurse's career stages. Of utmost importance are the many competencies a nurse must be validated on. If healthcare expects to have positive translational outcomes, then the educational methodologies must match the level of complexity. Simulation offers nurses a unique opportunity to be immersed in a realistic environment and reflect on their work. Moreover, utilizing simulated scenarios for competency validation allows multiple competencies to be managed in one scenario.

References

1. American Nurses Association. Nursing: scope and standards of practice. 3rd ed. Nursebooks.org; 2015.
2. Wright D. The ultimate guide to competency assessment in health care. 3rd ed. Minneapolis, MN: Creative Health Care Management, Inc.; 2005.
3. Crofts JF, Bartlett C, Ellis D, Hunt LP, Fox R, Draycott TJ. Management of shoulder dystocia: skill retention 6 and 12 months after training. Obstet Gynecol. 2007;110(5):1069–74.
4. Bergero C, Hargreaves L, Nichols A. Collaborative healthcare immersive learning dynamic: transitioning to simulation-based learning. Clin Nurse Spec. 2012;26:42–7.

5. Waterval EM, Stephan K, Peczinka D, Shaw A. Designing a process for simulation-based annual nurse competency assessment. J Nurses Staff Dev. 2012;28(6):274–8.
6. ANPD. ANPD-Association for nursing professional development 2021 (Available from: https://www.anpd.org/).
7. Harper MG, Maloney P. Nursing Professional Development: scope and standards or practice. 3rd ed. Chicago, IL: Association for Nursing Professional Development; 2016.
8. Kennedy JM, Nichols AA, Halamek LP, Arafeh JM. Nursing department orientation: are we missing the mark? J Nurses Staff Dev. 2012;28:24–16.
9. The Joint Commission. The Joint Commission 2021 (Available from: https://www.jointcommission.org/).
10. Anderson LW, Krathwohl DR, Bloom BS. In: Anderson LW, Krathwohl D, Airasian PW, et al., editors. A taxonomy for learning, teaching, and assessing : a revision of Bloom's taxonomy of educational objectives. New York: Longman; 2001.
11. McGaghie WC, Issenberg SB, Cohen ER, Barsuk JH, Wayne DB. Translational educational research: a necessity for effective health-care improvement. Chest. 2012;142(5):1097.
12. Alexander M. NCSBN National simulation study. Deans Notes. 2014;36(1):1–2.
13. Institute of Medicine. To err is human: building a safer health system. Washington, DC: Institute of Medicine; 2000.
14. McGaghie WC, Marco FP. The science of learning and medical education. Med Educ. 2014;48(2):106–8.
15. Jeffries P. Simulation in nursing education: from conceptualization to evaluation. 3rd ed. New York, NY: Lippincott Williams & Wilkins; 2020.
16. Knight LJ, Gabhart JM, Earnest KS, Leong KM, Anglemyer A, Franzon D. Improving code team performance and survival outcomes: implementation of pediatric resuscitation team training*. Crit Care Med. 2014;42(2):243–51.
17. Good S, Schneider M. Meeting the challenges of nursing staff education. Nursing 2021. 2018;48(8):16-17.
18. Cant RP, Cooper SJ, Lam LL. Hospital nurses' simulation-based education regarding patient safety: a scoping review. Clin Simul Nursing. 2020;44:19–34.

31 Simulation for Emergency Nursing

Rebecca Weiss

Introduction

Emergency Departments (EDs) and the staff that works within them are critical focal points for the healthcare system. ED staff are faced with many challenging situations due to the unpredictable and varied cases encountered every day. As a specialty, Emergency Nurses require a focused and detailed orientation program. The orientation program for Emergency Nurses may vary based on the patient population they care for and the courses offered by the healthcare organization. Emergency Departments are also known for having high turnover rates, leading to a disproportionate number of novice nurses to expert nurses [1].

Emergency nurses are known to be "the jack of all trades" in that they often encounter various patient scenarios and must be well-versed in many different procedures and acute disease processes. Therefore, there are many opportunities to incorporate simulation within the Emergency Department to help educate and maintain competency for staff. Simulation provides nurses the opportunity for hands-on practice to become more proficient at performing skills related to an unfamiliar topic, situation, or process. When simulation was first introduced in the Emergency Department is hard to ascertain, but clinical simulation for healthcare providers can be traced as far back as the eighteenth century [2]. However, simulation is an integral part of an ED nurse's role and training. Courses through the American Heart Association (AHA), like Basic Life Support and Advanced Cardiac Life Support, include simulation as part of the curriculum and are typically requirements for ED Nurses. ED nurses also have to be prepared for low-occurrence or high-risk situations like mass casualty, sexual assault, pediatric codes, moderate sedation, and so much more. All of the previously mentioned scenarios require hands-on training and forms of simulation to grasp the concepts being taught fully.

There is a vast amount of opportunity for the use of simulation in the Emergency Department due to the nature of the patient population, fast-paced work, and critical care environment. Literature supports the use of simulation in the Emergency Department and has been shown to decrease nurse anxiety and increase nurse self-efficacy [3].

The Emergency Nurses Association (ENA) is an **American professional organization that represents emergency nursing**. The ENA was founded in 1970, consists of 40,000 members, examines issues relevant to emergency care, publishes professional guidelines, and issues a peer-reviewed journal [3]. Currently, the ENAs Trauma Nursing Core Course (TNCC) [4] and Emergency Nurse Pediatric Course (ENPC) both incorporate simulations to practice scenarios in a controlled environment and apply concepts to meet learning objectives.

Background

For this chapter, the use of simulation for moderate sedation and sepsis will be detailed. The use of simulation in moderate sedation and sepsis can be designed in many ways, showing the vast possibilities for simulation in the clinical setting. Moderate sedation is a high-risk procedure that was identified as needing its own course because many new staff in the ED were not comfortable with the nursing interventions needed and documentation that was required for moderate sedation patients. The need for moderate sedation education presented itself in a few ways. Through an educational needs assessment survey, the ED nurses felt uncomfortable and unsure of the documentation expectations, especially newly hired nurses. Experienced staff nurses voiced concerns that the new hires were having difficulty anticipating needs and

Supplementary Information The online version contains supplementary material available at https://doi.org/10.1007/978-3-031-31090-4_31.

R. Weiss (✉)
Allegheny Health Network West Penn Hospital, Pittsburgh, PA, USA
e-mail: rebecca.weiss@ahn.org

J. M. Kutzin et al. (eds.), *Comprehensive Healthcare Simulation: Nursing*, Comprehensive Healthcare Simulation,
https://doi.org/10.1007/978-3-031-31090-4_31

critically thinking through a moderate sedation procedure. Lastly, chart audits supported the staff requests in that there were many required components within the electronic documentation missing which raised potential patient safety and regulatory concerns.

The healthcare system identified in this chapter followed the SEP-1 measure outlined by the Centers for Medicare and Medicaid Services (CMS) [5] for sepsis care. Compliance with sepsis bundles of care, per the measure, is hard to maintain within a busy, urban Emergency Department. Rather than providing the bundle information in a lecture format, simulation was used to enhance the education and allowed thought processes to be physically demonstrated and verbalized. For example, reinforcement of the 3-hour bundle for the SEP-1 measure was able to be completed throughout the sepsis simulation, as each station contained a different component of the measure. If a group struggled on a key learning point, the facilitator was able to address that during debrief and reinforce the education.

Sample Cases

Moderate Sedation

Moderate sedation is a procedure that requires critical thinking. From a clinical standpoint, there are many things that could go wrong during the procedure, leading to an unstable patient that needs immediate life-saving interventions. From a regulatory standpoint, there are clear documentation expectations that need to be followed. In a busy Emergency Department, nurses can find it difficult to properly prepare, assess, and document the interventions for a moderate sedation procedure. The purpose of creating a moderate sedation course was to ensure all ED RNs were more knowledgeable of the medications used, could identify and place airway adjuncts, and understood the nursing guidelines behind moderate sedation, including the required documentation.

After all Advanced Cardiac Life Support (ACLS) Initial Provider courses, students took an hour break and then came back to the classroom for a moderate sedation course. This two-hour course included a presentation from a clinical pharmacist who shared the types of sedation agents commonly used, the drug doses and frequencies, and reversal agents. A Clinical Registered Nurse Anesthetist (CRNA) taught airway management and airway adjuncts used during moderate sedation, and a clinical educator discussed the documentation requirements and nursing guidelines required by regulatory bodies. The learners then participated in a simulation exercise to pull together all the knowledge learned.

The ED leadership ensured that all new and current ED staff were enrolled in the course over a two-year span. After the first two courses, which were run once a month, the class was opened up to staff from other areas that require moderate sedation training, such as the Pre-Anesthesia Care Unit (PACU), Intensive Care Units (ICUs), and procedural areas such as the Catheterization Lab. There was a pre and post-test for learners to evaluate knowledge retention as well as a course evaluation to make sure that staff felt the content provided was appropriate and useful to their practice. The course is now a routine part of orientation, and enrollment has remained steady over the past 3 years.

Sepsis Escape Room

Emergency Department nurses are no strangers to sepsis and the necessary interventions for quality care. Emergency Medical Services (EMS) personnel transport more than 50% of all sepsis cases to the ED, so EDs are a priority location for sepsis education and awareness [6]. However, some nuances within the SEP-1 measures are challenging to convey, and they could make a difference in patient outcomes or hospital sepsis compliance rates. A short presentation, e-mail, or in-person discussion were not viable education modalities to validate learning in an engaging way. For Sepsis Awareness Month, a low-budget sepsis escape room was created to address some of the commonly missed components in the SEP-1 bundle and engage staff in a way that was fun and memorable. Escape rooms can be a form of simulation as it engages learners physically and offers professional and educational development in an engaging way [7]. However, the critical thinking components, as well as the pressure of time and correctness, are still present, similar to what is experienced in high-fidelity simulation.

Sample Curriculum #1: Moderate Sedation

Course Creation

A moderate sedation course was created to incorporate an interdisciplinary approach as well as a simulation exercise linked to the learning objectives. Often when an area for education is recognized, it is commonly incorporated into a course or nursing orientation. However, the lack of hands-on practice or clinical experience to apply knowledge hinders the attempt to educate and enhance the retention of knowledge [8].

Buy-in was needed from key stakeholders, including executive nursing leadership (Director of Nursing), as well as the Director of Organizational Development, Nursing Education, and Research. An interdisciplinary approach was important, so anesthesia and pharmacy were also contacted and agreed to help teach the course. Once the content, time frame, and speakers were finalized, the proposal with learning objectives was sent to the stakeholders for approval. Once approved, the nurse managers in the hospital were notified of the course, and they were provided the dates and times for course sign-up. This was paid time for the staff nurses, and the moderate sedation course was required during the nurse's orientation.

Pre-Work

The learner was required to electronically complete a 10-question pre-test survey prior to coming to the course. The pre-test, which included questions related to medications, airway adjuncts, and documentation requirements, only provided a score to the learners and did not provide the correct answers. This was done intentionally because we wanted to be able to compare pre-course and post-course scores. After the course, the learner took the same test to assess if learning had occurred. In the first 3 months, the average pre-test score was 4.8 out of 10 points; the post-test had an average score of 9 out of 10 (n = 24). The comments from the nurses about the course were positive, and the moderate sedation audits showed an improvement in nursing documentation in real moderate sedation cases in the clinical setting. This has the potential to improve quality patient care and meet the requirements of regulatory bodies like The Joint Commission. The Joint Commission (TJC) is an independent, not-for-profit group in the United States that is an accrediting body and sets standards for healthcare organizations. This course met the requirements for TJC as it provided initial comprehensive education for this high-risk procedure done in a specialty setting. Nurses in the ED then have an annual competency related to moderate sedation to maintain competency in the skill.

Course Content

This moderate sedation course was held after a brief break and completion of ACLS Initial Provider courses. The learners had already participated in the Megacodes and were familiar with the manikin and the simulation process. The learners were first presented with airway adjuncts and airway management techniques from a CRNA within the hospital. Next, the learners were presented with a hands-on opportunity to touch and practice the skills of inserting oropharyngeal and nasopharyngeal airways. They also received reinforcement on the proper bag-valve-mask technique. The learners then engaged in a presentation from a clinical pharmacist who discussed sedation medication indications, side effects, doses, and reversal agents. During this phase, the learners were given a few case studies to apply the information that was learned. Lastly, a clinical educator presented the scope of nursing practice for moderate sedation, the needed assessment and equipment, as well as the documentation requirements. Examples of recent moderate sedation chart audits were presented for learners to identify what was missed or what was correct about the charting.

Then, learners participated in a simulation to tie all the aspects that were just learned together. We found that the optimal group size was no larger than 4. Suppose there were more learners, two or more scenarios were conducted, and the other participants that were not active in the scenario were documented on clinical laptops that were set up in a training domain. The group in the simulation was completing the pre, intra-, and post-assessments as well as carrying out orders and ensuring a "timeout" was completed. Those not actively in the scenario were navigating the training domain and documenting the critical pieces of the assessment. At the end of the simulation, a debrief occurred where documentation, assessment, and interventions were discussed as a group.

For the first group participating, the facilitator asked for a "team lead." The team lead was the primary RN in the scenario and the first one that walked into the room. When the team lead determined that additional help was needed, they indicated so, and the other participants in that group joined and participated in the scenario. For example, one scenario focused on a frail elderly patient that required moderate sedation for a hip reduction. Other examples included sedation for cardioversion in a young adult, and another involved a middle-aged patient that had sleep apnea. The scenario was read, and the team leader approached the patient and started to prepare for moderate sedation. Soon after interacting with the patient, the team lead called in the other group members to assist. Member roles should be clear and established by each other during the scenario. Examples of roles during the simulation included a person to document, medication administration, airway management/assessment, and/or a "float" participant in helping oversee and ensure nothing was missed.

Some of the expected observed actions for this simulation are:

- Primary RN hands-off other patients to another nurse (received in the report that the RN has three other patients)
- States there is a lack of suction set up in the room
- Documented appropriately (vitals, consents, pain score, level of consciousness, medications given and doses, etc.)
- Receives consent for the physician to review with the patient
- Completes "time out" prior to start
- Prepares medications, including the reversal agents
- Performs patient assessment related to vitals, oxygen saturations, airway management, and level of consciousness

- Chooses appropriate dosing and medication choice (physician initially orders inappropriate medication dosing)
- Performs assessment post moderate sedation and documents assessment

Debrief

Once the learners met most of the learning objectives for the scenario, or the scenario went over 5 min, the simulation was halted, and the debrief started. The facilitator began the debrief by asking the group that participated in the simulation to identify things that went well, followed by what they think could have gone differently or if anything was missed. The facilitator then asked those that were documenting if there was anything that was missed for the purposes of documentation to promote group discussion. The facilitator ends with the whole group discussing what would have happened next if the scenario had kept running and opens it up to the group to discuss and validate learning. The participating group and the documentation group then switch so that each group has the opportunity to interact with the simulator and the documentation training domain during the course. This process continues until everyone has had an opportunity to participate in an active role in the simulation. Following the session, all of the learners are asked to complete a course evaluation prior to leaving the simulation center.

Simulation Curriculum #2: Sepsis Escape Room

Sepsis is a commonly seen condition in the Emergency Department, and most ED nurses are comfortable with the expected treatment for these patients. However, many nurses needed to be made aware of some of the small details in the Sep-1 Measure, and these details can affect patient outcomes and compliance rates. To engage staff, the hospital Sepsis Coordinator was trying to think of a unique way to engage staff during Sepsis Awareness Month. During one of the Sepsis Committee meetings, a member suggested using an escape room concept to educate staff.

The escape room was low-budget, costing about $20 in total. These costs included:

1. Five (5) boxes with holes for padlocks
2. Five (5) locks (4 padlocks and one combination)
3. Four (4) magnet picture frames
4. Three (3) blank 15-piece puzzles

The folders, papers, and lamination were provided by the education department, so the cost was minimal. The escape room was held in a room with multiple tables and chairs, a manikin in a bed, and a Zoll defibrillation monitor. There was also a keyboard and a coffee cup placed in the room as these two items had riddles attached to them that helped direct participants to hidden keys. An electronic virtual assistant was also in the room for the learners to interact with and ask questions for one of the clues.

Escape Room Start

Prior to beginning, the participants were oriented to the room, allotted 30 min to *escape*, and were provided the general directions for the escape room. For example, the participants were told the locked boxes should be opened in the order they are labeled, one through five. A timer for the activity was started as soon as the first or "start" folder was handed to the learners.

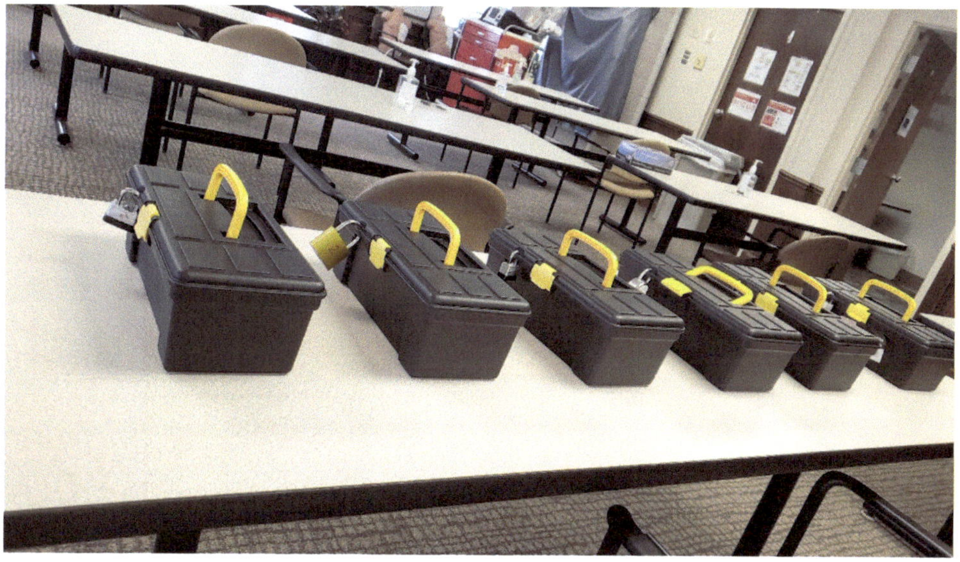

The lockboxes were placed in order, one through five. There was a sixth box, a box with a combination lock, that learners were told they would use at some point in the scenario.

The learners were then handed the Start folder, which included de-identified screenshots of a physician's History and Physician (H&P) as well as vital signs and labs over a 6-hour time span. The learners were asked to identify "time zero" for this sepsis patient. There was a slip of paper in the start folder that stated, "When time zero is identified, find the Blue colored folder for the next step." A blue (can be any color) folder was placed on the other side of the room on a table.

Within the blue folder, the learners were given three slips of paper, each with a different time on it, and under the time was a question. The times on the slips of paper were the "time zero" options for the learners. The learners picked the time zero paper that was agreed upon and asked the question that was printed on that piece of paper to the virtual assistant. The virtual assistant provided an answer with a number. For example, the learner chose one piece of paper with an agreed-upon time zero and read out loud, "How many people died of sepsis in 2018?". The numbers (answers) that came from each question correlated with three envelopes taped to a wall within the room. The numbers on the envelopes were the answers the virtual assistant gave to the participants for each of the three questions. There was only one correct answer, so if the participants picked the wrong time zero, they asked the wrong question, went to the wrong envelope, and saw that there was a clue that said, "TRY AGAIN." The spacing in the clues was incorrect and translated to "TRY AGAIN." One envelope had a correct answer with the riddle "TH EKE YISU NDE RSAM," which translated to "THE KEY IS UNDER SAM." The participants went to Sam (the manikin), turn him, and there they found the key to the first box.

Box 31.1

Learners found four 4 × 6″ clear magnets that have cultures, antibiotics, lactate, and fluids in the text, with one word on each magnet. Learners had to place the three-hour bundle in the correct order and place it on the whiteboard. CALF (Cultures, Antibiotics, Lactate, Fluids)—was an acronym the hospital used for the three-hour bundle and was the correct order. The facilitator told the participants how many were correct out of 4 in each attempt. Once the learners had all four in the correct order, they ran over to get a clue from the facilitator. In this scenario, it was a riddle for coffee, where they would find the key under a coffee cup, but any riddle or hints can be used here. The key hidden under the coffee cup opened Box 31.2.

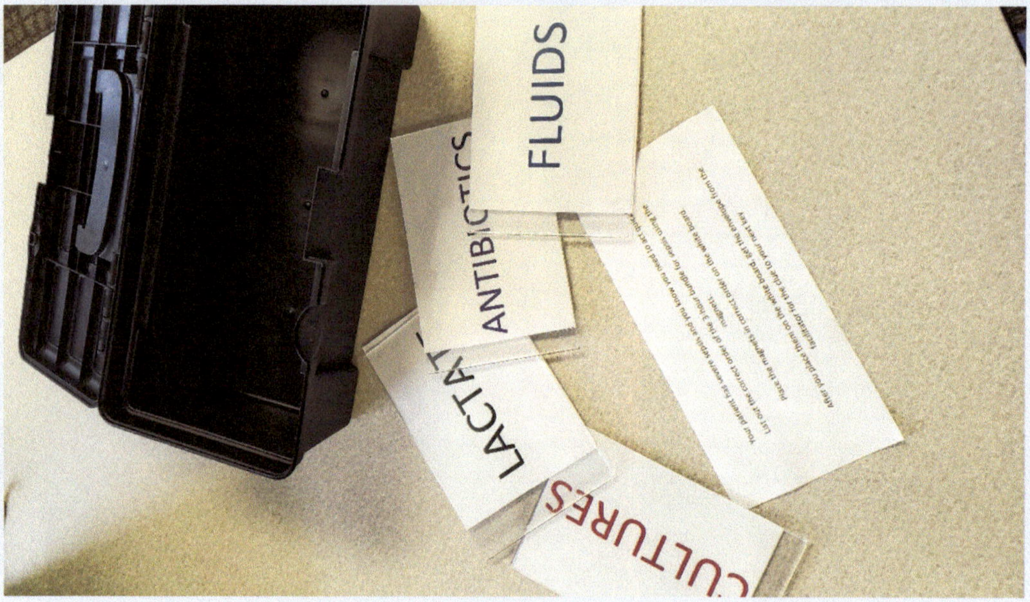

The magnets with the components of the 3-hour bundle for sepsis and the directions.

Box 31.2

Learners found in the box a pair of blood culture bottles and three 100 mL "antibiotics," which were mini-saline bags labeled with various antibiotic names. A piece of paper with directions was also included. The learners were asked to take the blood culture bottles and place them in the correct order of draw (aerobic bottle first then anaerobic bottle second). Each blood culture bottle had a number on it. They were also required to place the three antibiotics in the correct order in which they should be given. The antibiotic bags also had numbers on them. This was to reinforce monotherapy and combination therapy antibiotics in the SEP-1 measure. The participants were then asked to take the number on the first antibiotic, the number on the second culture bottle, and the number on the first culture bottle and list them on a piece of paper that was included in the box. The participants had to realize the numbers were the sequence for the combination lock to open the next box.

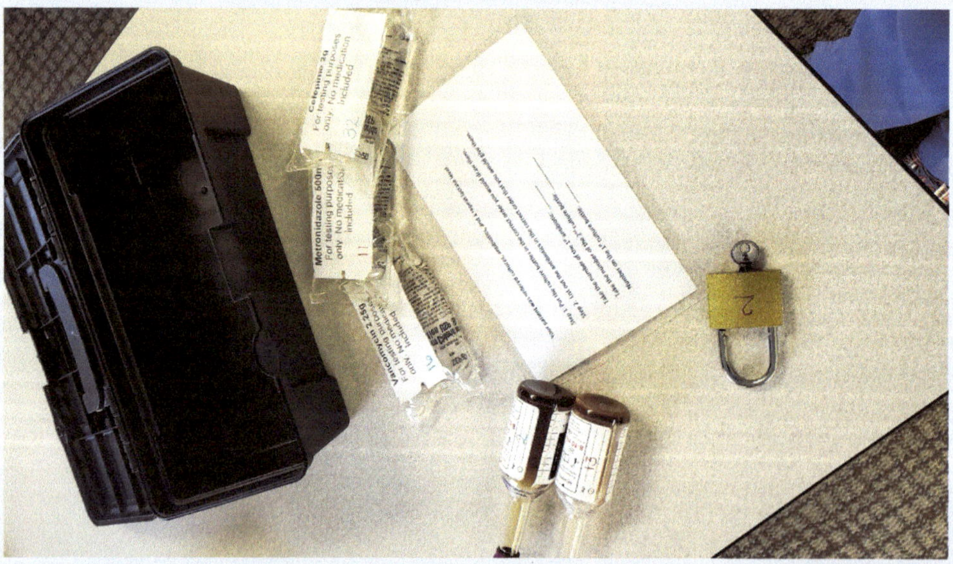

The second box had three fake antibiotics (made with 100 cc normal saline bags with fake labels) and a set of blood cultures. Notice that the blood culture bottles and antibiotics had numbers on each of them to allow the learner to get the lock combination.

Combination Lock Box

Learners opened the combination lock box and found a paper directing them to another set of vitals and labs. The labs showed persistent hypotension and a lactate level greater than 4, which per the SEP-1 measure, required a 30 mL/kg fluid bolus. Learners were directed to three orange folders on a table that had three different interventions printed on the front: (1) 20 mL/kg fluid bolus, (2) 30 mL/kg fluid bolus, and (3) vasopressor. Within each folder were loose puzzle pieces that created a 12-piece puzzle. Each puzzle had a message written on it, and the participants had to put the puzzle together in order to read the message. The participants picked the folder they thought was the right intervention and completed the puzzle. Two of the folder's puzzles spelled out "try again," and the correct one, the 30 mL/kg fluid bolus, stated something along the lines of "Use the repeat lactate level to find your next key (Row/Chair)." For example, the repeat lactate provided in the labs was 4.2, so under the fourth-row, second chair of the room, they found an envelope that provided the key for Box 31.3 within it.

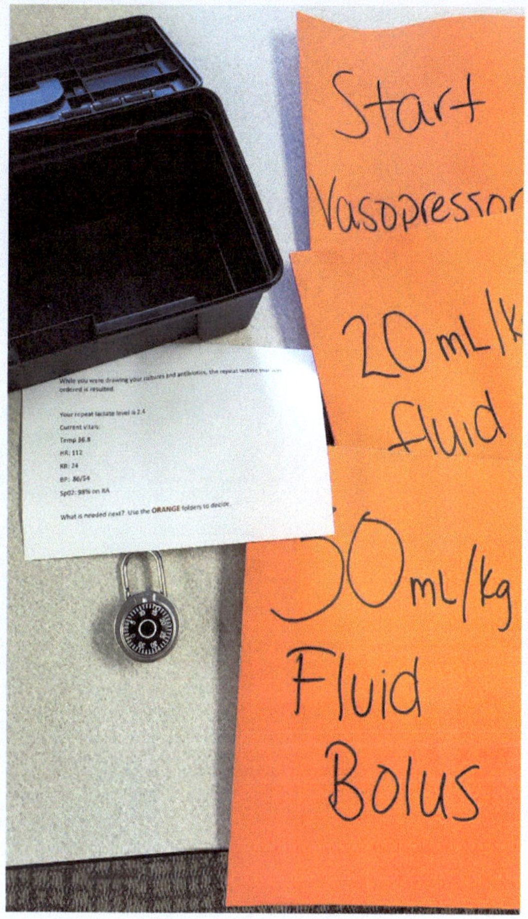

The combination lock box contained the piece of paper only giving the vitals and labs. The orange folders were on a table in the room. The learners then had to run to the folders and, using the data on the paper, figure out which folder had the correct intervention.

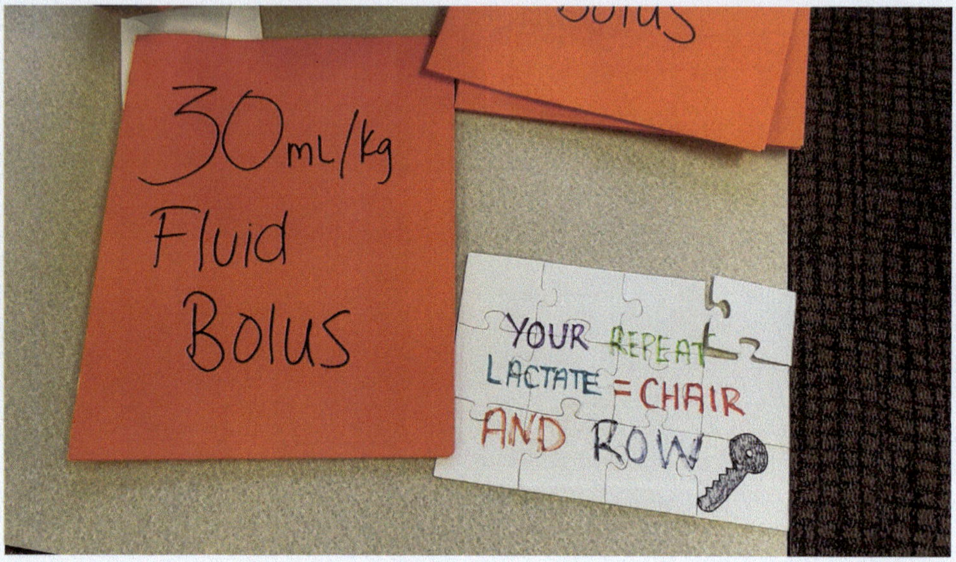
30mL/kg
Fluid
Bolus
YOUR REPEAT
LACTATE = CHAIR
AND ROW

In the correct folder, the learners would find this puzzle directing them to the next key for Box 31.3. The other folders also had puzzles, but they spelled out "TRY AGAIN."

Box 31.3

The learners took the key found under the chair and opened Box 31.3. The learners found a riddle to the next key. This can be any riddle, but in this example, one was used for a keyboard.

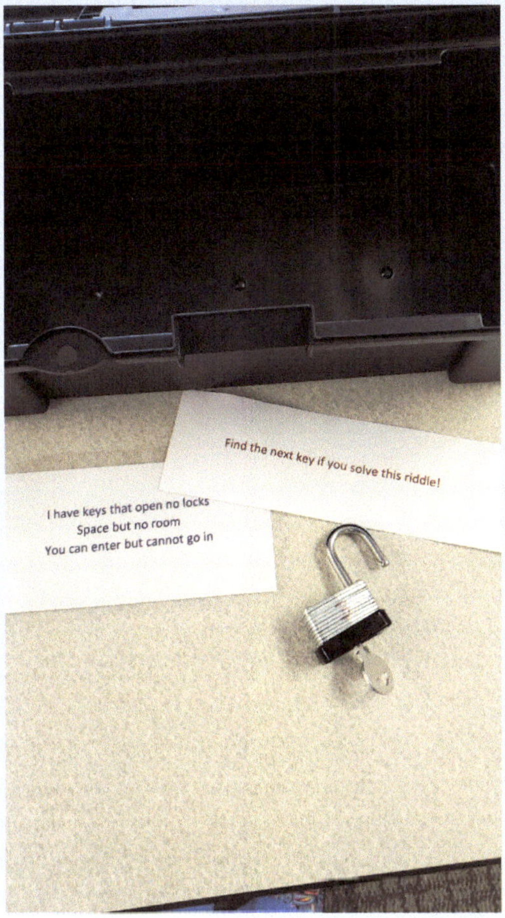
Find the next key if you solve this riddle!
I have keys that open no locks
Space but no room
You can enter but cannot go in

Once the learners figured out the riddle, they would find the key to box four under the keyboard in the room.

Box 31.4

Box 31.4 had a sepsis article related to incidence and mortality, a blacklight, and a worksheet with four multiple-choice questions. The article had words highlighted with a special highlighter that could only be seen when a blacklight was used. The participants were directed to answer the multiple-choice questions (answers A through D) and then find each correct answer's letter within the article using the blacklight. Once the letter was found in the article, the participants were directed to take the letter to the left of the correct answer letter and write it down in the code box.

For example, a multiple-choice question answer was "A." So, within the article, a word with an "a" in it was highlighted that had the desired letter to the left of it to spell the code word (the code word in this example was Zoll). This process was repeated for the three other letters from the multiple-choice worksheet. Once the code word was deciphered, learners ran to the Zoll, where they found the key underneath it to open the last box, Box 31.5.

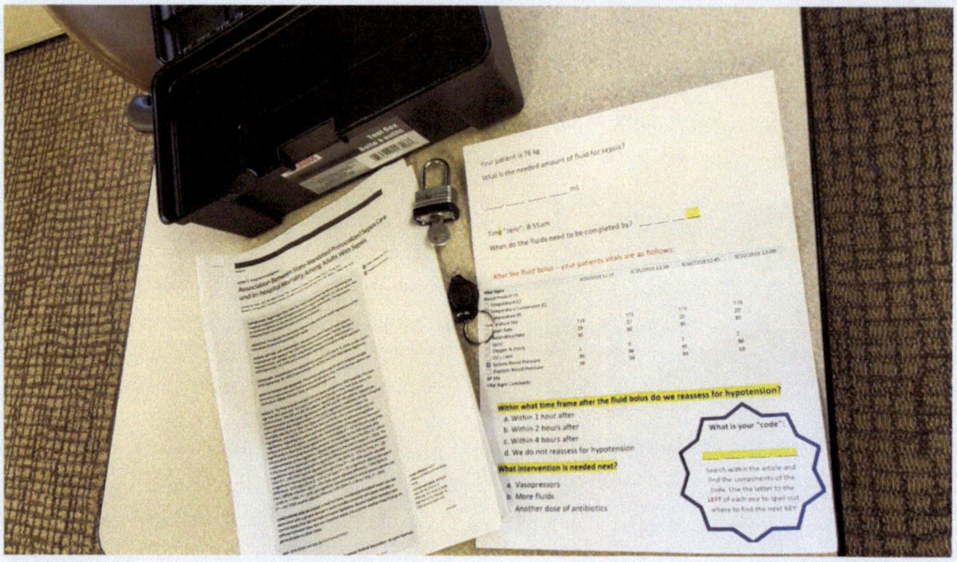

The worksheet, blacklight, and article were used for the scenario. All of the directions were on the worksheet. This box took the most amount of time for learners.

Box 31.5

The learners were provided one slip of paper in this box, directing them to pick the correct way to call a sepsis response code at the hospital. The learners found a table in the room with many small slips of paper with multiple answers on them, only one slip being correct. Together, the participants sifted through the slips of paper, and once the correct one was found, one person ran the paper up to the facilitator. Once the facilitator confirmed it was correct, he/she stopped the timer and announced that the group had escaped the room!

Debrief

After the group completed all the tasks in the escape room, the facilitator led a debrief with the participants. The debrief allowed for a discussion focused on the items the group had difficulty understanding or discovering and was an opportunity for the participants to ask questions and give feedback. An escape room allowed learners to apply specific education from the SEP-1 measure in a fun and engaging way. The variety of topics and approaches for an escape room are vast and can be applied to any escape room. While not a traditional way to practice simulation, an escape room can offer similar approaches, objectives, and outcomes [7].

Integrating into Existing Education

Instead of finding additional time for RN simulation, incorporating simulation within existing content, classes, or competencies was an innovative way to meet the educational need of a busy healthcare organization. If it is a skill that can be demonstrated, simulation provides a more engaging learning environment versus a didactic presentation only.

For moderate sedation, after a small break, the course was added after the hospitals' ACLS initial provider course. This expands the simulation seamlessly because instead of having the learner come in two separate times, the learner takes a break after ACLS class and then comes back to the classroom for a separate 2-hour course to incorporate moderate sedation education and simulation practice. Having a moderate sedation class on the same day as ACLS is also strategic in that the content is similar, and simulation is already incorporated in the ACLS mega codes. ACLS and moderate sedation education is similar in that nurses who complete moderate sedation need to be ACLS certified per the hospital policy. Also, ACLS skills are needed in moderate sedation in case there are changes in the patient's condition (bradycardia, hypoxia, arrhythmia, airway management). Moderate sedation can be incorporated into annual competency education as well.

Sepsis could be added to any curriculum within an ED RNs expected learning. The sepsis escape room could be placed in courses like RN Residency, Emergency Nurse Course, Orientation programs, or even a department education day. Often sepsis is taught in a lecture format, and it is hard to engage learners in such a detailed, difficult disease process to understand. By incorporating hands-on experience and/or simulation, the learner can apply the knowledge in a meaningful way, and learners are more likely to retain or remember the information compared to a slide presentation [9].

Lastly, moderate sedation and sepsis can be placed in an ED Education Day for staff. An ED Education Day is a day of learning for ED RNs that consists of topics that are either identified by the staff through a needs assessment or data showing an opportunity or need. Creating a separate time and day dedicated to RN education provides an opportunity to be creative in the education modalities, including the use of simulation and department-specific examples. Other suggestions for topics in which simulation can be incorporated within an ED Education Day include sexual assault, arterial line setup, sepsis, orthopedic splinting, mass transfusion or blood product administration, use of the cardiac defibrillator, pacing, a code or crisis, donning and doffing, and difficult conversations.

Challenges and Solutions

Planning

When planning educational programs, it is important to consider initial barriers such as staffing. A well-planned curriculum will only be successful if attendance is adequate. Engaging leadership early and obtaining their buy-in when planning and scheduling staff for simulation programs is crucial to the success of any program to ensure staff are prescheduled and attend the simulations. Leaders can set the expectation that attendance is expected or make the training mandatory depending on the topic and setting.

Barriers

One common barrier is the need for more excitement for simulation from the learners. This may be due to anxiety-producing simulation sessions in previous educational environments, a failure to create a safe learning environment, or a fear of dolls/manikins. For these reasons, it is essential that the facilitator ensure a psychologically safe environment, utilize small group sizes to help foster interaction and a connection with each learner, and set clear expectations so everyone feels safe, is clear on objectives, and can engage in the hands-on experience. Although objectives are created at the course inception, they can be tailored to the group depending on experience and the area where the nurses work. For example, if a group is mostly ancillary staff participating in a cardiac arrest simulation, the scenario should be altered to meet the learning goals and objectives for that specific group. The goal is to have the learners practice a scenario that is congruent with their surroundings and role expectations.

Another barrier, often seen in smaller facilities, is the need for more availability of technology and resources. If a high-fidelity simulation is not an option in a facility wanting to present a course focused on moderate sedation simulation, it would be important to brainstorm ways the change in a patient's condition or vital signs can be portrayed and still produce urgency and critical thinking with minimal prompting. A solution for this could be to create various large poster boards with vitals and specific assessment details that are produced after an observed learner intervention. The use of the internet and pulling up various images and sounds during the simulation can also be used as a substitute for high-fidelity simulation, as could the recording of actual patient care monitors being manipulated by a vital sign generator. The advent of tablet-based vital signs generators is also a cost-effective way to increase realism during simulation sessions without the use of a high-fidelity simulator.

Debrief

Debriefing a simulation exercise is as important as the simulation exercise itself. Walking the group through a "prebrief" is important so the learners are aware of the technology available and what to expect during the simulation. Examples of setting expectations are walking the group through what the manikin can and cannot do, when/if the facilitator will be called upon for anything during the scenario, objectives of the simulation, and expectations of those not actively participating. Post-debriefing is the time to reinforce the simulation learning objectives and discuss both the things that went well and any opportunities for improvement. Debriefing can also pose a difficult or awkward time if the facilitator needs to be properly prepared. Some learners want to go right to what they did wrong or blame the technology for why they did not perform well. Blaming the simulation equipment should rarely happen if the participants have been well prepared and briefed regarding clear expectations of the simulation equipment and experience. For the learners that want to focus on what went wrong at the start of the debriefing, it is important to reinforce that the debriefing will start with what went well and then any missed opportunities and thoughts on what they might do differently next time. It is important to ensure the debrief does not turn into a facilitator-led lecture but rather a time of reflection on the main learning objectives and what happened in the simulation. Although the simulation scenario might be short, all learners should leave the debriefing experience with at least one key take-away.

Interface with Regulatory Bodies

Simulation is an engaging teaching modality that has the potential to improve practice and policy and procedure compliance. The Joint Commission (TJC) sets standards that can be reinforced during simulation. Moderate sedation education for those that will be performing it is a TJC requirement. Simulation not only provides necessary education on the topic, but hands-on education can reinforce hospital policies and procedures and provide the opportunity for nurses to demonstrate competency.

Also, sepsis education can help improve quality patient care to ensure that the 3- and 6-hour bundles are being met. The increase in sepsis education and awareness can also help contribute to hospital Centers for Medicare and Medicaid Services (CMS) compliance rates for fallouts and met measures. CMS compliance rates are posted on websites like "Hospital Compare," which has the potential to impact a patient's willingness to seek care at a healthcare organization if rates are low. In the health consumer culture today, positive patient outcomes and experiences in an organization can impact a hospital's reputation and patients' willingness to seek care there.

Scenario Examples

Most of the high-fidelity simulation used within this organization was supported through the Winter Institute for Simulation, Education, and Research (WISER) Center, part of the University of Pittsburgh Medical Center (UPMC) and the University of Pittsburgh [11]. Some hospitals, including the one discussed in this chapter, have their own simulation rooms/areas where these sample cases took place. The cases below include a moderate sedation simulation, a decompensating patient needing intubation, and a sepsis patient that needs the 3-hour bundle started.

Summary

Emergency Department nurses must be prepared for many low-occurrence, high-risk situations that require hands-on training and simulation to fully grasp the concepts being taught. The use of high-fidelity simulation to teach these high-risk situations, like moderate sedation, can help participants apply the learned concepts through hands-on experience. Creating a different form of simulation, like a low-budget escape room, allows learners to immerse themselves in the content and encourages learning in an exciting new way.

References

1. Hesse C, Emergency Nurses Association. Executive synopsis: emergency nurse retention. Des Plains, IL: ENA; 2016. Available from: https://www.ena.org/docs/default-source/resource-library/practice-resources/other/emergency-nurse-retention-executive-synopsis.pdf?sfvrsn=b8b1a708_4
2. Chiniara G, Crelinsten. A brief history of clinical simulation: how did we get here? In: Clinical simulation: education operations, and engineering. Academic Press; 2019. p. 3–16.
3. Boyde M, Cooper E, Putland H, Stanton R, Harding C, Learmont B, Thomas C, Porter J, Thompson A, Louise N. Simulation for emergency nurses (SIREN): a quasi-experimental study. Nurse Educ Today. 2018;68:100–4.
4. Emergency Nurses Association. Trauma nursing core course. Des Plains, IL: ENA; 2020. Available from: https://www.ena.org/education/tncc
5. Missouri Hospital Association. Fact sheet: SEP-1: early management bundle, severe sepsis/septic shock; 2020. Available from: https://www.mhanet.com/mhaimages/Sepsis_FactSheet.pdf.
6. Sepsis Alliance and National Association of Emergency Medical Technicians. Sepsis and EMS survey. Sepsis Alliance; 2019. Available from: https://www.sepsis.org/sepsis-and-ems-survey/.
7. Diaz D, Clapper T. Escape rooms: a novel strategy whose time has come. Simul Gaming. 2021;52(1):3–6.
8. Berger JD, Kuszajewski M, Borghese C, Muckler VC. A quality improvement project using high-fidelity simulation training to improve clinical knowledge among critical care transport nurses. Clin Simul Nursing. 2018;14:54–60.
9. Kutzin JM. Escape the room: innovative approach to interprofessional education. J Nursing Educ. 2019;58(8):474–80.
10. Emergency Nurses Association. Coaching guide for the lantern award application. Des Plains, IL: ENA; 2020. Available from: https://www.ena.org/docs/default-source/about-us/awards/coachingguide76ce1814acc3470e91598c7c14d3198f.pdf?sfvrsn=154f6faf_0
11. Winter Institute for Simulation, Education, and Research. Simulation template. Pittsburgh, PA; 2020. Available from https://www.wiser.pitt.edu/.

32 Simulation for Those Caring for the Obstetric Population

Holly Champagne

Background

Nurses working in maternal-child settings require developing clinical skills specific to the population they serve. These skills include knowing how to provide treatment during rare and emergent events. Some of these events are unique to pregnancy, such as management of a precipitous birth, preeclampsia, eclamptic seizures, obstetric hemorrhage, shoulder dystocia, and amniotic fluid embolism (anaphylactic syndrome of pregnancy). Maternity nurses work as part of a clinical team, including obstetrical, neonatal, and anesthesia providers. Teams must be prepared prior to the occurrence of an emergency. Simulation allows nurses and their colleagues to practice clinical and team communication skills without the risk of harming either the mother or her fetus. Simulation is also beneficial as an adjunct to performance improvement and educational initiatives.

Obstetrical simulators have a rich history. In the late 1700s, Madame Angelique le Boursier du Coudray used a device she called "the Machine" to teach midwives in France how to manage the delivery of an infant [1, 2]. Images of this device look similar to a modern-day training pelvis and newborn mannequin often used in the simulation. The Budin-Pinard simulator was created in the late nineteenth century for use by obstetricians. This model included a wooden female torso and thighs, which could accommodate a uterus made of pliable natural rubber [3]. The uterus could contain a fetal cadaver and liquids to simulate amniotic fluid [3]. Additional parts for this model included a bladder, perineum, labia, and an abdomen, each of which could be replaced when needed [3].

Obstetrical simulators available today include high-fidelity mannequins, which can deliver an infant and be programmed to present a variety of birth complications. Newborn high-fidelity mannequins are available in term and pre-term models. Task simulators are available for obstetric-specific training, such as cervical exams or the management of a birth complicated by shoulder dystocia. Some models specific to shoulder dystocia allowed a simulated infant to pass through the pelvis and provide a measurement of the amount of pressure placed on the neonatal neck. Models and devices are also available to represent cervical dilation, fetal heart rate rhythms, and abdominal palpation for Leopold's maneuvers. Infant models range in complexity, but at a minimum, most can receive lung inflation and chest compressions.

In-person simulation training is used to augment the practicing nurse's clinical experiences in labor, delivery, and postpartum settings. This is necessary as limited student nurse hours in this area may not allow the student or novice nurse to view a birth or develop experience in this setting. Virtual reality has been proposed as a future step in the simulation of learning for clinicians [4]. This type of learning includes "game type" interaction with a computer program as well as training with augmented reality and visual headsets [5]. Electronic simulation programs can provide additional exposure to obstetric and neonatal scenarios that might not be encountered during the student nurse's clinical rotation.

Interface with Regulatory Bodies

The Joint Commission is an organization that provides accreditation services to healthcare facilities. Accreditation is linked to payment by insurers, including the United States Centers for Medicare and Medicaid Services. The Joint Commission set standards for the care of women who experience an obstetric hemorrhage, severe range hypertension, or preeclampsia. These standards include a requirement to demonstrate that drills are conducted annually or more frequently to evaluate system issues associated with the care of women experiencing either condition [6]. Additional

H. Champagne (✉)
Kaiser Foundation Hospital, Roseville, CA, USA
e-mail: Holly.A.Champagne@kp.org, Holly@pchampagne.com

J. M. Kutzin et al. (eds.), *Comprehensive Healthcare Simulation: Nursing*, Comprehensive Healthcare Simulation,
https://doi.org/10.1007/978-3-031-31090-4_32

requirements include participation by a multidisciplinary team and performing a debrief as part of the drill [6]. Using simulation is not an absolute requirement as part of these standards. However, simulation can assist in evaluating systems issues that act as barriers to patient care and allow for a multidisciplinary approach to providing the care needed for these high-risk conditions.

Best Practices

A Lucille Packard Children's Hospital Stanford team began leading multidisciplinary perinatal education in a simulated delivery room in 2002 in the Center for Advanced Pediatric and Perinatal Education (CAPE) [5]. They continue to offer training to individuals and teams in managing obstetric emergencies and skills for briefing and debriefing events. The American Academy of Family Physicians (AAFP) offers training in Basic Life Support in Obstetrics™ (BLSO) and Advanced Life Support in Obstetrics™ (ALSO) programs [7]. These programs use simulation to practice basic skills such as delivery and neonatal resuscitation and advanced skills in managing bleeding and shoulder dystocia. The CAPE and AAFP

programs also provide instruction to individuals who can then provide the training to their facilities or academic institutions.

The Kaiser Permanente healthcare system instituted simulation training due to findings outlined in the IOM Report, To Err is Human: Building a Safer Health System [8]. Obstetrical units in particular, created interdisciplinary perinatal patient safety teams designed to review clinical events and promote best clinical practices. These teams identified opportunities for improvement in teamwork training for high-risk or problem-prone clinical issues. Improvement in interdisciplinary clinical and team communication resulted from the yearly practice of simulated critical events.

General Preparation Guidelines

The content in this section will provide information about some general approaches to preparing for obstetrical simulations. This type of preparation may benefit any simulation but is particularly well-suited to simulations that will be repeated many times to train large multidisciplinary teams. During preparation, it is important to determine the key learning outcomes for the training. This is often linked to the participants' experience, or lack thereof, with the expected standards. The following is an example of a program that initially had a simple patient scenario based on the learning needs of our clinical staff in our maternity units.

In 2014 our facility decided to implement standards related to the timely treatment of severe range hypertension in pregnant women. The standards included accurate measurement of the patient's blood pressure, a repeat of the blood pressure within a specified interval, notification of the obstetric provider, receiving an order for appropriate antihypertensive medication, then administering the medication, and assessing the patient's response to the medication and risk for preeclampsia. The simulated patient never progressed to a more complicated clinical condition. We learned during our initial trial of the simulation that most of our obstetric providers needed to familiarize themselves with the antihypertensive orders available in our electronic medical record (EMR) system. We then included a "sample patient" in our EMR so the providers could practice finding and entering the orders for antihypertensive medications and magnesium sulfate.

This seemed like an easy scenario, and sometimes our participants would say, "Is this all that's going to happen?". However, it was important in integrating the workflow and establishing role expectations for timely treatment of severe range hypertension. Our concurrent audits of patient treatment at the time showed significant and ongoing compliance for this treatment, which is associated with lowering the risk of maternal morbidity. Many years after the initial training, our simulation team members present a much more nuanced and complex presentation of a patient with preeclampsia, as we know that our timely treatment of severe range blood pressure is a hard-wired practice at our facility. We learned that it is important to determine the skill level that will need to be developed during the training. I also learned not to underestimate the complexity of our participants' tasks.

Pre-reading

The importance of pre-reading or the discussion of key points prior to simulation is an important part of gaining trust among participants. Pre-reading allows participants to have cognitive knowledge about the scenario. In general, clinicians wish to be prepared for simulation and to avoid looking foolish or ignorant about the standards of clinical practice. Pre-preparation also allows participants to engage in an informed discussion during the debriefing. It can enhance team communication by promoting a shared mental model regarding the clinical skills practiced during the simulation.

Some components to consider including in the pre-reading are professional organization statements, evidence-based practice guidelines (EBP), and standards for communication techniques. Clinical environment review may include the need for room safety, such as stating the standards for emergency equipment readiness, such as oxygen, suction, and the availability of emergency supplies. It is important to know how to lower the head of the bed quickly and the location of the backboard in order to perform adequate chest compressions during a maternal code blue. However, nurses and obstetric providers may to be refreshed on these seemingly simple items.

Including images of where items are located and how to operate equipment such as the bed, or the defibrillator, sets the team up for success during simulation. We found that the nurses often knew how to locate or operate some of the equipment, but the obstetric providers needed to learn this information. By including images in the pre-reading, all participants are aware of this information, and thus reduce the amount of time we need to spend presenting this information as part of the orientation to the room or during the debriefing. We prioritized the hand's-on practice of lowering the bed or locating specific items in an emergency cart so that all team members could assist during the simulations in the patient care setting.

Providing information on EBP guidelines and summarizing policies or professional practice guidelines allows individuals to mentally prepare for the emergencies that will be presented. Many obstetric providers appreciate having the original documents available for perusal as well. Examples of documents to consider are the American College of Obstetricians and Gynecologists practice bulletins related to the topic, American Heart Association basic life support guidelines, or recently published relevant medical or nursing literature. Also helpful is to list examples of expected teamwork principles, such as TeamSTEPPS® communication techniques [9]. It is important to make any job aids or algorithms available to the clinical team following the training so that they may be used to support bedside patient care.

Training Considerations

Locating a training space is an important initial step in planning for simulation. A simulation center with dedicated staff to manage the simulator and computer programs allows the trainers to focus on observing the participant's actions and communication. We do not have access to a simulation center. Our preference is to run scenarios in-situ for several reasons. Practicing scenarios in the obstetric units reduces the resistance the clinicians sometimes express about the scenario's reality. We sometimes discover barriers to efficient practice and opportunities to improve patient care by training in the clinical setting. For example, our postpartum patients stay on a floor above that of the labor and delivery operating room (OR). The team determined that one of the initial steps in response to an obstetric hemorrhage in a postpartum patient would be to bring a gurney to the room to facilitate transportation to the OR. Practice in situ allowed for this discovery, which would not have necessarily been discovered if the practice had been held in a simulation center. Confer with your fellow trainers prior to creating the pre-reading materials. Review the training goals, and obtain feedback from a representative of each discipline present during the training. We routinely solicit input from nurses, obstetric providers, physicians, certified nurse midwives, and anesthesia providers. They provide feedback on the goals and expected outcomes, and can suggest literature relevant to the clinical scenario.

When possible, use the training to reinforce any best practices adopted by your facility. We incorporated "emergency checklists" once they became available to our specialty. The simulation allowed us to reinforce this best practice and let our clinicians become more familiar with the content related to the obstetric emergency we were simulating.

Consider performing a dry run of your simulation with your fellow trainers if you teach with others. Include clinical staff in the practice training and solicit their feedback. This allows the training team to identify any possible difficulties with the equipment, scenario, or length of the simulation and debriefing, e.g., perhaps not meeting the allocated time for training.

We use a few standard procedures that have facilitated participant learning and participation. One standard is to create poster-sized images of key training materials as reference materials for debriefing. Examples include a copy of an eclampsia management algorithm, images of maneuvers used to relieve shoulder dystocia, and a copy of a facility-specific algorithm related to the timely assessment and treatment of severe range hypertension.

The advantages of the posters are twofold. One is that some learners need to process verbal information more effectively or hear the trainer. The learners can look at the poster and more easily follow the discussion. A second benefit is that using a standardized reference also reinforces the "standard work" of the participants related to the emergency.

An example is using the eclampsia management algorithm in the Hypertensive Disorders of Pregnancy toolkit HypertensiveDisordersofPregancytoolkit [10]. The algorithm lists the medications following the patient's first, second, and third eclamptic seizure. Magnesium sulfate is listed as the agent to be used for the first two seizures, followed by a consideration of several other medications following the third seizure. This sequence has prompted discussion among our obstetric and anesthesia providers about which medications to use, the rationale for use, and how to differentiate between a patient having a seizure from a seizure disorder and one associated with preeclampsia. The visual display on the poster board of the recommended treatment sequence helps the team develop a shared mental model about actions to take when eclampsia occurs. It is important to keep copies of the references used during training readily available in the clinical setting as reminders of the facility's standard work for the specific patient condition.

Another standard procedure employed during training is the use of observer checklists. Sometimes more trainees are present than are needed to participate directly in the simulation. We request these extra participants act as "skilled observers" and provide them with checklists. Checklists include the key actions required in the scenario. For instance, in a maternal code blue, actions include calling for help, timing from the time of pulselessness to determine when to deliver the infant, and bringing in the crash cart, among many others. In this checklist, there is a requirement to "time" when maternal pulselessness begins to provide feedback to the participants during debriefing. The observer also notes the length of time there are pauses in chest compressions, which can be discussed in light of basic life support guidelines for cardiopulmonary resuscitation (Appendix A).

Another checklist was created for observation related to TeamSTEPPS techniques, such as the use of SBAR, the establishment of a leader, and "check back" and "call out" behaviors (Appendix B). A final example of a checklist was designed to heighten awareness of team communication with the patient during an emergency and highlight items that might be associated with the patient having long-term persistent negative thoughts related to the experience. Items on that checklist included "communication too detailed/technical," "experience of the body in stressful positions," and "limited privacy." During debriefing, the team discussion would highlight the role each team member could play in keeping the patient informed of the care provided. This checklist helped build awareness of the need to follow up with the patient after an emergency and debrief the event with the patient and her family (Appendix C).

During debriefing the checklist, observers are asked to review what actions were performed or missed. There are several advantages to using checklists in this manner. One is that it allows the "observers" to participate in the debriefing and add their observations. The leader of the debriefing can rely on the checklist items to act as a prompt for the key points to be reviewed. Using the standardized checklist also lessens the risk that feedback may be perceived as personal criticism of the participants. Appendix D provides an example of a checklist designed for use during a shoulder dystocia simulation and debrief.

A final general training consideration is to prepare to run complex scenarios twice or to identify specific skills that may need repetition by all participants. For example, in running shoulder dystocia simulations, usually, one nurse would apply suprapubic pressure to the "pelvis" during the scenario. It became apparent that while the maneuver was described during pre-reading and demonstrated during the simulation, each nurse benefitted from practicing the skills. Following the shoulder dystocia scenario debrief, it was set as an expectation that every nurse who worked in labor and delivery would demonstrate how to apply suprapubic pressure. Similarly, each obstetric provider was required to practice the rotational maneuvers with the training pelvis. The participants universally agreed that demonstrating the skill increased their feeling of confidence in being able to act correctly in an emergency.

The trainees benefit from repeating the scenario following a debrief when there are complex scenarios with multiple disciplines and many steps. Our standard practice is to run a maternal code blue simulation twice. Maternal codes are rare in obstetrics, and simulation can highlight practice gaps. Commonly individuals delay initiating chest compressions, turning on the defibrillator, displacing the uterus, and delivering the infant within 5 min of maternal pulselessness. These gaps can result in the participants feeling disappointed in their performance. It was extremely well-received when this particular simulation was run a second time. The improved performance is apparent to all participants, and this re-run reinforces the key learning points for this simulation.

The Role of Debriefing

Solely one or two clinicians rarely manage the care of complex clinical situations in the obstetrical area. A few steps taken during simulation can benefit many clinical team members practicing as a group. Leadership in obstetric emergencies often migrates from the primary nurse to an obstetric provider and frequently occurs without a formal handoff. Debriefing allows the team to discuss the "leader" role, who has it, when the leader changes, and who assumes leadership when multiple physicians are responding to an emergency.

Critical event team training uses simulated experiences to promote teamwork and communication as part of perinatal safety initiatives [11]. Developing a shared mental model regarding the roles and expectations of non-nurse clinicians is critical in providing seamless care during an emergency. The following example is one experienced by this author when leading a simulation of a maternal code blue. Anesthesia providers, physicians and nurse anesthetists, respond to a code blue on the maternity units and thus participate in the team training. During the code, the anesthesia provider usually asks for intubation supplies. Most maternity service unit nurses need more experience assisting with emergency intubation. They would generally grab the largest intubation tube available and hand it to the provider, who would pause to indicate the tube was much too large. Comments included, "I do not need to intubate a horse (or an elephant)," and "Get me another tube." During the debrief, the team discussed this and suggested that the anesthesia provider request a specific size. However, an innovative solution presented itself when during one scenario, a nurse pulled out the entire tray of intubation supplies, brought it close to the anesthetist, and allowed that clinician to select the correct size. As a team, we could suggest this as a best practice and disseminate the learning through subsequent simulations.

During shoulder dystocia, the provider often performs several maneuvers to alleviate the impacted shoulder. Sometimes the provider "narrates" the maneuvers being performed. This narration helps those who can hear but not see the maneuvers. The narration allows everyone in the room to share a mental model of the care provided. If observed, this "narrating care" behavior can be called out during debriefing, and often those present remark on the usefulness of that behavior. The concept of "narrating care" can be discussed, even if not observed, as a model for keeping the team informed.

A technique that assists participants in integrating learning from the simulation is to ask each participant to name one thing, a "nugget," that they will take from the scenario and apply to practice. They are told that it may be something new or that reinforces something they already practice. This exercise provides insight into each participant's experience of simulation, allows each clinician a chance to reflect on the training, and through reflection, reinforces the one "nugget" for the learner. The trainers benefit from this exercise by listening to the responses and thus determining if the desired learning outcomes were met.

Outcomes Observed

Obstetric critical event team training simulations have improved our facility's patient outcomes and team performance. Audits revealed improvement in the timely administration of antihypertensive medication to patients with severe range hypertension. Over several years improvements were noted in the early recognition and treatment of obstetric hemorrhage. These improvements led to ongoing work related to communication about the need for blood products and developing a streamlined blood bank process to obtain and administer blood quickly in an emergency. Obstetric and anesthesia providers and nurses report improving team communication, especially in providing (or requesting) an SBAR and identifying the leader in an emergency. Nurses report improvement in communication as more providers "narrate" their care.

One particular outcome improvement related to simulation has been the use of a routine communication strategy during Cesarean delivery. The entire body of a newborn is usually delivered in less than 1 min following the uterine incision. Multiple factors may result in a prolonged extraction of the infant, including the size or the position of the fetal body or head. In order to improve communication among the surgeons, surgical techs, nurses (circulator and nursery nurses), and anesthesia providers in the operating room, some standards were proposed to improve communication. This included calling for additional personnel to assist if the delivery might take longer than anticipated. Interdisciplinary teams practiced a simulation in a "fake" operating room, where the team practiced communicating the time since incision, calling for help, and having the surgeons practice a variety of maneuvers that facilitate delivery. The anesthesia member's role was to ask if uterine relaxation agents would be needed. The nursery team was alerted to call for additional resources if resuscitation needed. This simulation improved communication and standardized each team member's role during the delivery of the infant. Ultimately the timeliness of recognition and treatment of emergencies, and communication among the clinical team members, have led to improvements in patient care in our obstetric units.

Sample Scenario: Severe Range Hypertension and Eclampsia

An example of a simulation that can be modified for varying types of learners is one related to treating severe range hypertension and an eclamptic seizure. Recognition and timely treatment of severe range hypertension and eclampsia are associated with reduced maternal morbidity [6]. The learning needs related to this topic vary predictably by the learner's experience, or lack thereof. Novice learners, generally clinicians new to maternity care, generally lack knowledge related to treatment standards, including timely notification of the obstetric provider and the need to administer antihypertensive agents within 30–60 min of confirmatory blood pressure. They also may not assess the patient for symptoms of preeclampsia. The learners often do not anticipate that the patient may be at risk for eclampsia and the patient will therefore require the administration of magnesium sulfate to reduce the risk of seizure. They often need more knowledge about anticipating what might occur next and the expected roles of the obstetric and anesthesia providers. Experienced clinicians often benefit from a "refresh" of the information, including fine-tuning the response time, communication among team members, and reviewing eclampsia medication management (see Table 32.1).

Preparation for simulation for either group would include pre-reading or a lecture on treatment guidelines of severe range hypertension, when magnesium sulfate is required, and management of an eclamptic seizure. The equipment for this simulation includes a manikin or actor, oxygen mask, yankauer suction (or entire suction set-up), and training medications. If possible, have a patient "arm," either part of the manikin or an artificial arm, with an intravenous (IV) needle and dressing in place prior to the start of the simulation. The medications available for this scenario should include having an IV mainline solution, an IV dose

Table 32.1 Learning needs for assessment and management of maternal severe range hypertension and eclampsia

Novice learners	Experienced learners
Accurate positioning of the patient and size and placement of the blood pressure cuff	All the novice skills were practiced sequentially, anticipating the need for treatment and lab work
Repeat the blood pressure within 10–20 min	Work as part of a multidisciplinary team
Timely notification of the obstetric provider of the severe range blood pressure ≥ 160/110	Differentiate among treatment modalities for a patient with an underlying seizure disorder and eclampsia
Administration of the appropriate antihypertensive medication within 60 min of the confirmatory blood pressure. (Placement of Intravenous access versus PO medication option)	Refer to magnesium sulfate administration guidelines in the setting of multiple seizures. Discuss when use of benzodiazepines or anti-convulsants might be needed
Assessment for symptoms of preeclampsia	Focus on use of teamwork communication skills: SBAR, check back, closed-loop communication
Management of eclampsia: prioritizing keeping the patient's airway open, preventing patient injury	Discuss the role of the leader
Recognition of the need for magnesium sulfate administration	Use of facility-specific emergency checklists

of magnesium sulfate, and a vial of IV hydralazine or IV labetalol. It is useful to have scenario-specific job aids printed and available in handouts or enlarged into a poster format for use during the simulation. For this scenario, it is helpful to have the guidelines for treating severe range hypertension and eclampsia management available for reference during the debrief.

Both teams benefit from having name tags to identify the roles. Assign roles for a minimum of an obstetrical provider, primary nurse, supporting nurse, and nurse leader, such as a charge nurse or manager. Provide vital signs on a display stand or flashcards, with the instructor verbalizing a few symptoms that indicate the presence of severe features of preeclampsia. A manikin (either a half-torso or a high-fidelity simulator) can begin to "seize" a few minutes after providing symptoms such as a headache and visual disturbances and a blood pressure ≥ 160/110 mmHg. The fidelity of the seizure is inconsequential; e.g., one can shake the torso for 1–2 min. What matters is the sequence of treatment, communication among, and roles and responsibilities of the "team members," the ability to follow management algorithms, and a verbalized understanding of the key clinical concepts. The simulation may last less than 10 min, with the debriefing lasting 10–20 min.

While brief, this simulation allows the participants to quickly identify the gaps in their skills and understanding of this potentially high-risk situation. Novice learners generally remark on how limited their understanding of the roles of the other team members, including nursing leaders (charge nurses or managers). They often do not know what type of order to request from the provider for acute blood pressure treatment or the need to assess for symptoms of preeclampsia. There is an acknowledgment that they "know" the symptoms and treatment, but when faced with the admittedly low-tech "seizing" manikin, they freeze and forget what to do. Fortunately, this is a very simple scenario to run again. The second run-through allows the participants to apply their new skills and to feel successful about their actions.

Integrating into Existing Education

Lectures related to new or modified concepts related to pregnancy, the postpartum period, or newborn care benefit from the addition of simulation. Consider the educational outcome goals. Is this about a process or communication? Does it require high fidelity? Would it benefit from adding greater complexity or visual cues?

Skills considered beginner, such as providing basic life support (BLS), require modification when provided to a pregnant woman. Consideration for uterine displacement and timely delivery of the infant to save the mother's life takes on a new perspective when coupled with BLS training. Simulation in this scenario requires participants to begin a timer at the time of pulselessness and actively displace the uterus to promote blood flow to the heart to meet the standards of care per the American Heart Association [12].

The addition of low-fidelity simulation, or task trainers, can assist in planning for new equipment, processes, or communication standards. New equipment deployments, such as neonatal warmers, intravenous pumps, defibrillators, operating room equipment, fetal or vital sign monitoring equipment, personal protective equipment standards, or electronic healthcare record documentation, can benefit from simulated scenarios. Use of new or updated standards, such as neonatal resuscitation, emergency checklists, treatment of hemorrhage, severe range hypertension and preeclampsia, blood product pickup, and medication use, provide an opportunity to walk through the indications to look for systems issues or potential obstacles to use. New or altered physical space, such as a novel or refurbished delivery room or operating room space, presents an opportunity to determine workflow and communication barriers.

Practicing clinicians appreciate and value the opportunity to practice for an upcoming complex case. For instance, delivering higher-order multiples, such as quintuplets, may require a modified delivery space. The simulation provided care coordination and delineated roles among the obstetric, nursing, neonatal, and anesthesia teams when preparing to deliver quintuplets. The multidisciplinary team members practiced preparing for an emergency Cesarean section and possible complications such as hemorrhage or the need for a hysterectomy.

Several years ago, the Kaiser Permanente Northern California _____ facility implemented maternal and infant skin-to-skin bonding immediately following Cesarean delivery. An interdisciplinary team reviewed the literature and developed a protocol. Before implementation, a small group of clinicians ran brief simulations in the operating room (OR). A team of labor and delivery and nursery nurses, an obstetrician, and an anesthesiologist participated. One staff nurse acted as the mother by lying on the OR table. We used an infant manikin to simulate a newborn. The team walked through the delivery steps, including the initial handoff to the nursery providers at an infant warmer and then the infant placement with the "mother." The anesthesiologist remained at the head of the OR table, with a surgical drape blocking the simulated sterile field.

This simulation revealed some limitations in our protocol and allowed us to correct these gaps. For instance, the anesthesiologist determined that cardiac leads would be better placed in an alternate position so the mother could hold the infant on her chest without the infant being placed on the leads. The nursery team found ways to support the mother holding the infant and determined that the nurse needed to remain at the mother's side if the mother became nauseous or faint.

Since then, our teams have walked through multiple mini-simulations to determine the best workflows. Most recently, simulation allowed for the practice of the distribution and donning of personal protective equipment during the initial days of the COVID-19 pandemic when the teams lacked experience in providing emergent care for pregnant women with this illness.

Challenges and Solutions

Common barriers to the simulation include the lack of dedicated training space, lack of access to a high-fidelity maternity manikin, lack of financial support, and lack of a shared mental model regarding the benefit of simulation. Using a dedicated space that simulates a labor and delivery room or operating room suite, with a "pregnant" high fidelity manikin and support staff who can facilitate and video-tape the simulation, is ideal.

Simulation can occur in an existing hospital room or classroom space with some modifications. This author's team used a video camera feed attached to a television to provide a view of the simulation when only a very small procedure room was available. The training space only had room for the "patient," two nurses, and an obstetric provider. The video feed allowed observers outside the small room to participate "virtually" in the simulation. The participants who viewed the training remarked that being outside the room allowed them to discuss the key learning points without disrupting the simulation.

The training team co-opted a family waiting room and placed a hospital bed in the space when the patient census prevented using a labor room. While it did not resemble a labor room, the essential equipment (labor bed, infant warmer, and delivery supplies) provided sufficient cues to the clinicians practicing in the simulation. The waiting room has been used as a virtual operating room as well. The room had a large metal table, surgical drapes, and instruments placed in it to replicate an OR. Our anesthesia department even provided a training anesthesia machine. While the room lacked access to surgical gasses and suction, the presence of the machinery and instruments allowed the room to feel like an operating room.

To simulate pregnancy, a standard adult high-fidelity manikin can be modified with a pillow or infant manikin strapped to the inside of the manikin's abdomen. The basic life support torso can be adapted to use if the training goals do not specifically need to result in a simulated delivery. Similarly, a pelvis with a newborn can be used with a female actress to simulate a precipitous birth, hemorrhage, or shoulder dystocia.

Some core equipment is useful in simulating frequently encountered scenarios in the maternity population. Having an infant manikin, fake blood (tempera paint already diluted and stored in an intravenous solution or rigid plastic containers), a vital signs display, sample fetal heart rate tracing, resuscitation equipment, training pelvis, blood pressure cuff, imitation medications, and role cards can support many obstetric emergencies. The advantage of this approach is that the equipment is easy to maneuver and transport and can quickly simulate a patient encounter with visual cues.

The following are some approaches to facilitate more challenging scenarios: place an infant manikin into a "uterus" created out of a fabric sack or cut into a sports ball; use a foam sports ball to simulate a boggy uterus; use a squirt bottle to express fake blood during a hemorrhage; collaborate with the blood bank to develop artificial "blood products". The National League for Nursing Simulation Innovation Resource Center provides an example of a manikin adapted for a simulated emergency Cesarean section and has been used successfully [13]. A hospital clinical technology department likely has a fetal heart rate rhythm simulator to calibrate a fetal heart rate monitor which can also be used for clinical training. It can be used to create an audio or visual recording of various fetal heart rates.

Challenges related to lack of financial support and lack of a shared mental model regarding the benefit of simulation may be more difficult to resolve than acquiring training equipment or space. Numerous articles have been published on the relationship of simulation to team training, improvement in communication, and patient safety in the obstetric setting [14, 15]. Highlighting the benefits reported in the literature may provide an effective strategy for securing support for the routine use of simulation.

Many clinicians practicing in the maternity setting experienced simulation as part of their pre-licensure or certification training and are familiar with the benefits of team training. It is important to demonstrate the benefits of specialty-specific training to those in leadership and those with non-clinical backgrounds. Often the exposure to the clinical team interactions to save a simulated patient's life is enough to obtain leadership support for this type of training. Identification of a spokesperson for each clinical specialty involved in caring for the perinatal patient (certified nurse midwife, nursing, obstetrician, pediatrician, anesthesia provider), who can provide examples of how interdisciplinary training prevents maternal and neonatal morbidity and mortality, may garner needed support to finance attendance at simulation training.

Summary

Simulation supports the needs of novice and expert learners in caring for pregnant and newly delivered women and their infants. It allows clinicians to assess for quality and safety issues related to high-risk conditions without putting the patient at risk. Training with simulation results in the interdisciplinary team interacting and communicating with each other freely while practicing and perfecting approaches best suited to keeping the patient safe.

Additional Resources for Severe Maternal Morbidity Related Simulations

The California Maternal Quality Care Collaborative (CMQCC) (https://www.cmqcc.org) offers free access to their toolkits, which were developed to prevent and manage maternal mortality and morbidity conditions. Two of the toolkits provide sample simulation training scenarios. These toolkits provide evidence of clinical best practices, and the simulations were designed specifically for these high-risk conditions.

- Improving Health Care Response to Obstetric Hemorrhage, a California Maternal Quality Care Collaborative Toolkit, 2022 https://www.cmqcc.org/resources-tool-kits/toolkits/ob-hemorrhage-toolkit, includes three obstetric hemorrhage scenarios and guidelines for the simulation and debriefing.
- Improving Health Care Response to Hypertensive includes scenarios related to severe range hypertension, preeclampsia, and eclampsia.

Appendix A: Recording Sheet—Code Blue, OBLS

✓		Comments
	Recognition of Unstable patient	
	Called for help	
	Recognize Code Blue	
	Call Code Blue	
	Chest compressions begun	
	Crash cart to room	
	Backboard under patient	
	Airway open	
	Bag/mask ventilation	
	Uterine displacement	
	Defibrillator in AED mode	
	Defibrillator pads placed	
	Scene "cleared" prior to shock	
	Shock delivered	
	Maternal intubation	
	Discussion of need to deliver infant	
	Call for pediatric team	
	Scalpel in surgeon's hand	

Timing:

Time that patient became pulseless:

Time that compressions began:

Time that decision to deliver infant made:

Time of infant delivery:

Goal: less than 10 s interruptions in compressions:

How many times were there >10 s in chest compression interruptions?

Appendix B: TeamSTEPPS Behavioral Skills

	1° RN	OB/ CNM	Chg/ ANM	Anesthesia	Helper RN
Scenario 1:					
✓ **By Whom**					
SBAR from primary RN to first responder	Comment:				
SBAR to Provider					
SBAR as other team members arrive					
	By Whom				
Leader identifies self	**1° RN**	**OB/ CNM**	**Chg/ ANM**	**Anesthesia**	**Helper RN**
As individuals arrive, they announce their names and roles	**1° RN**	**OB/ CNM**	**Chg/ ANM**	**Anesthesia**	**Helper RN**
Call out: *Topic:*	**1° RN**	**OB/ CNM**	**Chg/ ANM**	**Anesthesia**	**Helper RN**
Call out: *Topic:*	**1° RN**	**OB/ CNM**	**Chg/ ANM**	**Anesthesia**	**Helper RN**
Closed loop communication: *Topic:*	**1° RN**	**OB/ CNM**	**Chg/ ANM**	**Anesthesia**	**Helper RN**
Closed loop communication: *Topic:*	**1° RN**	**OB/ CNM**	**Chg/ ANM**	**Anesthesia**	**Helper RN**
Scenario 2:					
✓ **By Whom**					
SBAR from primary RN to first responder	Comment:				
SBAR to Provider					
SBAR as other team members arrive					
	By Whom				
Leader identifies self	**1° RN**	**OB/ CNM**	**Chg/ ANM**	**Anesthesia**	**Helper RN**
As individuals arrive, they announce their names and roles	**1° RN**	**OB/ CNM**	**Chg/ ANM**	**Anesthesia**	**Helper RN**
Call out: *Topic:*	**1° RN**	**OB/ CNM**	**Chg/ ANM**	**Anesthesia**	**Helper RN**
Call out: *Topic:*	**1° RN**	**OB/ CNM**	**Chg/ ANM**	**Anesthesia**	**Helper RN**
Closed loop communication: *Topic:*	**1° RN**	**OB/ CNM**	**Chg/ ANM**	**Anesthesia**	**Helper RN**
Closed loop communication: *Topic:*	**1° RN**	**OB/ CNM**	**Chg/ ANM**	**Anesthesia**	**Helper RN**

Appendix C: Obstetric Emergency Simulation Observation Worksheet—Experiences Which May Benefit from Patient/Family Debrief (Content adapted from Hall [16][a])

Check if present	Physical discomforts[a]	Patient remarks	Comments
	Pain		
	Experience of body in stressful positions		
	Restriction of movement		
	Environmental discomforts[a]		
	Exposure to sounds (monitors, alarms, etc)		
	Limited privacy		
	Lack of personal clothing		
	Lack of personal space		
	Exposure to needles		
	Exposure to blood		
	Experience of private areas being touched		
	Experience of private areas being seen by staff		
	Emotional Discomforts[a]		
	Fear for own life		
	Fear for life of fetus/infant[b]		
	Feeling anxious		
	Feeling powerless		
	Feeling vulnerable		
	Concern about quality of care		
	Feeling numb or detached		
	Communication[a]		
	Communications too detailed/ technical		
	Communications too quick/ confusing		
	Communications too vague		
	Communications too infrequent		
	Communications too frequent		

[a] Hall [16, 17], Harris and Ayers [18]
[b] KP ROS addition

Appendix D: Shoulder Dystocia Recording Sheet

- RN makes sure step stool is in the room/available
- Bed was broken down if risk factors present (or as soon as possible once SD recognized)
- All staff watching perineum for possible "turtle sign"
- Recognition of shoulder dystocia (i.e. provider "calls out" the emergency to room)
- Shoulder code called to operator
- Apgar timer started

- McRoberts done
- OB Provider indicated to RN the direction to apply pressure (i.e. "towards the window" or "towards the door")
- RN uses step stool or otherwise positions self correctly for suprapubic pressure
- Suprapubic pressure applied
- Other maneuvers used:
  - Posterior arm
  - Woods screw
  - Rubin
  - Gaskin
- Provider calls out what maneuvers they are attempting
- OB provider calls out to stop suprapubic pressure/maternal pushing while maneuvers done
- Second provider announces his/her arrival in the room, attempts maneuvers
- Time called out during event
  - 30 s
  - 1 min
  - 1.5 min
  - 2.0 min
- Provider announces the need to move to the OR if SD extends past 2 min
- TeamSTEPPS communicationKey "call outs" performed
- SBAR given to incoming staff
- Closed loop communication (check backs)

References

1. Moran ME. Enlightenment via simulation: "crone-ology's" first woman. J Endourol. 2010;24(1):5–8. https://doi.org/10.1089/end.2009.0423.
2. Gardner R, Raemer DB. Simulation in obstetrics and gynecology. Obstet Gynecol Clin N Am. 2008;35(1):97–127. https://doi.org/10.1016/j.ogc.2007.12.008.
3. Owen H, Pelosi MA 2nd. A historical examination of the Budin-Pinard phantom: what can contemporary obstetrics education learn from simulators of the past? Acad Med. 2013;88(5):652–6. https://doi.org/10.1097/ACM.0b013e31828b0464.
4. Austin N, Goldhaber-Fiebert S, Daniels K, Arafeh J, Grenon V, Welle D, Lipman S. Building Comprehensive Strategies for Obstetric Safety: Simulation Drills and Communication. Anesth Analg. 2016;123(5):1181–90. https://doi.org/10.1213/ANE.0000000000001601.
5. McGrath JL, Taekman JM, Dev P, Danforth DR, Mohan D, Kman N, Crichlow A, Bond WF. Using virtual reality simulation environments to assess competence for emergency medicine learners. Acad Emerg Med. 2018;25(2):186–95. https://doi.org/10.1111/acem.13308. Epub 2017 Oct 11
6. California Maternal Quality Care Collaborative. Preeclampsia toolkit. https://www.cmqcc.org/resources-tool-kits/toolkits/preeclampsia-toolkit, 2014. Accessed 21 January 2021.
7. Stanford Medicine. OB Simulation Program. https://www.stanfordchildrens.org/en/service/pregnancy-newborn/ob-simulation-program (2021). Accessed 24 Jan 2021.
8. American Academy of Family Physicians. Advanced life support in obstetrics (ALSO®). https://www.aafp.org/cme/programs/also.html (2020). Accessed 21 Jan 2021.
9. Kohn LT, Corrigan JM, Donaldson MS, editors. To err is human: building a safer health system. Washington, DC: National Academy Press, Institute of Medicine; 1999.
10. Agency for Healthcare Research and Quality. TeamSTEPPS® Strategies & Tools to Enhance Performance and Patient Safety. https://www.ahrq.gov/teamstepps/index.html (n.d). Accessed 30 January 2021.
11. Arafeh J. Update: Simulation-Based Training. J Perinat Neonatal Nurs. 2017;31(4):286–9. https://doi.org/10.1097/JPN.0000000000000288.
12. The Joint Commission. R3 report issue 24: PC standards for maternal safety. https://www.jointcommission.org/standards/r3-report/r3-report-issue-24-pc-standards-for-maternal-safety/, 2021. Accessed 21 Jan 2021.
13. Halamek LP, Cady RAH, Sterling MR. Using briefing, simulation, and debriefing to improve human and system performance. Semin Perinatol. 2019;43(8):151178. https://doi.org/10.1053/j.semperi.2019.08.007. Epub 2019 Aug 10
14. Panchal AR, Bartos JA, Cabañas JG, Donnino MW, Drennan IR, Hirsch KG, Kudenchuk PJ, Kurz MC, Lavonas EJ, Morley PT, O'Neil BJ, Peberdy MA, Rittenberger JC, Rodriguez AJ, Sawyer KN, Berg KM. Adult Basic and Advanced Life Support Writing Group. Part 3: Adult Basic and Advanced Life Support: 2020 American Heart Association Guidelines for Cardiopulmonary Resuscitation and Emergency Cardiovascular Care. Circulation. 2020;142(16 Suppl. 2):S366–468. https://doi.org/10.1161/CIR.0000000000000916. Epub 2020 Oct 21
15. National League for Nursing. Emergency Cesarean section IPE simulation: homegrown solutions. http://www.nln.org/sirc/sirc-homegrown-solutions/emergency-cesarean-section-ipe-simulation, 2021. Accessed 21 January 2021.
16. Hall, M. (2015). Experience of medical trauma scale (EMTS). Retrieved from http://safehealthcareforeverywoman.org/wp-content/uploads/2016/09/2-Response-Experience-of-Medical-Trauma-Scale-MFHall.pdf
17. Hall, M. (2015). Recognizing signs of acute stress disorder in postpartum women in the hospital setting. Retrieved from http://safehealthcareforeverywoman.org/wp-content/uploads/2016/09/3-Recognition-Recognizing-Signs-of-Acute-Stress-Disorder-in-Postpartum-Women-in-the-Hospital-Setting-MFHall.pdf
18. Harris R, Ayers S. What makes labour and birth traumatic? A survey of intrapartum "hotspots". Psychol Health. 2012;27:1166–77.

Neonatal Simulations

33

Christine Broome

Background

The relationship between the Neonatal Intensive-Care Unit (NICU) and healthcare simulation is one that has been in place for many years. Seventeenth-century Roman Empire soldiers documented using human torso replicas and cloth dolls to teach midwives to deliver and resuscitate newborns. In the early 1900s, military personnel, hospitals, and nursing schools began to simulate pediatric and neonatal scenarios with the first life-sized manikin called the "Martha Chase Hospital Doll." The first infant-size Chase manikin was used in 1911 at the Hartford Hospital Training School for Nurses [1]. During the 1960s, the Resusci Anne manikin was developed and used as a training aide for mouth-to-mouth resuscitation. It was shortly followed by the Baby Anne manikin, used specifically for infant cardio-pulmonary resuscitation practice [2].

In 1969, the first realistic training simulator was introduced, featuring: respirations, heartbeat, pulses, blinking eyes, and other realistic features. However, the simulator was not well received due to cost and a deep-rooted bias toward needing real patients for training [2]. Approximately ten years passed before simulation-based training was consistently utilized in neonatal education. After this period, resuscitation simulation began to lay the groundwork for neonatal simulation, demonstrated by two programs in particular, Neonatal Resuscitation Program (NRP) and Helping Babies Breathe (HBB).

NRP started in the 1970s as a 6-module series, the Neonatal Education Program, developed by Dr. Ron Bloom, MD, and Cathy Cropley, RN. This program, supported by the American Academy of Pediatrics, formed the bases of the future NRP. Representatives from the academy and American Heart Association jointly committed to developing a training program to teach neonatal resuscitation to have a trained provider at every delivery [3]. It was not until 1980 that NRP linked traditional didactic and test learning with simulation scenarios to provide a safe environment for medical personnel to master high-risk deliveries. The NRP's partnership with simulation revealed improved team communication and delivery outcomes. The first NRP training session that included simulation was launched in November 1987 [4].

In the 1990s, advanced simulators began to appear in nursing simulation education by introducing affordable, high-fidelity simulators that demonstrated palpable pulses, audible physiologic sounds, and vital sign monitoring, adding realism to simulations and providing realistic feedback to the learner, ultimately increasing learner engagement. Improvement in scenarios, task-trainers, and simulators moved neonatal resuscitation education from a traditional skills laboratory into high-fidelity simulation [5]. With this shift, in 2000, Halamek et al. [6] began to bridge the gap between the traditional NRP structure and simulation-based education, adding realistic simulation resuscitation scenarios to the training course. The program eventually spanned across the United States, then internationally. Today NRP continues to educate over four million healthcare professionals with state-of-the-art interactive education, simulation, and debriefing [3].

Helping Babies Breath (HBB) is an evidence-based educational initiative to teach neonatal resuscitation techniques in resource-limited areas, developed in 2010 by the AAP in collaboration with the World Health Organization. The key concept of the program is the Golden Minute. Within the Golden Minute, a birth attendant must identify the steps after birth to evaluate the baby and stimulate breathing. The curriculum is designed with an innovative neonatal simulator, graphic learning materials, and content tailored to address the major causes of neonatal death in low and middle-income countries. Laerdal Global Health collaborated with national and international health organizations to produce training

C. Broome (✉)
Neonatal Intensive Care Unit, John Muir Health, Walnut Creek, CA, USA
e-mail: Christine.Broome@johnmuirhealth.com

J. M. Kutzin et al. (eds.), *Comprehensive Healthcare Simulation: Nursing*, Comprehensive Healthcare Simulation,
https://doi.org/10.1007/978-3-031-31090-4_33

color graphic icons outlining three simple care paths and illustrations that draw attention to critical decision points in resuscitation, stressing the need to initiate ventilation no later than the end of the first minute after birth. A neonatal simulator (NeoNatalie™) is provided to trainers to help guide the decision-making and management of the newborn, who may range from healthy and crying to needing advanced care [7].

The success of simulation in resuscitation led NICUs to use simulation in other areas of practice, such as bedside procedures, transport, process evaluation, response-time improvement, and a number of high-risk, low-frequency patient scenarios. Today hospital administration, medical staff, and nursing leaders continue to dedicate time and resources toward simulation and its benefits. Growth in Neonatology and its workforce has expanded the need for neonatal simulation to tackle increased demand for trained personnel to handle high-pressure, high-risk patient situations. With an influx of personnel into the workforce, junior practitioners compete for the training opportunities needed to manage such situations. Decreased opportunities to perform these critical skills have diminished expertise and increased medical practice errors. Today simulation remains a solution to providing proper education on skills required to manage neonatal patients. Both experienced and new personnel practice delivery resuscitation, endotracheal intubation, central line access, and chest tube placement within a structured simulation and debriefing environments that avoid patient risk [8].

Recently a link has been established between ineffective communication and neonatal morbidity and mortality. The Joint Commission, a global driver of quality improvement and patient safety in health care, indicated that 75% of reported neonatal deaths and serious neonatal morbidity could have been related to ineffective communication. To improve outcomes, recommendations were given to conduct neonatal and obstetric clinical drills to prepare staff for high-risk events, followed by debriefings to evaluate team performance and identify areas for improvement [9]. Prior to this report, the emphasis on neonatal simulation was narrowed to improving cognitive and technical skills, which alone are insufficient when managing critical neonatal cases under intense stress. Since these recommendations, behavioral skills such as communication, leadership, situational awareness, and mutual support are standard in neonatal and obstetric simulation.

The history of simulation in neonatology, partnered with the recommendations in literature to incorporate behavioral skills, has influenced neonatal educators and specialists to create simulation-based best practices and innovative curricula into standard education requirements. The following section will describe optional best practices in neonatal simulation to consider when providing education.

Best Practices

Innovation and research in neonatal simulation have broadened the ways in which simulation is used in the care of neonates. In addition to the common ways simulation-based education is used, neonatal units everywhere are developing innovative ways to implement simulation as a tool for education.

Simulation-based training can bridge the gap and allow new graduate nurses to practice safely before working with a real patient. New graduate nurses specializing in Neonatology face overwhelming didactic content and numerous specialized technical skills to transition to Neonatology. There are a few ways to make the education concrete [2]. Memorial Health System in Colorado Springs, CO, uses scenarios for the most common neonatal diagnoses, allowing the new nurses to use the nursing process while caring for an infant with a specific diagnosis. Sepsis, seizures, respiratory distress syndrome (RDS), and codes are just a few of the scenarios included. The didactic content is presented first, followed by scenarios on the same day. The new nurses are given a chance to make mistakes and learn from them in a safe learning environment without the repercussions of harming a real patient. They can use all of their senses and have a heightened awareness not present during traditional lectures.

The University of California San Francisco Benioff Children's Hospital Perinatal Outreach Program provides customized low-fidelity simulation classes to community-level hospitals, focusing on communication in team training during obstetric and neonatal emergencies. A mobile multidisciplinary team, including doctors, nurses, support staff, and educators, focuses on medical and nursing staff education scenarios to improve communication and perfect role requirements. A mobile in-situ simulation is a unique approach to outreach education that allows staff in the community settings opportunities to practice and prepare for emergencies within their personal equipment systems and working environment. Scenarios are videotaped, and confidential debriefs are conducted to identify system issues, share staff performance, and improve communication [2].

The nursing education department at Baylor University Medical Center in Dallas, Texas, uses a simulation model that moves the focus from skills lab to competency assessment. Each year, the education team identifies opportunities for nursing skill development and cultivates creative methods to demonstrate competency in those skills. Simulated scenarios are one of the methods nurses may choose to demonstrate competency. The education team develops simulation scenarios encompassing technical, interpersonal, and critical thinking skills. The staff member may either develop a realistic scenario for simulation or enroll in a developed scenario. Using this type of simulation-based learning to assess competency immersed the staff in a realistic clinical setting, allowing them to draw from personal experience, problem-solve, and immediately apply the knowledge to their clinical practice [2].

To improve relationships with families of neonates, Lucile Packard Children's Hospital in Palo Alto, CA, developed a simulation program focusing on shift-to-shift handoff of incidental family information and communication techniques that develop trust between nurses and family in a short time frame. Using their simulation lab, actual parents from their NICU Parent Advisory Group participate in scenarios that focus on parent education regarding the neonate's condition, medications, and expectations of care. Along with parents, bedside nurses and medical providers gather around the patient care simulator as medical conditions such as supraventricular tachycardia, respiratory desaturation events, and seizures are simulated. Care providers practice managing the condition while communicating with parents. The scenarios were followed by debriefs that met objectives specific to the medical condition and parent communication [2, 10].

Ongoing standards of simulation in Neonatology also focus on skill retention. Studies have shown a significant loss of skill as early as two months after NRP [11]. In addition, senior, more experienced physicians and nurses often focus on proctoring skills instead of having the opportunity to practice themselves, potentially causing a reduction in proficiency. Follow-up sessions over shorter periods can improve learning retention, and concurrent simulations can be offered as an evidence-based approach to continued evaluation.

As a standard for ongoing practice improvements, hospitals have implemented ongoing in-situ simulations that offer total immersion, high-fidelity, and simulation scenarios on the neonatal unit. Examples include Leicester Royal Infirmary, where two physicians and two nurses (junior and senior) attend each session in their usual role. Simulation sessions lasting approximately one hour are offered with minimal disruption to clinical service. Sessions are offered in a safe, non-punitive environment to facilitate practice and open discussion. Scenarios are derived from common clinical scenarios designed to reflect previous participant feedback, national patient safety efforts, and internal clinical governance information. Scenario examples include meconium/persistent pulmonary hypertension of the newborn, pneumothorax, congenital diaphragmatic hernia, and delivery of extremely low birth weight (ELBW) neonates weighing under 1000 g. Following the scenario, teams debrief immediately with an advocacy-inquiry approach (combination of rigorous feedback with genuine inquiry) to discuss problems and concerns in an open and honest fashion. At each debrief, participants are asked to share the three most important things they gained during the simulation to solidify their learning.

Programs like those listed above have gained widespread increased attention in recent years, establishing simulation-based education as a future standard in Neonatology.

Sample Curriculum

Innovative examples begin to grow as the need for simulation moves beyond neonatal resuscitation. The remainder of the chapter will describe neonatal simulation-based education programs and examples successfully implemented in Neonatology. Each of the following sample curriculums uses simulation to evaluate the problem, determine the needs of the multidisciplinary teams, assess space and process, and improve teamwork and collaboration.

Sample Curriculum #1: Neonatal Transport Handoff–Critical Neonatal Transport

Neonatal transport teams are specially trained personnel who care for critically ill neonates in transport between different levels of care. Neonates that require a higher level of care are transported from one hospital to another in a transport rig (mobile incubator retrofitted with stabilization equipment) via ambulance, plane, or helicopter. Traditionally neonatal transport teams consist of a registered nurse (RN), a respiratory therapist (RT), a paramedic or an emergency medical technician, and sometimes a neonatal nurse practitioner or a physician. Teams require specialized handling and assessment skills to safely transport critical neonates due to their potential for rapid deterioration, especially when premature or extremely low birth weight.

To improve access to neonatal healthcare and higher levels of care, John Muir, an adult-centered community hospital, employed pediatric transport specialists to safely transport critically ill neonatal patients to its Level III NICU. Because the transport of neonatal patients is managed differently than pediatric patients, the transport team required intensive didactic training, technical skill practice, and transport rehearsals. The process of facilitating transport also needed to be evaluated, including transport initiation, communication, equipment, and timelines. The simulation was chosen as a practical tool to provide skill training and transport rehearsal while establishing the process and communications supporting the transport program. Through simulation, the neonatal transport team practiced newly learned skills, prompt assessment, interventions, and stabilization of acutely ill infants. A realistic scenario (Appendix 1) was created to rehearse responses to signs of clinical deterioration, develop effective communication skills, improve team performance, and determine process issues in a safe, realistic environment free from patient risk.

Before developing simulation-based education, didactic instruction and clinical preceptorships were offered to support the transport nurse's understanding of the specialized care required to manage neonates in transport. Numerous hours of observation, focused assessment, and proctored hands-on care allowed the transport nurses to acquire the technical skill needed to stabilize and transport sick neonates. Skills included intubation, line placement, rapid assessment, and stabilization.

Once preceptorships were complete, four consecutive simulation scenarios were developed for each stage of the simulation:

1. Transport center request for transport MD/MD (validate transport request process and call escalation)
2. Delivering hospital arrival and stabilization (practice handoff and stabilization guidelines)
3. In transit—transport rig (practice further complication response and escalation)
4. Arrival at receiving hospital (the final destination of the neonate, including handoff of all aspects of the case)

Each stage contained expected interventions and objectives for the learner to meet based on the requirements of the process or condition of the patient simulator as stated in the 'Neonatal Transport Scenario Guideline' (Appendix 1). All scenarios featured the critical care transport of a 1-hour-old, 750-g, 25-week gestation infant born vaginally at a newborn delivery hospital that was ill-equipped to manage care. The scenario began after receiving a request for transport from the delivery hospital to the Level III NICU for a higher level of care.

Three independent scenes were set up in various locations throughout the hospital to facilitate the simulation. (1) A simulation suite would be used to set up the delivery hospital's infant nursery, (2) a transport ambulance located in the hospital parking lot would be used to practice loading and unloading the patient in the ambulance transport rig, and (3) a Level III NICU patient room would be the final stop as the receiving hospital. The benefits of ending the simulation in the actual receiving hospital's NICU included evaluating the patient room space, transporting familiarization with the NICU layout, and accommodating equipment needs. In addition, staff from the receiving hospital observed transport handoff and safe transfer of the neonate from the transport rig to a warmed patient incubator for ongoing care.

To initiate the simulation, a physician phoned the receiving hospital to request transport through the Transfer Center, testing the interpretation of the patient's status and the escalation process. Objectives included the required relay of the patient's history, current status, reason for transport, immediate management of complications, and facilitation of a conference call with the partnering Neonatologist. The time of each call was recorded to determine the length of time between communication and the total length between initial request and departure.

During the scenario at the delivery hospital, the learners faced a patient simulator that was less than 1000 grams in weight in position on a radiant warmer bed in critical condition. The simulator was set up in accordance with the 'Transport Scenario Guideline' (Appendix 1). The simulator was intubated and appropriately connected to a ventilator; umbilical lines were unsecured and connected to fluid pumps. Vital signs were displayed on the monitor, and the simulator displayed chest rise, cyanosis, and weak movement.

Objectives and expected interventions included proper communication, thorough assessment, addressing immediate needs, recognizing risk factors, proper set up of the transport isolate and ventilator, proper transfer of medications and fluids, proper handling, and appropriate interaction with the family. During the transfer of the patient from the warmer to the transport isolate, a change in patient status was simulated, requiring the team to adjust appropriately to stabilize the patient prior to departure. Once complete, the transport team proceeded to the parking lot with the simulator secured in the transport isolate. All tubes and IV lines were connected to their correlating device and functioning appropriately.

The 'in transit' portion of the scenario included the setup of the transport ambulance with equipment needed to support neonatal transport, including oxygen, ventilator, IV pumps, and monitoring devices. The transport isolate with the simulator was secured in the ambulance for transport, initiating the second simulation scenario. During transport, the simulator status deteriorated, requiring rapid assessment, recognition of complications, and expedited intervention. Objectives included appropriate interventions for typical medical complications of a 24-week gestation neonate during transport, including hypotension, hypoglycemia, hypercarbia, and temperature instability, partnered with effective communication to facilitate treatment.

The final destination and last portion of the scenario was 'handoff to the receiving hospital.' The NICU patient room, previously set up with a warming isolate, is changed to include a patient monitor, patient bedside cart, and support equipment. A team, including a nurse, a neonatologist, and a respiratory therapist, greeted the transport team and patient simulator. The scenario objectives included relaying a proper history from the delivery team, reviewing patient status, sharing complications during transport and appropriate interventions, demonstrating proper handling and positioning, providing proper positive-pressure ventilation upon transfer, and correctly relaying medications and doses.

The simulation was followed by a debrief covering the objectives listed in the scenario (Appendix 1). Focus was placed on communicating a relay of vital information, proper handling of the preterm, recognition of complications, and expedited interventions. The neonatal team shared optional interventions with the transport team and clarified practice concerns. Communication between the support transfer center, physicians, and transport team was discussed in detail, and opportunities were identified.

'Time checks' were recorded and analyzed to reduce response time. Additional education was provided after debriefing to clarify the communication process, discuss other transport scenarios, and support technical skills.

Ongoing transport simulations continue quarterly at the receiving hospital to further streamline the initial transport request process. A patient scenario is presented each quarter to improve critical thinking and skill. Debriefing offers continual feedback on team training and communication.

Sample Curriculum #2: Standardization of Tools & Team Roles to Improve Delivery Resuscitation

The successful transition from fetal to neonatal life depends upon significant physiologic changes at birth. Although most newborns make this transition without assistance, many require resuscitative support in the delivery room.

Medical staff who are adequately trained in neonatal resuscitation should be readily available to perform NRP whether or not complications are anticipated. In all instances, at least one healthcare provider is assigned primary responsibility for the newborn infant. However, when resuscitation is required, teams must respond with the necessary skills to initiate resuscitation procedures, such as positive pressure ventilation and chest compressions. Standard recommendations in neonatal resuscitation are that teams assign roles and responsibilities prior to delivery, communicate effectively, establish leaders, maintain situational awareness, and mutually support one another during the resuscitation. Much of the success in the neonate's transition and long-term outcome depends on the communication and care the clinicians provide during resuscitation [12].

In addition, standardized equipment that is routinely checked and functioning properly should be available at every delivery. Although there is consensus on the resuscitation of newborns, there needs to be standardization on how resuscitation equipment should be organized, leading to difficulty and inefficiency in retrieving the right equipment during resuscitation. Simulation proved useful in determining a standardized strategy for equipment set-up and standardized roles to reduce task saturation.

The neonatal delivery team at Kaiser Permanente identified the need for resuscitation skill practice, team training, and standardization of their neonatal crash cart. Observation of a series of resuscitation simulations and a formal needs assessment revealed the opportunity to improve the skill level of the support staff that did not regularly attend deliveries. Hands-on skills, team training, role establishment, and standardization of the code cart were determined as necessary for improving resuscitation outcomes. Bi-weekly simulation courses were used to implement these best practices.

The Clinical Nurse Specialist in the NICU determined hands-on skills for the course after observation of previous simulations and employee surveys. Skill sessions included a review of umbilical line set-up, epinephrine preparation, MRSOPA (an airway management technique used in NRP *including Mask adjustment, Repositioning of the airway, Suction, Open mouth, Pressure increase, and Alternative airway*), compression-breath coordination, and communication handoff. Umbilical line kits were created to practice quick assembly and priming. Medication reference cards were created in collaboration with the Neonatologist and Pharmacy team, displaying weight-specific medication doses, endotracheal tube size and placement depth, and umbilical line placement depth. Learners were given time to practice drawing emergent medications referencing the medication cards. (Appendix 2).

The second section of the class included a brief review of TeamSTEPPS® communication tools (an evidence-based teamwork system to improve communication and teamwork skills among healthcare professionals) followed by communication practice sessions. TeamSTEPPS® visual aids were used to prompt the learner and guide communication. Communication tools were practiced streamlining handoff between nurses and physicians during a critical resuscitation.

Roles cards and delivery prompts were created with the help of the Advanced Life Support (ALS) nurses that regularly attended deliveries. The role cards and delivery prompts would help guide the resuscitation teams through the steps of NRP and to define responsibilities based on their physical location around the resuscitation bed. Roles cards posted on the warmer focused on equipment preparation, timely completion of tasks, and clear communication to allow the physician leader to rapidly assess and maintain situational awareness during resuscitation. Learners were placed in role spaces and shown posted role cards. (Appendix 3). Teams practiced movement around the bedside, preparation of equipment, and chest compression-breath coordination.

Standardization of neonatal delivery code carts included researching best practices and coordinating with the Code Blue committee in the hospital. A streamlined cart was developed based on evidence-based practice (Appendix 4). Five new code carts were purchased, and supplies were stocked according to the steps of NRP. They were color coded to match roles and coordinated with the airway, breathing, and circulation steps of NRP [13]. Carts were displayed for approximately two months in the neonatal unit for nurses to become familiar with prior to simulation. During the simulation-based education course, the code carts were reviewed, and learners were allowed time to familiarize themselves with the contents.

The final portion of the course consisted of two simulations. The first simulation scenario was of a basic neonatal resuscitation beginning with delivery and ending with endotracheal intubation. The second simulation scenario was a more substantial code that began with delivery and ended with epinephrine administration and volume management. Simulation scenario guidelines were provided to simulation instructors for use during each class (Appendix 5). Each simulation was followed by a debrief and an opportunity for reflection. Learning points were applied to the second simulation, also followed by debriefing.

Each simulation-based education class began with the completion of a survey to determine the student's current state of knowledge (Appendix 6). These surveys helped determine pre-existing conceptions of resuscitation, confidence in NRP skills, the learner's role during deliveries, and the average number of deliveries attended yearly. The course concluded with a post-evaluation (Appendix 6). This helped the simulation and education team determine the effectiveness of the skill session, simulation-based learning, and future needs.

The neonatal simulation program and course continued for approximately 1 year, allowing each nurse to attend two 2-hour simulations annually. The content for both attendance periods remained the same, providing repeated opportunities to review the objectives. One full year of neonatal simulation revealed improved confidence in the learner's ability to perform the skills needed for resuscitation, communicate effectively during delivery resuscitation, and perform in their designated roles during resuscitation.

Sample Curriculum #3 Neonatal Surgical Bedside Procedure

Simulating complicated bedside procedures in the NICU can help teams improve skills, communicate effectively, and determine required support. Surgical bedside procedures, in particular, require evaluation of needed space, facilitation of several layers of team communication, determination of needed equipment, and patient and staff safety management. To avoid potential complications when performing surgical procedures at the bedside, a NICU team collaborated with Operating Room (OR) staff and neonatologists on a complicated simulation scenario to provide the best care possible during critical surgical procedures.

Critically ill neonates in the NICU often require surgical procedures. Traditionally neonates are transferred to the main OR outside the NICU, increasing the risk of complications. Complications such as harmful changes in heart rate and blood pressure, dislocation of endotracheal tubes, loss of vascular access, and hypothermia cause significant morbidity, which may alter the outcome in these already compromised patients [14]. To avoid harmful events during transport, selected surgical procedures are performed in the NICU at the patient's bedside. Neonatal surgical procedures performed at the bedside include emergent procedures such as drain placement for bowel perforation or ligation of a patent ductus arteriosus when the critical level of the patient does not allow transfer to a standard OR. Bedside surgical procedures may also be considered for critical immobile neonates due to intubation or extreme prematurity [15].

Traditionally, only Level III and IV NICUs are approved to perform surgery at the bedside, pending accreditation by the individual state involved. Level III NICUs may apply to perform higher-risk surgeries after state approval. In order to gain approval, a specified number of designated surgeries must be performed within a required time frame, causing a high-priority need for nursing education, process and space evaluation, and team training. Simulation of these objectives provided John Muir's Level III NICU the opportunity to educate several OR nurses and collaborate with the NICU to support surgical bedside procedures.

The education experience provided offered not only opportunities to evaluate space and process. However, it began to lay the foundation of communication for the future of the neonatal surgical program by breaking down communication barriers and establishing standard mutual support.

Space and Process Evaluation

To evaluate the NICU's space and process for surgical procedures at the NICU bedside, key personnel gathered in a NICU patient room similar in size and shape to most standard rooms in the NICU to evaluate needs. Operating room (OR) team members directly involved in the simulation were invited to the bedside, including a surgeon, circulating nurse, scrub tech, surgery charge nurse, and surgical educator. The NICU team included a neonatologist, two registered nurses, neonatal CNS, and a neonatal respiratory therapist. Needed equipment for surgery was moved into the NICU patient room to determine the layout of equipment and personnel in the room during a surgical procedure. Considerations included room for ventilators and incubators, ample space for sterile fields, surgical equipment, and care providers. Furniture was removed, and doors were adjusted to accommodate the procedure, focusing on sterility, adequate space, and proper communication and charting. Time was spent reflecting on potential complications and the movement in the room to accommodate the patient's crisis. The team simulated equipment set-up and opening of sterile fields to further determine the order in which the team would need to facilitate set-up to maintain sterility and safe patient care. Once the layout was determined, maps were created as a reference for future training, simulation, and patient procedures. Visualizing the entire set-up offered perspective on future education and team training needs.

Nursing Education and Team Training

Often when Level III NICUs are applying for surgical licensing, it is within a hospital system that is predominantly adult focused. Pediatric surgeons and anesthesiologists are available to perform the surgery. However, the supporting personnel (NICU nurses and OR nurses) require education and collaboration to bridge the gap between the two units. NICU nurses are traditionally unfamiliar with OR procedures and practices, while OR nurses and technicians are unfamiliar with a neonate's specialized needs and potential procedures. Collaboration around the simulation and bedside procedure plan improved trust and understanding of roles, further establishing a cohesive team.

Education for NICU and OR teams began with a didactic course on neonatal surgical patients, common surgeries performed, pre-and post-operative care of the neonate, complications, and outcomes. Education was previously provided to NICU surgical nurses through both didactic presentations and preceptorships. The CNS offered education for the OR nurses during skills days, tours of the NICU and OR were provided, and common equipment requirements were covered.

To determine the learning needs for surgical procedures in the NICU, representatives from both teams were again placed in the room with surgical equipment previously set up to assess needs. The discussion covered the process from start to finish, identifying the needs of both teams as the process moved forward. Education opportunities were recorded for future simulation-based education courses. Team communication and handoff requirements were discussed and also documented for future training. The result was a detailed outline of all moving parts of a neonatal surgical procedure and a list of requirements for future simulation-based education classes that would teach the OR team and NICU team about the program. A simulation scenario was developed to be followed during each simulation (Appendix 7).

Simulations would be scheduled monthly and directed toward three NICU RNs, three OR RNs, and two Surgical Technicians. Simulations would take place in situ at the start and end of the day shift to accommodate the schedule of the neonatologists and surgeons. Occasionally, the Neonatal CNS and OR Clinical coordinator would play the role of the Neonatologist or Surgeon if unavailable.

The scenario begins with a direct request for "emergent drain placement" in the NICU for a patient with suspected perforation of the bowel. The surgeon is notified, and a consultation is requested. The simulation is broken down into the following stages:

1. Surgeon arrival & consultation
2. Surgeon & OR Charge nurse communication
3. OR team arrival in the NICU
4. Patient preparation
5. Patient induction
6. Procedure
7. Post-procedure

Each stage contains required steps to complete all aspects of the simulation and, ultimately, the patient's procedure. Participants are given a checklist (Appendix 8) to keep them on task. These checklists were created to guide practitioners as they prepare equipment, prepare the patient, monitor the patient throughout the procedure, and manage post-procedure care. Checklists were procedure specific and laminated for ongoing simulations and real patient procedures.

Follow-up would cover the following objectives:

1. Validate the checklist as a guide for task completion and staff communication during a surgical bedside procedure in the NICU
2. Practice team communication, response time, set-up, patient preparation, induction, and monitoring during a surgical bedside procedure in the NICU
3. Analyze response time between the following markers in a surgical bedside procedure in the NICU:
   (a) Procedure decision to OR/NICU team huddle
   (b) OR/NICU team huddle to patient induction
   (c) Patient induction to procedure
4. Provide education to NICU and OR nursing staff and technicians regarding surgical procedures performed at the bedside in the NICU.

'Time check' recording was planned to analyze opportunities to improve response time, set-up time, patient induction time, and decision-to-incision time. Ideas and opportunities to improve team communication, fine-tune the checklist, and streamline practice would also be recorded, followed by additional education after debriefing to clarify the process, detail the patient's condition, expand upon post-operative care needs, and discuss prognosis.

Process establishment and practice of surgical procedures at the bedside, partnered with team simulation education, provides the opportunity for NICU and OR teams to collaborate in the care of critically ill neonates with effective communication and adequate response times. As surgery continues and education is provided, teams will complete evaluation forms of each surgical procedure at the NICU bedside and standard OR. Thus far, the NICU has seen reduced critical incidences and improved communication during surgical procedures and continues collaborating on complicated cases.

Sample Curriculum #4 Neonatal Delivery of Multiples

Multiple gestation pregnancies, or "multiples," are pregnancies with three or more fetuses. Multiple gestation pregnancies present a significantly increased risk for fetal, neonatal, and maternal complications or potentially complete pregnancy loss. Perinatal morbidity and mortality increase without extra care during antenatal, especially when complications are not addressed promptly [16].

Outcomes for multiple-gestation pregnancies are primarily related to gestational age at delivery and the number of fetuses. The higher number of fetuses, the higher rate of premature births or the higher the risk of intrauterine growth restriction. Due to the potential for extreme prematurity and complications, delivery of multiples, especially triplets or higher, can be challenging for the delivery teams. Several quick interventions are necessary to stabilize a preterm baby, requiring multiple highly skilled experts to facilitate the delivery. If the preterm baby needs a full resuscitation, including medications and chest compressions, the number of delivery personnel quickly increases to 4–5 providers [16].

In addition, the amount of equipment required to deliver multiples can also be challenging. Each neonate is delivered onto a radiant warmer containing much resuscitation equipment, monitoring technology, and emergent intervention supplies. Delivery rooms must be large enough to accommodate the mother and her delivery team and a full team for each neonate. In the rare case when multiple gestation pregnancies reach five or more babies, a significant amount of planning must be done to prepare for the delivery and provide a safe transition for each baby.

Expert tertiary centers can positively influence the outcome of multiples with diligent monitoring, thorough planning, adequate staff, and a multidisciplinary approach. Planning involved in the delivery of quintuplets includes determining needs such as delivery location, equipment, personnel, supporting disciplines, timing of delivery, and understanding all potential complications. The neonatal team must consider additional details such as the type and number of providers needed for each baby, provider roles, appropriate space required during delivery, equipment allocation, and consistent communication across the teams. In partnership with the medical team, Neonatal Educators and CNSs have a particular system-level perspective on the details needed to plan the delivery of multiples and the skill needed to provide delivery guidelines, outline equipment needs, and plan and facilitate simulations to improve staff collaboration.

Simulation can be key in planning and executing such a large undertaking. Organizing staff and walking through the plan helps the team visualize the delivery space and equipment location to avoid potential barriers. Evaluating the delivery plan step-by-step offers opportunities to share solutions regarding communication and safety. Simulations offer staff time to practice the delivery plan and determine solutions to complications.

Simulation-based education to support the planning for such delivery should include early communication between the Obstetric and Neonatal teams if the multiples deliver prematurely. Teams should share the progression of the pregnancy and the status of each baby and discuss delivery options to ensure a safe transition for the family. Both teams should consider the number of providers needed for each mother and baby and create staffing plans to accommodate the day.

Determination of the Neonatal team should be based on the potential gestational age of the neonates and associated risks. Preterm deliveries of multiples less than 28 weeks should consist of a team of neonatologists, delivery nurses, and respiratory therapists for each multiple if one or all need significant resuscitation, including intubation, line placement, and emergency medications. Neonatal teams should consider backup personnel for the ongoing stabilization of this type of patient.

When determining the appropriate location in the hospital to deliver multiples, especially when premature, the neonatal team should consider the space required for several resuscitation warmers, emergency crash carts, monitors, ventilators, and adequate procedural working surfaces. This may only sometimes be facilitated in a delivery room. The team should consider other options nearby and facilitate the transfer of the neonate from the delivery room to an adequate place for resuscitation.

In addition to space and equipment, staff must be assigned a specific role during delivery. Once delivery is imminent, many staff must arrive at the hospital quickly, gather for role assignment, efficiently move to their assigned delivery space, and collaborate regarding the resuscitation. A plan for consistent communication must be established. This may include regular updates to the staff about the patient's status and the delivery timing, relaying information between the delivery team and the resuscitation team, communication between resuscitation teams once multiple units have arrived, and communication with supporting disciplines.

One example of using simulation to plan for the delivery of multiples took place in a non-profit Level III NICU. Simulation in this circumstance helped the teams establish a plan for delivering quintuplets, educate staff on the process, and establish effective communication during the delivery. Five babies were born via cesarean section and quickly moved into the NICU for resuscitation.

Initial collaboration to determine the needs for the quintuplet delivery began as a tabletop discussion to help map out the current process of delivery and needed changes required to accommodate the demands of delivering multiples. Independently, perinatal leaders and neonatal leaders met to discuss concerns and ideas to help facilitate the delivery. Once an initial framework was created, the teams collaborated in simulation simultaneously to perform a gap analysis.

Neonatal challenges were as follows:

1. Determination of where to deliver and resuscitate.
2. Equipment and room set-up
3. Process documentation for quick reference on the day of delivery
4. Facilitation of repeated simulations

Initially, the neonatal team needed to determine where the delivery should take place, what supplies and equipment were needed, and how many team members per neonate would be required. Team differentiation, role assignment, and communication before delivery, at the start, and during resuscitation would also need to be defined.

After walking the space of the Labor and Delivery operating room suite, the team determined that delivery should occur in the operating room closest to the NICU. However, the resuscitation of the neonates would occur in the NICU to ensure adequate space for five, possibly six, simultaneous resuscitations.

A delivery team was assembled to determine resuscitation space in the NICU, including one neonatologist, one delivery nurse specialist, two bedside nurses, and one respiratory therapist. The team gathered around the warmer, simulated a basic resuscitation, and measured the necessary space. Some additional considerations were revealed; a need to accommodate ventilators, IV pumps, and larger bedside monitors. Teams considered how they could move around the patient during resuscitation with these additional equipment not traditionally in a resuscitation space. In addition, the team determined the potential to set up a sixth bed space in the event that there was an additional baby. Once the space for delivery was determined, additional supplies for resuscitation were gathered, placed in kits, color-coded, and labeled "Baby A" thru "Baby F". Included in the kits were colored vests for staff to wear during the delivery that correlated with the baby teams. Additional color coded items included umbilical clamps, medications, chest X-ray plates, and documentation.

After weeks of collaboration, the plan was ready to be further tested using simulation. Guidelines and bedside checklists were created for ongoing simulation and future delivery. Each checklist and guideline was tested, changed, and re-tested until clear. Guidelines and checklists included the following:

1. *Staff Mobilization Plan*: A large concern in the delivery of multiples is mobilizing a large number of staff quickly. This guideline demonstrated the steps the charge nurse required to socialize the immediate pending delivery and begin mobilizing staff. General steps included leadership notification, staffing guidelines, notification for outside disciplines, location of contact numbers, assignment of delivery leader roles, and staff arrival guidelines. (Appendix 9).
2. *Team Check-in and Role Delineation*: This checklist provides delivery lead and personal role descriptions. It provided the delivery facilitator with a color-coded check-in list of delivery personnel and team assignments to correlate with each baby team (Appendix 10).
3. *Bedside Delivery Team Checklists*: Each color-coded checklist provided steps for the delivery team to perform, including team arrival check-in, resuscitating set-up, team organization, pre-delivery huddle, and steps once delivery begins (Appendix 11)

Over 60 nurses attended simulations over 2 months to ensure all staff potentially involved had been trained. Simulations were structured with the following stages:

1. Pre-delivery (organize staff intake/assign roles/equipment set-up/pre-resuscitation huddle)
2. Delivery (delivery nurse preparation, cord clamping, transfer, and resuscitation)
3. Communication (pre-delivery, during delivery, and escalation of needs)

Thirty resuscitation personnel were assigned to this single delivery. The simulation began by lining up staff in a dedicated staging area outside the door of the NICU. As resuscitation staff walked into the NICU, they were given a team assignment (A-E), handed role cards by the delivery facilitator, and sent to the assigned bedside, where they were asked to open the delivery kits, set up for supplies for delivery, put on their color-coded vests, and begin a pre-resuscitation huddle.

The second stage of the simulation was the delivery of the quintuplets. The delivery nurse left their assigned team and gathered in the operating room to don sterile gowns, gloves, and hats for the delivery. Obstetric personnel assisted the delivery nurses with sterile gowns and gloves. Delivery nurses then lined up to receive each baby individually (Appendix 12).

Simulation dolls were crafted with umbilical cords and connected placentas. The dolls were placed inside individual sacks emulating a placenta. Five dolls and placentas were placed in a large sack, emulating a uterus (Appendix 13). A simulation volunteer tucked the large bag under a cloth stomach band to simulate the pregnancy (Appendix 12). This provided the opportunity to simulate the cutting of different layers of anatomy during a cesarean section. During each simulation, the uterus was cut, babies were extracted, cords were clamped with color-coded clamps, and handed off to the delivery nurse assigned to that specific baby. Delivery nurses carried the simulation dolls down a short hallway of the operating room, into the NICU, to their appropriate bed space, where their resuscitation team was waiting.

During the delivery, a liaison in the operating room relayed the delivery time to the delivery coordinator in the NICU so the resuscitation teams could start their Apgar timers. Low-fidelity resuscitation began as each baby was brought into the NICU. Teams relayed additional needs during resuscitation to the delivery coordinator for communication and escalation practice.

Intense delivery planning and repeated simulations took place over approximately two months while awaiting the delivery of quintuplets. Approximately 100 learners went through a simulation between the neonatal and perinatal departments. The quiet, controlled environment that existed during resuscitation measured success. Team members responded quickly to the call for help, used checklists to organize their practice, communicated efficiently and effectively, and performed the necessary tasks to deliver each baby in the safest way possible. After the delivery, staff expressed significant similarities between the simulations and the actual delivery, further solidifying simulation as the best solution to evaluate needs, determine plans, and educate personnel on the delivery of multiples.

Integration into Existing Education

The above samples have demonstrated simulation-based education as an effective tool to improve processes and supplement bedside education in the neonatal setting. Simulation-based education incorporates psychomotor and cognitive activities required for good clinical decision-making and practice [17] while immersing the learner in a familiar environment. Continually assessing healthcare providers in their working environment offers further opportunities to improve processes and potentially patient outcomes. Leadership and educators are challenged to avoid traditional education plans and instead integrate simulation experiences into a curriculum to achieve optimal learning as active participants. Active participation in a safe and controlled environment allows the learner to receive immediate feedback in a continual loop not found in traditional education and is congruent with adult learning theories [18]. Learning is provided by educators and specialists trained in learning theory and debriefing, further improving their experience.

An essential component needed to integrate simulation-based education in neonatology is debriefing. Facilitating a successful debriefing session is critical to the student's successful reflection and knowledge acquisition. For this reason alone, nursing education, particularly neonatal nursing, should be quick to embrace this invaluable tool.

Further considerations for integrating simulation into existing education is the opportunity to incorporate pre-and post-assessment inquiry to evaluate the learning level of participants and potential improvement. Regularly scheduled simulations should allow time for adequate debriefing that offers honest discussion and inquiry. Providing these ongoing simulations in situ allows providers to work together in their work environment with tools and familiar team members.

In addition, there is an opportunity for greater collaboration between units using simulation and improved links with obstetric, pediatric, and surgical within their hospital network and across other systems statewide and nationally. Collaboration efforts should focus on sharing resources, disseminating good practices, facilitating research collaborations, and determining the direction of future developments.

Another consideration for integrating simulation in neonatal nursing is incorporating simulation training into their new neonatal employee education programs. Many high-risk nursing activities put the patient at risk until these skills have been perfe. As novicwhenexpert programs are developed, high-risk activities should be identified and taught. Traditionally, these activities are not practiced until an actual patient need arises. Providing simulation training opportunities, such as endotracheal tube insertion and securement, inserting intravenous and central catheters, changing intravenous solutions, assisting with the umbilical line insertion, and positioning patients for x-ray and lumbar punctures, would provide frequent education and practice opportunities to perfect their skills [19].

In addition, more experienced nurses may also benefit from simulated scenarios prior to caring for severe, medically complicated, and fragile patients. Opportunities include the transfer of an ELBW infant into a skin-to-skin position on the mother while maintaining endotracheal tubes and umbilical arterial lines and avoiding a disorganized developmental state for the growing brain. Other examples include fragile care of the pulmonary hypertensive neonate to avoid alteration in oxygenation or care of the neonates requiring extracorporeal membrane oxygenation (ECMO). This treatment uses a pump to circulate blood through an artificial lung back into the bloodstream.

Simulation may also be used to educate neonatal nurses on proper communication with parents or other team members. Creating scenarios that prompt communication around the bedside between families and care providers provides the opportunity for all involved to understand communication barriers and misunderstandings and broaden the understanding of challenging ethical issues in the NICU [10].

The future is an opportunity for simulation to become a standard in training specialized neonatal personnel, such as the activities shared in this chapter, including activities in transport, deliveries of multiples (triplets, quadruplets, and upward), neonatal surgery, code response improvement, and emergency evacuation. Other basic opportunities include golden hour deliveries, weighing and changing linen, medication titration, and assisting with chest tube insertion and set-up. These activities can be practiced as a team in a simulation setting to help perfect the technique before it is performed on a patient.

Challenges and Solutions

Challenges to implementing neonatal nursing simulation are numerous. Similar to adult simulation programs, neonatal programs report challenges in cost, time, technical issues, and instructor requirements. The most common difficulty found in the literature was the cost linked to both low- and high-fidelity simulation. Most full-functioning simulators cost between $30,000 and $175,000, increasing with more complex technology and not including hardware and software maintenance. Though low-fidelity manikins of around $5000 may still be inaccessible to nursing units due to budgetary constraints [20].

Technical issues are frequent and can arise unexpectedly during scenarios. Proper maintenance of simulation equipment and reliable technical support from the manufacturer can alleviate most problems. However, low-fidelity backup options such as handwritten monitor cards or readable prompts can be a reliable alternative to maintain the integrity of the simulation when technology is not cooperating.

In addition, other high-cost equipment is needed to set the simulation scene, such as incubators, resuscitation warmers, ventilators, and positive pressure delivery systems. Using this equipment in simulations requires storing simulation equipment or cleaning patient equipment used for simulation and a large amount of space to facilitate certain types of simulation [21]. Depending on the unit's acuity, equipment and patient rooms may not be available during simulation despite the cost invested in planning and facilitating. Leaders should be urged to designate simulation education equipment and space to avoid financial loss.

The cost associated with nursing hours is also high. The time associated with simulation classes is traditionally between 2–4 hours. Nurses are paid their hourly rate, including shift differential, if applicable. The cost can be substantial depending on the total number of learners per session. Time for simulation is often taken from patient-care budgets, causing staffing challenges and a lack of nursing and physician availability.

Additional barriers include the training of simulation personnel. Simulations require educators to be trained to use technical equipment, develop patient scenarios, conduct research on best practices, and design education competencies. In addition, formal debriefing training should be offered to support the educator in complex debriefings, where emotions may be high.

There is also a cost associated with the number of instructors required to facilitate a simulation. One instructor may be sufficient to manage a small class with a low-fidelity simulator, while 2–3 instructors may be necessary for a larger or high-fidelity simulation. In either situation, simulation attendance is traditionally low to maintain the realism of a live event. Therefore, more sessions are required to cover the entire staff, equating to an increase in the number of instructor hours dedicated to the course [21].

Many hospital units are turning to in-situ simulation to alleviate the cost and space requirement. This also has less impact on service provision and is more cost-effective, as staff are not removed from their work environment for a whole day to train at a high-fidelity simulation center. Instead, the training can occur while staff remain at work, providing the learners with a familiar environment and saving costs [22].

To mitigate equipment, personnel, and support challenges, many hospitals are turning to partnerships in simulation across their network or with other systems. This shares the cost of simulation, debrief-trained instructors, and equipment needed to facilitate a scenario. Many hospital networks employ highly skilled simulation experts to create scenarios, construct simulations, simulate the scenarios, and organize debriefs. Simulation facilitators collaborate with the content experts in each unit to provide a learning opportunity specific to their area of expertise.

A large barrier to simulation programs in nursing is a lack of staff and leadership support. Though often staff members, such as nurses, are interested in simulation education, they are often confined to their scheduled hours. They must dedicate their time to projects such as simulation education. Leaders are vital in allowing nurses and other staff members to participate in simulations within their normal work commitment. Simulation can help healthcare organizations provide safe, effective patient care. Leaders should help reach these goals by leading the charge for continual improvement through simulation.

Lastly, one of the challenges in further implementing simulation-based education in neonatology is the need for more research supporting the positive impact of simulation-based education on patient outcomes. Though many dispute the delay in the widespread implementation of simulation-based education in neonatology until after valid studies are in place, the vulnerability of neonates partnered with limited opportunity for practice makes simulation an attractive option for neonatal care providers. Most recent publications on neonatal simulation programs suggest that simulation education can increase safety, decrease errors, and improve clinical judgment and skill. In addition, research supports simulation education in developing self-confidence, collaboration, and teamwork [23] yet does not reveal specific evidence correlating neonatal patient outcomes to simulation-based education. Studies that address this correlation are few, include a small number of participants, and have various study designs. Yamada et al. [11] researched the impact of standardized communication techniques on errors during neonatal resuscitation simulation. The neonatal simulation study revealed a trend toward decreased error rate, decreased time to initiation of positive-pressure ventilation, and decreased time to initiation of chest compressions, suggesting a future improvement of outcome for the neonate.

According to a systematic review completed by Rakshasbhuvankara and Patole [24], the opportunity exists to conduct large randomized control trials assessing clinically significant outcomes with simulation-based education. The review proposed new trials to evaluate the efficacy of resuscitation and the quality of resuscitation to patient outcomes. Appraisal of efficacy included evaluating post-resuscitation temperature, pre- and post-delivery blood gas pH, and post-delivery amplitude-integrated electroencephalogram. Evaluation of resuscitation quality suggested appraisal of video recordings of real-life resuscitation steps in the delivery room by two independent reviewers. Shortly following this recommendation, the California Perinatal Quality Care Collaborative (CPQCC) began "Simulating Success." The collaborative was designed to help NICUs implement simulation-based neonatal resuscitation training programs at their hospitals to improve resuscitation team performance during deliveries and reduce neonatal morbidity and mortality. Fifteen sites across California and Oregon participated in recording simulations and reviewing debriefs. Each hospital following data submitted to CPQCC both before and after simulation program implementation [25]. Data collected by CPQCC includes markers listed in Rakshasbhuvankar review. Since the start of the collaboration, several hospitals have begun implementing the simulation and debriefing techniques suggested in hopes of providing efficient and effective resuscitation to improve neonatal outcomes.

Future neonatal simulation studies should link actual clinical performance and team training to neonatal outcomes. Research to further bridge this gap will only advance the number of uses of simulation-based education to prepare staff, promote safety, and reinforce standards [26].

Interface with Regulatory Bodies

Though simulation-based education has room to integrate in many areas of neonatal education, it has established itself as a standard throughout the world as a tool required to maintain certification in neonatal resuscitation. The Neonatal Resuscitation Program (NRP) is a standard accepted method for neonatal resuscitation certification using didactic, electronic, and live simulation. However, despite the skills learned during NRP certification, studies demonstrate that the skills learned in NRP typically last for as little as 6–12 months. In order to provide safe, proficient resuscitation, it is vital for hospitals to offer providers the opportunity to practice resuscitation more frequently.

Several hospital systems with a neonatal intensive care unit employ NRP instructors to maintain nursing and physician certification within their hospital environment. In addition, many hospitals offer ongoing simulations to physicians and nurses to satisfy the number of hours required for residents by the Accreditation Council for Graduate Medical Education (ACGME) and the Residency Review Committee (RRC). These hours are a challenge for pediatric residents to meet, as guidelines allow a maximum of 400 hours in critical care, with only a small percentage of those hours in Neonatology. Due to the restriction of time allowed to spend training in a pediatric environment, residents need to be given more opportunities to practice emergencies. This, partnered with competing nurse practitioners and attending hospitalists, decreases procedural opportunities for residents and risks their accreditation [27–29].

Providing NRP certification in the hospital system, partnered with ongoing neonatal simulation, offers nurses, residents, physicians, and therapists the opportunity to certify in NRP while continually practicing high-risk, low-volume scenarios that help to sharpen technical skill, decision-making, and team performance [30].

Summary

Neonatology has a special need for simulation-based education due to the critical nature of neonatal patients. Neonatal healthcare providers require adequate training to handle this delegated population to avoid deficiencies that cause the majority of fatal errors, deviations from recommended practice, and poor patient outcomes. Simulation provides an option for patient practice to ensure that providers remain competent in activities that would otherwise be too dangerous to practice on patients.

Simulation in neonatal education has been well established by implementing the Neonatal Resuscitation Program and the Helping Babies Breathe Program. The success of simulation in resuscitation led the way for simulation implementation in practice areas such as bedside procedures, transport, process evaluation, response-time improvement, and several high-risk, low-frequency patient scenarios. Recommendations for incorporating behavioral skills such as communication, leadership, situational awareness, and mutual support into neonatal simulation-based education has further established simulation as a tool to promote effective education.

Neonatal units across the country and worldwide continue to use simulation-based education as a best-practice solution for education. Best practice solutions include the identification of neonatal complications, providing outreach education in the form of mobile in-situ simulation, demonstrating skill competency, performing shift-to-shift, and understanding communication techniques for staff and parents. Advanced curriculum demonstrating how to support transport facilitation, delivery and code cart processes, implementation of surgical bedside procedures, and delivery of multiples are only a few ways neonatology may use simulation-based education to support learning and process development. Additional innovative programs that have been implemented or may be considered include pre-and post-assessment inquiry, transferring ELBW infants into a skin-to-skin position, family communication, ethical training, transport, deliveries of multiples, neonatal surgery, code response improvement, and emergency evacuation. Other basic opportunities include golden hour deliveries, weighing and changing linen, medication titration, and assisting with chest tube insertion and set-up.

Nurse and physician leaders should be challenged to collaborate with educators, clinical nurse specialists, and simulation experts to avoid traditional education plans and integrate simulation experiences into a curriculum to achieve optimal learning as active participants, including hands-on experience and debriefing. Though this may be partnered with challenges such as cost, time, technical issues, and instructor requirements, solutions are creative, including low-fidelity simulators, in-situ training, hospital or department partnerships, and further leadership support.

Maintenance of regulatory simulation-based education to certify neonatal resuscitation providers and accredit graduate medical and residency students should remain a standard in neonatal simulation while looking for innovative ways to advance simulation. The future state of neonatal simulation should include future research to link actual clinical performance and team training to neonatal outcomes. Research to further bridge this gap will only advance the number of uses of simulation-based education to prepare staff, promote safety, and reinforce standards. Future innovation in simulation may also open doors to virtual reality that immerses the learner in scenarios by using aids such as smartwatches and accelerometer-based devices that calculate rate and depth values for feedback during chest compressions to enhance the quality of compressions.

The choice to use simulation-based education in neonatology is supported in research and often welcomed in the NICU. The simulation uses techniques that immerse the learner in patient scenarios, improving skill and enhancing working memory. In neonatology, simulation is an excellent choice to determine care processes, improve team collaboration, and provide education because it allows the staff to learn from one another and receive direct feedback on their practice. The scenarios discussed in the chapter showed innovative ways in which nurse specialists and educators can work with staff and supporting disciplines to develop working teams, evaluate space and practice, and provide education through simulation and debriefing.

Appendix 1 Neonatal Transport Scenario Guideline. Includes 4 scenarios transitioning the neonate from transport request to arrival at the receiving hospital. Objectives noted

SCENARIO: NEONATAL TRANSPORT

Scenario: 25 weeks gestation, 750 at birth, Level I to Level III Transport
Target Trainees: Transport RN & Transport RT

TRANSPORT CENTER CALL MD/MD	
Patient Description	**One-hour old, 25-week, male infant born vaginally at a delivery center. G1P1 pregnancy complicated by placenta abruption. Infant received 3 minutes of CPR in the Delivery Room, Apgar 0/2/5/7. Contacted by delivering hospital for transport to receiving hospital for higher level of care.**
Report given	ETT: 2.5 secure @ 6.5 lip VENT: - 54% FiO2 - PC/PS 12 - Peep 5 - Rate 35 Heart Rate: 148 Respiratory Rate: 62 Oxygen saturation: 90 Cuff Blood Pressure: 34/18 (26) Temp: 36.5
DELIVERY HOSPITAL ARRIVAL	
Arrival at Delivery Hospital	**Upon arrival at Delivery Hospital, infant on Panda warmer, temp probe in place. ETT secured via Neobar, patient on ventilator. IVF infusing via UAC/UVC. OGT secure and to gravity. RN, RT, and Pediatric Hospitalist at bedside providing care.** Weight: 750g UVC: Dextrose 10% @ 2 ml/hr UAC: NS @ 0.7 ml/hr OGT: 6F to gravity MEDS: Ampicillin 75mg currently infusion, Gentamicin to follow VENTILATOR: 60% FiO2, PC/PS 12, Peep 5, Rate 35 Heart Rate: 142 Respiratory Rate: 60 Oxygen saturation: 87 Mean Arterial Pressure: 21 via UAC Temp: 35.9 Glucose: 44, 2ml/kg bolus ordered, f/u due in 30 minutes CXR revealed proper placement of ETT. Amp x 1 complete, Gentamicin 3mg IV currently infusing CXR for tube placement is pending. Arterial ABG: Upon admission 7.17/80/40/20/-6

Expected Interventions/ Objectives	□ Face to face discussion with pediatric hospitalist to obtain brief history and current status □ Perform initial assessment □ Evaluate ventilation settings, review labs and vital signs □ Adequately secure UAC/UVC □ Recognize hypothermia and implement corrective steps □ Recognize normal BP range for gestational age and discuss plan for treating hypotension □ Transport isolette set-up for 25-weeker □ Transport isolette ventilator set-up □ Medication transferred with appropriate rates, double-checked □ Proper handling during transport □ Maintain stable VS □ Safely move patient to transport isolette □ Depart after updating family
Progression	**Upon transfer to transport isolette, infant desaturates and becomes bradycardic.** Heart Rate: 79 Respiratory Rate: 80 Oxygen saturation: 57
Expected Interventions/ Objectives	□ Quickly recognize need for re-intubation □ Successful intubation verified with pedi-cap, equal bilateral lung sounds □ Secure ETT □ Prepare for departure from unit
IN TRANSIT – TRANSPORT AMBULANCE	
Transport Ambulance	Infant deteriorates Mean arterial pressure: 20 via UAC transducer Follow-up ABG: 7.21/75/50/26/-6 Follow-up blood glucose: 35 Temperature: 36.1
Expected Interventions/ Objectives	□ Address Hypotension if not already completed □ Recognize hypoglycemia and treat appropriately □ Recognize hypercarbia and treat appropriately □ Maintain stable temperature □ Appropriate communication to facilitate treatment

RECEIVING HOSPITAL ARRIVAL	
Arrival at receiving hospital	Infant stable ETT: 2.5 secure @ 6.5 lip UVC: Dextrose 10% @ 2.5 ml/hr UAC: NS @ 0.7 ml/hr OGT: 6F to gravity MEDS: Amp and Gent complete VENT: - 40% FiO2 - PC/PS 12 - Peep 5 - Rate 45 Heart Rate: 148 Respiratory Rate: 48 Oxygen saturation: 91 Mean Arterial Pressure: 27 via UAC Temp: 36.7 Glucose: Follow-up 72 Arterial ABG: Follow-up 7.26/55/80/27/-4
Expected Interventions/ Objectives	☐ Relay history to neonatal team ☐ Review labs, ventilation status, and current status ☐ Recognize potential complications of transport ☐ Correct positioning of transport isolette in relation to the patient room set-up ☐ Proper handling during transfer to giraffe isolette ☐ Demonstrate proper PPV if necessary ☐ Correctly relay medications does and rates
End Scenario	Infant safely transferred to Giraffe isolette in the NICU with adequate handoff

SCENARIO SET-UP – DELIVERY CENTER (SIMULATION LAB)	
Room Configuration	Appearance of a Well Baby Nursery • Panda Warmer • Ventilator • Delivery code cart in position • Monitor
Equipment	• Panda Warmer – Heat on, T-piece resuscitator set 20/5, 85mmHg suction connected with 8f catheter, intubation box below • Ventilator – settings • Pulse oximeter, EKG leads connect to functioning monitor, sat probe, UAC transducer • Med-Fusion pumps x 3: UAC fluids + transducer, gentamicin via medline, • Plum pump x 1: D10% via tubing with trifurcate connection • Infant bedside cart • Stethoscope

Simulator	Preterm Annie • Circumoral cyanosis • PPV via T-piece resuscitator in progress • HR below 150 • Saturations 88-92 • UAC/UVC infusing fluids – sutured only • UAC transducing: maps 26
Simulator Deterioration	• Heart Rate: 79 • Respiratory Rate: 80 • Oxygen saturation: 57 • Absent breath sounds • No chest rise
Roles	• Delivery Center: Pediatric Hospitalist, RN1, Respiratory Therapist • Transport Team: Transport RN, Transport RT
SCENARIO SET UP – TRANSPORT AMBULANCE	
Room Configuration:	• Transport rig • Rig • Infant Transport Isolette with ventilator and monitor • Blended Oxygen • Pumps
Equipment	• Transport Isolette • Simulation monitor • Simulator – turned off
Roles	• Transport Team: Transport RN, Transport RT
Simulator Presentation	• Preterm Annie • Transport ventilator • HR above 140 • Saturations 88-92 • UAC/UVC infusing fluids – sutured only • UAC transducing
SCENARIO SET-UP – NICU PATIENT ROOM	
Room Configuration:	• NICU Patient Room • Giraffe Isolette • Ventilator • Monitor • Patient bedside cart

Equipment	• Giraffe Isolette – Heat on, T-piece resuscitator set 17/5, 85mmHg suction connected • Ventilator – PC/PS 12, Peep 5, Rate 40 • Pulse oximeter, EKG leads connect to functioning monitor, sat probe • Med-Fusion pumps x 3: UAC fluids + transducer • Plum pump x 1: Stock HA via tubing with trifurcate connection • Infant bedside cart with intubation box on top • Glucometer • Stethoscope
Roles	• Delivery Center: Pediatric Hospitalist, RN1, Respiratory Therapist • Transport Team: Transport RN, Transport RT
Simulator Presentation	• Preterm Annie • Transport ventilator • HR above 140 • Saturations 88-92 • UAC/UVC infusing fluids • UAC transducing

SIMULATION DAY LOGISTICS	
Location	1st WCMC FLOOR SIM CENTER (Behind the Cafeteria, across from the Lab)
1:00 – 1:15	INTRODUCTION / SIMULATION PLAN
1:15 – 1:45	SIM: DELIVERING HOSPITAL
1:45 – 2:15	SIM: TRANSPOT RIG
2:15 – 245	SIM: NICU ARRIVAL
2:45 – 4:00	DEBREIF / DISCUSSION

Appendix 2 Delivery code medication card sample. Each set included 9 cards with medication dosing, ETT size and depth, umbilical catheter size, and volume dosing. Cards were created in 500 g increments from 500 g to 4000 g with the addition of a 750 g card

NEONATAL RESUSCITATION:		750 grams (0.75 kg)
TUBES/LINES		
ETT SIZE:		2.5mm
ETT DEPTH:		6.75 cm
UMBILICAL CATHETER SIZE:		3.5F
ENDOTRACHEAL TUBE EPI	DOSE	VOLUME
EPINEPHRINE: (0.1 mg/mL)	1 mL/kg	0.8 ml
INTRAVENOUS EPI	DOSE	VOLUME
EPINEPHRINE: (0.1 mg/mL)	0.3 mL/kg	0.2 ml
VOLUME EXPANDER (0.9% NS, PRBC)	10 mL/kg	7.5 ml

Appendix 3 Standard resuscitation warmer set-up with role cards and delivery guidelines

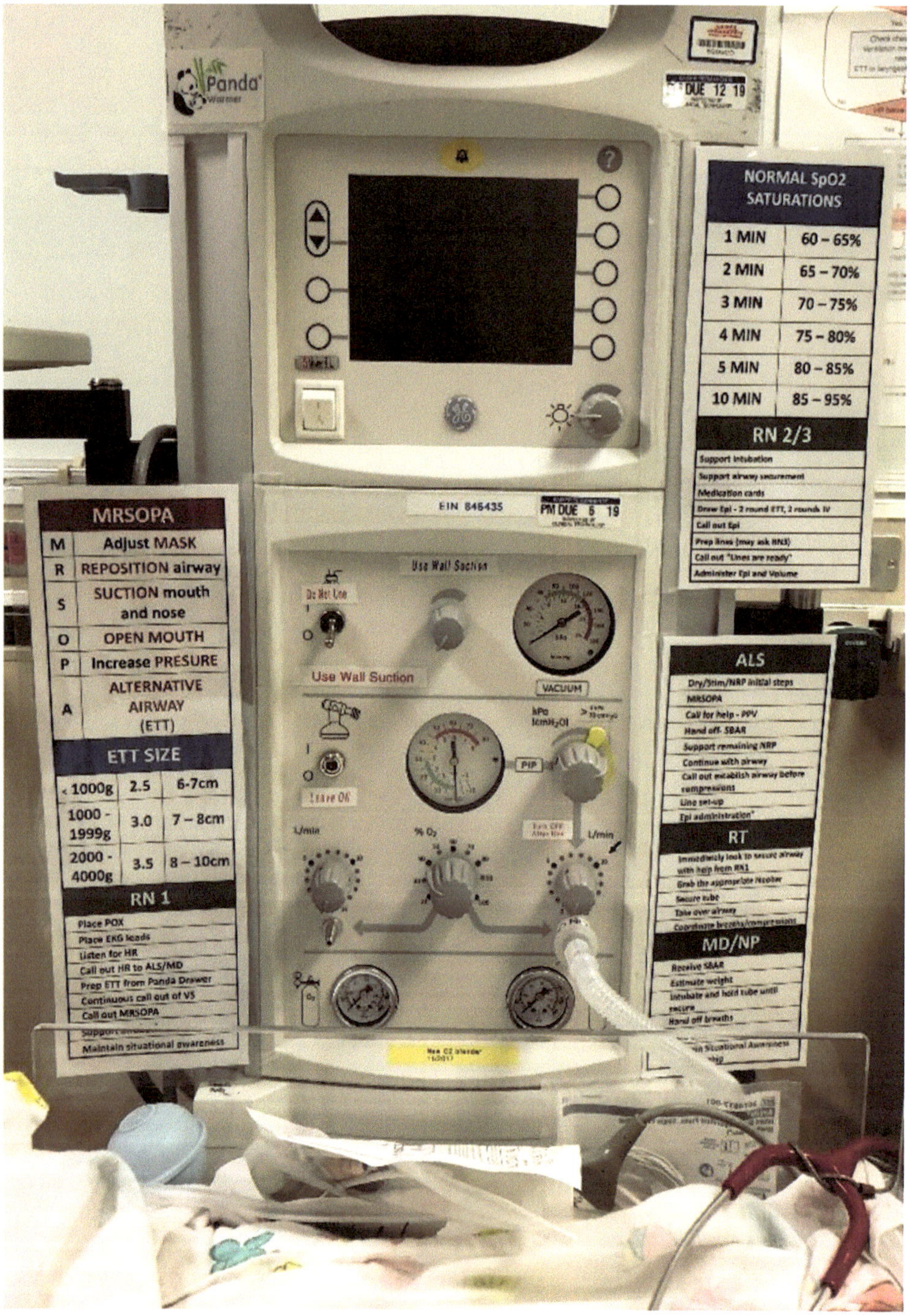

Appendix 4 Standard delivery cart, organized by Airway, Breathing, and Circulation

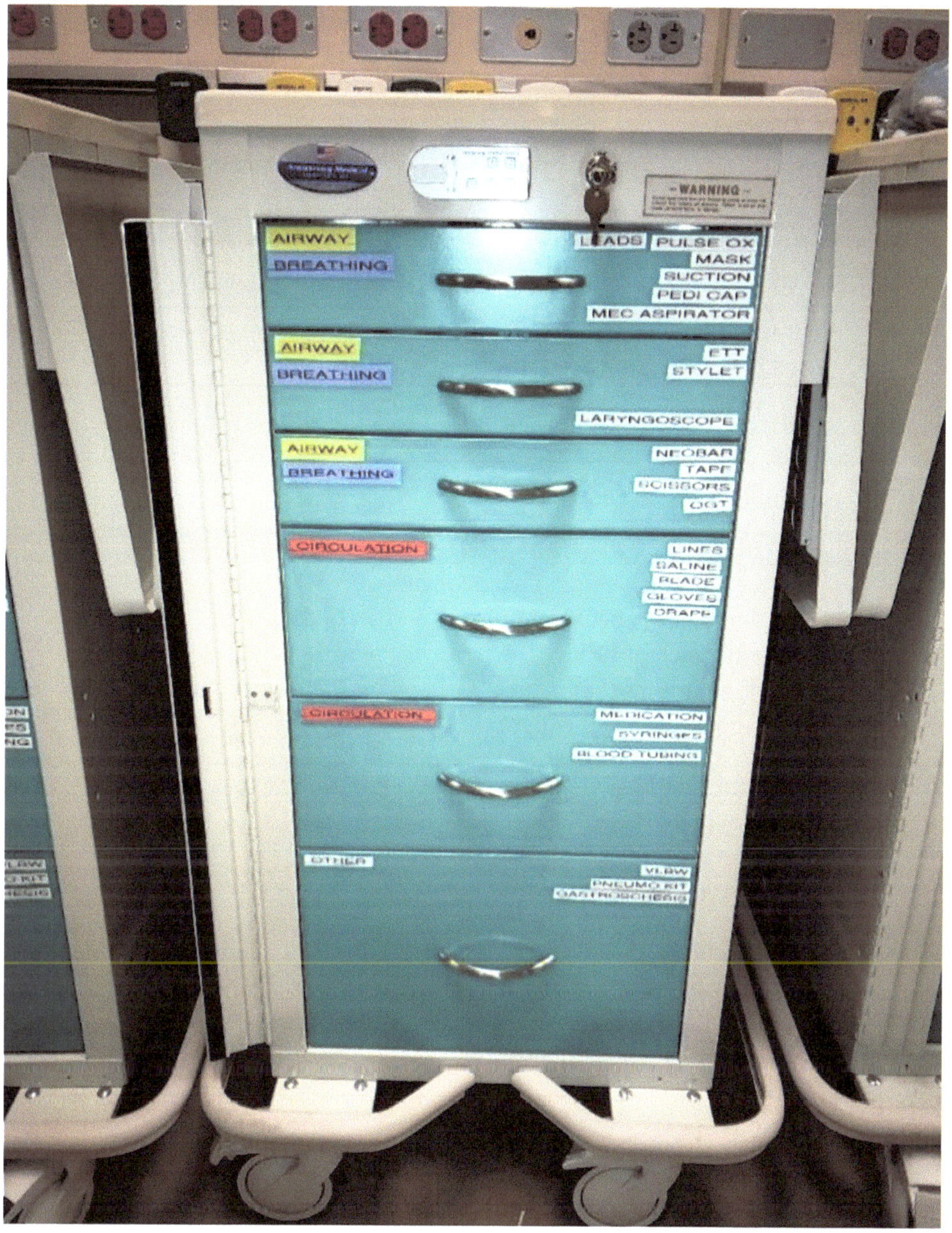

Appendix 5 Delivery resuscitating rolls and code card simulation guideline. Includes scenarios objectives, set-up, logistics, roles, and debriefing. Objectives noted

SCENARIO: DELIVERY RESUSCITATION ROLES & CODE CART

Scenario: 40-week infant, 3.8kg at birth, critical delivery
Target Trainees: Advanced Life Support RNs, NICU RNs, Neonatologists, & RTs

SCENARIO OVERVIEW	
Name:	Stat c-section, decelerations, decreased variability, and fetal bradycardia
Patient Description:	40-week infant, mom G1 P1, uncomplicated previous c-section. Laboring x 15 hours. Estimated weight 3.8 kg.
Target Trainees:	MD, ALS RN, Shift Leader, RT
Anticipated Duration:	10 minutes
LEARNING OBJECTIVES	
Cognitive:	• Effects of bradycardia on a neonate. • Differentiation between primary and secondary apnea • Significance of PPV • NRP algorithm • Consider estimated weight
Technical:	• Warmer set-up • MR SOPA • Intubation prior to compressions • Resuscitation medications
Behavioral:	• Adequate brief – including role establishment • Establish leader • Call out-check backs • Maintains situational awareness

SCENARIO SET-UP	
Room Configuration:	• Labor and Delivery OR • Warmer off • Delivery code cart in position
Equipment:	• Pulse Oximeter, EKG leads • Bulb suction • T-piece resuscitator • Intubation supplies (Miller 01 and handle, 3.5 ETT, stylet, pedi-cap, stethoscope, securement devise and tape.
Simulator Presets:	Term size simulator: • Delivered via c-section • HR below 100, baby floppy • No delayed cord clamping • Remains apneic on the warmer, HR 65, sat 60% Equipment set-up • Have equipment and warmer available but not set-up (trainees to turn on warmer, prepare leads, check T-piece, set pressures, prepare intubation equipment, bulb suction, set-up blankets)
Patient Chart Contents (if necessary):	N/A
Demonstration items needed in Debriefing Room (if necessary):	• Debrief using video • NRP Algorithm • Target O2 sat card
SCENARIO LOGISTICS	
Expected interventions:	• Pre-brief and role assignment • Discuss potential volume and medication dosing for estimated weight • Appropriate set up of warmer and selection of supplies • Warm, dry, stimulate • Check HR • Place pulse oximeter • Check for breathing • Initiate PPV • Place EKG leads
Likely progression:	• PPV for 30 seconds does not increase HR (remains at 65 bpm) and baby remains apneic • Increase O2 to 100% • Need to start MR SOPA

	• MR SOPA does not increase HR (remains in 60s) • States need for intubation • Successful intubation, positive pedi-cap color change and visible chest rise. HR increased to above 100
Expected endpoint:	• HR remains above 100, • Sats stabilize based on minute of life chart • O2 adjusted appropriately
Distractors:	None
Additional/optional challenges:	None
ROLES	
Confederate Roles:	Simulation instructor gives patient description
Trainee Roles:	• MD • ALS RN • Shift Leader • RT
DEBRIEFING POINTS	
Cognitive:	• Effects of bradycardia on a neonate • Primary vs secondary apnea • Significance of PPV to increase HR • Significance of intubation prior to potential compressions • NRP algorithm • Estimated weight in relation to potential medications
Technical:	• Appropriate warmer set-up • Steps of MR SOPA • Intubation and airway stabilization • Resuscitation medications
Behavioral:	• Adequate brief – including role establishment • Establishment of a leader and support of the leader to maintain situational awareness. • Consistency in call out-check backs

Appendix 6 Pre-and post-survey question for Delivery Resuscitation Roles and Code Card Simulation

What is your role? ALS/RN/RT/MD (circle one)					
What is that average number of deliveries that you attend per year?					
When was the last time you attended a delivery?					
Before Simulation	**Disagree Strongly**	**Disagree Slightly**	**Neutral**	**Agree Slightly**	**Agree Strongly**
I am confident in attending deliveries?					
I am confident in speaking up during critical situation?					
I am confident drawing up epinephrine?					
I am confident in setting up umbilical lines during NRP?					
I am confident in performing the steps of MRSOPA?					
I feel there are clear established roles when I attend a code?					
I am confident that the leader on your team is well supported during a code?					
I am confident in my ability to support my team during a code?					
After Simulation	**Disagree Strongly**	**Disagree Slightly**	**Neutral**	**Agree Slightly**	**Agree Strongly**
I am more confident in attending deliveries?					
I am more confident in speaking up in a critical situation?					
I am more confident in drawing up epinephrine?					
I am more confident in setting up umbilical lines during NRP?					
I am more confident in walking through steps of MRSOPA?					
I feel this course has established clear roles for critical situations?					
I am more confident that the leader on my team will be well supported during a code?					
I am more confident in my ability to support my team during a code?					
Please provide at least two learning that you plan to apply to your practice.					
What barriers do you perceive that might impact your ability to make these desired changes?					
What components would you like to see repeated in the future?					
Suggestions for ways this program could be made more useful to improve practice and performance.					

Appendix 7 Surgical bedside procedure in the Neonatal Intensive Care Unit. Scenario includes logistics, simulator set-up, surgeon/NICU RN/OR RN tasks and communication, patient induction/surgery/and post procedure objectives, followed continued simulation-based education plan. Objectives noted

SCENARIO: SURGICAL PROCEDURE IN THE NICU

Scenario: 25 weeks gestation, 75 grams at birth, Spontaneous Perforation

Target Trainees: NICU RNs, OR RNs, and OR Techs

INITIAL SIMULATION LOGISTICS	
Location	**NICU ROOM 25**
Goal	**Provide opportunity for OR and NICU teams to come together to test the current response time, process, and checklists for urgent/emergent surgical bedside procedures in the NICU.**
Date/Time	**June 2, 2020**
10m	**INTRODUCTION / SIMULATION PLAN**
30m	**SIM: CALL FROM SURGEON TO OR CHARGE RN**
	SIM: TEAM PREPARATIONS
	SIM: IN ROOM SET-UP
	SIM: INDUCTION & PROCEDURE
	SIM: CLOSING & DEBRIEF
30m	**SIMULATION DEBRIEF**

SIMULATION SCENARIO & SET-UP	
Patient Description	**25-week, 750g male. Previously stable for gestation. Ventilated via ETT, UAC/UVC lines secure infusing TPN/IL, NPO, OGT secure draining dark green, voiding, no stool since birth.** Patient presents with an acute onset of abdominal distension and hypotension. No signs of abdominal wall erythema, crepitus, or induration. A black-bluish discoloration of the abdominal wall is noted, which extends into the groin. Left-lateral decubitus revealed pneumoperitoneum
Simulation Set-Up	**NICU preterm infant simulator is in a giraffe warmer, temp probe in place, humidity 80%. ETT secured via Neobar, patient on ventilator. IVF infusing via UAC/UVC. OGT secure to gravity draining dark green. Discoloration to left right lower abdomen. RN and RT at bedside providing care.** ETT: 2.5 secure @ 6.5 lip VENT: HFOV 54% UVC: HA D10% @ 2 ml/hr UAC: NS @ 0.7 ml/hr Monitor settings: -Heart Rate: 168 -Respiratory Rate: n/a -Oxygen saturation: 89% -Cuff Blood Pressure: 30/18 (23) -Temp: 36.5

SURGEON ARRIVAL & CONSULTATION	
Begin Scenario	**Decision to perform Penrose Drain Placement for spontaneous intestinal perforation**
Expected Interventions/ Objectives	☐Face to face discussion with neonatologist to clarify symptoms and confirm diagnosis ☐Call to Operating Room Charge RN to request NICU bedside procedure: Penrose Drain Placement

SURGEON & OR CHARGE COMMUNICATION	
Report given to OR Charge RN	**25w, 750gram preterm baby needing immediate: Penrose drain placement for spontaneous intestinal perforation.**

Expected OR Interventions/ Objectives	☐Establish team: Circulating RN and Tech
	☐Place surgery on the OR schedule
	☐Check 'preference card' to ensure appropriate equipment
	☐Ensure verification of consent matches the consent to operation
	☐OR team to bring the following to the NICU
	  ☐Bedside procedure cart
	  ☐Bovie
	  ☐Head light
	☐Communication NICU arrival time

Expected NICU Interventions/ Objectives	☐Establish team: Patient RN, NICU Surgery RN, Neonatologist, Respiratory Therapist, Pharmacist ☐Consent to operation complete – unless emergency ☐Complete NICU bedside procedure checklist ☐Contact pharmacy for assistance with induction medications ☐Distribute surgical caps and masks ☐Close appropriate doors ☐Remove non-essential visitors ☐Remove hanging decorations around bed ☐Wipe down high-touch surfaces

OR TEAM ARRIVAL IN NICU	
Brief Team Huddle	**Brief team huddle including (Surgeon, Neonatologist, NICU RN, OR RN, Tech, RT, and Pharmacist) to discuss any concerns or missing supplies. Confirm preparedness and state plan.** (TIME CHECK)
Set-Up OR Team	☐Bedside cart as sterile table ☐Bovie ☐Cut-down Tray ☐Lighting – headlamp or NICU procedure light

Set-Up NICU Team	☐Place procedure sign on door ☐Additional suction set-up specifically for surgery ☐Remove excess furniture ☐Arrange bedside cart to be used by scrub tech ☐Provide warm saline ☐Position baby for right-sided drain – collaborate with RT ☐Move lines away from surgical area ☐Ensure medication lines are accessible ☐Place blood pressure cuff if necessary prior to placement of the sterile field ☐Temp probe properly place throughout procedure ☐Provide a workstation on wheels for the OR
Pharmacy/ Medications	☐Verify induction medications with Neonatologist ☐Double check medications with NICU RN ☐All medications to be supplied by the NICU

PATIENT PREPARATION / PATIENT INDUCTION	
OR TEAM	☐Place Bovie ☐Prep surgical site ☐Drape baby with clear drape ☐Set-up surgical instruments and drain devices
NICU TEAM	☐Scan and administer induction medications – all medications to be supplied by the NICU ☐Double check medications with NICU RN ☐Fentanyl on pump ☐Monitor patient response ☐Monitor vital signs

PROCEDURE	
OR / NICU TEAMs	☐Assist surgeon as needed ☐Monitor vital signs ☐Maintain temperature ☐Maintain fluid therapy ☐Manage complications

POST PROCEDURE CARE	
OR TEAM	☐Instrument count ☐Safely remove surgical drape ☐Clean surgical site ☐Closing debrief

NICU TEAM	☐Assist with drape removal and surgical site cleansing ☐Maintain thermoregulation ☐Closing debrief

CONTINUED EDUCATION SIMULATIONS	
Location	**NICU ROOM 25**
Goal	**Provide ongoing education for OR and NICU teams to practice established processes, checklists, and timing urgent/emergent surgical bedside procedures in the NICU.**
Date/Time	**Monthly: Every 4th Monday of the month (0730 & 1400)**
Duration	**20-30 minutes including short debrief**
Objectives	☐Collect Data ☐OR arrival in the NICU ☐Time to incision ☐Time to closure ☐Practice with OR procedure checklist ☐Practice with NICU procedure checklist ☐Evaluate room set-up and space ☐Observe surgical field set-up and positioning opportunities ☐Observe time-out ☐Calculate and administer induction medications ☐Response to complications ☐Observe closure & count ☐Practice post-op huddle
Additional Needs for Simulations	☐Soft band surgical marking (to avoid pen) ☐NICU cheat sheet ☐OR cheat sheet ☐Solidify physician and staff availability for initial simulation ☐Schedule NICU staff for simulations (TLs and Surgery RNs first) ☐Send initial simulation invite ☐Establish re useable materials for simulations ☐Create competencies for OR and NICU staff

Appendix 8 Surgical bedside procedure checklist

NEONATAL BEDSIDE SURGICAL PROCEDURE CHECKLIST	
OPERATING ROOM	**NICU**
☐ Confirm decision to perform bedside procedure with Neonatologist & Surgeon)	
	☐Face to face discussion with neonatologist to clarify symptoms and confirm diagnosis ☐Call to Operating Room Charge RN to request NICU bedside procedure (report specific procedure)
PRE-SURGERY PLANNING & EQUIPMENT	
OPERATING ROOM	**NICU**
☐Establish team: Circulating RN and Tech ☐Place surgery on the OR schedule ☐Check 'preference card' to ensure appropriate equipment ☐Ensure verification of consent matches the consent to operation ☐OR team to bring the following to the NICU ☐Bedside procedure cart ☐Bovie ☐Head light ☐Communicate arrival time to NICU Charge	☐Establish team: Patient RN, NICU Surgery RN, Neonatologist, Respiratory Therapist, Pharmacist ☐Consent to operation complete – unless emergency ☐Complete NICU bedside procedure checklist ☐Contact pharmacy for assistance with induction medications ☐Distribute surgical caps and masks ☐Close appropriate doors ☐Remove non-essential visitors ☐Remove hanging decorations around bed ☐Wipe down high-touch surfaces
OR TEAM ARRIVAL IN NICU & SURGERY SET-UP	
OPERATING ROOM	**NICU**
☐Brief team huddle including (Surgeon, Neonatologist, NICU RN, OR RN, Tech, RT, and Pharmacist) to discuss any concerns or missing supplies. Confirm preparedness and state plan. (TIME CHECK)	
☐Bedside cart as sterile table ☐Bovie ☐Cut-down Tray ☐Lighting – headlamp or NICU procedure light	☐Place procedure sign on door ☐Additional suction set-up specifically for surgery ☐Remove excess furniture ☐Arrange bedside cart to be used by scrub tech ☐Provide warm saline ☐Position baby for right-sided drain – collaborate with RT ☐Move lines away from surgical area ☐Ensure medication lines are accessible ☐Place blood pressure cuff if necessary, prior to placement of the sterile field ☐Temp probe properly placed throughout procedure ☐Provide a workstation on wheels for the OR

PHARMACY/MEDICATIONS	
OPERATING ROOM	**NICU**
	☐Verify induction medications with Neonatologist ☐Double check medications with NICU RN ☐All medications to be supplied by the NICU

PATIENT PREPARATION / PATIENT INDUCTION	
OPERATING ROOM	**NICU**
☐Place Bovie ☐Prep surgical site ☐Drape baby with clear drape ☐Set-up surgical instruments and drain devices	☐Scan and administer induction medications – all medications to be supplied by the NICU ☐Double check medications with NICU RN ☐Fentanyl on pump ☐Monitor patient response ☐Monitor vital signs

PROCEDURE	
OPERATING ROOM	**NICU**
☐Assist surgeon as needed ☐Monitor vital signs ☐Maintain temperature ☐Maintain fluid therapy ☐Manage complications	

POST PROCEDURE CARE	
OPERATING ROOM	**NICU**
☐Instrument count ☐Safely remove surgical drape ☐Clean surgical site ☐Closing debrief	☐Assist with drape removal and surgical site cleansing ☐Maintain thermoregulation ☐Closing debrief

Appendix 9 Neonatal Staff Mobilization Plan for delivery of multiples

INITIATES PHONE CALLS

❑ Call the Neo phone and ask thay they call the Attending On-Call
❑ Call NICU Manager and Neonatal CNS
❑ Contact NICU RT. RT will contact RT Mgr
❑ Contact staffing office: Request Code-Q Delivery at hoc be sent to all NICU nurses
❑ Assign 2 NICU Staff to warm call RN's listed in the Quintuplet Binder (See Red box below)
❑ Give instruction packets attached to this sheet to staff making calls
❑ Call Pharmacy for Epi kits & fluids/meds
❑ Call Blood bank and Radiology for heads-up
❑ Place yellow signs on NICU door and on the door outside NICU bed space #10

SET-UP STAGING AREA

❑ Table @ Bed #10 is the Staging Area - All staff will check in there
❑ Uncover White Board on wall. Dry Erase Pens located on board
❑ Line up medication bins across table in order
❑ Pharmacy to bring up Epi, place at bedside
❑ Get Curosurf Kits from the bottom shelf of the med refridgerator, place in appropriate baby bins
❑ When remaining meds arrive from pharmacy (ie, TPN, UAC fluids, Amp/Gent, Eyes/thighs) place in baby bins on staging table
❑ When needed distribute medications accordingly

STAFF CALL INSTRUCTIONS (Assign & Skip to "WHEN STAFF ARRIVES")

CALL GUIDELINES

❑ Use Volunteer Phone List (attached) to these instructions to begin calling
❑ Contact Unit Assistants on phone list attached
❑ Place warm calls to RNs on phone list attached
- Call those signed-up on day of delivery first (Quintuplet sign-in binder on staging table)
- Then call the remainder of staff on the phone list attached
- Fill in Call log to keep track of staff
- If leaving a message, ask staff to return calls to the NICU Main #, not staffing

RECEIVE 'AVAILABLE' CALLS

❑ Calls will be coming into the NICU Main number
❑ 2 Staff members to receive 'available' calls
❑ Determine ETA of arriving staff and place on Call Log
❑ Continually communicate with Assistant Manager/Delivery Facilitator

WHEN STAFF ARRIVES

❑ Establish Liason to remain in OR from first time-out through all deliveries (Possible ALS E) (Assign phone & place number on white board)
❑ Establish NICU Liason for bed communication and APGAR start time (Assign phone & place number on white board)
❑ Assign staff to Delivery Team A, B, C, D, or E. Assign in order of Role
- Distribute NEO, ALS, 1st RN, 2nd RN & RT (The goal is to spread the team evenly across babies as they arrive. Consider that we may be short some roles.)

❑ Place name on white board under appropriate team column
❑ Hand them a Role Card based on their assigned role- Role Cards are in the manilla envelope
❑ Send them to the bedside to follow the checklist instructions, including...
- Put thier vest on, open their delivery kit, set-up for delivery, establish their resusitation roles.

FACILITATE DELIVERY

❑ Once teams are established, begin huddle
❑ Gather all team members around NICU Assignment Board
❑ Review Delivery Plan:
- OR Liason to facilitate scrub, sterile blankets, communicate with NICU Liason, & hand-off baby
- NICU Liason will announce start of APGAR timer for each bed & relay critical delivery info
- Delivery Facilitator will direct each baby's path into the NICU & remain in contact with Liasons

❑ Determine readiness: Beds set-up, equipment checked, roles assigned, & baby receiver chosen
❑ State that Pharmacy, Blood Bank, Radiology & Leadership are aware and ready for delivery
❑ Moms status/baby status
❑ Concerns?
❑ Please communicate with call-out/check-bacl and be awareness of noise in the NICU
❑ Send baby receivers to OR with OR Liason

Appendix 10 Neonatal Team Check-In and Role Delineation in the delivery of multiples

ASSIGNMENT CHECK-LIST					
TEAM CHECKLIST	BABY A	BABY B	BABY C	BABY D	BABY E
Bring Delivery Bins to bedside					
Deliver Supply Carts to bedside					
Clipboard @ bedside					
Staff available					
--MD					
--ALS					
--RN					
--RN					
--RT					

# OF EACH	NEEDED PERSONNEL	ASSIGNMENT
1	Delivery Facilitator (Phone)	Initiates Phone Calls Set up Staging Area Organize delivery teams as staff arrives Remains available to facilitate organization of delivery tasks and personnel Facilitate Huddle before delivery Direct Baby Receivers to appropriate bed during delivery Triage Gather group for huddle
1	OR Liason (Phone)	To remain in OR throughout delivery Assist in delivery organization and gowning Relay critical delivery related information Communicate APGAR start time to NICU Liason Remain available for additional baby or delivery support as necessary
1	NICU Liason (Phone)	To remain in NICU throughout delivery Initially identify privacy issues and curtain off parents in NICU Start @ Bedspace 11, Baby A - relay critical delivery information and APGAR start time Move to Bedspace 12, Baby B - relay critical delivery information and APGAR start time Move to Bedspace 14, Baby C - relay critical delivery information and APGAR start time Move to Bedspace 15, Baby D - relay critical delivery information and APGAR start time Move to Bedspace 16, Baby E - relay critical delivery information and APGAR start time Remain available for potential Baby F Remain available for additional help when needed
5	Neonatologist	1 Neonatologist/bedside if possible Plan to scrub-in for delivery or assign ALS to scrub Determine resusitation roles and responsibilities Maintain awareness of other resusitation efforts if there is a shortate of Neonatologists
5	ALS Nurse	1 ALS/bedside Assist in resusitation If baby is stable, check in with Delivery Facilitator to potentially help with other resusitation efforts
5	RN	2/ bedside Assist in resusitation If baby is stable, check in with Delivery Facilitator to potentially help with other resusitation efforts
5	Respiratory Therapist	1/ bedside Begin warming vents upon arrival Remain available for resusitation If baby is stable, check in with Delivery Facilitator to potentially help with other resusitation efforts

Appendix 11 Neonatal bedside delivery team checklist for the delivery of multiples

BABY A

Set-up		
TO DO	Location	Description
☐ Locate Delivery Bin	Under Giraffe @ Bedside or	All supplies needed for
☐ Obtain Resuscitation Med Packet	Pharmacy brining up - Facilitator will call	Epinephrine, NS, Stopcock/fluid transfer
☐ Obtain Curosurf kits	Medication fridge in the green room	Curosurf, Multiuse catheter kit, 3ml syringe
☐ Choose Emergency Drug Sheets	In Delivery Kit	By estimated weight - choose appropriate
☐ Post Critical Hour checklist	Delivery Kit	
☐ Locate Mayo Tray	Bedside	May be used to set-up lines
☐ Consider Computer workstation	Bedside WOW or Nurses	

Arrival of Team		
Item	Location	Description
☐ Distribute vests accordingly	Delivery Bin	According to role
☐ MD ☐ RN ☐ ALS ☐ RN ☐ RT		
Don GREEN vests	Delivery Bin	Located in Delivery Kit
Assemble delivery supplies	Delivery Bin	Packages are labeled by need
Confirm readiness with Facilitator & follow additional instructions.		

Team Organization

- ☐ Check-Equipment
- ☐ Double check supplies
- ☐ Assign resuscitation tasks
- ☐ MD/ALS - Determine who will scrub for OR
- ☐ Establish Leader
- ☐ Await Huddle with all quintuplet members
- ☐ Consider Bio break (Pee)

Final Huddle

- ☐ Gather entire Quint Team for final huddle
- ☐ Voice last minute concerns
- ☐ Identify back-up plan

Delivery time

- ☐ MD/ALS in OR during time-out until delivery of baby
- ☐ Resuscitation team awaits Liaison call to start APGAR timer
- ☐ Await arrival of Baby A

Appendix 12 Delivery room simulation consisting of both delivery personnel and infant resuscitation personnel awaiting the delivery of quintuplets. Simulation dolls crafted with cords and placentas are wrapped in a cloth stomach band to simulate the cutting of each layer of anatomy during a cesarian section

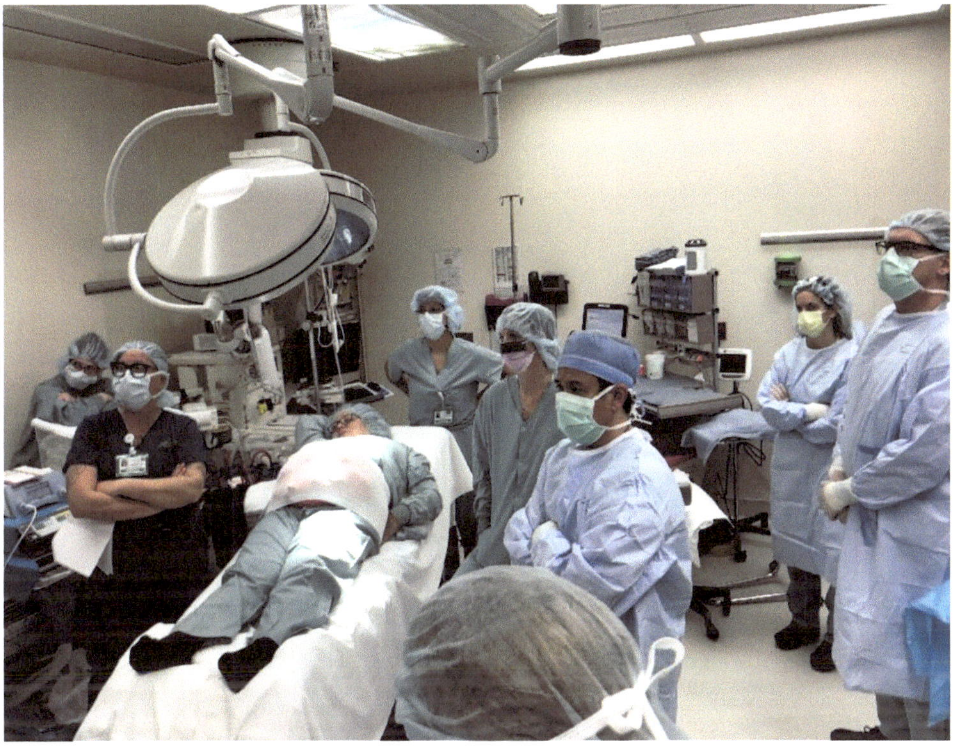

Appendix 13 Simulation dolls crafted with umbilical cords and placentas to simulate cutting cords for the delivery of quintuplets

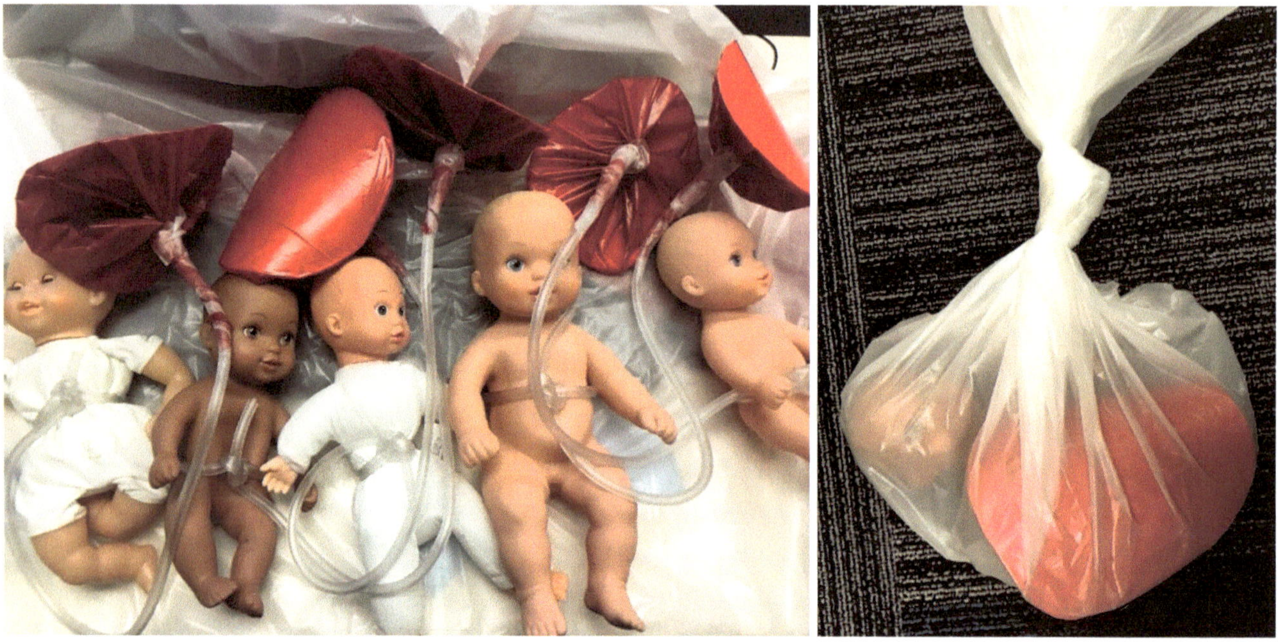

References

1. Owen H. Simulation in healthcare education: an extensive history. Springer International Publishing; 2018.
2. Pilcher J, Heather G, Jensen C, Huwe V, Jewell C, Reynolds R, et al. Simulation-based learning: it's not just for NRP. Neonatal Netw. 2012;31(5):281–8.
3. American Academy of Pediatrics. NRP History. services.aap.org. Available from: https://services.aap.org/en/learning/neonatal-resuscitation-program/nrp-history/.
4. Arnold J. The neonatal resuscitation program comes of age. J Pediatr. 2011;159(3)
5. Lateef F. Simulation-based learning: just like the real thing. J Emerg Trauma Shock. 2010;3(4):348.
6. Halamek LP, Kaegi DM, Gaba DM, Sowb YA, Smith BC, Smith BE, et al. Time for a new paradigm in pediatric medical education: teaching neonatal resuscitation in a simulated delivery room environment. Pediatrics. 2000;106(4)
7. Singhal N, Lockyer J, Fidler H, Keenan W, Little G, Bucher S, et al. Helping babies breathe: global neonatal resuscitation program development and formative educational evaluation. Resuscitation. 2012;83(1):90–6.
8. Halamek LP. Simulation and debriefing in neonatology 2016: mission incomplete. Semin Perinatol. 2016;40(7):489–93.
9. Preventing infant death and injury during delivery. Sentinel Event Alert. 2004;30:1–3. Available from: www.jointcommission.org/assets/1/18/SEA_30.PDF
10. Peterson E, Morgan R, Calhoun A. Improving patient- and family-centered communication in pediatrics: a review of simulation-based learning. Pediatr Ann. 2021;50(1)
11. Garvey AA, Dempsey EM. Simulation in neonatal resuscitation. Front Pediatr. 2020;8:59.
12. Salih ZN, Draucker CB. Facilitators of and barriers to successful teamwork during resuscitations in a neonatal intensive care unit. J Perinatol. 2019;39(7):974–82.
13. Chan J, Chan B, Ho HL, Chan KM, Kan PG, Lam HS. The neonatal resuscitation algorithm organized cart is more efficient than the airway–breathing–circulation organized drawer: a crossover randomized control trial. Eur J Emerg Med. 2016;23(4):258–62.
14. Valentin A. Faculty Opinions recommendation of safety of intrahospital transport in ventilated critically ill patients: a multicenter cohort study*. Faculty Opinions – Post-Publication Peer Review of the Biomedical Literature, 2013.
15. Al-Bassam AR, Mallick MS, Jado AM. Surgical procedures performed in the neonatal intensive care unit on critically ill neonates : feasibility and safety. Ann Saudi Med. 2008;28(2):105.
16. Kaur J, Pandit SN, Gade MP. Unbelievable, yet true….spontaneous quintuplets! J Obstetr Gynecol India. 2014;65(4):271–2.
17. McNeal GJ. Simulation and nursing education. ABNF, Assoc Black Nursing Faculty Inc. 2010;21(4):78.
18. Yaeger KA, Arafeh JMR. Making the move. J Perinatal Neonatal Nursing. 2008;22(2):154–8.
19. Sharma A. From evidence to implementation: Introducing neonatal simulation to a tertiary neonatal center in the UK. Open J Pediatr. 2013;03(01):10–6.
20. Birkhoff SD, Donner C. Enhancing pediatric clinical competency with high-fidelity simulation. J Continuing Educ Nursing. 2010;41(9):418–23.
21. Lindamood KE, Weinstock P. Application of high-fidelity simulation training to the neonatal resuscitation and pediatric advanced life support programs. Newborn Infant Nursing Rev. 2011;11(1):23–7.
22. Fawke J, Cusak J. Neonatal simulation—training a workforce for the future. Infant. 2017;7(1)
23. Palmer E, Labant AL, Edwards TF, Boothby J. A collaborative partnership for improving newborn safety: using simulation for neonatal resuscitation training. J Continuing Educ Nursing. 2019;50:319–24. https://doi.org/10.3928/00220124-20190612-07.
24. Rakshasbhuvankar AA, Patole SK. Benefits of simulation-based training for neonatal resuscitation education: a systematic review. Resuscitation. 2014;85(10):1320–3.
25. Simulating Success. California perinatal quality care collaborative. 2019. Available from: https://www.cpqcc.org/improvement/previous-projects
26. Hansen J, Bratt M. Competence acquisition using simulated learning experiences: a concept analysis. Nursing Educ Perspect. 2015;36(2):102–7.
27. Surcouf JW, Chauvin SW, Ferry J, Yang T, Barkemeyer B. Enhancing residents' neonatal resuscitation competency through unannounced simulation-based training. Med Educ Online. 2013;18(1):18726.
28. Bradley P. The history of simulation in medical education and possible future directions. Med Educ. 2006;40(3):254–62.
29. Malmström B, Nohlert E, Ewald U, Widarsson M. Simulation-based team training improved the self-assessed ability of physicians, nurses and midwives to perform neonatal resuscitation. Acta Paediatr. 2017;106(8):1273–9.
30. Hoshino D, Hensley C, Lewis K, Frazier M, Domenico R, Burley M, et al. Evaluating the use of high fidelity simulators during mock neonatal resuscitation scenarios to improve residents' confidence. SAGE Open Med. 2018;6:2050312118781 95.

Simulations for Pediatrics

34

Kimberly Bilskey and Tara J. Lemoine

Background

In hospitalized settings, pediatric resuscitation efforts often involve an interprofessional team that is tasked with a multitude of demands on the technical side and communication skills that are all necessary to achieve the best possible patient outcomes. There is often a need for more expertise and confidence in these situations, directly related to the limited opportunities in pediatric clinical experience to hone the necessary skills in caring for these patients. The gap in real-life clinical exposure can be mitigated using simulation-based training if designed and deployed correctly. Relying on only real-life events to develop these skills is undesirable and does not facilitate an optimal or safe environment for patients or the healthcare team. A robust pediatric simulation program provides a viable solution to train individual providers and teams in pediatric centers and institutions that focus primarily on adults but may also care for pediatric patients.

Simulation-based training can provide additional opportunities to practice clinical skills across pediatric clinical care and environments. The clinical work in pediatrics covers a broad spectrum of age, size, specific physiology, and disease presentation in each area. The complexity of pediatric medicine can create a unique challenge for healthcare providers caring for these patients. Pediatric simulations are often centered on the low volume of high-risk situations to support the education of healthcare teams and individual healthcare providers. A robust, well-designed simulation curriculum can be utilized to create an optimal milieu for training and education conditions. Specific focus on team training in these low-volume events in the pediatric clinical setting can include trauma, cardiac and respiratory emergencies. Additional simulation training for staff and teams can focus on lower acuity situations in clinical scenarios where communication skill sets are equally meaningful to develop competent providers.

Trauma is the leading cause of morbidity and mortality in the United States in pediatric patients [1]. Pediatric injured patients have a higher death rate within the first 24 hours of arrival at a hospital than adults [2]. The lifesaving procedures that pediatric trauma patients require immediately following injury are infrequently executed, yet they require a highly skilled interprofessional team. Because of the limited number of pediatric traumas in many hospitals, emergency department teams may not have the skills necessary to treat these patients. This can significantly impact the morbidity and mortality of pediatric trauma patients, as 1/3 of errors that lead to the death of trauma patients occur during the initial emergency care period. The most frequently reported shortcoming in pediatric training is trauma education [2]. Studies on interprofessional simulation-based pediatric trauma training have shown favorable results. Participants report increased confidence, preparedness, and understanding of their role [3].

Sepsis is another condition in pediatric medicine that is a low volume but has a high risk of disastrous outcomes if not recognized and intervened promptly [4]. Recognition of pediatric sepsis and adherence to treatment guidelines is typically associated with a robust clinical background and years of experience [5]. Simulated cases focused on early recognition of pediatric sepsis, treatment of pediatric septic shock based on guidelines, and interprofessional communication in deteriorating patients is associated with enhanced team performance [6]. Combining an interprofessional healthcare team and a simulated patient in septic shock allows learners to work on interprofessional skills such as communication and clinical skills focused on managing sepsis.

This movement from a silo classroom style training to an interprofessional experiential training methodology has several hurdles as healthcare providers face new training, education, and learning methods. The barriers centered on

K. Bilskey (✉) · T. J. Lemoine
Valley Children's Healthcare, Madera, CA, USA
e-mail: kbilskey@valleychildrens.org;
TLemoine@valleychildrens.org

J. M. Kutzin et al. (eds.), *Comprehensive Healthcare Simulation: Nursing*, Comprehensive Healthcare Simulation,
https://doi.org/10.1007/978-3-031-31090-4_34

communication when interfacing with multiple healthcare team members are addressed and magnified in a simulated experience to impact patient care and outcomes positively.

Crisis Resource Management (CRM) refers to principles dealing with cognitive and interpersonal behaviors that contribute to optimal healthcare team performance [7, 8]. While the root of CRM began in the aviation industry decades ago, it has infiltrated the healthcare industry in every type of clinical practice extending from pre-hospital care through the continuum of medicine in the hospitalized setting. Simulation-based training (SBT) has been positioned to teach the CRM skills of team leadership, interpersonal communication, and decision-making during high-stress events.

Best Practices

An estimated 80% of medical errors leading to death result from communication breakdowns and the failure of team dynamics [9]. Teams typically consist of core teams merged with contingency teams. Core teams provide direct care to the patient in a unit-specific area and are familiar with the patient and the clinical environment. Contingency teams, on the other hand, are comprised of team members from various specialty areas within the hospital that come together to manage a patient during a time-limited emergent event. This could be pediatric-trained healthcare providers helping with a pediatric patient in a primarily adult emergency department or pediatric intensive care healthcare providers assisting in a pediatric acute care unit. The convergence of these interprofessional teams in crisis or emergent situations can be challenging as they attempt to navigate complexities of communication and different skill sets [10]. These healthcare providers represent all disciplines of healthcare professions that are needed to provide the best and safest care. Whether this is a code team or a pediatric trauma team, the interdisciplinary group needs to work seamlessly and communicate effectively. The ultimate goal of collaborative practice, including nurses, technicians, pharmacists, respiratory therapists, and physicians, is arduous at times. There are a multitude of factors that create barriers to optimal team performance and negatively impact patient care. In a dynamic situation, professionals do not function in a silo but rather work together toward a common goal with their professional skill sets [11]. The interplay of the technical skill set across the different professions and the non-technical communication demands of a team during a high-acuity pediatric crisis can be challenging. Interprofessional training is gaining recognition as a method to combat communication gaps and barriers to delivering effective care during an emergency or medical crisis. The rapidly changing combinations of team members responding to a crisis lends itself to even more obstacles that may negatively impact the delivery of safe medical care. Code teams are staffed differently, with each shift creating an exponential number of permutations of who may be responding to an urgent patient need. Crisis Resource Training with these teams is essential for improving the team function and dynamics to lead to a successful patient outcome. Simulation is a known mechanism for creating optimal conditions for team crisis training focused on these low-volume high-risk events in the pediatric clinical setting. It can include disaster, trauma, cardiac and respiratory emergencies. Gathering an interprofessional group of core and contingency team members to engage in a simulated environment allows them to hone their skills while gaining insight into the duties of other roles [10].

If designed correctly, simulation-based training can include cases that focus on teamwork, leadership, and communication with various healthcare provider team combinations. These simulation exercises facilitate staff development and function as a tool to educate on crisis resource management and interprofessional understanding. The creation of a psychologically safe learning environment in simulation is one of the essential elements of having a successful curriculum. Another crucial piece is learner engagement, as they must be able to make mistakes and ask questions freely in this environment. Any worry about performance disclosure, performance review, reporting to directors, or judgment from other participants must be eliminated within the learner cohort. Scenario content is especially important as it must be linked to crisis resource management principles and interprofessional learning domains.

Scenario content can focus on communication and other non-technical skills imperative in pediatric resuscitations. Given the urgency and lack of opportunity for reflection or team debriefings, the focus on non-technical skills, such as closed-loop communication or priority clarification, may not be addressed in real-life situations. In the simulation environment, the time can be directed at team communication patterns and the complex dynamics of high-performing individuals and teams. A spotlight on technical skills can also be narrowed down within a simulation to allow for the repetition required for competency.

The selection of a location for SBT that facilitates a realistic environment mirroring typical resources and personnel is also vital. This may be done in a simulation center or situ utilizing a functional clinical environment. Using a clinical environment as an in-situ or replicated clinical space within the simulation center can trigger the engagement necessary to practice in simulation. Maneuvering within the real clinical space can create such a sense of reality that teams suspend their disbelief and work as if they do in a real environment. While in the actual space, workflow, equipment, and process issues can be identified and mended to achieve optimal patient care. For example, the absence of trauma supplies or transport equipment will become a focal point when the simulation is delivered in situ in the trauma bay.

In-situ means that the location of the simulation is in the real patient clinical care areas [12]. In-situ simulations must consider many factors before initiation, given their integration into the physical clinical care environment. The Emergency Response team (ERT) full system activation scenario is conducted in-situ on an Acute Care unit, starting with a core team of health care providers on shift providing direct patient care. These specific types of simulations are valuable to allow the discovery of institutional processes that may need improvements or change. The benefits of time pressure, latent safety threats, knowledge gaps, and procedural failures in the clinical spaces will be elucidated. This level of reflection and practice change cannot typically occur in the simulation lab space because it cannot accurately mirror the clinical environment with 100% accuracy. Participants are in their native clinical space where they normally care for their patients and can maneuver in their environment, overcoming barriers to clinical care. The contingency team members who need to become more familiar with this clinical space must work through those surroundings in real time.

In-situ simulation allows for the actual equipment, supplies, staffing plan, and testing of the ERT activation system and routes to the room being utilized. Barriers to real patient care can be identified during these events, such as how hospital construction can delay the team's arrival times or reveal equipment malfunction. Process and education opportunities for improvement can be highlighted through in-situ simulations during the debriefing to narrow performance gaps unrelated to participant knowledge, skill, or communication.

The debriefing process with skilled faculty well-versed in simulation pedagogy helps facilitate the reflective learning process. During a well-structured debriefing that promotes a robust discussion, an environment is explored to identify performance gaps and solutions to those opportunities. The facilitator leads the debriefing in a fashion focused on reflective practice for enhanced performance of both individuals and team performance. Faculty team members trained in the best practices of simulation are the core of programs and necessities in delivering an effective simulation curriculum.

Consistency of education and skill among the simulation faculty is inherently valuable as there is a relationship between increased learner outcomes and faculty with higher levels of training.

Faculty development is a crucial element that must be considered, as less than 50% of simulation faculty have received formalized training from experts in the simulation community by attending classes or workshops [13]. Executing a well-designed pediatric-specific simulation focused on crisis management and having measures of enhanced performance requires precise planning for a successful delivery.

Pediatric simulation has several unique elements to consider before deploying a simulation exercise. The nature of pediatrics inherently means a wide range of ages and sizes, from pre-term neonates to adolescents. In addition, there is large variability in differing sizes of equipment required to care for this patient population depending on the simulation exercise, health care team, and their specific area of focus within pediatric medicine. For example, a neonatal team cannot be tasked to perform a neonatal resuscitation on a toddler-size manikin or use equipment unavailable in their subset of pediatric medicine. Within the scope of manikin selection, there must be attention to the appropriate size, functionality for clinical states, and the software elements of physiological variables that can be displayed. For instance, if the simulation requires the ability to see an arterial wave of blood pressure, attention must be paid to selecting the equipment that can appropriately display that information to the learners. The adequate selection of manikin size with the necessary physical characteristics to emulate what is seen is imperative in real life to promote realism and enhance learning. The commercially available simulators for pediatrics, whether as task trainers or high technology simulators, each has various features and characteristics. It is essential to have a deeper knowledge of which simulators can produce certain functional states required, as well as their limitations both of the physical mannequin and the monitor display. The key differences between adult versus pediatric simulators continue to change as there are rapid changes in simulation technology and improved function of simulation equipment over time. Infant and child-specific task trainers are available for learning to perform various pediatric-specific procedures, including lumbar puncture, chest tube placement intubation, or vascular access. Certain software for vital sign displays and cardiac rhythm generators can have specific pediatric settings with ranges of vitals that emulate pediatric-specific clinical findings, while others generally used in adult simulation do not fully capture pediatric vital sign parameters. There is a wide spectrum of pediatric-specific simulation devices that assist learners in understanding anatomy, physiology, and medical conditions seen in pediatric medicine. The awareness of differences between pediatric and adult mannequin simulators and task trainers is important when developing curriculum and objectives. The other element is to ensure that all the granular aspects of clinical care specific to pediatrics in terms of supplies for procedures such as airway intubation, defibrillation, and intravenous catheter placement are specific to pediatrics. These details should reflect what is utilized in real life for the specific size of the span from neonatal to pediatric adolescent patients. It is crucial to spend time exploring the functionality of the various models to ensure that the optimal simulator or task trainer is chosen all the additional elements of clinical supplies are accurate and accessible to meet the educational needs of healthcare providers and teams.

Sample Curriculum

Scenario 1: Pediatric Sepsis Code

The scenario occurs at a freestanding children's hospital in a Pediatric Acute Care unit in an actual patient room. However, it can be simulated in an Emergency Department or Critical Care space with some modifications. A pediatric manikin is set up in the room as a patient would be with all the equipment typically available. Scenario objectives include:

1. Recognize and treat septic shock in the pediatric patient
2. Demonstrate activation of ERT
3. Prioritize care of the pediatric patient in septic shock
4. Use Crisis Resource Management skills
5. Recognize and treat PEA

This curriculum was developed to provide an in-situ simulation opportunity for the interprofessional hospital-wide Emergency Response Team (ERT). The ERT is made up of healthcare professionals from more than 15 departments within the hospital. The scenario offers multiple learning objectives and layers of complexity as interprofessional within the core Acute Care unit and contingency ERT arrive to participate. Scenarios are developed to include all healthcare team members so they can use their specialized clinical, teamwork, and communication skills during the simulation experience.

The scenario begins in a simulated acute care clinical space with a core team acute care nurse assessing a 5-year-old patient admitted from the Emergency Department.

The patient's vital signs are clinically supportive of shock with tachycardia and hypotension based on age normal values.

The time to recognize the patient's clinical state as abnormal is documented, as well as the time to notice the patient's clinical deterioration. Observation of who the team contacts for additional support, which response system within the hospital is chosen, the process used for activating response teams, as well as the time it takes for team arrival, are all tracked as a part of metrics performance. Activation of the ERT or the Rapid Response Team (RRT) are also options for additional support from contingency teams. The RRT typically consists of a Pediatric Intensive Care Unit (PICU) Nurse and PICU Respiratory Care Practitioner, unit-specific charge nurse, Pediatric Hospitalist, and Pediatric senior resident. Team members must respond to the bedside within 10 min of activation. The ERT is expected to respond immediately and consists of the members of the Rapid Response team and the additional fifteen other health care providers from various departments in the hospital. The scenario will continue based on the initial nurse's decisions to introduce the varying levels of the emergency response teams. The scaffolding effect of the code team members arriving happens organically, as this is often done in situ and announced without warning or as a simulated event across the organization. The ultimate purpose of the scenario is to activate the ERT and ensure that the process for activation is functional within that clinical space and that all team members who work clinically in that environment know the process to follow to engage that system. In order to engage the whole interprofessional team, the patient will continue to deteriorate until the nurse activates the ERT.

The members of the ERT arrive in waves with sequential involvement and start to participate in the scenario as they do in real life, creating the opportunity for communication and team leadership principles to be acted upon. As the patient continues to deteriorate, the team must recognize the patient is pulseless and in Pulseless Electrical Activity (PEA). As they complete a series of interventions outlined by the Pediatric Advanced Life Support (PALS) Guidelines, they work through all the elements of communication, teamwork, resource use, and situational awareness. If the team follows the correct guidelines, the scenario ends with the return of the patient's pulse and transfer to the PICU. If the team deviates from the guidelines, the patient will continue to deteriorate, and the scenario will be stopped prior to the patient's death. The debriefing process is used to dive deeper into the pertinent elements of refining the processes, whether technical or non-technical, to improve real patient care. These scenarios are performed monthly on all shifts to cast a wide net to learners. Increased transparency of process issues and knowledge gaps has led to increased simulation utilization for testing new processes before going live and filling in the gaps in knowledge.

Scenario 2: Interventional Radiology Suite Opening

The scenario takes place in a freestanding children's hospital before opening a new clinical Interventional Radiology (IR) suite. A pediatric manikin is placed in the IR suite and is situated as a patient undergoing a procedure that would be performed within that clinical space.

Scenario objectives include:

1. Demonstrate proper procedure for activating the ERT
2. Demonstrate proper emergency management of complex patients using PALS guidelines
3. Identify equipment gaps
4. Identify process gaps within the Interventional Radiology Suite.

This curriculum was developed to provide an in-situ simulation opportunity to identify latent safety events and process gaps in a newly opened procedure area for patients requiring invasive procedures in interventional radiology. The scenario offers multiple process objectives and complexity layers to include all healthcare team members within the ERT. There is a specific focus on ensuring access to the newly opened IR suite and its readiness for patient care emergencies for the core team.

The scenario begins in situ with a medically complex 11-year-old patient undergoing a Gastrojejunal tube exchange in the IR suite. The initial participants are the staff of the IR suite who are normally assigned to work in that clinical environment. The simulated patient is placed on monitors for vital signs and repositioned for the procedure. The simulated patient quickly deteriorates and has a pulseless cardiac arrest due to hypoxia from the upper airway obstruction that occurred due to repositioning. The IR team will intervene and activate the ERT within their clinical space and respond to the patient's medical needs. The initial core team within the suite consists of the Interventional Radiologist, the IR nursing staff, and the IR technician. The scenario ends after the initiation of PALS guidelines by the core IR team and documentation of the presence of the contingency team who form the ERT. This simulation focused on ensuring the healthcare team within a remote location had the necessary skills for resuscitating a deteriorating pediatric patient and engaging additional support across the hospital. These uncommon events in an isolated clinical space also present a complex interface full of communication hurdles. Do IR staff members know how and where to get help? Do members of the ERT know where the new IR Suite is located? Do they know where their emergency equipment is located? Using simulation to identify these process gaps and communication issues within the interprofessional team setting is crucial for patient safety. This process simulation highlighted several gaps in the algorithm. First was having seamless access to the correct equipment, such as an end-tidal carbon dioxide monitor and nitrous oxide tanks. Second was the ability of the ERT to find remote hospital locations. Finally, was the situational awareness of the deteriorating patient when staff are still acclimating to a new clinical area. Executive hospital leadership was immediate. Notified of the missing equipment and lack of door badge access to the ERT, which was rectified within 24 h.

The debriefing process is imperative to evoke change and spotlight the issues that need to change for patient safety. During the debriefing, the necessity for continued and more frequent simulations prior to patient use was highlighted. As a result, these scenarios are now performed at the onset of opening new clinical areas and then on a regular annual basis in remote locations across the hospital.

Scenario 3: Pediatric Trauma

The scenario occurs in a Trauma Bay within an Emergency Department with all the equipment typically available, such as oxygen, suction, airway cart, code cart, IV supplies, wound care supplies, and medication pumps. The pediatric manikin is utilized, and moulage is applied to replicate a trauma patient with realistic injuries matching the patient in the scenario. This scenario requires a simulated laceration on the forehead and an open femur fracture, with blood applied to mimic active bleeding.

Scenario objectives include:

1. Establish well-defined trauma team roles once the team arrives
2. Perform C-spine stabilization
3. Recognize signs and symptoms of increased intracranial pressure
4. Demonstrate appropriate preparation of Rapid Sequence Intubation medications
5. Demonstrate proper administration of appropriate medications for intracranial hypertension

This curriculum was developed to provide an in-situ simulation opportunity for the interprofessional Trauma Team as they receive an unstable trauma patient. The scenario offers multiple learning objectives and layers of complexity as interprofessional Trauma Team members arrive in response to an unstable, injured patient. The complex physiology unfolds throughout the scenario challenging participants to prioritize and re-prioritize the needs of their dynamically changing patient. Providers are arriving at different times, which has the potential to create communication gaps and breakdowns and complicate these situations.

Scenarios are developed to include all healthcare team members so they can use their specialized skills during the simulation experience.

The scenario begins in-situ in the triage area of the Emergency Department with the arrival of a 6-year-old male who suffered a head and leg injury during a fall down a staircase. The patient's vital signs and assessment are clinically supportive of activating the Trauma Team, composed of over 15 interprofessional team members with specialized training to care for pediatric trauma patients. The core emergency department team will continue to assess the patient and perform interventions based on the patient's needs while the trauma team members arrive to assist. The wave layering of participants into the scenario mirrors the real-life experience of different arrival times in a trauma situation of the team. The patient continues to deteriorate and demands the deployment of the algorithmic approach of Advanced Trauma Life Support. Figure 34.1 shows the trauma lead physician intubating the simulated patient. The simulation experience unfolds to engage the learners' technical and non-technical skills. The complexity of layers requires advanced communication skills in a crisis with a large cohort of health care team members. The focus on trauma moves from stabilizing the patient's airway and interventions for treating increased intracranial pressure to transfer to the Operating Room. The process of moving unstable trauma patients within the hospital is also simulated as a unique set of workflows that should be evaluated aside from

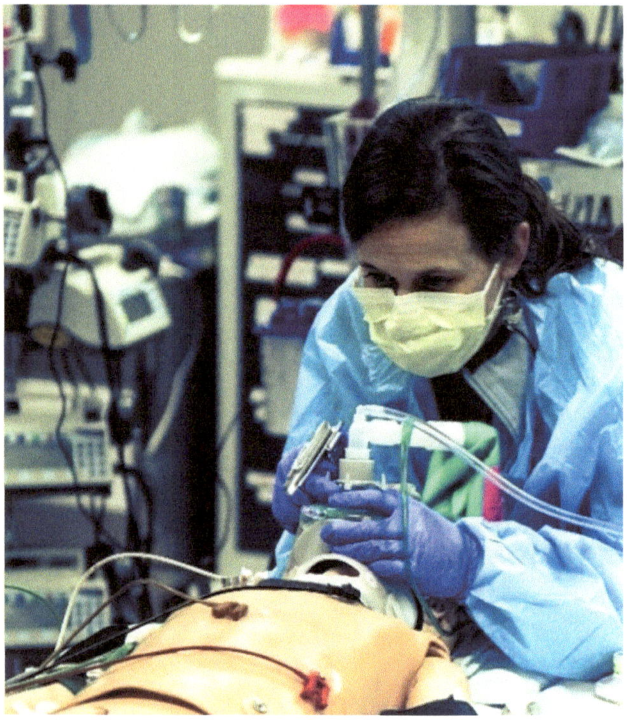

Fig. 34.1 In-situ trauma simulation

the clinical elements. The debriefing process illuminates the communication breakdowns within the interprofessional team and the system failures that could reach a real patient. These scenarios are conducted monthly and annually in a 4-h off-shift training format.

Scenario 4: Extracorporeal Life Support (ECLS) Activation

The scenario occurs in an Intensive Care Unit with all the equipment typically available, seen in a critical patient, such as intravenous access, vascular access, endotracheal tube, ventilator, and multiple lines of actively infusing medications. The pediatric manikin and a paired vital sign monitor reflect data seen in a critical care setting to replicate a critical care patient with the necessary intravenous access lines, a ventilator, and running intravenous medications.

Scenario objectives include:

1. Test the design and flow of the ECLS activation process
2. Demonstrate adherence to the ECLS activation script
3. Demonstrate timely execution of ECLS support
4. Demonstrate adherence to intrafacility transport checklist

Extracorporeal Life Support is a technologically complex endeavor having a known high-risk low, volume profile with no established guidelines or standardized process for educating an interprofessional team [14]. This technology is used to support patients in cardiac or respiratory failure when they have failed all other options in medicine. The critical nature of their illness demands higher technology and support, which can occur anytime without warning.

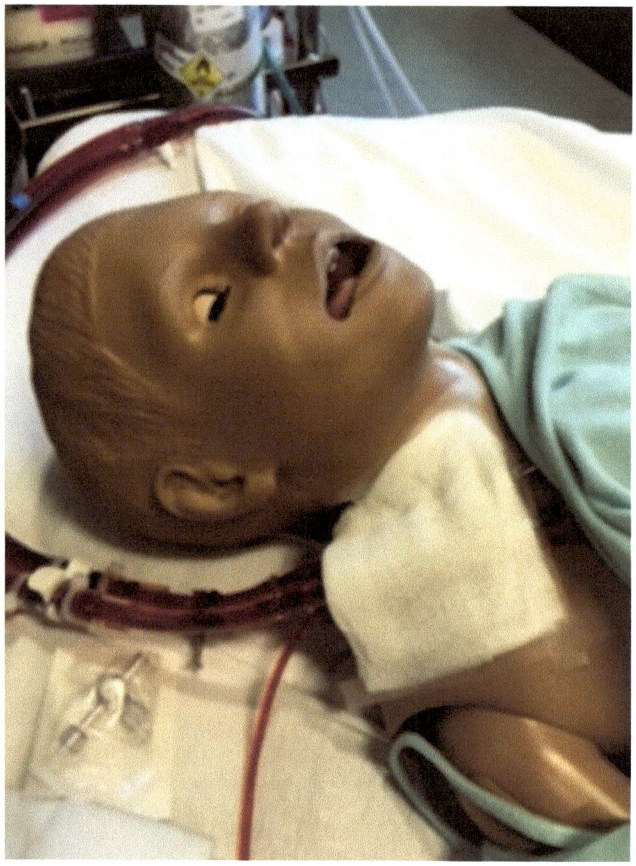

Fig. 34.2 In-situ ECLS activation simulation

Pioneering the frontier of building a new ECLS program and offering a new service line within a hospital requires innovative training to develop a competent interprofessional team and mitigate safety threats. A simulation curriculum can facilitate a safe environment to improve the delivery of ECLS care and communication for the interprofessional team.

With simulation, more time is spent in the active learning phase allowing for improved retention of knowledge, clinical skills, and behavior skills imperative to ECLS program initiation and development. A team-based approach ameliorated the new process for better patient care and best practice for a new program by having all team members of this extremely complex procedure present to provide feedback. For example, having a wide-scoping understanding of each of the team members, their roles, and their challenges helped build a more cohesive team with open lines of communication. There was a better understanding of all the moving elements that must happen in tandem for this ECLS process. Figure 34.2 shows a simulated patient with ECLS cannulas in place and attached to the pump.

The simulation experience is carried out before the new clinical service line is opened and regularly as the system and people change within the organization. Based on these simulation events, there were highlighted errors of technical failure on paging systems within the operating room, lack of elevator space for the large equipment transfers, absence of surgical equipment and resources within an intensive care unit, and patient room ergonomics. Based on these findings, the ECLS program generated changes to the paging system plan, created a road map for which bank of elevators are always used for ECLS patients, and a more robust array of medical equipment in the supply room specific to ECLS. These simulation experiences facilitated fundamental changes to patient safety elements in the areas of technical knowledge, system processes, and team communication.

Integrating Into Existing Education

The current didactics and classroom learning system often does not translate to clinical practice. Replacing some of the lecture time in existing classes with simulation is a budget-neutral method to increase exposure to simulation and provide a learning environment that has a maximum positive impact on patients and providers. Specific course offerings that meet criteria in size, duration, and educational objectives are augmented by simulation-based learning. For example, sepsis education to acute care nursing orienteers is now done in part as a didactic lecture, then supplemented with an immersive simulation in divided groups by the simulation team with faculty support by the clinical educators. The time spent for the course remains the same, with simulation replacing more lecture time to facilitate additional learning with attention to budgetary limitations.

Additionally, trauma team members have their focused lecture series and then engage in simulation-based training within a specific time frame that allows traditional learning and simulation. The benefits of simulation are widely recognized, and using this modality with regularity allows departments to include simulation activities in their annual budgets and move their programming from the classroom to the simulation experience replacing a lecture with a simulation. For example, a didactic on intubation and airway management is moved to both static simulation training with a task trainer and a dynamic simulation with a high-fidelity manikin who required intubation. Replacing two-dimensional lectures with hands-on experiential learning creates a more impactful medium for adult learners. Additionally, performing simulations with participants on shift is another way to expand program activities and continue to develop the healthcare members individually and in teams. The execution of in-situ simulations must have careful preparation to ensure staff availability; situational awareness of budget-neutral simulation is particularly appealing to organizations with budget restrictions and can facilitate support from executive leadership as they see the value in having additional education for their staff that does not create additional organizational costs. Changing the landscape of how education is delivered into a dynamic experiential solution is the ultimate goal for future learners and our patients.

Challenges and Solutions

Developing an interprofessional scenario requires multiple stakeholders to ensure the content expertise for scenario development. The cohort organized for simulation development is crucial for accuracy and realism. The cohort will vary depending on the subject matter of your simulation scenario. Subject matter experts representing all roles anticipated to be involved in the simulation should be included to provide valuable insight into their role and apply the best evidence-based practice.

The overarching objective of the simulation and a clear brief for each participant's role should be articulated to facilitate full team engagement and create an optimal learning environment. Adequate time for debriefing should be allotted and led by a trained simulationist, given the inherent value of this phase of simulation-based learning. This time allows for reflection and discussion and is often where the most learning occurs.

Scenario development with the identification of subject matter experts can be time-consuming and challenging because of the time commitment to creating a functional scenario that incorporates best practices. Finding interprofessional experts for developing simulations can be difficult, especially if there is limited knowledge of simulation or time constraints within a particular organization, such as the amount of time budgeted for staff education. There are often many subject matter experts within healthcare centers and organizations, but they may lack a simulation background lens to create scenarios. With support from the simulation team, identification and engagement of interprofessional subject matter experts can provide support for scenario design guidance and adherence to simulation best practices. Additionally, financial support from the simulation program or individual departments may be required to provide paid non-clinical time for administrative costs for the expertise surrounding scenario development from institutional content experts. Simulation Programs must consider budgetary needs for faculty content expert support within each budget cycle.

Once the scenario is created, another challenge may arise with the competing time during clinical shifts for health care providers and possible interference with clinical demands required for an in-situ on-shift simulation. Fully engaging the interprofessional team in the simulation means that there is additional energy focused by all to buffer their absence from real patient care to participate in the scenario. Novice participants in simulation have extra time to adjust to this new method of training and rely on the facilitators to ensure that it remains a safe, protected, and productive learning environment. A culture shift from lecture-based learning to hands-on learning must occur as simulation becomes the primary learning modality, specifically when focused on crisis resource management. Administrators, educators, and all stakeholders will have to collaborate to support team training and acknowledge the limitations of antiqued learning modalities. The movement outside of silo education to the interprofessional training milieu is focused not on the individual but on the improvements in patient care that will be seen due to team performance [8].

Simulation space can be a limiting factor depending on what options are available within individual institutions. Some programs have expansive dedicated simulation spaces, while others are limited to temporary options such as licensed clinical bed spaces, outfitted non-clinical spaces, or only in-situ opportunities [12]. Programs must adjust and navigate what is available and build their scenarios to fit their specific organizations. For example, suppose everything must be done in situ because of a lack of dedicated space. In that case, scenarios must fit into certain clinical areas in licensed beds and be able to be carried out with those limitations. If there is a dedicated space, then planning and scenario development will be different, as maneuvering around a licensed bed space is no longer a concern. If neither of those options is available and the simulation can be done in a modified non-clinical space, then planning for what is achievable in that milieu.

While there are benefits to conducting simulations in-situ, there are challenges that must be considered carefully before deciding to move forward with a simulation in-situ. On-shift staff participants, current stressors on the medical system, and unit-specific matters must be fully vetted before beginning. While simulation-based training is important, it must not deter real patient care or add a burden on the system that would create negative implications for staff. There must be a delineation between stressing the system to promote improvement versus penalizing or distracting the experience to staff. Adequate space and safety for patients hospitalized receiving care must be considered as well; utilizing the team for a simulation-based training event should not distract from real patients. Additionally, the used clinical space should be as remote as possible from real patients so the process and debriefing are not disturbing to staff and patients.

Due to the involvement of multiple units in all the simulations, charge nurses determine that the Unit can accommodate the simulation based on patient numbers, acuity, and competing patient demands. Other contingency team members, such as the house manager and supervisors, were included in the discussions to maintain patient safety. Whether this discussion involves the house manager, charge nurse, attending physician, or staff supervisors, the pulse on all the patient care areas can be adequately accessed. Time constraints can be honored by limiting the length of the simulation and debriefing. Each simulation can be preplanned for an ideal time for optimal learning and engagement with contingency plans if there are competing priorities. For example, if clinical demands exist for real patients and the planned time is 30 min, then accommodations can be made for impactful learning in a shorter time block. Being flexible with time planning and respecting time limitations will facilitate more opportunities for simulation events and participation from the learners.

Other potential challenges include the technical aspects of the human simulators and the additional equipment needed to implement the clinical scenario. There are concerns about the portability of simulation equipment and malfunctions of simulators outside of the simulation lab space. Ideally, testing the high-fidelity equipment before the actual simulation helps identify any issues surrounding technical failure or limitations within that space. The preparatory work of vetting these logistics may take additional time but yield a better simulation experience for the learners. There are medical supplies to be dealt with, as having all the available and necessary simulated medications or supplies results in enhanced realism for participant engagement. Including a detailed list of scenario-specific supplies and their accuracy relative to the unit or service area where the simulation will occur helps ensure everything is readily available. The safety risks of having simulated medical equipment in a real patient area that could be inadvertently used on a real patient require diligence to ensure all simulation supplies are properly marked and removed at the end of the event. There is additional cleaning of equipment used during the scenario in that environment to mitigate infectious risk so that it is left ready for patient care.

Simulation programs should create a contingency plan for adjusting the timing, location, and even cancellation of in-situ simulations. An estimated 10–15% of in-situ simulations will not occur due to census or acuity-related issues within the organization [12].

Planning logistics focused on simulation location, timing of the simulation, and backup planning for alternative solutions are essential to the success of any simulation program.

Interface with Regulatory Bodies

Extracorporeal Life Support Organization (ELSO) is an international association of healthcare organizations created to promote comprehensive interprofessional collaborations to develop and evaluate novel therapies [15]. Guidelines for training healthcare providers must be referenced when creating initial and ongoing training of ECLS specialists for adult and pediatric ECLS programs. These guidelines help establish a standardized process across different intuitions and countries for both pediatrics and adults to ensure optimal care is delivered to patients. The established training infrastructure will be the same footprint for all organizations providing this service line. Specific requirements for "water drills," which are low-fidelity simulations, are outlined in their guidelines. They include how to change major equipment like the oxygenator, heat exchange, and bladder, as well as less complicated components of the circuit like the raceway and pigtails, and checking pump head occlusion in a reasonable time. The recommendation for new ECLS centers is to repeat the "water drill" training until the specialists are competent. For ongoing training, the simulations occur at least every 6 months. Increased frequency is at the center's discretion, depending on their specific training needs based on patient volume [16]. For centers in California that are part of the California Children's Services (CCS) Program, there are specific requirements for "water drills" that align with the ELSO guidelines [17].

Conclusion

Simulation-Based Training geared to elevating the Crisis Resource Management skills of health care providers specific to pediatric emergencies is a modality to help improve patient outcomes. The potential safety impact for pediatric patients is limitless with this mode of education and training. This form of simulation offers an additional platform to improve the system and the providers. Whether the simulation is focused on interprofessional team training to train and help people evolve in the mastery of crisis resource skills or integrate a new clinical service line or space into an organization, this deliberate practice improves performance, confidence, and skills by providing an experiential safe learning environment.

References

1. Cunningham RM, Walton M, Carter PM. The major causes of death in children and adolescents in the United States. N Engl J Med. 2018;379:2468–75. https://doi.org/10.1056/NEJMsr1804754.
2. Swendiman A, Sharoky C, Russell K, Goldshore M, Blinman T, Nance M. Life-saving interventions in pediatric trauma: a national trauma data bank experience. J Trauma Acute Care Surg. 2019;87(6):1321–7.
3. Weiss S, Alhazzani W, Flori H, Nadel S, Schlapback L, Tasker R, et al. Surviving sepsis campaign international guidelines for managing septic shock and sepsis-associated organ dysfunction in children. Pediatr Crit Care Med. 2020;21(2):e52–e106.
4. McLaughlin C, Wieck M, Barin E, Rake A, Burke R, Roesly H, et al. Impact of simulation-based training on perceived provider confidence in acute multidisciplinary pediatric trauma resuscitation. Pediatr Surg Int. 2018;34:1353–62.
5. Jeffery AD, Mutsch KS, Knapp L. Knowledge and recognition of SIRS and sepsis among pediatric nurses. Pediatr Nursing. 2014;40:271–8.
6. Kessler DO, Walsh B, Whitfill T, Dudas RA, Gangardharan S, Gawel M, for the INSPIRE ImPACTS Investigators. Disparities in adherence to pediatric sepsis guidelines across a spectrum of emergency departments: a multicenter, cross-sectional observational in situ simulation study. J Emerg Med. 2016;50:403–15.
7. Howard SK, Gaba DM, Fish KJ, Yang G, Sarnquist FH. Anesthesia crisis resource management training: teaching anesthesiologists to handle critical incidents. Aviat Space Environ Med. 1992;63(9):763–70.
8. Cheng A, Donoghue A, Gilfoyle E, Eppich W. Simulation-based crisis resource management training for pediatric critical care medicine: a review for instructors. Pediatr Crit Care Med. 2012;13(2):197–203.
9. Joint Commission on Accreditation of Healthcare Organizations. Sentinel event statistics, June 29, 2004. Available at: www.jcaho.org/accredited+organizations/ambulatory+care/sentinel+events/sentinel+event+statistics.htm.
10. Babiker A, Hueesini ME, Al Nemri A. Health care professional development: working as a team to improve patient care. Sudanese J Paediatr. 2014;14(2):9.
11. World Health Organization. Framework for action on interprofessional education & collaborative practice. Geneva: World Health Organization; 2010. Available from https://www.who.int/hrh/resources/framework_action/en/
12. Patterson M, Blike T, Nadkarni V. Advances in patient safety: new directions and alternative approaches. In-situ simulation: challenges and results. AHRQ Publication; 2018.
13. Paige JB, Graham L, Sittner B. Formal training efforts to develop simulation educators, simulation in healthcare. J Soc Simul Healthc. 2020;15(4):271–81. https://doi.org/10.1097/SIH.0000000000000424.
14. Thiagarajan RR, Laussen PC, Rycus PT, et al. Extracorporeal membrane oxygenation to aid cardiopulmonary resuscitation in infants and children. Circulation. 2007;116:1693 700.
15. Extracorporeal Life Support Organization. Welcome to ELSO. ELSO; 2020 [cited 2020 November 12]. Available from: https://www.elso.org/Home.aspx.
16. Extracorporeal Life Support Organization. ELSO Award of Excellence. ELSO; 2010 [updated 2010 February; cited 2020 November 12]. Available from: https://www.elso.org/AwardofExcellence/BeforeYouApply/ELSOGuidelines.aspx.
17. Department of Health Care Services. Provider standards. Department of Health Care Services; 2020 [updated 2018 April 26; cited 2020 November 12]. Available from: https://www.dhcs.ca.gov/services/ccs/Pages/ProviderStandards.aspx.

Simulations for Critical Care Nursing

35

Tara J. Lemoine, Kimberly Bilskey, and Rebecca Weiss

Background

The current landscape of modern medicine focuses on patient safety and is fueled by the 1999 Institute of Medicine report To Err is Human: Building a Safer Health System [1].

This landmark paper forced the acknowledgment of failures in the healthcare system that resulted in unnecessary morbidity and mortality of hospitalized patients. The estimates of medical errors resulting in hospitalized patients' deaths approach about 98,000 each year [2].

Patients in the critical care environment are at an even higher risk based on the complexity of their illness, the technology or equipment necessary to save their lives, and human factors in a busy and distracting environment.

There is evidence that the error rate in the Intensive Care Unit (ICU) setting is about 1.7 errors per day, and almost all suffer a potentially life-threatening error at some point [3]. Additionally, there has been a shift within the critical care nursing workforce. Growing numbers of graduate nurses or nurses with no critical care experience are being hired to staff these complex, high-risk environments [4, 5]. The combination of lack of experience and absence of practice readiness compromises assessment and intervention skills necessary to function in this complex clinical milieu. The knowledge and performance gaps have the potential to negatively impact patient outcomes.

T. J. Lemoine · K. Bilskey (✉)
Valley Children's Healthcare, Madera, CA, USA
e-mail: TLemoine@valleychildrens.org;
kbilskey@valleychildrens.org

R. Weiss
University of Pittsburgh Medical Center Shadyside,
Pittsburgh, PA, USA
e-mail: Rustr@upmc.edus

Best Practices

Simulation-based training (SBT) is optimal for education in this high-risk convoluted clinical setting to improve competency. Simulation also lends itself nicely as a potential strategy to address the issues of behavioral performance, situational awareness, and communication skill sets necessary for the optimal functioning of a healthcare provider within the ICU setting. If designed correctly, simulation-based training can replicate the ICU setting and focus on medication errors, high-risk, low-volume procedures, deteriorating patients, and communication. These simulation trainings can facilitate staff development extending from a nursing focus to interdisciplinary training to function as another tool to optimally reinforce practices needed in critical care settings.

The timing of these simulations can be done both throughout the orientation phase with novice providers until past the licensure phase for continued professional development. Tiered skill acquisition or phased orientation models have been described as improving new hire onboarding practices in critical care by steadily increasing nurse responsibility, patient load, and experiences.

Likewise, these interactive dynamic education sessions can also be deployed as part of ongoing clinical practice to provide additional complex layers of technical and non-technical skills in the ICU setting. Executing a well-designed critical care simulation focused on error prevention, early error recognition, competency-based performance, and interprofessional team training requires focused planning for a successful delivery.

The creation of a psychologically safe learning environment in simulation is one of the essential elements of having a successful simulation. Establishing a psychologically safe space positively influences learning and contributes to participants having better recall, performance, and engaging in self-correcting behaviors [6]. Learner engagement, well developed and relevant curriculum content is especially

J. M. Kutzin et al. (eds.), *Comprehensive Healthcare Simulation: Nursing*, Comprehensive Healthcare Simulation,
https://doi.org/10.1007/978-3-031-31090-4_35

important to facilitate education that can translate to enhanced learning with improved patient care and outcomes [7]. Well-designed simulations and a clear overview of expectations establish a framework to support the learners in a positive simulation experience. The debriefing process with skilled faculty is the best practice for delivering an effective simulation curriculum and creates the best opportunity to change the healthcare provider's behavior. Consistency of education and skill among the simulation faculty is inherently valuable as there is a relationship between increased learner outcomes and faculty with higher levels of training [8]. Static or dynamic simulation can be used with either task trainers for procedural skills to replicate and hone psychomotor technical skills. Equally useful are high or low-fidelity manikins that can function for individuals needing to practice specific elements or for an experience that is a complete process seen in the ICU. For example, a task trainer simulating the standardized intubation process or a central line dressing change can impact learning and skill performance equally. Hybrid simulations involve combining a standardized patient (SP) into a simulation exercise with either a task trainer or other elements. A hybrid ICU scenario might incorporate an SP with a difficult end-of-life discussion with a high-fidelity simulator requiring extubation and palliation of pain control in an emotionally complex environment [9]. Each type of simulation has a place within the critical care educational milieu serving to create a higher-performing individual and team.

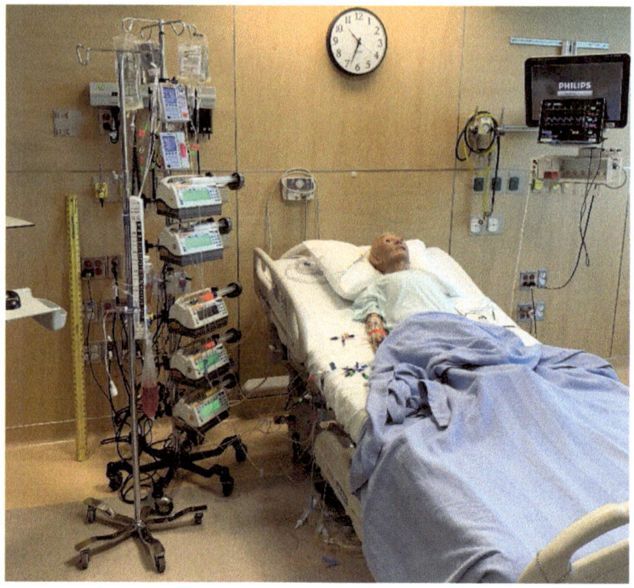

Fig. 35.1 Room of errors

Sample Curriculum

Scenario 1: Pediatric Neuro Patient ICU Room of Errors

The scenario occurs in a Pediatric Intensive Care Unit (PICU) in an actual patient room with all the equipment typically available for a post-operative neurosurgical patient. A pediatric manikin is set up in the room with multiple invasive lines for central and arterial access, medication infusions, and an external ventricular drain (EVD). The simulation team embedded twenty (20) patient safety errors for the participants to identify during the scenario. (Fig. 35.1).

Scenario objectives include:

1. Recognize and communicate all 20 embedded patient safety errors.
2. Identify deviations from established care standards in the post-operative management of the neurosurgical patient.

This curriculum was developed to provide an in situ simulation opportunity for the PICU nurses to identify errors that diverge from the standard of care, ultimately creating patient safety risks [10].The estimates of medical errors resulting in death or morbidity are known factors in the ICU [11]. Pediatric patients are not excluded from these statistics, and those in the pediatric critical care setting are complex, medically fragile, and even more at risk of medical errors. Prior to the development of this simulation curriculum, there was no educational modality within our PICU education that focused on the multitude of safety elements associated with the complexity of care for this specific patient population. Direct feedback to nursing leadership, PICU educators, and reports from our patient safety alert system focused on safety issues in this patient cohort were drivers of rethinking an educational plan moving forward.

This scenario presents multiple safety elements based on physician order errors, poor communication, absence of knowledge of essential policies, and complex equipment interface. The nurse participants spanned a wide range of experience, from novices, with less than a year of PICU experience, to veteran nurses with over 30 years of experience. The nurses underwent the presentation of a bedside handoff report of the patient in a typical format. They also had access to the simulated patient's electronic health record (EHR) with written physician orders to follow and acknowledge as in the real clinical environment.

They were given specific instructions to only identify the errors and not correct anything to ensure that each participant had the same experience. Participants were given a fixed time frame to maneuver through the room, look through the electronic medical record, and examine the simulated patient. During this exercise, they were instructed to verbally identify any error they felt was present either in the clinical report, EHR, patient room, patient equipment, or on the simulated patient. At the end of the scenario, all embedded errors were transparent to the participants and discussed in the debriefing process. Each error in the room was chosen based on the frequency in which they were seen during real patient care, and each one had a high probability of reaching real patients. Using simulation focused on error exposure and recognition heightens the vigilance of healthcare providers and is a meaningful tool to impact patient safety.

Scenario 2: Pediatric Neurological Patient Assessment

The scenario occurs in a Pediatric Intensive Care Unit (PICU) in a patient room with all the standard equipment available. A standardized patient was in the room with simulated invasive lines for arterial and venous access and medication infusions.

Scenario objectives include:

1. Complete a full neuromuscular and neurovascular assessment
2. Demonstrate the use of documentation in the electronic health record
3. Identify signs and symptoms of postoperative complications of a spinal fusion procedure
4. Identify communication pathway for provider notifications

This curriculum was developed to provide an in situ simulation opportunity for the PICU nurses to perform a neuromuscular and neurovascular assessment on a patient that can interact dynamically. The nurses underwent the presentation of a bedside handoff report of the patient in a typical format. They also had access to the simulated patient's electronic health record (EHR) with written physician orders to follow and acknowledge as in the real clinical environment.

A standardized patient (SP) was used for the learners to perform a physical exam, identify a physical assessment abnormality and document that process in the EHR. The use of SPs in the pediatric critical care realm for simulation training in physical assessment is a novel concept to help expand the training depth and enrich the learners' experience. This exercise focuses on diagnostic skills necessary to work at the bedside in the ICU.

Scenario 3: Pediatric Spinal Fusion Surgery with Loss of Signals

The scenario occurs in Free-Standing Children's Hospital Operating Room (OR) with all the equipment typically available. A pediatric manikin is supine on the OR table with a spine model placed over the manikin's posterior torso. The simulation team then sets up the OR suite just as it would be in real life. (Fig. 35.2).

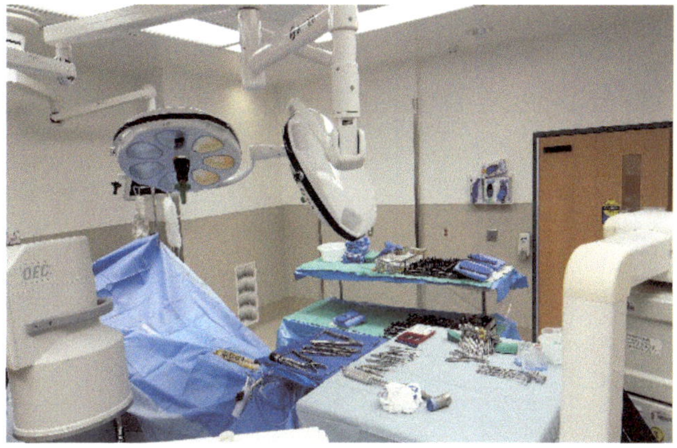

Fig. 35.2 Spinal fusion surgery

Scenario objectives include:

1. Demonstrate use of Crisis Handbook: Loss of Spinal Cord Signals Checklist
2. Demonstrate clear and concise interprofessional communication

This curriculum was developed to provide an in-situ simulation opportunity for the operating team to utilize the crisis handbook. The crisis handbook is an institution-specific catalog of twenty-two high-risk clinical events where distinct processes will be followed in the operating room, cardiac catheterization laboratory, or any remote anesthesia location. The clinical staff established this checklist in the operating room consisting of nursing, anesthesiology, and registered nurse first assistants and technicians. The focus is on utilizing medical equipment, personnel, and an algorithmic approach to crises unique to this clinical milieu. For example, local anesthetic toxicity, malignant hyperthermia, and the loss of evoked potentials are included in this handbook. Access to the handbook is readily available in the operating room core space. It is introduced during orientation to the OR staff but not routinely accessed or used for training purposes. Before this experience, there was no dynamic educational opportunity to operationalize these algorithms and evaluate their feasibility, staff knowledge, or competency. These have been implemented in real life and refined over time based on actual patient experiences where the process did not fully lend itself to preventing harm or was not a time-sensitive effective approach. The established operating room staff training curriculum now includes simulating the scenarios in the crisis handbook rotating throughout the calendar year.

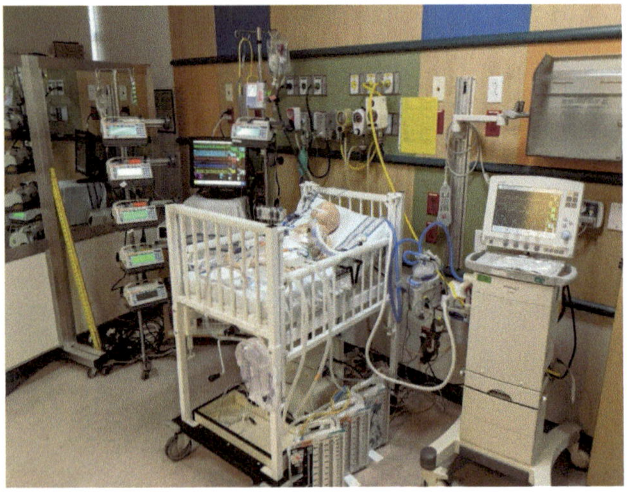

Fig. 35.3 Pediatric cardiac patient

Scenario 4: Post-Operative Care of the Pediatric Cardiac Patient

The scenario occurs in a Pediatric Intensive Care Unit (PICU) in an actual patient room with all the available equipment. An infant manikin is set up in a crib with multiple invasive lines, chest tubes, medication infusions, and a ventilator. (Fig. 35.3).

Scenario objectives include:

1. Identify invasive lines in immediate post-operative cardiac patients
2. Utilize invasive lines for medication administration
3. Recognize dysrhythmias of post-operative patients

This curriculum was developed to provide an in-situ simulation opportunity for PICU nurses on cardiac orientation. Historically, these nurses would individually complete a case study on one of their patients by the end of their orientation. Adding this simulation experience in their initial education allows all the orienteers to experience the same complex patient scenario. They interface with a critically ill patient in a safe learning environment that leads to open discussion. These experienced PICU nurses will spend approximately 7–9 shifts alongside an expert cardiac intensive care nurse learning to care for pediatric post-operative cardiac patients. This simulation opportunity begins their journey down a complex path that requires strong critical thinking and clinical skills.

Scenario 5: Pediatric Respiratory Failure

The scenario is an in-situ simulation that takes place in a PICU. An infant manikin is set up in a crib with BiPAP.

Scenario objectives include:

1. Demonstrate room safety checks
2. Recognize side effects of Precedex
3. Recognize respiratory failure in the pediatric patient
4. Prepare for intubation
5. Administer medications for intubation
6. Prepare code medications
7. Administer code medications

This curriculum was developed to provide an in-situ simulation opportunity for novice PICU nurses and respiratory care practitioners to work with their interprofessional team, including the PICU intensivist, to care for a medically unstable infant. Participants typically have less than 2 years of experience in the PICU and have had limited exposure to these events limiting their competency in these real-life situations.

Scenario 6: Simulation in Adult Critical Nursing Clinical Orientation

In one hospital, a tiered skill acquisition model comprises four phases to onboard and orient nursing staff selected for the adult critical care areas. There is complete transparency in the orientation process detailing the four phases on the new hire's first day. On the initial day of onboarding, the new hires are informed of the simulation-based competency and the need to complete it to come off orientation. The simulation requires a pass rate of 80% with a subsequent remediation process if the minimum competency is not met based on standard passing scores.

The phases are executed in a rolling format over time for programmatic purposes. In the third phase, the new hire critical care nurse is introduced to escalating numbers of high acuity and complex critically ill patients. The direct result of more complex physiology and critical illness translates to demanding more advanced nursing care skill sets and knowledge. The necessary skills are often high-risk interventions such as emergent intubation, cardiopulmonary resuscitation, and advanced monitoring with invasive physiologic measuring devices. The goal of the third phase is to facilitate the acquisition of skills, knowledge, and confidence in the critical care environment. To progress to the fourth or last phase in orientation, the newly hired critical care nurse must complete an in-person simulation-based competency evaluation. The simulation competency consists of replicated patients and clinical experiences that mimic the expected experiences during the new hire's orientation. Successful completion of this simulation demonstrates that the new hire is ready to move on to the last phase of orientation as a critical care nurse. The unit nurse educator completes the simulation with the new hire using the rubric to grade each learning objective (Appendix A). If the oriented fails the simulation, based on the established objective scoring criteria, then they remain in the third phase of orientation with clear learning objectives to cover while waiting to undergo remediation. The remediation process is established, and the orientee repeats the simulation exercise 1–2 weeks later with the same scoring mechanism.

The intensive care unit educators and members of the ICU leadership designed the simulation case studies. Clinical preceptors were queried about the most common tasks and skills that new critical care nurses struggle with during orientation. The main learning objectives expected of a nurse just completing orientation were the primary focus of the simulation. The assessment was approximately 90 minutes and included 12 overarching topics. The 12 topics were spread into two patient cases, each with two to three learning objectives embedded. In addition, the unit educator worked with the Director of Informatics of the hospital to create a simulated electronic patient chart that included labs and orders to facilitate the realism of the scenario. This electronic charting also served to allow nursing documentation throughout the simulation experience. The simulation was typically scheduled on a day when the nurse was scheduled for a clinical shift, and they participated during clinical hours. The space was either an empty licensed patient room within the intensive care unit or the simulation lab. The rooms were set up the same way so each participant had the same experience. In addition to the nurse oriented, the educator or representative from unit leadership was present and served as the evaluator during this process. The nurse educator trained the unit leadership on completing an evaluation by having them observe one full simulation experience. Then the nurse educator watched them complete one to be signed off. The nurse was oriented to the physical space, the purpose of the simulation, and the objective numerical system used for grading. They were not given the grading rubric before the simulation but were given the topics that would be reviewed when they first started on the unit in their department orientation binder.

The equipment in the room included a low-fidelity manikin, a defibrillator, oxygen delivery devices, electrocardiogram electrodes, and an arterial line invasive monitoring system. A formatted script was read with specific prompts, followed by directed questions focused on the nurse's follow-up action plans. If this simulation occurred within the ICU, the orientee is prompted to maneuver through the unit and obtain all the necessary equipment to follow through with the assigned task or intervention. The orientee articulated where to find equipment within their respective ICU if the simulation exercise is delivered within the simulation lab. Using the simulated electronic patient chart, the orientee was expected to complete specific documentation and review orders or labs as indicated throughout the scenario. After completion of the simulation exercise, there was a debriefing process reviewing the performance of the individual elements. During the debriefing, there was full disclosure about moving into the fourth phase of orientation or a remediation process that would occur over the following 1–2 week cycle. If a remediation plan was implemented, ongoing dialogue occurred with the ICU leadership, orientee, and preceptor to focus on salient elements identified as not meeting competency during the simulation assessment.

In the trial of this tiered skill acquisition model, 15 nurses participated in the phased orientation and simulation evaluation. Thirteen of the fifteen passed the simulation assessment on the first attempt, and only two required a remediation process. Feedback from the new hires at the end of the process validated that despite this process causing some performance anxiety, it was impactful for the external validation of skills and enhancing self-confidence. This needs further validation, and we plan to continue to study this with future cohorts to increase our sample size.

Integrating into Existing Education

There needs to be more than the current system of classroom didactics or brief on-the-job experiences to translate to clinical practice skills in the intensive care unit setting. This may be a side effect of differences in learning styles or variability of clinical exposure precluding a consistent knowledge set among more novice staff. Transitioning the traditional practice of lectures into interactive simulation can be challenging but is a needed change to increase the simulation footprint within healthcare systems. The content and objectives have already been developed for these classroom sessions, and by manipulating the content, it can evolve into a simulation format using a multitude of modalities. A more contemporary learning platform to deliver consistent and relevant education will also be more palatable for the new generation of healthcare providers as simulation has become part of the fabric of their pre-licensure education [12]. Given budget constraints, adopting hands-on experiential learning may facilitate a more financially solvent plan for expediting competency-based training and ensuring consistency of knowledge and skill acquisition across the interprofessional team. Additionally, performing simulations with participants who are working but on orientation is another way to expand program activities and continue to develop the healthcare members. Orientees did not need staff to cover their assignments during simulation because they were extra. The in-situ simulation training concept is paramount in the ICU settings where the interprofessional team performs optimally with consistent, focused training on mastery of communication and individual skills. Changing the landscape of how education is delivered into a dynamic experiential solution is the ultimate goal for our healthcare teams, individuals, and the safety of our sickest and most complicated patients.

Challenges and Solutions

Developing an interprofessional simulation curriculum requires multiple stakeholders to ensure the content expertise for scenario development. In the ICU domain, accuracy and realism are demanded as deviation from a legitimate environment can confuse learners. Subject matter experts with representation from each discipline must be involved and should be included at the onset. There is often limited bandwidth for individuals who might be champions of this simulation-based work or want to contribute their expertise but are faced with limited simulation knowledge. While the interdisciplinary approach allows valuable insight into the development of a simulation exercise, time constraints can be overcome with asynchronous work. Objectives for each role should be identified to ensure during the debriefing process, the facilitated learning process will create either full team engagement or individual skill competency. This type of initiative means acknowledging the limitations of antiqued learning modalities and shifting the resources to simulation [13]. A content expert in simulation can provide optics on objectives to ensure standards are met consistently for simulation-based education. Once the scenario is created, another challenge may arise with the time demands required for an in situ on-shift simulation.

In situ means that the location of the simulation is in the real patient clinical care areas [14]. An estimated 15–30% of in situ simulations will not occur due to census or acuity-related organizational issues [15]. Our institution has a similar rate of cancellations. About 25% of our in-situ simulations across the organization are aborted. Attempts to mitigate this include planning more in-situ simulations during lower census months based on seasonal changes in pediatric medicine with a consistent decline in our average daily census. Additionally, our planning has shifted to investigating when we have more resource staff available, the number of staff on orientation, and trainees on shift who can fully participate. To deliver the learning experience in the face of a cancellation, we pursue offering the same activity within a month's rotation. In-situ simulations must consider many factors before initiation, given their integration into the real physical clinical care space. Based on the fast-moving pace and dynamically changing clinical nature of the ICU, there is an even higher chance that planned simulations must be aborted for patient care responsibilities. Given the knowledge of in situ training requirements, the administrators, educators, and all stakeholders will have to collaborate to support the use of on-shift team training. Those canceled events could create an unbalanced knowledge and performance gap for those engaging in a simulation. Repeating these simulations at another time may require additional resources, time, and engagement by the educators. While there are benefits to conducting simulations in situ, there are challenges that must be considered carefully before deciding to move forward. On-shift staff participants, current stressors on the medical system, and unit-specific matters must be fully vetted before beginning. Adequate space and safety for hospitalized patients must be considered such that a simulation-based training event is focused on real patient care. Additionally, the clinical space should be as remote as possible from real patients so the simulation and debriefing do not disturb patients, families, or staff engaged in patient care. Time constraints of staff should be honored by balancing the execution of the simulation experience versus patient care duties. Other potential elements to consider include the technical aspects of the human simulators and the additional equipment needed to implement the clinical scenario. There can be issues with the portability of simulation equipment and malfunction of simulators outside of the simulation lab space that should be investigated in advance. A few safety elements need a codified plan to ensure the simulated medical equipment is properly marked and removed from the real clinical space. There must also be a process to have the space cleaned and readied for real patients that mitigate both the infectious risk and delay in patient access. Simulation programs should create a contingency plan for adjustment in the timing, location, and even cancellation of in situ simulations.

For those simulations within a designated simulation space, this may be a limiting factor depending on the options available within individual institutions. Some programs have expansive dedicated simulation spaces, while others are limited to temporary options such as licensed clinical bed spaces or outfitted non-clinical spaces.

Simulation in a non-clinical space has some limitations on the level of reflection and practice change that is challenging to translate in the clinical space. By using the actual equipment and supplies, there are improved learning and engagement capabilities. The benefit of having a readily available outfitted space can always be noticed as a consistent, steady opportunity for education.

Summary

Critical care nursing and medicine are constantly evolving with an increased demand for an elevated skill set and competency. The shift in educational opportunities to simulation-based education is focused on preparing healthcare providers to deliver safe high, quality medical care. There are now a myriad of simulation applications to enhance the performance in technical and non-technical skills specific to the ICU setting. Meeting the needs of the learners planning around venue, modality, and impact are all issues that require careful consideration. Simulation with a specific focus on the ICU can accelerate proficiency, expertise, and focus on the most fragile and complex patients.

References

1. Kohn LT, Corrigan JM, Donaldson MS. To err is human: building a safer health system. Washington: National Academy Press; 1999.
2. Joint Commission American Hospital Association. Sentinel Event Alert 19, 2001.
3. Pronovost PJ, Thompson DA, et al. Defining and measuring patient safety. Crit Care Clin. 2005;2:1–19.
4. Morris LL, Pfeifer PB, Catalano R, Fortney R, Hilton EL, McLaughlin J, Nelson G, Goldstein L. Designing a comprehensive model for critical care orientation. Crit Care Nurse. 2007;27(6):37–57. https://doi.org/10.4037/ccn2007.27.6.37.
5. Bortolotto SJ. Developing a comprehensive critical care orientation program for graduate nurses. J Nur Prof Dev. 2015;31(4):203–10. https://doi.org/10.1097/NND.0000000000000139.
6. Aranzamendez G, James D, R. Toms finding antecedents of psychological safety: a step toward quality improvement. Nurs Forum. 2015;50(3):171–8.
7. Harvey A, Bandiera G, Nathens A, V. LeBlanc impact of stress on resident performance in simulated trauma scenarios. J Trauma Acute Care Surg. 2012;72(2):497–503.
8. Cason M, Sessions LC, Nemeth L, Catchpole K, Bundy D. Components of team science-what contributes to success? J Interprofessional Educ Pract. 2019;18(100298):1–8. https://doi.org/10.1016/j.xjep.2019.100298.
9. Howley LD. Standardized patients. In: Levine AI, DeMaria S, Schwartz AD, Sim AJ, editors. The comprehensive textbook of healthcare simulation. New York: Springer; 2013. p. P173–90.
10. Dauphin J, Atkinson S, et al. Medication errors room: a simulation to assess the medical, nursing, and pharmacy staff's ability to identify errors related to the medication-use system. J Eval Clin Pract. 2016;22(6):906–17.
11. Rothschild J, Landrigan C, et al. The critical care safety study: the incidence and nature of adverse events and serious medical errors in intensive care. Crit Care Med. 2005;33(8):1694–700.
12. Konia M, Yao A. Simulation-a new educational paradigm? J Biomed Res. 2013;27(2):75–80. https://doi.org/10.7555/JBR.27.20120107.
13. Cheng A, Donoghue A, Gilfoyle E, Eppich W. Simulation-based crisis resource management training for pediatric critical care medicine: a review for instructors. Pediatr Crit Care Med. 2012;13(2):197–203.
14. Patterson M, Blike T, Nadkarni V. Advances in patient safety: new directions and alternative approaches. In: Situ Simulation: Challenges and Results, vol. 3; 2018.
15. Lairamore C, Reed C, Damon Z, Rowe V, Baker J, Griffith K, et al. A peer-led interprofessional simulation experience improves perceptions of teamwork. Clin Sim Nur. 2019;34:22–9. https://doi.org/10.1016/j.ecns.2019.05.00.

Process Improvement Simulations for Nursing

36

Kathleen Laffoon

Introduction

Process improvement (PI), often called system integration, is about identifying, analyzing, and improving existing work processes to enhance performance, meet best practice standards and improve quality [1]. Healthcare PI simulation offers an opportunity to improve team performance, highlight the need for system changes, streamline processes, test and improve procedure guidelines and identify areas that could lead to patient safety issues [2, 3]. PI simulation and system integration goals include fewer errors, reduced waste, improved productivity, streamlined efficiency, and improved patient safety and outcomes.

Background

Process improvement has its roots in manufacturing hundreds of years ago. Henry Ford was the first person to successfully integrate the process at his assembly line manufacturing plant in Highland Park, MI [4]. Ford's 1913 fabrication process allowed vehicles to be assembled within days rather than weeks. However, his system lacked the ability to change. In the 1930s, the Toyota Corporation improved on Ford's process. It introduced self-monitoring machines to ensure low cost, better variety, high quality, and rapid throughput times to respond to fluctuating customer requests [4]. The Toyota Production System evolved into Lean, a popular means of eliminating "waste" from organizational processes. The system centered product flow and sequencing through their entire process instead of focusing on individual machines and their performance. Toyota's Lean thinking has been replicated worldwide, encouraging business leaders to adapt their tools and principles beyond manufacturing and into healthcare [4]. In the mid-1980s, Motorola introduced the Six Sigma system that focused on improving quality [5]. Six Sigma is based strongly on other quality approaches, such as Total Quality Management (TQM) and Quality Improvement (QI). Today, methodologies such as Lean, Six Sigma, TQM, A3 Process, and Plan-Do-Study-Act (PDSA) are PI and QI tools that view systems from different perspectives to add value to organizations, improve efficiency, and decrease errors. Process Improvement simulations run parallel to many processes outside of healthcare; these are easily adapted to resolve an unlimited array of procedures, activities, and practices uncovered through inquiry, root cause analysis, and error reporting. Regardless of the methodology, PI is important in reducing errors and underlying hazards and improving existing systems.

Best Practices

It has been over 20 years since the Institute of Medicine's landmark publication "To Err is Human: Building a Safer Health System." [6]. Two decades later, medical errors remain a serious concern. The patient safety movement has evolved into numerous safety and quality initiatives designed to reduce diagnostic errors, improve team communication and set safety expectations to prevent patient harm [6]. Simulation provides an ideal opportunity to replicate processes and examine these threats before harm occurs. It can also serve as a tool for encouraging a safety culture through norms set in a simulated environment [3]. PI simulation can be used for various best practices, including improved systems thinking and identifying latent safety threats [7]. Latent safety threats can be identified during in-situ simulations or tabletop exercises that lead participants through a real-life event in a safe, simulated environment. These latent threats would normally be evident once you attempted to implement the procedure [2]. During an in-situ PI simulation, for exam-

K. Laffoon (✉)
Center for Learning and Innovation, Scripps Health, San Diego, CA, USA
e-mail: Laffoon.Kathleen@scrippshealth.org

J. M. Kutzin et al. (eds.), *Comprehensive Healthcare Simulation: Nursing*, Comprehensive Healthcare Simulation,
https://doi.org/10.1007/978-3-031-31090-4_36

ple, it may be revealed that a vital piece of equipment resides behind a locked cabinet that is not readily accessible, or the group discovers that some members of the resuscitation team do not have key card access to enter a locked unit where the cardiac arrest is happening. These situations could be quickly remedied if identified as part of a PI simulation.

PI simulations that focus on teamwork and communication issues are a best practice for reducing errors resulting from inadequate, poor, or missing communication among the team. Simulation can also be beneficial for rehearsing and improving team performance. Research has shown that healthcare teams better understand individual roles and communicate better during trauma events after participating in the simulation [8]. In the obstetric community, communication problems were the main causes in 72% of perinatal death or permanent disability cases, with organizational culture noted as a barrier to effective communication in 55% of cases [9]. Researchers at the University of Minnesota demonstrated that comprehensive interdisciplinary team training using simulation-based interventions resulted in a 37% improvement in perinatal morbidity scores [10]. Training goals that focus on developing interprofessional teamwork, a reorganized approach to high-risk situations, and improving team dynamics have been linked to greater confidence in team members and fewer communication-related errors [11].

Sample Curriculum

Implementing a new process or workflow requires teamwork, collaboration, clear communication, and strong leadership. In a 125-bed suburban medical center in California's Central Valley, clinical educators led an interprofessional group of healthcare providers in a Labor and Delivery (L&D) unit to implement several newly established critical event protocols and algorithms. The protocols included common obstetrical emergencies such as eclamptic seizure, postpartum hemorrhage, shoulder dystocia, and neonatal resuscitation. Caring for complex obstetric patients required collaboration from a diverse group of providers; for example, the shoulder dystocia simulation included obstetric and neonatal nurses, respiratory therapists (RTs), obstetricians and nurse midwives, anesthesiologists, and neonatologists. Participants were provided new critical events checklists/algorithms for review before the simulation, and a team leader was identified for each drill. A pre-brief was conducted with the team to review the steps in the shoulder dystocia algorithm, discuss best practices, identify team members/leaders, and conduct a walk-through of the L&D suite to survey the location of pertinent emergency equipment and supplies. A review of the birthing manikin's operation was also demonstrated, and participants were allowed to practice obtaining vital signs and review the simulated cardiorespiratory monitor. Performance objectives for the simulation included:

1. Recognize maternal/fetal compromise and call for additional help (i.e., OB Tech/runner, infant resuscitation team, secondary provider(s), secondary nursing support, etc.).
2. Record the length of shoulder impingement by initiating a timer as soon as shoulder dystocia is announced to the team.
3. Utilize a critical events checklist to guide and record interventions.
4. Use closed-loop communication to collaborate with the team and call out the length of dystocia at 1-min intervals to maintain situational awareness.
5. Obtain emergency equipment within 2 min of request.

The simulation was conducted with a high-fidelity obstetric manikin that could simulate shoulder dystocia. Alternatively, the simulation could be conducted using a partial task trainer and a standardized patient. The patient was a 28-year-old gravida 2 para 1 at 40 weeks, 3 days, with gestational diabetes and a history of a vaginal delivery 3 years ago. Her last labor was 16 hours long and was complicated by shoulder dystocia; the infant weighed 9 pounds, 8 ounces, and suffered a fractured clavicle at birth, all risk factors for shoulder dystocia with subsequent deliveries. During the simulation, participants were told that she had been in labor for 6 hours and was fully dilated, pushing, at +3 station, indicating that the fetus' head was close to delivery. As the simulation began, the fetal heart rate (FHR) showed a Category 2 tracing, with a baseline of 140 beats per minute (bpm), with moderate variability and variable decelerations during pushing, down to 90 bpm. The FHR returned to baseline quickly after each contraction. This type of FHR pattern is typical during the pushing phase of a mother's labor and is not overly concerning. The midwife delivers the infant's head, but the shoulders become impacted in the maternal pelvis, and delivery is obstructed. As time elapses during shoulder dystocia, the situation becomes more urgent. Additional personnel are called to assist. Using the shoulder dystocia critical events checklist as a guide, the team must quickly progress through maneuvers designed to dislodge the impacted fetal head and ensure a safe delivery for the mother and the baby. These maneuvers are called out in order and with their degree of success or failure. After several minutes, the infant is delivered and handed to the neonatal resuscitation team, and the simulation is called to an end.

Debriefing this emergency process included a simulation summary and a discussion of what went well and what could be done differently next time. During the debrief, there was a review of team collaboration and human factors that may have affected the prompt delivery of the infant, clarification of the team leader, and whether the correct stakeholders were present and had the information they needed to perform their duties. The critical event checklist was compared to the events that unfolded during the scenario, revealing gaps in the process. This led to a relocation of the critical events binder in the room to make it more accessible to the team leader, a streamlined protocol to reduce redundancies in the checklist, and a clearer process for calling for additional help. The team leader also identified workflow issues with obtaining the correct equipment, and the group suggested the leader relocate to the foot of the bed to improve communication and delegation. All these workflows and QI processes were practiced multiple times with different team members until they became high functioning and proficient.

Integrating into Existing Education

Existing training for healthcare providers takes on many forms, such as instructor-led training, online or eLearning, self-guided education, and a hybrid of these models. For example, the American Heart Association (AHA) has various basic and advanced adult resuscitation training options. When integrating this training into the hospital setting, simulation educators must be creative when educating staff from different departments and aware of the participant's experience level. Existing evidenced-based resuscitation education can be augmented with in-situ and simulation lab experiences to meet the needs of various learners. This chapter will describe two examples of PI simulation integration into resuscitation education.

Example #1: Maternal Cardiac Arrest Simulation

Maternal cardiac arrest (MCA) is a rare and devastating obstetric emergency; maternal and fetal well-being depends on the speed and proficiency of resuscitation procedures [12]. Collaboration during this infrequent event requires coordinated efforts from an interprofessional group of caregivers, including obstetrics, anesthesiology, and neonatal team members who must have a shared mental model. Depending on the hospital's patient population and level of care, many obstetric and neonatal nurses will never experience this alarming patient complication. However, this does not exclude them from being prepared for this emergency if it does occur. Team training and in-situ drills are an important part of this training.

A mid-sized hospital conducted a series of in-situ simulations to prepare the staff for a potential maternal arrest. As a requirement of their work setting, all L&D nurses at the hospital received standard American Heart Association training in Advanced Cardiac Life Support (ACLS) and neonatal resuscitation. The ACLS training contained minimal education on MCA, and since this is such a rare occurrence, most nurses never applied this original training in actual patient care. Conversely, neonatal nurse education focused on neonatal resuscitation and excluded the mother's care entirely. Previous provider education was varied, with some midwives and obstetricians certified in Basic Life Support (CPR) and a handful of anesthesiologists with basic or advanced life support. A few anesthesiologists had been involved in an MCA event, but none of the obstetric or neonatal caregivers had experienced this complication.

Support from the management team was vital to the success of these drills that were conducted unannounced and on the L&D and postpartum units. Resistance from department leaders was a barrier to the training as they perceived this as an unnecessary interruption in their workday and did not believe it would ever happen in their unit. Simulation champions were recruited from nursing and physician groups to overcome reluctance and increase participation. Intensive care unit (ICU) nurses, who are experts in ACLS, were also included in this training. The ICU staff expressed confidence in their ACLS skillset except in the obstetric setting, with many reporting that they were quite nervous about working with pregnant patients and had rarely been to the maternal child departments before.

Building on their basic and advanced life support training, the curriculum included a pre-teach on the risk factors and causes of MCA, medical management, and team communications training. Storyboards, educational posters, and evidenced-based research were placed on the units for 2 weeks before the drills began for self-study. A summary of this information was reviewed during the pre-brief prior to each drill. The staff were informed that MCA drills would occur on their units but were not given specific dates and times. The simulations were planned on all three shifts in L&D and postpartum, approximately twice weekly for 10–12 weeks or until competency was achieved. This required the commitment and flexibility of multiple stakeholders over a long period of time. Several variations of the basic MCA scenario were created to educate intrapartum and postpartum teams about the causes and risk factors, and presentation varied with the timing and location of the MCA simulations. Objectives for this training included:

1. Recognize maternal unresponsiveness/change in status and activate maternal code blue to obtain help.
2. Initiate basic life support interventions within 30 s of maternal collapse.
3. Advanced life support and neonatal resuscitation teams will respond within 3 min.
4. A physician with scalpel privileges will arrive at the bedside within 3 min and initiate a perimortem Cesarean Section within 4 min of arrest.
5. Understand the rationale of performing delivery in the location of cardiac arrest instead of relocating to the operating room.
6. Communicate and delegate clearly and effectively with the team, using SBAR and closed-loop communication.

Based on these objectives, a self-created checklist was used to determine if PI measures were met. These interventions were scored as Met, Partially Met, or Not Met. The results from each drill were shared during debriefing and with department leaders. This provided a framework for the necessary changes. This tool can be recreated in any setting by utilizing a similar approach.

The first several MCA simulations exposed numerous knowledge, workflow, and performance gaps; it was eye-opening how poorly the teams performed and reinforced the need for continued training. For instance, most L&D nurses were only proficient with basic life support tasks and could not operate the defibrillator easily. The ICU nurses did not know the layout of the L&D and postpartum units and had never worked with the staff, impeding their collaboration and communication. It was unclear who should be the team leader as the obstetricians were most knowledgeable about the patient, but the anesthesiologists were more skilled with advanced life support.

As workflow issues were revealed, new processes were implemented and communicated to the group. After several weeks of drills, the team started to function more cohesively, and the new workflows, role assignments, and timed interventions improved. After several weeks of drills in L&D, these were moved to the postpartum unit, and the process started all over again with modified scenarios, new team members, and updated objectives. However, much of what was put in place in L&D also applied to postpartum, and the team started learning from and with each other.

After more than 15 MCA bi-weekly drills, the interprofessional team was performing competently, and the frequent simulations were stopped, with the plan to drill quarterly to maintain competency. Another MCA drill was held 3 months later, and the team performed well. The following day, the inevitable happened, a pregnant patient presented awake and alert but with significant shortness of breath, cardiopulmonary instability, and severe fetal distress. She was rushed to the operating room for a cesarean delivery due to fetal distress. The mother was arrested on the operating table just after the infant was delivered. The anesthesiologist took control of the situation calmly but with authority. Advanced resuscitation measures were implemented quickly and efficiently, but despite their best efforts, the mother did not survive; the baby was healthy. A critical incident debriefing followed shortly after. During this debriefing, participants expressed confidence in their previous training and remarked how grateful they were to have simulated the MCA in the months prior. Providers noted the coordination of care, team communication, and the seamless transitions between ACLS interventions. Department leaders and staff, who never thought this would happen in their unit, were stunned by the outcome. Autopsy results later revealed that the patient had a lethal, non-obstetric complication that was untreatable. While the outcome was suboptimal, the caregivers felt vindicated in providing the patients the best, most organized care possible. However, future drills were placed on hold to allow staff time to heal and regroup and not induce further trauma. Six months later, leaders requested another drill to keep everyone current. This was done in-situ, and it was obvious that some skills had been forgotten, but this was quickly remedied. Yet again, another real-life MCA event occurred within 24 h of the drill. However, this time both the patient and infant survived. The lessons learned from these cases reinforce the need for regular team training and process improvement.

Example #2: Code Blue Documentation in the Emergency Department

Experienced nurses transitioning to work in a new specialty require training on their new units' tasks, processes, and workflows, even if they were proficient in their previous specialty. Nurses transitioning to work in the Emergency Department (ED) at Scripps Health in San Diego, CA, have at least 1 year of experience or a recent graduate from the RN New Grad program. In the 12-week program, nurses developed the necessary knowledge and skills to care for the demanding and varied population of ED patients. They may or may not have experience with adult resuscitation in their previous department, and the documentation requirements are different in the ED. Resuscitation training for nurses in the ED transition program included eLearning, ACLS training, EKG interpretation, and a cardiopulmonary instability/arrest simulation. During the Coronavirus pandemic, all in-person simulations were halted, and simulation training took place virtually via an online platform. Even in normal circumstances, training for these new ED nurses revealed a knowledge gap with real-time computerized documentation during an arrest or rapid response event. A PI simulation was created to fill this gap to supplement their transition program training.

The dilemma of recording real-time interventions during a code blue or rapid response event lies with the rapidly changing environment inherent in these incidents. While it is possible to simulate a cardiac arrest so that participants can document the same interventions in real time, it is not easy to be consistent with repeated simulations, different learners, and many simulation facilitators. To reduce the inevitable variation in real-time simulations, a video was created with educators demonstrating correct ACLS interventions during a simulated code blue, with a pre-determined course of events. This code blue video was then shown to the transition program trainees, and they used it to document concurrent interventions in the electronic medical record (EMR) playground as events unfolded in the video. This code blue video is also used to train other caregivers throughout the organization and is available on a shared intranet site for easy access.

The first step in augmenting the existing training was creating the code blue simulation video. We developed the simulation with the following objective:

1. Recognize essential elements of a cardiac arrest and sequentially document all critical interventions into the Code Narrator flowsheet in the EMR so accurate information is chronicled.

During the simulation, the recorded resuscitation was played back for participants, who would then use the details from the case to document the care that occurred. The simulation used a high-fidelity manikin with integrated physiologic monitors and a laptop to control changing EKG patterns and vital signs. The video was taped in the simulation center in a room set up to mimic a bay in the ED. The scenario involved an adult male patient presenting to the ED with complaints of chest pain while doing yard work. He exhibited increasing chest pain, became unresponsive, and his cardiac rhythm showed pulseless ventricular fibrillation. The standardized participant nurse must recognize the arrest, call for help, and initiate chest compressions, and the team will follow ACLS guidelines to resuscitate the patient. The simulation was filmed using two cameras: one centered on the patient and care team and the other on the defibrillator screen. These two views were later superimposed on one another during editing, so the interventions corresponded with rhythm changes and shocks, providing the viewer with the necessary data to document all interventions concurrently. The video was created in multiple takes so that the timing of each event was accurate and flowed smoothly.

Once the video was finalized, subject matter experts used the video to document all the interventions in the computerized Code Narrator flowsheet to create an "ideal" record. Multiple simulated patients were created in a safe training environment within the EMR to allow trainees to document them during the simulation without affecting real-time documentation on inpatients. On the day of training, participants were given instructions on logging into the training environment in the EMR and accessing their patient's computerized charts. A previous review of the Code Narrator flowsheet helped them to locate the medications and interventions that might be documented during the event. The code blue video was shown, and trainees had to document 24 interventions over the 10-min resuscitation.

Following the simulation, the correct documentation was reviewed with the trainees, and this was compared to their own documentation made during the video playback. Debriefing included discussing their thoughts, feelings, and frustrations with documenting concurrently during the simulated code. Participants were probed on strategies for becoming more proficient and barriers to using the Code Narrator flowsheet during a real code or rapid response event. They shared their observations about team collaboration, role assignments, closed-loop communication, and any suggestions for next time. Lastly, they were asked to share how they could use this experience to add to their traditional ACLS training and apply it to their everyday practice.

Challenges and Solutions

Many barriers can impede successful PI simulations and system integration. When adding or expanding simulations into an existing program, many healthcare organizations discover that the cost of simulation technology and training simulation educators can be challenging. The high cost of purchasing simulation equipment, including high-fidelity manikins, audio-visual equipment, and soft goods such as disposable medical supplies and moulage, can be prohibitive. Most healthcare systems seek grants and donations and use a staggered purchase approach to overcome these barriers. Expired or outdated supplies can be procured from a hospital's central supply department and reused in the simulation center if labeled "for simulation use only" to prevent their use on actual patients. Suppose actual clinical supplies or medications are used during an in-situ simulation. In that case, these should be replaced quickly so the unit has the necessary supplies for patient care and to prevent any adverse outcomes from their absence. For example, crash cart medications used during a simulation must be proactively resupplied with a fully stocked cart so that lifesaving medications and supplies are always available.

The lack of dedicated staff and limited time and availability to devote to simulation can be mitigated by utilizing students, interns, volunteers, and non-clinical staff to assist with administrative tasks, and they can be taught to run simulation equipment and act as standardized patients. Some organizations allow those with minor work-related injuries to work temporarily in a non-clinical setting, such as an education department or simulation lab if they have medical clearance to do so. This untapped staffing resource can enhance a simulation center's personnel roster, even if it is a provisional solution.

Simulation equipment can be low fidelity or inexpensive to be effective. The use of partial task trainers, low-fidelity manikins, and repurposed equipment can lower the cost of running a simulation program. Organizations developing their program should explore alternate sites for performing PI simulation, such as an unused room or office, previously closed unit, classrooms, conference rooms, and in-situ locations. For example, a neonatal resuscitation drill can be done with a low-cost toy doll placed on a classroom table or an unused nursery location. Storyboards, paper signs, and pictures can be used to replicate the changing patient status instead of using integrated physiologic monitors. There are also many free or low-cost computer applications that can be downloaded onto a smartphone or computer tablet to simulate vital signs. When using simple and low-fidelity equipment for a simulation, it is important to obtain a fiction contract with the participants so they understand the limitations of the environment and agree to engage as if the situation were real. For instance, the lack of realism that participants may encounter when injecting medications into a manikin requires a suspension of disbelief which is a necessary part of all simulations; each learner must do their own part to make the simulation meaningful [13]. Tabletop exercises and case studies are other low-cost alternatives to in-situ or simulation lab drills and can be very effective for PI simulation training.

The development of current and future simulation educators is vital to the success of any simulation program, but it can be time-consuming and overwhelming to inexperienced educators. With a formal program in place, leaders can assess the current competency of their staff and create a faculty development plan. There are many frameworks for faculty development and assessment. The California Simulation Alliance (CSA) Model uses Patricia Benner's novice-to-expert theory to describe the steps for instructor training. [14]. Faculty need to be assessed for their experience, training, debriefing skills, scenario development, and innovation in simulation.

There are many resources for a novice or inexperienced simulation educator to gain the necessary training. Leaders should start with a review of available organizational websites and their associated conferences, such as the Society for Simulation in Healthcare and their International Meeting on Simulation in Healthcare and SimOps conferences, the National League for Nursing Simulation Innovation Resource Center, the International Nursing Association for Clinical Simulation and Learning and Drexel University's Certificate in Simulation. Numerous publications and scholarly journals support the professional development of simulation educators and operation specialists; these are readily available in print and online. Most importantly, advocating for simulation experiences to be incorporated into existing curricula and cultivating new simulation educators involves a needs assessment of current training practices and a review of barriers. Some anticipated challenges may include a lack of training, the belief that it is not a useful teaching method, a lack of funding or staffing, and a lack of experience [14]. A strategy to overcome these challenges is to identify educators who have shown an interest in being trained in simulation or those who are novices in simulation but wish to expand their skills. Experienced and certified simulation educators must mentor and train these new staff. This should be done in a safe and supportive environment; role modeling positive behaviors, demonstrating effective scenario development and debriefing techniques, allowing the new learner to engage at their own pace, and providing real-time feedback will help the learner grow and develop into an experienced simulation educator [15].

Simulation educators must also understand PI methodologies and processes. Simulationists must be able to use PI and QI tools such as failure modes and effects analysis (FMEA), RCAs, Lean, Six Sigma, and other processes discussed earlier. PI simulation is an excellent way to partner with quality/safety/risk managers to ensure high-quality, safe learning opportunities. Integrating these tools into PI simulation to investigate errors in their workplace will help ensure that these processes are used consistently throughout an organization. Sentinel events or near misses can be reconstructed in the safe environment of a simulation lab to prevent dangerous situations from reoccurring; this is best achieved when simulation educators are familiar with PI concepts and methodologies [16].

Interface with Regulatory Bodies

Regulatory agencies and professional organizations dictate accreditation requirements and clinical practice guidelines. Hospitals may describe how they will meet these standards in their written policies. In addition, they may seek accreditation and national recognition for meeting additional requirements, such as trauma center designation or stroke center certification. To achieve Stroke Center Certification, for example, hospitals must meet a rigorous set of requirements set by the AHA and American Stroke Association; this requires standardized care processes, a reduction in variation, and a low risk of complications when care is provided consistently [17]. Developing a highly reliable team of medical professionals that can effectively care for stroke patients' needs requires coordination of care and adherence to a variety of performance measures, several of which involve patient assessment and administration of thrombolytic therapies within a specific time frame. Anecdotally referred to as "door-to-needle time," this performance standard can be measured and practiced with team training. A PI simulation on improving door-to-needle time is the perfect opportunity to examine the rapid progression of the stroke patient from admission to diagnosis and, ultimately, treatment. Simulation provides a means to remove barriers and fill gaps in this high-risk, problem-prone process to achieve a door-to-needle time of 2 h or less. This requires a complex interaction between many departments and health professionals. This process is best simulated in-situ to reveal choke points during the transfer of a stroke patient from one department to another, collaboration of caregivers from different specialties, and the timely administration of intravenous thrombolytics. Information from these simulations can then be used as supportive data to show adherence to the core measures for stroke certification. Failure to meet each measure could result in an unsuccessful certification application.

Major emergencies, crises, and natural disasters have become more frequent during recent decades, with a widespread effect on countries, states, and local communities. Regulatory agencies and global organizations such as the World Health Organization (WHO), the Federal Emergency Management Institute (FEMA), and municipal governments advocate for developing Mass Casualty Incident (MCI) plans for schools, houses of worship, the healthcare community, and emergency managers at all levels [18, 19]. This is an important public health issue that can result in an even greater loss of life if governments do not prepare for these crises. Effective management of an MCI requires a coordinated effort across a wide variety of sectors. A key strategy shared in these plans is a strong recommendation for team training, MCI drills, and field exercises to test, monitor and evaluate processes to ensure effective training and education [19]. These PI simulations can be scaled up or down, depending on the level of community involvement desired and the number of agencies involved. This training can be conducted in various settings, including workplaces, schools, and healthcare institutions. Tabletop PI exercises with multiple stakeholders are logistically easier to conduct and offer an effective means to test knowledge, systems integration, and interprofessional collaboration [19]. This strategic planning can result in a better understanding of the threats and challenges of an MCI, assess and mitigate vulnerabilities, test response procedures, plan for recovery, and stay prepared for future disasters [18].

Sample Cases

A unique approach to PI simulation is using an unfolding simulation to train interprofessional preceptors at Scripps Health, a large healthcare system in San Diego, CA. Unfolding simulations evolve, typically following the progression of the same patient through their continuum of care, from an acute condition to its resolution or the point of chronic but stable illness. Participants encounter new information with each simulation that helps them develop problem-solving and decision-making skills to address each situation [21]. This unfolding simulation curriculum integrates both PI (human performance) and QI (work processes).

When using an evolving simulation to train preceptors, the focus is on building what they know, how they interact with their trainees, and promoting critical thinking rather than developing specific technical skills. We redesigned the preceptor training program to be interprofessional and included both didactic and simulation training. The new preceptor training program included a 30-minute eCourse, a 4.5-hour didactic class, and a 4-hour simulation. All courses were approved by the California Board of Registered Nursing and for Respiratory Care Practitioners in California for contact hours. An existing 30-minute eLearning course provided a foundation of knowledge before the in-person training. The eLearning included concepts of adult learning, the Educator-Coach process, strategies to elicit critical thinking, and characteristics of an effective preceptor.

Building on the eLearning, during the instructor-led training, participants were taught principles of learning styles, managing conflict, communicating to promote critical thinking, giving feedback, evaluating competency, and managing difficult situations with trainees. Small group exercises and several self-created tools were incorporated into activities on conflict resolution, the art of questioning, critical thinking practice, assessing competency, developing a coaching plan, providing feedback, and completing weekly, mid-point and final evaluations. Role plays, and videos were incorporated as teaching methods to provide variation.

Following the in-person didactic training, class participants gathered the next day at the simulation lab to apply the information learned. To train these new preceptors, a fictional case study was presented as a framework for the progressive simulations. This case study included a brief biography of the fictional preceptor, trainee, and the patient they have been assigned to care for. While knowledge of the patient's clinical diagnosis and medical condition was not essential to this training, it did provide context for the preceptor/trainee relationship. The simulations were intentionally designed to be interprofessional rather than nursing-centric, so this training could apply to the many types of clinicians who precept new hires or experienced employees training in a new specialty. Registered Nurses, Occupational Therapists, Physical Therapists, case managers, and surgical and ultrasound techs have been trained with this curriculum from specialties such as medical/surgical, maternal child, ED, operating room, ICU, and case management departments. A key aspect of PI team training is interprofessional collaboration and caregiver communication. The Joint Commission reported that communication and teamwork issues were the most common contributors to both unexpected deaths and injuries [20]; improving the communication, coaching, and feedback between the trainee and preceptor are the goals of this training.

Following the didactic portion, participants were brought to the simulation center at the hospital's Magnet-certified facility, where they practiced applying the principles learned in the classroom during a 4-hour progressive simulation session. This non-traditional unfolding simulation includes four scenarios that build on each other. The first scenario introduces the participants to the fictional preceptor and trainee working on a medical/surgical unit caring for a homeless woman admitted recently in a hyperosmolar hyperglycemic state and a severely infected foot. This first scenario is composed of a series of case studies that the new preceptors must use to assess their trainees' conflict and learning styles. As the case studies unfold, additional details are provided on the patient's compromised medical condition so that the participants can practice communication principles with one another. Prepared videos are used as a facilitation technique to demonstrate examples of appropriate and improper mentoring; small group role plays, and a group debriefing provides an opportunity to practice these difficult conversations.

Following the case study scenario, participants move on to the second simulation. This simulation will be a scripted role-play of a disorganized and distracted trainee. Participants are assigned roles that may be the same as their clinical roles in real life. Roles included in this simulation include the patient, preceptor, trainee, respitaroty therapist, desk clerk, provider, and X-Ray technician; because these roles are flexible, they can be replicated in almost any setting by choosing the roles that apply to an institution or work setting. Participants are only asked to perform tasks they are already competent in. They all receive coaching from the facilitator and a sample script to follow. Objectives in this scenario include:

1. Fosters accurate clinical judgment/critical thinking while guiding the trainee in determining the priority level for competing tasks.
2. Assists trainee to determine appropriate resources for assistance based on the patient's need.
3. Implement coaching tools to assist trainees with identified needs/gaps in performance.

This unfolding simulation follows the same patient presented in the first scenario/case study. The trainee is easily flustered, disorganized, and overwhelmed from the very beginning of the scenario. New grads and employees transitioning to a new role frequently struggle with prioritization and assessment skills. Developing organizational skills will help the trainee be more efficient and reduce potential errors. Improving prioritization and assessment skills is a dynamic process measured at multiple points as the trainee grows throughout their mentorship period. Written feedback tools, discussed later in this sample case, gauge progress and areas of weakness so that PI and QI can be continually assessed.

It is well established that simulation can improve team communication and reveal latent safety threats inherent in many healthcare processes. In this second progressive scenario, the preceptor helps the trainee refocus and reprioritize to manage the patient's hypoglycemia by reviewing a decision tree which is provided as a handout. Participants are reminded that the focus is on collaborative communication, improved patient safety, and the development of critical reasoning rather than how to manage the clinical situation. The clinical state is merely a vessel to provide a framework to work within. It does not matter that the patient is hypoglycemic; the focus is on how to help the trainee problem-solve and prioritize. As the trainee acquires better prioritization skills, she will become more resourceful and able to see the bigger picture. These are essential skills of any clinician.

As this role play progresses, the trainee refocuses, gradually becoming more confident in her abilities; she leaves the preceptor in the room with the patient to obtain medication to manage the patient's hypoglycemia. However, on her way to the medication room, she encounters a series of pre-planned interruptions that distract her, mimicking real life. These multiple distractions cause the trainee to lose focus again, and she fails to administer the appropriate medication timely, resulting in the preceptor intervening to prevent harm to the patient. The scenario ends with the preceptor and training regrouping away from the patient to discuss the next steps.

Applying newly acquired communication skills occurs with the group debriefing, including developing training goals and a coaching plan. Debriefing prompts include a review of techniques to help focus the trainee, a discussion on how to encourage critical thinking, how to guide without taking over, and how to protect the trainee from making critical mistakes that could impact patient care. Simulating these crucial conversations can improve interprofessional teamwork, which leads to better team dynamics and fewer communication-related errors. PI simulations like this one, which focus on human performance and teamwork, can also improve patient safety.

The unfolding simulation continues with the third scenario, using the same patient. The patient has been hospitalized for 2 weeks, and her blood glucose has stabilized. Unfortunately, she has developed hospital-acquired pneumonia and a worsening infection in her foot. This scenario uses a high-fidelity manikin for the patient instead of the standardized patient in the second scenario; the patient will slowly deteriorate with signs of impending sepsis but will not become critically ill. The standardized participant/trainee in this scenario is privately coached by the facilitator to purposefully make mistakes and act insecure and uncertain about the clinical picture so that the preceptor must coach her in decision-making. The preceptor is given a communication and critical decision-making tool introduced during the didactic class to assist her with Socratic questioning of her trainee. The trainee must improve their clinical reasoning and critical thinking as these skills are linked to improved patient safety and fewer medical errors. The preceptor's role of protector is highlighted in this scenario to demonstrate the importance of giving and receiving constructive feedback and establishing a safe environment for asking questions. When the preceptor/trainee dyad has a psychologically safe relationship and open to feedback, common goals can be expressed, and the direct impact of their actions and/or inactions are reflected in better patient outcomes.

The objectives include:

1. Integrate questions and prompts to assist the trainee in understanding and managing the situation.
2. Guide the trainee by reflecting on the deteriorating situation and subsequent learning needs.
3. Facilitates problem-solving and critical thinking and is available to answer questions.
4. Applies a safe level of autonomy to allow for professional growth while still providing guidance and support.

The scenario starts with a vague and incomplete handoff from the previous shift to the preceptor and trainee. As often occurs in real life, the assessed clinical picture is more serious than what was reported by the off-going nurse. The preceptor must ask multiple questions to guide the trainee into recognizing the deteriorating situation without giving the answers directly. The trainee determines that sepsis is the likely diagnosis, and she must call the provider. This SBAR report is purposefully riddled with missing information, as can occur with a novice nurse, and the preceptor must guide clinical reasoning and problem-solving to intervene appropriately. Once a plan of action is established, the scenario is called to an end. The focus continues to be on improving critical thinking, decision-making, and team communication, not managing sepsis. Observation checklists can be provided to those not actively participating if the group is large. Written at a mid-level for learners, this scenario can be flexed to increase complexity for high-level learners or simplified for novice or non-clinical participants.

Debriefing this scenario includes acknowledging the clinical pictures presented and applying that to true-to-life situations. Debriefing prompts also include discussing the trainee's ability to detect clinical changes and how to guide clinical reasoning without taking over. The degree of autonomy to give new trainees is often subjective and will differ with each person, so this is a good time to explore when to "cut the apron strings" to allow more independent practice while still protecting them from harm. Strategies for providing various degrees of supervision can be examined and guidelines set for future supervision and progressive independence as competence develops. This is a good example of continuous QI as progress is evaluated incrementally over their training period, and plans are made to address behaviors, attitudes, communication concerns, and psychomotor skills that do not meet standards.

Lastly, the group comes together for the final scenario, which includes a case study and role plays on providing feedback and evaluation. Evaluation tools presented in the didactic class are again reviewed, and the group discusses how and when to provide feedback. Effective evaluation tools include cognitive, psychomotor, and affective skills to appraise human performance and adherence to work processes/policies. Providing effective feedback and honest observations are important PI and QI strategies to improve the trainee's performance. Without knowing how to improve specifically, the trainee will not grow professionally, and bad habits/shortcuts may develop; patient safety is threatened, and errors occur. Accurate and detailed feedback shows the trainee where their strengths and weaknesses lie so that performance standards can be met and new goals set each week to ensure progress. As learning goals are met, the trainee becomes more proficient, and the close mentoring and supervision gradually lessen.

Learning to evaluate the trainee accurately and effectively is the final step in becoming an excellent preceptor. The storyline of this progressive simulation continues: The preceptor and trainee have been working together for several weeks and are at the mid-point of the training period. A summary of the trainee's progress is provided, and a video is shown to demonstrate an evaluation discussion between the preceptor and trainee. Using the concepts shown in the video, participants work in small groups to complete weekly and mid-point evaluation forms. Performance gaps are discussed, and a remediation plan is created to address those gaps. Participants share their learnings with the larger group and how they rated the fictional trainee's accomplishments, behaviors, communication concerns, educational goals, and strategies for a successful transition to independent practice. These PI and QI learnings are then incorporated into the trainee's precepting plan so that the trainees will become safe, high-quality, independent patient care providers.

The evolving nature of this progressive simulation case lends itself to examining the dynamics between the preceptor/trainee team. It can provide opportunities to problem-solve and mentor new employees in situations that mimic real life. The flexible modality provides the platform to immerse participants in experiences or situations they will likely encounter in their first few months of mentoring a new employee [21]. The challenges of inefficient workflows and processes that affect multiple audiences can also be easily explored and their potential solutions tested.

Course evaluations and participant feedback provided PI and QI suggestions for improvement for this multi-faceted preceptor program. The evaluation tools were updated to provide more clarity and easier completion, including the ability to complete them electronically. All materials and resources from the program were placed on a shared intranet site for quick utilization and reference. Previous attendees and leaders recently requested advanced preceptor education to enhance their core training. This led to the creation of monthly 1-h supplemental preceptor classes that include how to conduct difficult conversions with your trainee, practical tips to help your new grad succeed, and how to help your trainee successfully transition to practice once the initial training period is over. These are held virtually and include an open discussion forum where new and veteran preceptors can collaborate with one another on current challenges they are experiencing. Response to the supplemental training will be reevaluated in 6 months to determine if additional or new topics are needed.

Summary

Performance and process improvement simulations can address the many processes, systems, and communication errors inherent in healthcare today. Team training is an important component of PI simulation as staff collaborate with various professionals in the acute care setting. These PI and QI simulations can expose knowledge gaps, workflow issues, and inefficient systems that impede safe patient care. There are creative ways to incorporate PI simulation, including resuscitation and preceptor training, new forms or processes such as a critical events checklist, program certification readiness, disaster preparedness, and the analysis of poor patient outcomes.

References

1. White S. What is process improvement? A business methodology for efficiency and productivity. CIO. 2021. https://www.cio.com/article/3433946/what-is-process-improvement-a-business-methodology-for-efficiency-and-productivity.html.
2. Rider A, Schertzer K. Quality improvement in medical simulation. Ncbi.nlm.nih.gov. 2021. https://www.ncbi.nlm.nih.gov/books/NBK551497/.
3. Gaba D. The future vision of simulation in health care. Quality and Safety in Health Care. 2004;13(suppl_1):i2–i10. https://doi.org/10.1136/qshc.2004.009878.
4. A Brief History of Lean. Lean.org. 2021. https://www.lean.org/WhatsLean/History.cfm.
5. Reid C. A brief history of the process: from the industrial revolution to today. Process excellence. Network. 2021; https://www.processexcellencenetwork.com/lean-six-sigma-business-performance/articles/a-brief-history-of-process-from-the-industrial-re
6. Haskins, J. 20 years of patient safety. Association of American Medical Colleges. 2019. https://www.aamc.org/news-insights/20-years-patient-safety.
7. Sanko J, Mckay M. Participation in a system-thinking simulation experience changes adverse event reporting. Simul Healthc. 2020;15(3):167–71. https://doi.org/10.1097/SIH.0000000000000473.
8. Munzer B, Bassin B, Peterson W, Tucker R, Doan J, Harvey C, et al. In-situ simulation use for rapid implementation and process improvement of COVID-19 airway management. Western Journal of Emergency Medicine. 2020;21(6):99–106.
9. Pronovost P, Holzmueller C, Ennen C, Fox H. Overview of progress in patient safety. Am J Obstetrics and Gynecology. 2011;204(1):5–10.
10. Riley W, Davis S, Miller K, Hansen H, Sainfort F, Sweet R. Didactic and simulation nontechnical skills team training to improve perinatal patient outcomes in a community hospital. Jt Comm J Qual Patient Saf. 2011;37(8):357–64.
11. Harwayne-Gidansky I, Panesar R, Maa T. Recent advances in simulation for pediatric critical care medicine. Intensive Care Med. 2020;8(4):147–56. https://doi.org/10.1007/s40124-00226-5.
12. Fischer C, Bonnet M, Girault A, Le Ray C. Update: focus in-hospital maternal cardiac arrest. J Gynecol Obstet Hum Reprod. 2019;48(5):309–14.
13. Lopreiato JO. Healthcare simulation dictionary. Rockville, MD: Agency for Healthcare Research and Quality; 2016. AHRQ publication no. 16(17)-0043
14. Waxman K, Telles C. The use of Benner's framework in high-fidelity simulation faculty development. Clin Simul Nurs. 2009;5(6):e231–5. https://doi.org/10.1016/j.ecns.2009.06.001.
15. Wilson L, Wittmann-Price R. Review manual for the certified healthcare simulation educator (CHSE™) exam. New York, NY: Springer Publishing Company, LLC; 2015.
16. Maxworthy J, Kutzin J. Quality improvement. In: Palganas J, Maxworthy J, Epps C, Mancini M, editors. Defining excellence in simulation programs. 1st ed. China: Wolters Kluwer; 2015. p. 49–63.
17. American Heart Association/American Stroke Association. Primary stroke center certification overview sheet. Heart.org. https://www.heart.org/idc/groups/heart-public/@wcm/@hcm/@ml/documents/downloadable/ucm_455522.pdf.
18. Federal Emergency Management Institute. IS-360: Preparing for mass casualty incidents. A guide for schools, higher education, and houses of worship. 2013. https://training.fema.gov/is/courseoverview.aspx?code=IS-360.
19. Guise J, Segel S. Teamwork in obstetric critical care. Best Practice & Research Clinical Obstetrics and Gynaecology. 2008;22(5):937–51.
20. World Health Organization. Mass casualty management systems. Strategies and guidelines for building health sector capacity. 2007. https://www.who.int/hac/techguidance/MCM_guidelines_inside_final.pdf.
21. Cato M, Cleary J, Reese C, Boese T. Unfolding simulation cases: purpose and process. In: Jeffries P, editor. Clinical simulations in nursing education. Baltimore, MD: National League for Nursing; 2014. p. 122–34.

Interprofessional Simulations

37

Lygia L. Arcaro and Richard L. Fidler

Introduction

Clinical simulation for healthcare education and training is a widely accepted platform for experiential learning. Clinical simulation commonly occurs in professional silos, where nurses train nurses and physicians train physicians, but this does not replicate how healthcare providers truly practice. Although there is a clear role for skills-based simulation to be profession-specific, higher-level application of simulation activities incorporates interprofessional participant groups that more closely resemble the healthcare delivery teams that reflect contemporary practice. As an integral part of skills-based training that may occur in silos, the concepts of interprofessional interactions in clinical simulations should be introduced to participants so they can be aware of the benefits of training the same way they practice. This should include content to improve communication, role delineation, and teamwork based on the crew resource management framework.

More recent clinical simulation strategies use simulation techniques as an integral part of quality management, patient safety, process evaluation, process improvement, and root cause analyses of untoward clinical events. The first half of this chapter will describe the uses of interprofessional simulations on a macro level for hospital activations, where new hospital systems, processes, and infrastructure are tested using clinical simulation as the vehicle for detecting latent threats to patient safety. A simple model for systems analysis using interprofessional simulations will be introduced in the second half of the chapter. This conceptual model will be presented as an unfolding case example used in the interprofessional implementation of an operating room designated for surgical care of COVID-19 patients as an example of a local-level change in practice.

L. L. Arcaro
VHA National Simulation Center, SimLEARN, Orlando, FL, USA
e-mail: Lygia.Arcaro@va.gov

R. L. Fidler (✉)
Director Advanced Fellowship in Clinical Simulation,
San Francisco VA Medical Center, San Francisco, CA, USA

Department of Physiological Nursing, University of California San Francisco, San Francisco, CA, USA

Background

According to the Department of Veteran Affairs, approximately 9.8 million Veterans used at least one of their Veteran benefits in 2017, and the VHA cared for approximately 6.1 million veterans [1]. Prior to 2012, and the planned opening of the VA Southern Nevada Health Care System, there had not been funded the construction of a Department of Veterans Affairs medical center since the West Palm Beach location was approved, built, and opened 17 years earlier at the end of the Gulf War. With more additional new construction or replacement VHA hospitals planned, identifying latent safety threats and hazards before patient occupancy became crucial. Herzer's five-phase framework for hospital activations was adapted to mitigate harm to any patient, staff, or visitors before opening a healthcare facility [2]. Uncovering hazards and systems defects prior to an untoward event should be a paramount concern for any new, replacement, or remodeled healthcare facility.

Herzer et al. defined a hazard as any event that could harm a patient and a defect as any clinical or operational occurrence that should not be repeated. Hospital activations is the term used by VHA/SimLEARN to test the physical spaces, equipment, processes, and workflows prior to opening for patient care services. The goals of activation evaluations should strive to uncover, reduce, or eliminate the risk associated with patient injury [2]. The five phases of the framework were categorized to:

1. Identify existing knowledge of hazards and defenses.
2. Anticipate what can go wrong.
3. Simulate the process.
4. Analyze hazards and defects.
5. Design a system to defend against hazards.

J. M. Kutzin et al. (eds.), *Comprehensive Healthcare Simulation: Nursing*, Comprehensive Healthcare Simulation,
https://doi.org/10.1007/978-3-031-31090-4_37

A Healthcare Failure Mode and Effects Analysis (HFMEA) was developed by the VHA National Center for Patient Safety to include the severity, probability, and risk of the hazards from the simulations to avoid any events after opening [3, 4]. The VHA's Vision, Principles, and Values for High-Reliability Organization (HRO) states that affirming the trust of Veterans and their families is paramount throughout the journey toward achieving zero harm and an unmatched experience. Using the Herzer model, the phases correlate to the principles and values the VHA holds in high regard. Phase 1, identifying existing knowledge of hazards and defenses, is an important aspect of achieving high reliability through deference to expertise (principle) when identifying existing knowledge of hazards and defenses and including and integrating the staff working around in-situ simulation. Clinical and non-clinical interprofessional front-line staff are cognizant of the care and services in the area. They are cognizant of the challenges and how to possibly solve them through recommendations of the tested categories of the simulations—equipment, staff, use of space, response to emergencies, and policies governing actions. The simulation activations team uses feedback and observations from the healthcare staff as recommendations for developing future curricula. A subsequent report is given to the medical center executive leadership team, combining the recommendations from the activation team and the employees who participated in the simulations directly or as observers.

Phase 2, anticipating what can go wrong, addresses anticipation of components of care delivery that may fail. To anticipate what can go wrong is the principle of preoccupation with failure. Simulation scenarios for expected patient care workflows are developed to test processes in the new location to determine additions and deletions to policies and procedures that will guide the staff once the building is occupied. The risk is also anticipated during this phase, and each staff member is considered a problem solver.

In-situ simulation occurs in Phase 3, simulating the process, demonstrating the High-Reliability Organization (HRO) principle of preoccupation with failure and the value of committing to zero harm. During this phase, hazards are uncovered by the staff during the simulation. Interprofessional observers record identified hazards or defects from the simulation, and the team leader may guide the simulation in a different direction based on the unfolding of the workflow's real-time results. Immediate debriefing takes place in Phase 4, analyzing hazards and defects. Once again, interprofessional staff closest to the tested workflow(s) will address opportunities for improvement and present possible solutions to decrease the risk level prior to patient occupancy. In addition to the observers, each staff member present must speak up and uphold this value continuing the HRO journey.

An important component of this phase is the use of the Failure Mode Effect Analysis (FMEA). Consistent with Herzer's (2009) framework, this step determines the severity, probability, and risk of the potential hazard identified during testing. A Patient Care Improvement matrix was developed using an already familiar document from the Department of Veterans Affairs National Center for Patient Safety. This allowed a description of the hazard and categorized the frequency, hazard rating, and acceptability of the hazard risk.

Lastly, Phase 5, the design system to defend against hazards, contains the mitigation plan developed to report findings and solutions consistent with accepted clinical practices and safety management. The plan contained strategies and efforts towards the components of the workflows tested: recommendations affecting equipment, staff, use of space and workflows, response to emergencies, and suggested policies for development.

Best Practices

Interprofessional Simulation for Process Evaluation and Improvement

In 2009 an Executive Decision Memo (EDM) was signed, creating a new organization under the VA Employee Education System. This new organization was called the Simulation Learning, Education, and Research Network (SimLEARN). However, in 2021 the name slightly changed to better reflect a realignment of SimLEARN under the Office of Healthcare, Innovation, and Learning. This organization is now known as the Simulation, Learning, Evaluation, Assessment, and Research Network, keeping the original SimLEARN acronym.

A decision was made to build a brand-new VA hospital in Las Vegas, Nevada. Hospital administration sought assistance in preparing staff and anticipating unforeseen hazards prior to patient occupancy. Before constructing the new facility, veterans were provided care through a joint venture with the US Air Force at the Mike O'Callaghan Federal Hospital in Las Vegas, Nevada. This new Las Vegas VHA facility would be an independent Department of Veterans Affairs hospital staffed with all VHA employees. The VHA had early adopters who used healthcare simulation for education; however, the concept of hazard mitigation via healthcare simulation was new to most employees. Education sessions were implemented prior to testing scenarios using SimLEARN employees as standardized participants and facilitators. One challenge to the employees was understanding the changes related to a brand-new building, new employees who have not previously worked for the VA, staff who had never worked together before, and the multiple expansive patient care locations. As a

High-Reliability Organization, the VHA used simulation to explore commonalities and differences in patient care from the old organization to the new with an understanding of the commitment to zero harm. Simulating patient care experiences provided the opportunity to highlight the upcoming new services provided to patients and helped teams to explore and plan how to mitigate potential errors.

Simulations were performed in numerous areas of the facility prior to the hospital's opening. Inside and outside the building, simulations traced patient processes, such as patients entering the facility on foot, those brought in by family members, and those brought by ambulance. All clinical and administrative service areas were used to test scenarios involving patients, staff members, family members, and visitors. The parking lots, administrative areas, and staff offices were not off-limits. The distinct processes tested focused on patient interactions, staff, and their workflows. Other factors affecting processes included new equipment and emergency responses. Diagnostic areas of the facility housing the CT Scanner, Laboratory, Radiology, or common locations such as the Cafeteria (called a canteen in VHA) and the Retail Store were used to simulate situations such as a patient in distress while their blood is being drawn, an employee suffering burns from the steam in the kitchen, a disruptive visitor raising their voice loudly while requesting service, and cardiopulmonary arrest and resuscitation.

Within the Herzer [2] framework, SimLEARN developed steps for a successful hospital activation, or Simulation Testing Phases, that includes the categories below known as the Hazard Identification and Mitigation Plan (HIMP).

- Planning—developing action plan, timeline, goals, and logistics with interprofessional subject matter experts.
- Pre-assessment—probing interprofessional subject matter experts for what new services, processes, and procedures are anticipated; questioning "what keeps you up at night" related to patient safety and care; creating FMEA.
- Testing/Assessment—simulation testing and case unfolding while assessing the environmental/other factors contributing to the simulation outcomes/results (equipment, staff, space, response to emergencies, and proposed policy enhancement/development). Interprofessional team debriefing; maintain FMEA.
- Evaluation—review and prioritize all results using a probability scale; assign priority risk levels to finish the FMEA and inform executive and senior leadership of results.
- Mitigation—determine what issues need improvement, such as systems redesign, process improvements, education, need for development, and/or changes to policies and procedures. Identify any team behaviors to strengthen individual and collaborative practice and socialization in a new organization and location.

Examples of Simulated Results (Taken from Several VA Locations Prior to Patient Occupancy)

Opportunity for improvement	Scenario(s)	Probing results/outcomes	Mitigation
Lack of long-range phone signal	Collapsed person in an extremely long hallway	Notification untimely for emergency	Cell phone signal booster Hall monitor Check the function of wall emergency call boxes
Questionable integrity of surgical instruments	Ophthalmology OR procedure	Procedure was stalled	Notify supply section Replace instruments Change vendor if indicated
Lack of emergency equipment	Person unresponsive in bus stop hut	CPR started timely waited for AED to arrive	AED in each police car Handoff AED to the next shift
Inform purpose of live phone number	Call for help from the parking lot	The parking lot helpline had no incidents after the simulation	Provide role description to workers and operator in case of emergency outside the building (unoccupied) Relocate the phone number when the hospital is operational
First-line medication not available	Person with nosebleed	Treatment delay	Review/update formulary specifically for the emergency department from an urgent care setting
Inform the end location of emergency buttons once activated	I pulled the emergency button during a walk-through of the clinic	Unclear who will answer the call for assistance/help	Alert appropriate staff internally/externally of procedure when emergency buttons are used or tested
Consider possible etiology for code blue	Allergic reaction leading to cardiac arrest	Choking patient in the canteen (cafeteria) dining area	Heart saver class Wall signs for steps in choking sequence
Collision points at hall intersections	Revealed during walk-through	Occupied wheelchair and supply cart moving at the same time Added to debriefing discussion	Install convex mirrors on walls
Child choking hazard	Revealed during a debriefing discussion from a pediatric code blue	Added to the debriefing discussion as a possible etiology of code blue	Remove decorative rocks in planters sitting on the floor

After invitations were sent from the Las Vegas VA Healthcare System, funding was made available, travel plans were confirmed, and the SimLEARN team prepared the schedule for simulation testing. The phases of planning and pre-assessment were completed, and the team was provided assignments and a general overview of each session, including the flow of the simulations. Once the simulation team arrived at the assigned location, interprofessional staff members from the unit were given introductions to the simulation team and introduced themselves. Prebriefing included information regarding healthcare simulation and various roles such as learner, standardized participant, recorder, and observer. The concepts of evaluation and hazard mitigation were explained to all participants to ensure their knowledge of the process. Consent forms were signed, and the simulation technicians were concomitantly setting the stage where the simulation would begin. Once debriefing was completed, the process was explained again, and questions were answered before moving to the next simulation.

Simulations described in this chapter were carried out in VA facilities prior to any patient occupying the facilities. Hospital staff participated in scenario testing using a combination of both high and low-fidelity manikins while uncovering risks and hazards according to Herzer's definitions [2]. For example, a long corridor was in the facility's basement where some hospital service offices were located. After setting up the simulation of a person lying on the floor in need of help, the team found the telephone system did not interact with the paging system, and the emergency box on the wall was not operational that day (after being operational earlier). Another simultaneous surgical scenario started at the check-in desk and followed the patient through the entire journey to the operating room. After the manikin was positioned for ophthalmic surgery, it was discovered that several brand-new surgical scissors were sticking at their hinges despite having been lubricated by the supply staff.

Simulations were not confined to inside the building and were performed outside in the parking lot or on the grounds as well. A cardiac arrest simulation was staged in a small enclosure with a bench, and two important results were obtained: not all the police cars patrolling the grounds had an AED (automated external defibrillator), and the emergency call button did not ring at the operator's location but rather rang at an extension in the free-standing VA warehouse. During a clinic walk-through and visually inspecting for emergency equipment, lights, and call buttons, staff who would be working in that area needed to know the location of the emergency buttons. When one member of the simulation team activated the emergency button, instead of VA police responding, two city police officers responded.

Considering the location of an emergency helps to determine possible etiologies of a standardized participant who simulates choking, which leads to an observed cardiac arrest. This was the simulation for the patient who was allergic to peanut butter in a candy bar being eaten in the cafeteria. Staff was encouraged to investigate all surroundings and begin anticipating "what ifs" while monitoring the environment before patients, visitors, volunteers, trainees, or others are finally allowed to enter a facility. Decorative rocks in planters were aesthetically attractive and could have been extremely dangerous to children in a waiting area; this was noted after a pediatric code blue simulation took place at the same location.

Debriefing after each scenario helped the simulation team gather interprofessional solutions to the hazards and risks uncovered and discussed. Interprofessional staff who participated in the simulation roles and worked in the area being tested shared with the simulation team:

(a) Concerns for any new services starting with the opening of the new location.
(b) Concerns for continued services and how to adapt to the new location.
(c) Challenges of many new staff having never worked together.

Suggestions made by the simulation team included education of the staff on any new policies needed or to be developed and the opportunity to re-simulate. Consultations with other subject matter experts were suggested or done when a level of expertise was absent on this team.

At the end of each episode of simulation testing, a slide presentation provided an overview of findings with a verbal presentation highlighting the most important findings to the senior leaders and other employees. Using the Patient Care Improvement Matrix allowed a description of the hazard, then categorized the frequency, hazard rating, and acceptability of the hazard risk. Leaders were immediately informed of the most severe hazards and risks, while others who were less severe were followed up with a written report.

Facility Level Application of Interprofessional Simulations--Applied Conceptual Model

Although clinical simulation has been established as an educational tool, this chapter focuses on interprofessional simulation for education, process evaluation, and systems probing. Clinical simulation as a tool and vehicle for process evaluation and improvement applies the strategies of clinical simulation in a similar method; however, the focus is not solely on educating the individuals or team. The focus is on the use of simulation for conducting SWOT (Strengths-Weaknesses-Opportunities-Threats) analyses [5]. Although some organizations adopt models or frameworks like LEAN or Six Sigma, these were designed for other industries and then

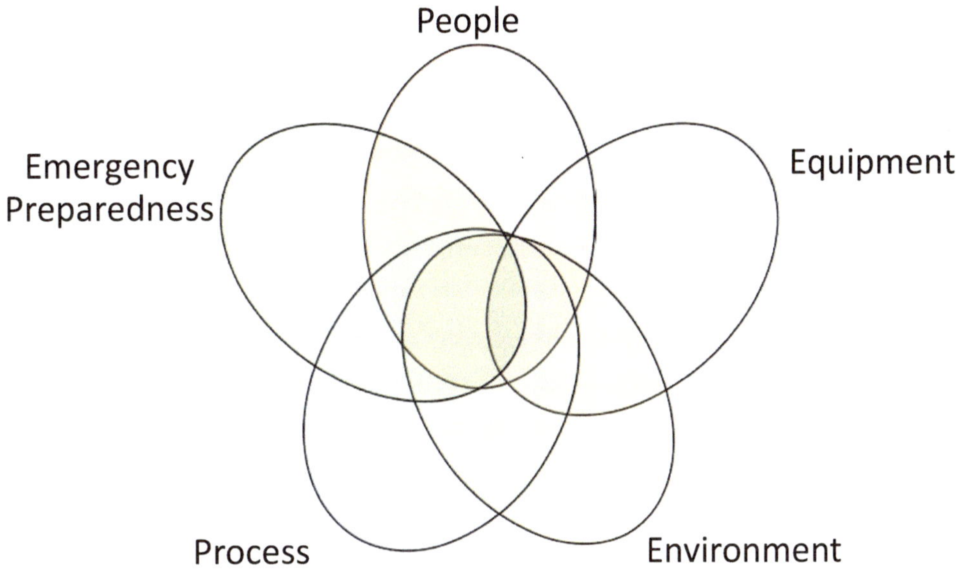

Fig. 37.1 PEEPEp model for continuous process evaluation

applied to healthcare [6–9]. With programs like LEAN and Six Sigma, a standardized curriculum provides some problem-solving framework, usually at a cost to the individual or the institution. These frameworks are sometimes criticized for being too superficial and not having industry-specific operational definitions available [6–8].

In this section, we will describe a conceptual model developed specifically for interprofessional healthcare processes and has been used successfully multiple times in process evaluation and continuous process improvement cycles. The conceptual model helps to organize the key elements of understanding a healthcare process, examining the interrelated components, and then applying iteratively to develop the process. We will first describe the elements of the model, then describe the real-world application of the PEEPEp framework as it was used to develop and establish a COVID-19-compliant operating room.

PEEPEp Model for Continuous Process Evaluation

Before understanding any process or phenomenon, it is important to have a strategy to organize, conceptualize, and understand the process containing all its components. The PEEPEp model is an easy-to-understand conceptual model for process evaluation and continuous process improvement. (Fig. 37.1). Although many believe a policy or procedure is a static document, optimization of clinical outcomes can be a simulation-based iterative evaluation of policies and procedures to incorporate new evidence. Interprofessional simulations allow exploration before implementing the new practices, and the interprofessional team can feel co-ownership of the policy and procedures developed from their input. The arrows surrounding the Venn diagram emphasize the continuous evaluative part of this conceptual model (Fig. 37.1).

In the following section, we will describe the application of the PEEPEp conceptual model to the development of a COVID-19-compliant operating room. The goals of developing this specialized operating room were to minimize contamination of the hospital, especially other operating rooms; minimize the risk of COVID-19 exposure to perioperative staff members; and maintain high-quality surgical infection prevention. Since the COVID-19 operating room could be used by any surgical specialty, multiple attending surgeons provided insight and participation in interprofessional simulations.

Sample Curriculum

COVID-Operating Room (OR) Development: A Case-Based Approach to Simulation-Based Process Evaluation and Improvement.

People

Although all the components of the PEEPEp model are crucial to successful processes, people are involved in every element of the PEEPEp model. Identifying all stakeholders from each of the five components of the PEEPEp model is important for interprofessional representation and input to optimize the output of the simulations. Scheduling all the key stakeholders together for interprofessional simulations at the same time is typically the biggest hurdle to overcome. This section focuses specifically on the involvement of clinical staff in directly delivering the healthcare service. Later, other care team members will be discussed as they relate to other components of the PEEPEp model. The learners/trainees/staff involved in each of the components of "environment," "equipment," "process," and "emergency preparation" will all be discussed in detail as each component of the model is presented and discussed.

All interprofessional simulations aimed at process evaluation and improvement require the right staff to be present to be successful. In creating a COVID-19 operating room, the clinical team of surgeons of various specialties, anesthesia providers, operating room nurses, and scrub techs were the right staff. Because there would only be one COVID-OR, all surgical specialties needed to be able to perform surgery in this space. Representatives from general, vascular, cardiothoracic, orthopedic, neurological, and podiatric surgery participated actively in the interprofessional simulations at all stages. To be successful, the simulations would have to produce a tangible output of a streamlined policy and procedure for the surgical care of the COVID-19 patient from preoperative evaluation through surgery and recovery. A stepwise progression ensued for the interprofessional simulations, with increasing levels of fidelity, set up, and analysis.

First, virtual meetings were conducted to create storyboards and tabletop-style interprofessional simulations that outlined specific clinical issues necessary to perform any surgery for any specialty. Several virtual tabletop simulations were conducted using hypothetical cases. The sample vignettes discussed were COVID-positive patients who needed to undergo cholecystectomy, lower extremity wound debridement, femur fracture for open reduction-internal fixation, and subdural hematoma evacuation.

Second, physical walkthroughs of the clinical spaces, examination of the minimum equipment sets for surgery, minimizing contamination risk moving COVID-positive patients through the hospital, and concerns regarding personal protective equipment (PPE) were addressed. Several iterations were developed during the walkthrough process explorations to identify barriers to success. These included patients coming from the emergency department (ED), the medical-surgical (MS) floor, and the intensive care unit (ICU) directly to the COVID operating room (COVID-OR). Input and buy-in were obtained from clinical nurse leaders and nurse managers in each patient care location, and they also sent staff who participated in the physical simulations.

Lastly, in-person simulations were conducted to test the process and systems developed. Each scenario was conducted using a high-fidelity manikin as the patient and the actual interprofessional team members performed their expected duties from preoperative evaluation, surgical setup, donning PPE, bidirectional communication between the healthcare team outside and inside the operating room, recovering the patient in the operating room, and finally delivering the postoperative patient to their destination unit. These simulations included documentation in the electronic health record under a test patient file. To test this process, a multi-departmental scenario was conducted. The scenario started with a COVID-positive patient who presented to the Emergency Department with altered mental status that required a CT scan of the brain and neurosurgical craniotomy for evacuation of a subdural hematoma. The scenario ended with the postoperative transfer of the patient to the ICU on a ventilator.

Equipment

In healthcare, equipment that is used for clinical care is often complex, requires training to operate, and may be specialized for just one procedure or task. Examples of specialized equipment are fluoroscopy for vascular surgery and cardiopulmonary bypass for cardiac surgery. Since many clinical processes in healthcare require a preparation phase, a procedural phase, a recovery component, and eventual disposition, the equipment that will be needed to support the patient intervention across all departments and phases of the process should be considered. The equipment interacts significantly with the other elements of the model to varying degrees depending on the state of process development. In the PEEPEp model, the equipment interacts with the people by training clinical staff to operate the equipment and biomedical engineering to maintain it. Equipment interacts with the environment since it will likely require electrical power, pipeline gases, physical space, and interaction with other pieces of equipment in the environment. Equipment will factor into the process component of the model to facilitate a procedure. For example, robotic surgery cannot be accomplished without the robot, and the robot as equipment in the PEEPEp model interacts with the people operating the robot, the environment where it occupies space and uses power, and is the major factor in the actual process of performing robotic surgery.

In our case example of creating a COVID-OR, interprofessional collaboration was expanded to involve biomedical engineering, which handles all the clinical equipment concerns for the facility, from ordering new equipment, maintaining current equipment, and repairing broken equipment. In this case, our process redesign to provide surgical care to the COVID-19-positive patient required the same equipment as standard surgical patients, without any modifications. Surgical instruments are sterilized using universal precautions by the sterile processing personnel, so no change was needed in the normal process for surgical instruments as equipment. The standard surgical table was an appropriate table for any procedure. It can be cleaned adequately for COVID care since it was designed to be cleaned to ensure operating room sterility anyhow. The same conditions apply to the fluoroscopy table needed for vascular surgery. The vascular surgery table is mobile, cleanable, and requires no modifications for COVID care. Sterile case carts and surgical kits also remained the same for care of the surgical COVID positive patient.

Anesthesia equipment, supplies, and the anesthesia machine required some modifications to the normal system. Because the anesthesia machine is clean but not sterile, it undergoes a different level of cleaning between cases. To minimize the contamination of the machine, large clear plastic equipment covers are used over the machine to eliminate any droplet contamination and minimize any aerosol contamination. The electronic touch screens that allow for controls of mechanical patient ventilation, as well as the monitoring screen that displays ECG, pulse oximetry, blood pressure, and capnography, were tested in simulations to ensure operability. Normally, anesthesia supply carts are fully stocked with medications, airway supplies, intravenous fluids, and other equipment are completely stocked. To minimize waste through contamination, anesthesia providers involved in the interprofessional simulations elicited opinions from their department and generated a minimum supply set. Once a COVID case is assigned to go to surgery, the anticipated equipment and supplies are added to the equipment cart, knowing that if not used, they would be disposed of at the end of the surgery. To facilitate retrieval of unanticipated supplies and equipment, a person outside of the COVID-OR serves as a "runner" or liaison between the isolation area and the rest of the hospital, underscoring the importance of interprofessional collaboration.

Environment

The environment is a very encompassing element of the PEEPEp model because this is the physical space where the people, equipment, and process convene to perform the procedure. In this case example of the COVID-OR, the environmental assessment began with ensuring that the physical space was large enough to accommodate the people, supplies, and equipment to perform the intended surgeries that we anticipated to be most likely to occur. Second, it was important to design an operating environment that allowed the perioperative team to provide care for the COVID positive patient without contaminating any other surgical environments or the rest of the hospital. It was also a major consideration in the design of the space to provide as safe a working environment for the perioperative team as possible, especially about the droplet and aerosol containment, air filtration and evacuation, and airflow directed at minimizing staff exposure to any infectious materials. The people involved in designing this environment included the interprofessional team of clinical perioperative staff, biomedical engineering, facilities engineering, patient safety, quality management, infection control, and executive leadership.

To maintain the surgical sterility of an operating room to minimize surgical site infection risk, operating rooms should never be made a negative pressure environment [10]. Normal operating rooms are positive pressure environments, with airflow entering the OR from the ceiling, creating a downward flow of filtered air inflow over the surgical field to move any airborne infectious particles away from the surgical field, and then evacuate the air through exhaust vents near floor level that filter the air as it is exhausted to the outside. A common misconception is that negative pressure spaces are the safest for aerosol-generating procedures, such as intubation. This is true for keeping people outside of the negative pressure space from being exposed to the airborne infectious materials; however, negative pressure rooms are totally reliant on the airflow and exhaust system of the environment to remove the infectious materials from the air. The providers in the negative pressure environment rely on airflow and circulation to remove the infectious material from the air. Many operating rooms are set to provide 12 to 15 air exchanges every hour, meaning that every 4–5 min, the air is moved out of the room and new filtered air is introduced. Providing a safe environment to provide optimal surgical outcomes requires a positive-pressure operating room, ideally surrounded by a negative-pressure antechamber to contain and evacuate airborne infectious material. Additionally, where feasible, it would be better to have a separate operating room away from the non-COVID surgical suites.

The environment component of the model includes the movement of people in space and the way the people interact with and use the equipment within the physical environment. The interaction of the environment with the clinical process, equipment, and people will move from one physical location to another. Evaluating the environments involved in a start-to-finish process is crucial to identifying latent threats to safety, quality, and throughput. For example, when testing a workflow process, it would be important to test whether an ICU bed can make a turn, fit through a doorway, roll over and door thresholds, and have electrical power at the destination. The contributions of the interprofessional team must be considered in identifying these barriers to success.

Process

Whether it is a basic process discussion with a tabletop simulation approach or a full high-fidelity evaluation of the process from the start through the finish, evaluating the process using interprofessional simulations can help to identify latent threats to patient safety, recognize barriers to meeting throughput challenges, and recognize issues among the interactions of people, equipment, and the environments prior to launching a program. Using clinical simulation strategies with interprofessional scenarios provides high visibility for a simulation program while also making a tangible contribution with a clear return on investment, where the output is a polished policy and procedures that have been tested and have staff buy-in since they were integral to the process.

Isolation precautions for other airborne transmitted diseases are already part of hospital processes for conditions like tuberculosis, but the highly infectious nature of coronavirus has enhanced the need for precautions related to contact, droplet, and airborne isolation. In this case, an example of creating a COVID-19-compliant operating room, knowing where these patients would be in the hospital and how they would be safely transported to the surgical suite, was critical. To understand the process, interprofessional simulations were created to anticipate and replicate the movement of the patients into the surgical suite from numerous situations in the facility. The use of simulation for systems-probing is becoming more commonplace for hospital activations, and this is a clear mechanism where a simulationist and simulation program can generate a tangible return on investment beyond education [11].

A series of interprofessional simulations occurred in the usual stepwise progression of a discussion of the proposed scenario, a tabletop simulation talking through the anticipated process, then a physical walkthrough of the process, with a physical simulation scenario occurring with the interprofessional team members. Interprofessional and interdepartmental simulations were conducted repeatedly between the ED and OR, the inpatient ward and OR, ICU to OR, and OR back to an inpatient unit, using an interactive data collection process to improve each subsequent scenario, sharing results with the participants. Although numerous process simulations were conducted to gauge system readiness, this section will focus on just one example.

As one example of a simulated process exploration scenario, a case of a known COVID-19-positive outpatient arrives at the emergency department complaining of abdominal pain, nausea, vomiting, and fever for 24 h with a known history of gallstones. Diagnostic testing in the emergency department reveals abnormal labs and ultrasound evidence of cholecystitis, and the patient is recommended for cholecystectomy. The interprofessional simulation begins in the emergency department (ED) with the ED team preparing the patient for transport and admission to the inpatient unit prior to surgery, following established infection containment protocols. The admitting surgical team sees the patient in the ED, writes admission orders, and arranges for an operating room and team. The ED staff transports the patient to the inpatient step-down unit. Interim debriefing is conducted to obtain participant feedback regarding mechanisms to improve efficiency, safety, and patient experience.

The inpatient step-down staff admits and assesses the patient and waits for the call that the OR is ready to take the patient. In the meantime, they implement the admission orders. Anesthesia sees the patient to complete their perioperative evaluation. In the meantime, the interprofessional OR team is setting up as they would normally. The multi-departmental aspects of the interprofessional simulation occurred simultaneously in all coordinated areas to replicate real-world service delivery. Once surgical instrumentation is available, anesthesia personnel have set up their equipment, and OR nursing has ensured readiness for surgery, a call is placed for the transport team to retrieve the patient from the inpatient ward and bring them directly to the COVID operating room. Direct observation of the transport process provided visualization of areas to reduce the potential for hospital contamination, possible safety issues for patient transport, and observation of timing for workflow analyses. A second interim debriefing is conducted to elicit areas for improvement in the process of getting the patient from the ward to OR.

Once the patient arrives in the operating suite following the COVID operating room policy, personal protective equipment (PPE) is donned, and the patient is moved into the COVID OR. Since the actual surgery is the same for COVID and non-COVID patients, the actual surgery is not simulated, and the scenario is fast-forwarded to anesthesia emergence, recovery, and transportation to an inpatient clinical area.

To facilitate the surgical process for COVID-19-positive patients, inpatient nurse leaders from each clinical area were present for the discussions and eventual simulations. Patient recovery from anesthesia and surgery is also an integral part of the process of surgery, so the post-anesthesia care unit nurses participated in the discussions and simulations as well. Due to the specific nature of caring for COVID-positive patients in surgery, infection control practitioners were included in the planning and implementation of the simulations to ensure the containment of infectious material, promote staff and patient safety, and consider equipment cleaning requirements. Biomedical engineering worked closely with the interprofessional team to anticipate challenges related to surgical instruments, specialized surgical devices, pipeline gases, and maintenance of equipment being moved into the COVID operative environment. Patient safety and quality management team members can provide helpful input after a draft of the policy and procedure is derived from interprofessional simulations. A final example of involving people is the involvement of executive leaders in reviewing final documents or processes once the interprofessional development team is confident the new policy and procedure are successful based on testing in simulation.

Emergency Preparedness

In many industries, preparation for emergencies that may arise is critical to operational readiness, and healthcare is no exception. Emergencies may be clinically patient-related, staff related, or they can originate from the environment or equipment. Using simulation helps uncover some of the interrelated ways that the people, environment, and equipment may interact to produce an emergency. Simulation is also a valuable tool for testing different approaches to emergency responses and can serve as the platform to develop educational curricula that address the emergency preparedness of the team.

In our interprofessional emergency preparedness systems probing and training scenarios, the emergency that was tested was a PPE failure with a battery depletion on a PAPR (Powered Air Purification Respirator) system. This emergency places the healthcare team member at risk for exposure to coronavirus, and the team must adapt appropriately by exiting the operating room, following partial doffing protocol including hand hygiene, and donning another PAPR system or using an N95 mask respirator.

Integrating into Existing Education

In most healthcare organizations, there are separate siloed departments for quality, safety, process improvement, and education. Simulation programs are frequently placed under education, and many education departments are sub-fragmented into nursing education and medical education. Although practicing nurses and physicians may have different educational requirements, there may be more similarities than differences. Simulation programs must be aligned with nursing or medical education and allocate resources in a preferential way to their respective affiliation; however, it should be considered that not aligning with a particular singular group may have significant administrative advantages.

When the clinical simulation has an intended use as a platform for more than education, there is an opportunity for the simulation programs to create a tangible return on investment that the administration will perceive positively. To bridge the entire facility or health system, alignment with administrative leadership is a logical placement for the simulation program in the organizational structure. Strategic placement of the Clinical Simulation Programs under the direction of the Executive Leadership Team allows the Clinical Simulation Program to operate more like a consultative service available to other administrative departments. This provides the opportunity for the Clinical Simulation Program to have leadership backing while still maintaining some degree of autonomy not beholden to any service, discipline, or profession. When the Clinical Simulation Program reports directly to facility leadership, simulation is visible and becomes an integral part of institutional problem-solving. This strategic positioning allows the Clinical Simulation Programs to gain a more comprehensive, big-picture view of the interrelationships of quality, safety, and education as they relate to process evaluation and process improvement goals.

When the Clinical Simulation Program functions within this structure, education becomes a component, not the sole objective of clinical simulation. As a related example to the COVID-OR development, the hospital needed to understand the current support, barriers to success, and opportunities for improvement for an emergency department to safely admit patients who require infectious isolation. The goal is to eliminate the risk of infection to emergency staff, receiving unit staff, and the entire hospital environment between the two clinical units. The premise of the scenarios is not to teach them how someone believes it should be done but rather to explore the process with interprofessional staff. The benefits that are achieved with this type of approach are multiple, including:

1. Explaining to staff that the simulation is about testing the process, not people, may make staff participants more willing to participate in the evaluation.
2. Staff who feel shared ownership of the process may be more likely to have increased adherence to the subsequently created policy and create stakeholder buy-in.
3. Staff with a sense of empowerment express concerns about the development process, which may affect a positive change.
4. Staff involved in the process develop a rapport with the simulation team as "partners in problem-solving."
5. Administration can capitalize on their staff's ideas and input without hiring outside consultants.

Summary

Interprofessional simulations can be used in many ways, including ensuring patient safety, quality of care, and continuous process improvement. High-Reliability Organizations and Healthcare Failure Modes Analyses were presented in the context of using clinical simulation strategies to implement these concepts through interprofessional simulations on both a national level for new hospital activations, as well as on a local level when developing, testing, and implementing a COVID-19 compliant operating room to maximize patient safety and throughput. The PEEPEp Conceptual Model was also presented as a pragmatic approach to using clinical interprofessional simulations to organize the implementation plan as a continuous component of the process.

References

1. https://www.va.gov/vetdata/docs/QuickFacts/VA_Utilization_Profile_2017.PDF.
2. Herzer KR, Rodriguez-Paz JM, Doyle PA, Flint PW, Feller-Kopman DJ, Herman J, et al. A practical framework for patient care teams to prospectively identify and mitigate clinical hazards. Jt Comm J Qual Patient Saf. 2009;35(2):72–81.
3. DeRosier JM, Hansemann BK, Smith-Wheelock MW, Bagian JP. Using proactive risk assessment (HFMEA) to improve patient safety and quality associated with intraocular lens selection and implantation in cataract surgery. Jt Comm J Qual Patient Saf. 2019;45(10):680–5.
4. Safety VNCfP. Healthcare failure mode effect analysis https://www.patientsafety.va.gov/media/hfmea.asp2021.
5. Rizzo A, Kim G. A SWOT analysis of the field of virtual reality rehabilitation and therapy. Presence. 2005;14:119–46.
6. Kuo AM, Borycki E, Kushniruk A, Lee TS. A healthcare Lean six sigma system for post-anesthesia care unit workflow improvement. Qual Manag Health Care. 2011;20(1):4–14.
7. Murphree P, Vath RR, Daigle L. Sustaining Lean six sigma projects in health care. Physician Exec. 2011;37(1):44–8.
8. Polk JD. Lean six sigma, innovation, and the change acceleration process can work together. Physician Exec. 2011;37(1):38–42.
9. Improta G, Cesarelli M, Montuori P, Santillo LC, Triassi M. Reducing the risk of healthcare-associated infections through Lean six sigma: the case of the medicine areas at the Federico II University Hospital in Naples (Italy). J Eval Clin Pract. 2018;24(2):338–46.
10. Spruce L, DeKay K, Burlingame B. AORN guidelines in the era of COVID-19. AORN J. 2021;113(3):225–34.
11. Gaba DM. The future vision of simulation in health care. Qual Saf Health Care. 2004;13(Suppl 1):i2–10.

Simulation in International Healthcare Environments: A Rural Perspective

38

Kirsty J. Freeman, Robert Amm, and Melanie Goode

Background

Rural healthcare workers, especially nursing staff, are expected to provide quality and timely critical care when the need arises. It is the expectation of the community when emergency care is required, that staff on shift are ready, available, and experienced to be able to perform competently. Equally, the National Health and Safety Quality Standards for which all healthcare facilities in Australia are measured against, demand the same level of care for all Australians no matter which healthcare facility they attend [1].

Nurses working in rural health services, such as the Indian Health Service (IHS) in the USA, and the West Australian Country Health Service in Australia, are health advocates for the indigenous populations. Nurses are looked upon within rural settings to be the clinical lead, often providing care when medical staffing is not available. Globally, the rural nurse becomes generalist in nature through filling the roles required to meet healthcare delivery. A study by Kidd, Kenny [2] investigating the experience of rural nurses working in rural Victoria, a region in south eastern Australia, found that almost half of the respondents reported a lack of confidence in providing emergency care, a key role when working in rural environments. The requirement to expand the rural nurses scope of practice was reinforced by Vanderspank-Wright and McMillan [3] in their qualitative study of critical care nurses working in the remote parts of Northern Canada. The authors found that this specialist group of nurses expanded their scope of practice to include skills such as respiratory therapy, and that these new skills enabled them to support emergency medicine teams, especially when mechanical ventilation is required. Such studies highlight the importance of educational opportunities that allow rural healthcare teams to not only maintain their clinical skills, but also broadening their scope of practice, where endorsed by governing bodies, to face the challenges of caring for rural communities.

As has been well documented throughout the chapters of this book simulation-based training is an essential tool to grow and develop the future and current nursing workforce. For healthcare simulation educators working in rural environments however, the delivery of appropriate continuing professional development present numerous challenges.

Challenges in Simulation-Based Education in Rural Environments

Three pillars underpin sustainable simulation programs—workforce; curriculum; and resources.

In January 2020 a group of passionate healthcare simulation educators from around the globe came together at the International Meeting for Simulation in Healthcare in San Diego to share experiences of creating sustainable simulation programs in rural environments. A plethora of challenges were identified by those wanting to leverage the benefits that simulation-based education offers healthcare providers (Table 38.1).

Workforce Challenges

Due to the small number of individuals that make up healthcare teams in the rural environment, healthcare simulation educators are often required to balance multiple roles from providing clinical care, taking on managerial roles, as well as meeting the educational needs of the organization. Being pulled in so many different directions can result in burnout, and decreased job satisfaction. Some rural communities have a transient population,

K. J. Freeman (✉)
The Rural Clinical School of Western Australia,
The University of Western Australia, Perth, Australia

R. Amm · M. Goode
Western Australian Country Health Service, Perth, WA, Australia
e-mail: Robert.Amm@health.wa.gov.au;
Melanie.Goode@health.wa.gov.au

J. M. Kutzin et al. (eds.), *Comprehensive Healthcare Simulation: Nursing*, Comprehensive Healthcare Simulation,
https://doi.org/10.1007/978-3-031-31090-4_38

Table 38.1 Challenges faced when creating sustainable simulation programs in rural environments

Simulation Workforce	Simulation Curriculum	Simulation Resources
• Maintaining staff balance due to competing clinical, managerial, and educational demands • Increased demand for faculty development due to a transient workforce with high turnover of staff • Educators need to be a jack of all trades—curriculum developer, simulation technician, content expert, facilitator, debriefer • seasonal clinical demands can result in large periods of time with no education • geographical isolation can impact access to faculty development opportunities such as workshops or conferences • access to content specialists to create and deliver education	• Tailored content to local context • Skilled faculty to design simulation experiences • Developing a curriculum that addresses both the clinical and behavioural skills required by small interprofessional teams • Integrating simulation-based education into the broader institutional curriculum • Providing dedicated time for educational activities • Ensuring the curriculum is accredited for CPD points • Face to face opportunities to complement the eLearning programs	• Availability of dedicated simulation teaching and storage spaces • Access to simulation equipment including task trainers, manikins, and consumables • Timely maintenance and repair of equipment • Lack of information technology support

resulting in a high staff turnover in the health workforce. In many sites the position of healthcare simulation educator is like a revolving door, with people moving in and out of the position often. This impacts the number of qualified staff available to facilitate simulation-based education and increases the demand for faculty development programs.

Whilst those working in metropolitan healthcare institutions are accustomed to working with a team of simulation faculty, it is not uncommon for those in rural sites to be a team of one or two. As a result they are required to coordinate and deliver all aspects of simulation activity from creating the content, scheduling, room bookings and rostering of staff, to briefing, facilitating, and debriefing the simulation, as well as managing the set up and tear down. It takes a highly skill educator to successfully complete all roles.

Whilst those in metropolitan environments are equipped to deal with seasonal impact on healthcare delivery, rural healthcare teams do not have the same number of human resources, which means during times of extreme weather events, clinical care is prioritized over education, meaning the education programs may be put on hold for a period of time.

Geographical isolation can often impact educators' ability to access faculty development activities that would enable them to build and develop their skill around simulation-based education. It can be very expensive to travel the long distances to attend conferences and workshops. However it is not just the financial impact on the individual or the organization for transport out of the rural community, but the time required to be away from work may require the need to backfill a position or role to ensure continuity of services, an added cost to the organization.

Curriculum Challenges

Curriculum challenges faced by healthcare simulation educators working in rural environments are unique to those in metropolitan environments. Whilst the opportunity exists to purchase generic simulation packages they do not always translate to the needs of rural healthcare. With unique patient presentations, healthcare teams need to customize content to the local context to ensure it is fit for the appropriate purpose.

As highlighted previously the rural healthcare team is predominantly made up of nurses, who are required to have an extended scope of practice in terms of both clinical and behavioural skills. It can be challenging for those working in rural environments to develop such a broad curriculum when they themselves may not be the content expert and securing such expertise can present challenges of their own.

With person-power a precious resource, scheduling staff to attend education so that clinical care is not negatively impacted can be challenging. Key to addressing this important issue is to simply ask the educational leadership team at each specific site what their preference is for scheduling. Early evening sessions, often with catering provided, have proven to be effective in some rural sites, with others requesting weekend. Whilst educator might be more familiar in delivery sessions to numerous learners at one time, in very small sites the learners may only be released one at a time, requiring the educators to tailor their teaching to this.

Registered healthcare providers around the world may be required by their accrediting bodies to maintain a specified amount of continuing professional development activity every year. It is essential therefore that simulation-based educational programs are accredited by the designated agencies so that staff can maintain the necessary licensure requirements.

Resource Challenges

The availability of dedicated teaching space, as well as simulation specific spaces, is often limited in rural hospitals. In situ or point-of-care simulation, which is simulation teaching activities that are conducted in the actual clinical environment, is often the default option due to the lack of dedicated teaching/simulation space. However, the unpredictable nature of healthcare delivery means that scheduled simulation sessions may be cancelled should the space be required for actual clinical care.

Simulation equipment, such as task trainers, mannequins, and consumables, can be difficult to source when working in rural environments. Finding a vendor that services rural communities can also be a challenge. Ensuring that equipment is fit for purpose is essential in the procurement process as some rural environments require simulation to be delivered in extreme temperature with varying levels of humidity. The extreme conditions can impact the functionality and lifespan of the resources. Should the items require annual servicing and repairs this can result in the item being out of service for an extended period as it is transported to and from rural areas, impacting planned delivery of education.

Solutions

The challenges faced by the healthcare simulation educators working in rural environments are unique and varied, and so too are the solutions. Three exemplars are described below as: addressing locally embedded solutions, telesimulation solutions, and hub and spoke mobile solutions. These options can be tailored to address specific challenges.

Locally Embedded Solutions

The first place to start when looking at locally embedded solutions for the simulation workforce is by building a culture within the organization that values simulation-based education. A top down, bottom up approach is essential for all staff to acknowledge the contribution that simulation-based education makes to both patient and clinician safety. As the delivery of healthcare simulation in rural environments differs to larger metropolitan based centre faculty development programs need to be tailored. A train the trainer faculty development program that provides skills the rural educator needs on the art of multitasking is essential if they are expected to be a team of one.

A solution to the issue of high staff turnover may include organizations investigating remuneration and other incentives that could decrease staff turnover. Staff that feel valued by their employer may experience greater job satisfaction and remain with the employer longer. Developing a community of practice for healthcare simulation educators that work in rural environments, linking educators with like-minded colleagues, providing a platform to share experiences can aid in the development of an educator's professional identity.

Common patient presentation types to be addressed in simulation sessions that would have benefit for the rural nurse include trauma, sepsis, pediatrics, obstetric emergencies, geriatrics, toxicology, acute coronary syndrome, and mental health. The opportunity to collaborate and strengthen links with partners internal to the organization, such as the safety and quality department, can help educators ascertain the curriculum needs of the organization. By identifying the most common clinical patient presentations to the hospital, simulation scenarios that meet clinical needs of the community can be prioritized. To meet the clinical demands of the rural nurse Table 38.2 outlines a list of core skills that can be addressed through simulation-based education.

Embedding simulation into the culture and daily practice of the organization can be achieved by starting small, designing simulation sessions that are short and sharp, taking

Table 38.2 Core skills that can be taught through simulation

Airway, breathing, circulation, disability, exposure (A to E) approach to the immediate assessment and treatment of critically ill or injured patient

- Systematic approach to primary examination of ED patients
- Reinforces common approach to an organised, structured approach to examining patients

Head to Toe exam

- Important expansion on A to E exam, especially in traumatic presentations

Basic Life Support (BLS)

- Bringing BLS into a structured simulation scenario emphasises recommended guidelines to approaching the critically unwell patient

Advanced Life Support (ALS)

- Defibrillation safety. In a team environment, simulation involving defibrillation galvanizes your team, which for a rural ED would be an intimate group of individuals
- Understanding ALS drugs used and their pharmacokinetic properties strengthens staff understanding of the ALS flowchart and its rationale

Airway management

- Basic use of simple airway opening and support techniques, and practicing implementation of these techniques in simulation scenarios provides empowering opportunities for nurses in basic airway management, not routinely practiced in rural settings

Ventilation

- Equipment—How to use and apply safely
- Ventilator—individualized to each ED, promoting a team approach to safe use through simulation encourages teamwork and communication
- Drugs used—especially in a controlled intubation setting, where rescue transport teams would require assistance to intubate patients for a safer transfer to tertiary centers

ECG assessment

- Using a simplified structured approach can empower nurses to effectively communicate their ECG interpretation, improving communication when escalating care

between 15 and 20 min out of their day and so endeavouring to not encroach on the delivery of patient care.

The opportunity to develop online platforms that enable the sharing not only of scenarios, but policies, templates, and other documents such as evaluation forms can make the transition to healthcare simulation educator less daunting when taking on a new role.

As highlighted earlier, one of the challenges faced in rural clinical sites is the availability of dedicated teaching spaces. Depending on the learning outcomes of the simulation session, ensuring a high degree of environmental fidelity is not always required. Healthcare simulation educators should be open to the idea of facilitating their simulation session in any available space, even utilizing the breakroom, depending on the requirements of the session.

In the rural environment the healthcare simulation educators will often also oversee the procurement of equipment. To help mitigate some of the challenges related to maintenance and repairs highlighted earlier, sourcing equipment that is robust, with as fewer moving parts as practicable will prove beneficial, especially if the items need to be transported. Working with vendors to access basic technical training will enable staff to troubleshoot onsite, potentially minimizing the need to transport equipment. Building partnerships with external agencies within a local community, such as colleges and prehospital care providers, opens the opportunity of sharing resources, not just simulation equipment, but also staff, teaching space and even curriculum (Table 38.3).

Table 38.3 Localized solutions for creating sustainable simulation programs in rural environments

Simulation Workforce	Simulation Curriculum	Simulation Resources
• Build the culture within the organization to support the value of simulation-based education, acknowledging the contribution it makes to patient and clinician safety • Develop a localized train the trainer program for simulation faculty development • Investigate remuneration and other incentives to decrease staff turnover • Develop a community of practice within the rural community, and with similar communities, to enable sharing of experiences and mentoring opportunities	• Strengthen links with internal partners such as safety and quality departments to ascertain curricula needs and to assist with measuring outcomes • Engage staff in the creation of content, increasing buy in. • Start small by designing sessions that are 20-30mins in length, so as not to encroach in clinical care delivery • Develop an online platform to enable the sharing of scenarios as well as forums for exchanging of ideas	• Environmental fidelity is not always required for effective learning • Procure equipment that is robust, and train staff to troubleshoot repairs onsite • Build partnerships with external agencies such as colleges/ universities and prehospital community providers to share resources

Telesimulation

To meet the needs of a diverse community of health care providers over a vast geographical space, education provision needs to be innovative, dynamic, and revolutionary. Australia is a vast country, with pockets of populations spread over many kilometres, isolated by distance, working environments, and local resources. Provisioning a specialist, equitable education program to health professionals, the majority of whom are nurses, is challenging and exciting. Utilising all possible means of education delivery has led to a program that harnesses and depends on a blended Tele-education program. Telesimulation, video conferencing (VC) education and more recently virtual reality (VR) telesimulation all working together to deliver a blended tele-education program.

Telesimulation is an emerging concept across the world. It has been defined as "a process by which telecommunication and simulation resources are utilised to provide education, training and/or assessment to learners at an offsite location" [4]. Within parts of Australia the emergence of telesimulation programs has been necessitated by the need for contemporary, equitable education delivery, regardless of location or resources. Working within an established telehealth system, education via the telecommunication network has been an enormous collateral benefit and ensures that the rural workforce is supported and developed within their own environments.

Rural healthcare setting varies greatly in size, both in relation to the size of the facilities and the size of the clinical teams, ranging from one or two practitioners to multiple. Within the healthcare workforce in Australia, over half are nurses and midwives. According to the Australian Institute of Health and Welfare [5] medical practitioner numbers fall from 143 full-time equivalent (FTE) practitioners per 100,000 population in major cities to 22 FTE per 100,000 in very remote areas. However, the reverse can be seen for nurses and midwives. There are more nurses and midwives per 100,000 population in very remote areas than major cities. Thus, highlighting the need for robust nursing and midwifery education in rural environments. Provisioning education to such a varied landscape requires significant skill and adaptability. Incorporating simulation-based education

(SBE) into rural facility's curriculums allows the rural clinicians to adapt their practice to their context, it increases credibility and realism for the learners, and enables experiential learning to happen [6]. According to Kolb's experiential learning cycle [7], immersing the learner into concrete learning experiences, facilitating the review and reflection phase to enable the learning to be meaningful and real, whilst allowing for the application of these learnings to the learners world [8] is a powerful motivator for adult learners [4]. This is achievable via telesimulation as the process is synchronous, happening in real time and the learnings are valid and relevant for the clinicians and ultimately for patient care and safety.

Enabling high quality, psychologically safe simulation practices in the rural context is multifaceted. SBE in this setting, encompasses skill acquisition, team dynamics and crisis resource management, as well as essential critical care skills such as basic and advanced life support, resuscitation, and trauma management. Focusing on high acuity, low occurrence situations is essential to avoid the degradation of essential skills, when the clinical environment may not provide enough regular exposure to these situations to maintain optimal skill levels [9, 17].

The telesimulation program has many similarities with face-to-face simulation training. The premise is the same, with essential components of SBE needing to be identified and addressed. For telesimulation to be a positive experience for the learner and the facilitator, it is vital that the learners are supported with the underpinning clinical knowledge and skills to be able to apply them in a clinical setting. Using a blended learning approach to educate and enhance clinical understanding, provides the scaffolding to develop and build a robust simulation education program via video conferencing modalities.

Rural practitioners thrive in an environment that is familiar and telesimulation promotes the notion of community learning. In small teams, with often limited physical resources, the concept of team is vital. Learning and practicing crucial skills together within their own environment has proven to be invaluable, both for team culture but also clinical confidence and patient safety [4].

Scenario based telesimulation education is the culmination of a comprehensive expert led education program delivered via video conferencing. By using a blended learning approach to deliver education content learners experience interactions with subject matter experts such as practical skills sessions, telesimulation demonstrations, and telesimulation based education (TBE). The term blended learning, in this context, is best described as a multifaceted approach to embed knowledge and understanding for key clinical concepts or approaches. For example an Advanced Life Support program Airway Module may encompass

- Didactic education sessions delivering expert content via video conference presentation
- Practical skill sessions enabling remote clinicians to practice along with an expert instructor in real time
- Simulation demonstration session, where the learners observe a simulated clinical scenario and discuss the learning opportunities

Clinical specialists/content experts deliver clinically focused education sessions using live video conferencing modalities. These sessions are designed to deliver current, evidence-based education to clinicians, wherever they are. Clinicians can access these education sessions from their local clinical facility or via a secure internet link from the comfort of home. These education sessions reflect similar practices within large facilities, such as teaching rounds, lunchtime teaching sessions, regular planned educational opportunities for the multidisciplinary team. Content is delivered via a didactic presentation, followed by an interactive two-way conversation between learner and educator, where questions are answered and experiences shared. These sessions are often recorded and added to a bank of e-learning resources, accessible at any time. This helps to ensure continuous shift workers have equitable access to education. These sessions can facilitate many attendees from one to hundreds, dependant only on the capacity of the technology.

Clinical specialist/ content expert based in the tertiary hospital can contribute to education sessions on topics such as those outlined in the table below (Table 38.4).

Table 38.4 Clinical expert topics of interest

- Cardiac
  - Cardiac anatomy and physiology
  - Common cardiac presentation
    ECG interpretation
  - Chest pain management/thrombolysis
- Paediatrics
  - Special populations
  - Common paediatric presentations
  - Rashes
  - Trauma
  - Non-accidental injury
  - Distraction therapies and family centred care
- Advanced life support
  - Overview
  - Algorithm management
  - Pharmacology
  - Defibrillation
  - Post resuscitation care
- Transfer and aeromedical retrieval
  - How to prepare the patient for safe transfer/aeromedical retrieval
    - By road
    - By air

Providing an opportunity for clinical skills teaching and acquisition has helped to fill the tool kit available for rural nurses working in isolation. Access to expert educators in rural areas is limited, often resulting in travel and time away from communities [9]. The overarching aim of the practical skills sessions are to provide theoretical and practical education for those essential skills that may have low frequency occurrence in rural areas. The skills identified to address the needs of nursing workforce include plastering, suturing, intra-osseous (IO) insertion, airway management /maneuvers, chest decompression and inter-costal catheter insertion, and chest drain management.

Skills sessions are smaller focused group education sessions, intentionally to allow synchronous learning, pausing, discussing, demonstrating, and facilitating a 'follow along' approach. Participants are scheduled to attend with colleagues from similar sized rural facilities, inviting conversation to evolve, where similar experiences can be shared. Nurses have reported feeling empowered and more confident with the skills addressed in these sessions, specifically plaster skills, suturing and IO insertion. All sessions are supported by pre-reading evidence-based education that supports organizational policy and procedures. Interprofessional learning is a strong focus of these sessions, as learning together enhances the community ethos which is vital within small clinical teams. It also promotes and supports the confidence and familiarity of the video conferencing modality for telehealth delivery of clinical care.

Specific skill assessment via the video conferencing modality for clinical skills are being explored with caution. Moving away from a competency-based assessment process, where a clinician is deemed competent on 1 day, to a system where nurses are driven to demonstrate skills, knowledge, and competency within their scope of practice and maintain currency is the current thinking. Achieving competency can be met in many ways. Competency has been defined as 'the effective application of a combination of knowledge, skills and judgement demonstrated by an individual in daily practice or job performance [10]. Studies have suggested that situational experience, such as that offered by SBE and telesimulation, helps to facilitate the movement of the learner from novice to expert, in line with Benner's theory [11, 12]. Jewer, Parsons [9] demonstrated that the modality of delivery, either face to face or remote did not have an impact on retention of skills, supporting reliability and learner satisfaction with remotely delivered education for skill development. Hence the layering and diversity of educational opportunities for rural clinicians helps to address not only moving the learner along the learning continuum, but also the different learning styles learners bring to the picture [13].

Delivering a blended learning program allows for a diverse, engaging program. The telesimulation demonstration sessions encompass the 'play along, learn along' ethos. Telesimulation demonstration enhances the learning of practical skills [13]. Skills such as airway maneuvers for adult and pediatric; pediatric basic life support; defibrillation; and difficult conversations, such as breaking bad news following a sudden death.

The demonstration aspect of the session requires preparation, both for the educator and the learner. The remote clinician learners need advanced notice of what will be required for the sessions such as equipment needed, how many team members are needed, etc. The sessions involve an overview of the relevant theory associated with the skill, a best practice demonstration, followed by a practice along with the educator. These sessions can be paused in real time and concerns or issues discussed as they arise, thus embedding the key learning points in a situational experience. These sessions are most valuable in a small group environment and help to lay the foundations for SBE via telesimulation.

The focus of the telesimulation based education (TBE) program is to move the learners from task training and skill acquisition to a transitional learning environment that is relevant and directly reflective of their current clinical environments. TBE supports the use of applied knowledge, which enhances the application of knowledge and skills in the real environment for both the individual learner and teams [14]. Having the capacity and technology to enable TBE contextualises and enhances concrete learning, moving from abstract concepts to learning or reflecting in action [8]. This concept, reflection in action, by Schon [15] is thought to be more congruent with real clinical environments, which are dynamic and ever changing and is reflective of the clinical reasoning cycle [16]. McCoy, Sayegh [4] highlight that telesimulation promotes the benefits of SBE beyond the confines of designated simulation laboratories within tertiary facilities or universities and into the learner's environment.

The overarching principles of telesimulation are directly reflective of SBE in the traditional sense. The key aspects of the simulation purpose, basic assumption, fictional contract, confidentiality, familiarization with equipment and environment, the pre brief, simulation, and debrief learning conversation are reviewed to protect the learner's psychological safety and comfort.

The session requires preplanning, negotiating appropriate timings, sharing of information for preparation of the team and the environment. The telesimulation expert facilitator requires an on-site, remote facilitator, to support the mechanics of the session. Ensuring the required equipment is available for example, manikins, defibrillators, rhythm box etc., is crucial. Fidelity is an important consideration here; costly high-fidelity equipment is not generally available within the rural environment. This can be organised if essential and couriered to the team, however working with low fidelity, often simulated patients, or basic CPR manikins is the reality of these sessions. Garland, Wilson [17] suggest that low fidelity simulation supports a safe learning environment and that the learning outcomes are not impacted or hindered by the fidelity.

These sessions are limited to single rural locations, or single locations with another location as an observer. The decision to host an observer site is individually assessed on each occasion. In some instances, the addition of an observer location is not appropriate for the team engaging with the TBE. New teams may not be comfortable with external observers or the TBE may be in response to a critical incident and in these circumstances psychological safety for the team is paramount. It is well evidenced that observing SBE is a valuable learning environment for those observing and is encouraged, when appropriate [6].

For the rural teams, the only member of the simulation that is remote is the telesimulation expert facilitator. The live, interactive component of the simulation happens within the team's clinical environment, engaging with the telesimulation facilitator in the same way that they may engage with a telehealth provider on a screen in their emergency departments.

During the session, all relevant clinical information is shared via screen sharing technology on large TV screens. This may include monitoring equipment, ECG's (EKG's), chest x-rays, blood work etc. All helping to add realism to the scenario and engage the reflection in action process. As with all simulation, it is possible to call a time out and address any essential concerns or safety matters in real time, synchronously, thus embedding the learning in real life concrete experiences. Immediately following the TBE a debrief learning conversation is facilitated. The value of the debriefing conversation post TBE cannot be underestimated. Evidence has demonstrated again and again the value and importance of the debrief learning conversation [18, 19]. These conversations require significant skill when conducted via video conferencing. Inclusion and engagement are often the most challenging aspects of debriefing with a remote team, having skilled facilitators who know and understand their clinical teams is vital.

This aspect highlights one of the many challenges when working within a TBE program, the limitations of skilled simulation educators who also have advanced skill within the telesimulation field. The other vital aspect is a thorough understanding of the challenges and working environments faced by clinicians working within rural facilities, clinical credibility amongst the learners is essential to enhance a close, trusting working environment.

Telesimulation based education is becoming increasingly accepted within Australia as an essential tool to enable SBE for all, regardless of geographical location or proximity to a designated simulation laboratory. Universities within Australia are using similar modalities to provision SBE within their facilities. Patient assessment via SBE is embedded as part of the final year nursing education and training. Nursing students engage in patient assessment SBE and the interactions are live streamed to a debrief room with the rest of the cohort and a facilitator. Live debriefing happens in real time and then the simulation event is posted, with the whole group. This is an example of observation learning in collaboration with experiential learning and prepares the Australian nursing workforce for working within environments where this approach is the norm.

Another exciting and developing learning environment within nursing education in the rural workforce is the use of Virtual Reality. Virtual Reality (VR) has been described as 'a technology that allows users to explore and manipulate computer-generated, real or artificial three-dimensional multimedia sensory environments in real time to gain practical knowledge that can be used in clinical practice' [20]. VR can enhance the experience for the learner by increasing interest, engagement, and authenticity, whilst supporting the experiential learning model [21]. VR for patient experience is well established and accepted. Examples include distraction therapy for children undergoing painful procedures or experiential tours through facilities at large referral hospital.

The leap for healthcare professionals is not far behind. In an experimental pilot program, a small sample of nurses engaged in a VR program designed to increase their understanding and skill in the facilitation of SBE. With the aim being to enable rural facilities to facilitate SBE face safely and effectively face to face, including TBE support when needed. This involved recording an immersive 360° video of a telesimulation event in a representative small rural facility. Embedding this video as the core learning allowed the development of a program via VR. The program was supported with a blended learning approach including core underpinning knowledge, presentations in small groups via VR, using goggles to display content, interacting in real time and placing clinicians from all over the rural landscape, virtually in the room together. VR allows for first person interaction via an avatar, sharing of ideas and discussions flow as if the learners and facilitator were in the same room [20]. Once the content and under pinning knowledge has been communicated over several sessions the participants watch the 360° immersive recording and the facilitator has the capacity to pause the recording and discuss learning opportunities as they happen within the scenario. Participants are then assigned a role, facilitator or participant and can practice/rehearse the debrief learning conversation in a safe, supported, and controlled environment. The VR facilitator, an experienced TBE facilitator can guide the conversation and give live contemporaneous feedback, thus enhancing the learning experience and supporting the reflection in action ethos. Whilst in its infancy this program has proven to be extremely exciting and in need of robust review and expansion.

Telesimulation as an educational modality is still in its infancy. Telesimulation based education is proving to be an essential tool within rural environments where location and resources are restricting factors. Enabling equitable educational opportunities for all clinicians regardless of location, must be the end goal. Telesimulation enables rich, relevant learning to occur, where the learner is. The need for travel is avoided, depleting the local workforce for educational opportunities is prevented and clinicians are kept in their communities. Networking and inter-facility collaboration have become apparent as enhancing relationships between geographically distant clinicians. Putting clinicians virtually in the room together enables sharing of stories and experiences and diminishes feelings of isolation. Situational learning in the clinician's clinical environment supports experiential, real world learning. Moving simulation 'beyond the walls of the simulation centre' [4] and enriching the educational journey for all nurses and interdisciplinary clinicians is cost effective, equitable and enables change management to happen in a timely manner [6, 8, 9, 13].

Limitations of telesimulation include access to high quality reliable video conferencing equipment, however within Australia's robust telehealth network, this is less of an issue. User /learner level of skill with the equipment can impact on the effectiveness of the interactions and the learner's experience of the intended education. Another significantly limiting factor is the number of simulation experts who also have expert level telesimulation, video conferencing experience. The ability to develop these skills is an area that needs to be explored and researched moving forward. Telesimulation will not and should not replace the rich environment of face-to-face simulation-based education, however for those learners without access to this essential education modality telesimulation based education is a significant shift in providing an equitable educational experience for all clinicians regardless of geographical location, with the ultimate aim of enhancing patient safety and outcomes.

Hub and Spoke Mobile Solution

As touched on previously, the healthcare teams working in rural communities look different to those of their larger metropolitan counterparts, relying heavily on General Practitioners and Nurses, with limited access to specialist physicians, surgeons, and critical care support. Whilst locally embedded and telesimulation solutions can be leveraged to meet the some of the educational needs of the rural clinician, access to advanced clinical skill simulation-based training remains challenging. Mobile simulation programs have been effective in the delivery of state of the art, hands-on simulation experiences to rural clinicians through a variety of modalities [22, 23]. The use of converted recreational vehicles or semitrailers, enables the transportation of a specialized simulation equipment and precious teaching spaces to regional communities. For geographically isolated communities however the use of this form of mobile simulation is not always a viable option due to the vast distances needing to be covered, therefore the third solution for those working in rural communities describes a hub and spoke mobile simulation-based education program that has been embedded in in the Kimberley region of Western Australia.

A "hub and spoke" model of healthcare simulation delivery is a model whereby a regional hub coordinates a program of activity and distributes simulation-based education to the network of spokes (Fig. 38.1).

Regional hubs coordinate the development of learning programs, usage, and research, but should not discourage local initiatives. Purchase of major infrastructure on a shared basis, and regional or national contracts for servicing of equipment may allow some economies of scale. Regional centres or even a national institute for health simulation could coordinate standards for simulation training programs and staff accreditation.

The hub and spoke model is unique in that it is not a uni-directional, instead as depicted by the multidirectional arrows in fig. 38.1, it is a multidirectional collaboration between partners. The aim of the regional hub is to support the needs of the rural spoke. This collaboration starts with the development of curriculum. Instead of dictating what should be taught, the regional hub works with the rural spoke to conduct a gap analysis, identifying the simulation-based needs not met through local or telesimulation programs. With the gap analysis the planning, coordinate by the hub simulation team, identifies the curricula content required. With access to a library of simulation scenarios, the hub can tailor the content to the unique requirements of the spoke—taking into account patient populations, human resources, and healthcare services available at the rural sire.

The next component of collaboration between the hub and the spoke relates to simulation faculty. Whilst it is important to ensure clinical experts are available to share their knowledge and skills, it is essential that the faculty are cognisant that care may be delivered differently in small rural clinical sites. Key is recruiting an interprofessional faculty that can be flexible in their teaching and application in clinical skills in what is often a resource poor environment. It is essential that the program faculty include local champions. Not only will these individuals assist external faculty to contextualize their content, they are often the sole individual that will remain at site to reinforce the learning of the program in the week and months after the external faculty leave.

As acknowledged earlier, teaching spaces in rural environments can be lacking, therefore the hub team can assist with sourcing alternate venues that might be suitable for simulation-based training. Sourcing a venue away from the

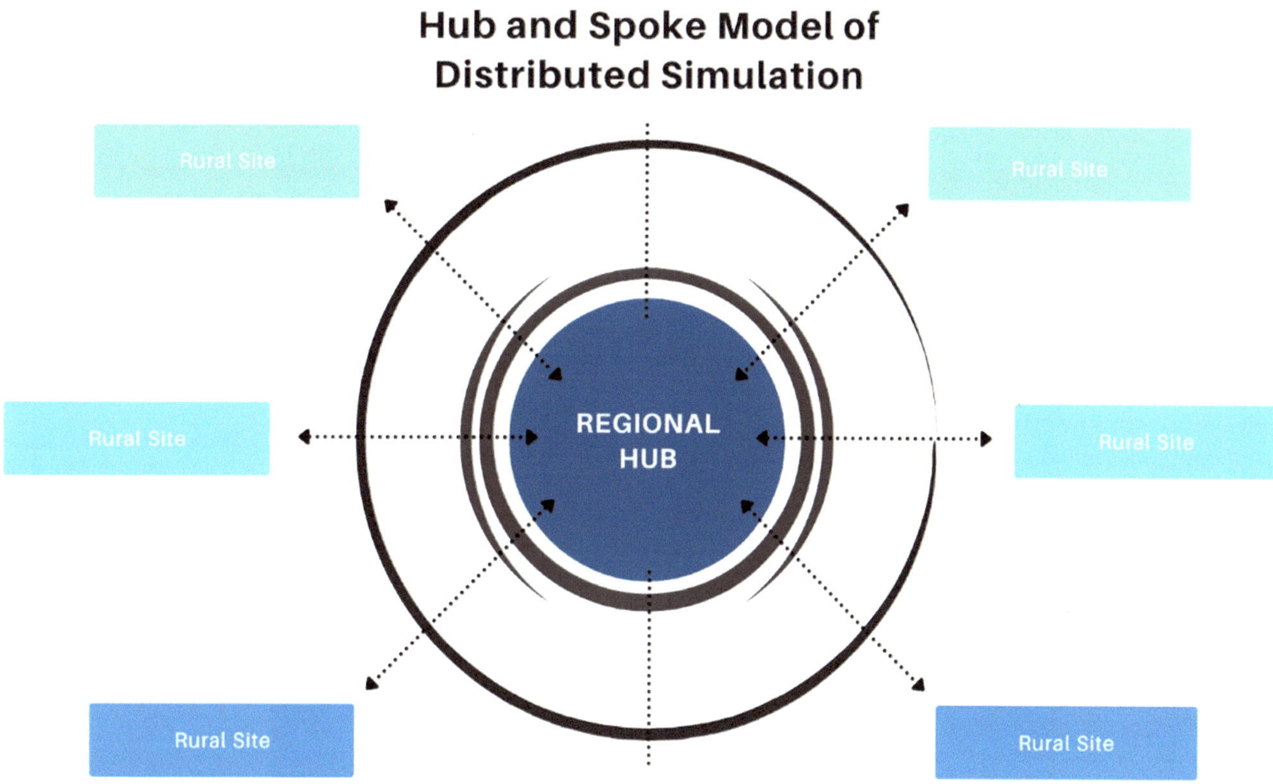

Fig. 38.1 Hub and spoke model of distributed simulation

clinical area also helps secure dedicated time for learners, who have the potential to be pulled back to the floor if colleagues know they are around. Collaboration between the hub and spoke in relation to clinical consumables is essential when planning locally delivered training. It is essential that the simulation program utilise the consumable and other clinical equipment available at site. Expecting the learner to train with equipment that they would not usually have access to can confuse the learner, impact their ability to effectively engage in current and future education if they feel it is not applicable to their current needs.

Another key component that the hub team can coordinate is the credentialing of the simulation program to ensure the awarding of continuing professional development credits for those who attend. It is these administrative tasks that rural teams may not have the time or knowledge to undertake. With much of the planning and logistics coordinated by the hub simulation team, the spoke lead is left to coordinate the scheduling to ensure learners are relieved of their clinical duties to attend the simulation program.

With funds from the Commonwealth Department of Health, the Emergency Medicine Education and Training program, led by Fellows of the Australasian College for Emergency Medicine (FACEMs), the hub and spoke model has been adopted in rural Western Australia to deliver educational content specifically for health care professionals responsible for providing emergency care to rural communities. This program provides simulation-based education and practical skills workshops, tailored to the needs of the local community, and in the last 3 years has educated over 1000 clinicians. The program aims to provide clinicians with the opportunity to develop their critical care skills and leadership in various clinical situations without having to leave town and thereby compromising continuity of care in finitely resourced areas. Through a combination of immersive simulation experiences, hot and cold case reviews where clinicians can openly discuss current or historical patient presentations, and clinical skills workshops, participants not only report increased confidence in critical care skills but also improved interprofessional team performance, particularly in the area of crisis resource management skills including leadership, teamwork and communication. Key to the success of the program is the use of an interprofessional faculty in building relationships with clinical staff at rural sites to encourage communication and trust. Evaluation of the program revealed that participants' value locally delivered, contextually appropriate educational opportunities that increase their knowledge, skills and attitudes in the delivery of emergency skills. The program also enables local staff to become trainers and therefore provide professional development to other local clinicians once the Simulation Education team has gone. This ensures that all clinicians can handle that "one-off" clinical emergency that occurs.

Conclusion

Providing clinicians with the opportunity to develop their clinical and leadership skills in various clinical situations, without having to leave town and thereby compromising continuity of care in finitely resourced areas, should be a priority for all rural communities across the globe.

The chapter has described the challenges face by healthcare educators when delivering simulation-based education in rural environments. Whilst some of the challenges may be similar to their metropolitan counterparts, the solutions need to be tailored to the local context to ensure a comprehensive, sustainable, locally embedded simulation-based education programs that will ensure patient safety and quality in geographically disparate communities.

By building the skills of local clinicians, patients in rural communities can feel confident that they have access to appropriate health care when required and has the potential to help ensure high levels of clinical competency with a highly mobile workforce.

References

1. National Safety and Quality Health Service Standards. Australian Commission on Safety and Quality in Health Care. 2nd ed. Sydney: ACSQHC; 2017.
2. Kidd T, Kenny A, Meehan-Andrews T. The experience of general nurses in rural Australian emergency departments. Nurse Educ Pract. 2012;12(1):11–5.
3. Vanderspank-Wright B, McMillan K. Critical care nursing north of the 60th parallel: a qualitative pilot study. Can J Crit Care Nurs. 2016;27(3):12–7.
4. McCoy CE, Sayegh J, Alrabah R, Yarris LM. Telesimulation: an innovative tool for health professions education. AEM Educ Train. 2017;1(2):132–6.
5. Australian institute of health and welfare. Health Workforce: Australian Government; 2020. https://www.aihw.gov.au/reports/australias-health/health-workforce.
6. Sprehe J, March AL, Wilson CB, Park HS. The effect of video-conferencing on code blue simulation training. Clin Simul Nurs. 2016;12(7):260–7.
7. McLeod SA. Kolb—learning styles; 2017. https://www.simplypsychology.org/learning-kolb.html.
8. Papanagnou D. Telesimulation: a paradigm shift for simulation education. AEM Educ Train. 2017;1(2):137–9.
9. Jewer J, Parsons MH, Dunne C, Smith A, Dubrowski A. Evaluation of a Mobile Telesimulation unit to train rural and remote practitioners on high-acuity low-occurrence procedures: pilot randomized controlled trial. J Med Internet Res. 2019;21(8):e14587.
10. International Council of Nurses. Scope of nursing practice decision making framework toolkit. Geneva: International Council of Nurses; 2010.
11. Benner P. From novice to expert. Am J Nurs. 1982;82:402–7.
12. Boman E, Levy-Malmberg R, Fagerström L. Differences and similarities in scope of practice between registered nurses and nurse specialists in emergency care: an interview study. Scand J Caring Sci. 2020;34(2):492–500.
13. Mikrogianakis A, Kam A, Silver S, Bakanisi B, Henao O, Okrainec A, et al. Telesimulation: an innovative and effective tool for teaching novel intraosseous insertion techniques in developing countries. Acad Emerg Med. 2011;18(4):420–7.
14. Wilkinson TJ, Smith JD, Margolis SA, Sen Gupta T, Prideaux DJ. Structured assessment using multiple patient scenarios by videoconference in rural settings. Med Educ. 2008;42(5):480–7.
15. Schon D. Educating the reflective practitioner. San Francisco: Jossey-Bass Higher Education Series; 1987.
16. Levett-Jones T. Clinical reasoning: learning to think like a nurse. Australia: Pearson; 2013.
17. Garland C, Wilson JA, Parsons MH, Dubrowski A. The application of low-fidelity chest tube insertion using remote Telesimulation in training healthcare professionals. Cureus. 2019;11(12):e6273.
18. Health. 2018. The 411 on debriefing in clinical simulation: How nursing simulations & debriefing create better nurses 2018. https://www.wolterskluwer.com/en/expert-insights/the-411-on-debriefing-in-clinical-simulation-how-nursing-simulations-debriefing-create-better-nurs.
19. Savoldelli GL, Naik VN, Park J, Joo HS, Chow R, Hamstra SJ. Value of debriefing during simulated crisis management: oral versus video-assisted oral feedback. Anesthesiology. 2006;105(2):279–85.
20. Kyaw BM, Saxena N, Posadzki P, Vseteckova J, Nikolaou CK, George PP, et al. Virtual reality for health professions education: systematic review and meta-analysis by the digital health education collaboration. J Med Internet Res. 2019;21(1):e12959.
21. Aziz A. Virtual reality programs application in healthcare. J Health Inform. 2012;9(1):305.
22. Smith SD, Thompson CE, Sims S. Adapting a nurse-managed Mobile simulation program to meet rural health nursing continuing education needs. J Contin Educ Nurs. 2020;51(2):82–6.
23. Martin D, Bekiaris B, Hansen G. Mobile emergency simulation training for rural health providers. Rural Remote Health. 2017;17(4):1–7.

Perioperative Simulation for Nursing

39

Jennifer C. Mendenhall, Anjanette Y. Pong, Marc Parent, and Cindy M. Blenis

Introduction

Simulation modalities that facilitate knowledge exchange, skill validation, and improved teamwork are well suited to the perioperative environment. The patient, on the day of surgery, is cared for by three different multidisciplinary teams who ideally provide safe, coordinated, patient-centric care in a fast-paced, highly technical, minutely orchestrated window of time. The multidisciplinary teams responsible for surgical patients include the pre-operative team, who prepares the patient for surgery; the intra-operative surgical team of surgeon, surgeon assistant, anesthesia provider, nurse, and surgical technologist; and the post-operative team, who "recovers" the patient. Perioperative is an all-encompassing term meaning pre, intra, and postoperative care of surgical patients.

Regardless of experience, professionals working in perioperative areas need to work well together, be familiar with multiple pieces of technical equipment, and communicate effectively within and between teams. Like sports teams who practice continuously, practice in the form of simulation of actual surgical events provides team members with opportunities to improve teamwork and communication. Simulation provides the opportunity for immersive experiential learning for both the individual and the team, with the goal of turning a team of experts into an expert team. However, to become experts, individuals must practice repeatedly, and simulation offers the opportunity to practice not only team skills but individual skills as well. In the surgical arena, surgeons must practice the technical skills of knot tying, laparoscopic procedures, and other fine motor skills necessary for success in the OR. Similarly, nurses working in the perioperative environment must be familiar with a wide array of skills. Nursing situations that lend themselves to the modality of simulation include:

1. Perioperative staff training for student nurses and novice nurses in a perioperative immersive clinical program, in preceptorships, or in a graduate training program such as the Association of Operating Room Nurses (AORN) Perioperative 101 [1]. Simulation provides a safe environment in which novice nurses practice skills such as creation and maintenance of a sterile field, gowning and gloving self and others, support of anesthesia during patient intubation, or practice skin antisepsis.
2. Practicing OR specific skills (ex., L&D skills related to childbirth complications)
3. Validation of knowledge, skills, and attitudes of experienced nurses new to the organization (pre-hire, onboarding, competency assessment).
4. Team training for experienced providers (ex., intra-operative cardiac arrest).
5. Learning complex surgical procedures (ex., conjoined twins' separation, multiple births).
6. Pilot testing new workflows (ex. Opening a new surgical suite).

Background

Anesthesia providers were early adopters of simulation, collaborating with the aviation community, especially in the realm of anesthesia crisis resource management as adopted

J. C. Mendenhall (✉)
Perioperative Services, Kaiser Permanente Northern California Patient Care Services, Oakland, CA, USA
e-mail: Jenny.C.Mendenhall@kp.org

A. Y. Pong
RN Magnet Program Coordinator, Kaiser Permanente, Oakland, CA, USA
e-mail: Anjal.Pong@kp.org

M. Parent
CommonSpirit Health, Roseville, CA, USA
e-mail: Marc.Parent@commonspirit.org

C. M. Blenis
Kaiser Permanente, San Leandro Medical Center, San Leandro, CA, USA
e-mail: Cindy.m.blenis@Kp.org

J. M. Kutzin et al. (eds.), *Comprehensive Healthcare Simulation: Nursing*, Comprehensive Healthcare Simulation,
https://doi.org/10.1007/978-3-031-31090-4_39

by Stanford [2]. In 2001, an anesthesiologist working for Kaiser Permanente, a large not-for-profit organization, helped lead the development of a Perinatal Patient Safety Program (PPSP) in response to the report "To Err is Human" [3] and the call for a decrease in preventable errors such as birth injury. This program was successfully pilot-tested prior to regional dissemination across Northern California. The elements of this program included human factors and critical events team training (CETT), using simulation as an educational tool. The initial project was funded by a large internal grant and included training all disciplines in the maternal child department at one Kaiser medical center (see appendices A, B). Initial intra-disciplinary team meetings were held around a table, and a special emphasis was put on hearing from a diverse group of representatives, from physicians to environmental services staff. The goal was to encourage everyone to have an equal voice, thereby flattening the hierarchy and encouraging a high-functioning team. The pilot program made a powerful impression throughout the organization, and the endeavor was translated to the perioperative setting. However, grant funding was not available, but the manikins purchased for the pilot were o used in a perioperative simulation program in 2001. In 2009, Kaiser purchased "families" of simulation equipment (adult male, female birthing simulator, and task trainer, child, and baby) for each of its 21 Northern California Medical Centers to encourage the adoption of simulation as an educational modality region-wide. Because of the long-standing perioperative simulation program, when perioperative crisis checklists were planned to be implemented in 2013, they were pilot-tested using simulation in the operating room at the Kaiser Permanente facility in which the simulation program originated. Because of the foundation laid for many years, the perioperative teams were familiar with critical event team and human factors training that utilized simulation. However, they needed to become more familiar with the perioperative crisis checklists (see Appendices C and D). Therefore, three simulation scenarios were conducted in situ in an operating room on a Saturday morning with a volunteer team. The three scenarios, all adult cases, were sepsis, cardiac arrest, and malignant hyperthermia (see appendices E, F). The participants included OR nurses, surgical technologists, and a Certified Registered Nurse Anesthetist (CRNA). The team participated in each scenario twice, the first time without the checklists, and then they repeated the scenario with the checklists. The scenarios were facilitated by two anesthesiologists, one a perioperative safety expert and the other a sepsis champion. Pre and post-surveys were completed by the participants, $N = 6$, which identified the perception that crisis checklists improved compliance with critical lifesaving interventions. A later survey completed after the checklist was implemented regionally of OR RNs and surgical technologists, $N = 122$, validated the results of the earlier survey. This result mirrored similar study results conducted by Harvard's Chan School of Public Health to study the effectiveness of OR crisis checklists when teams were trained to use them [4].

Future Considerations for Simulation

Facility instructors and clinical nursing are challenged to design innovative multimodal educational opportunities, including simulation, virtual reality (VR), augmented reality (AR), and perioperative learning experiences to prepare the next generation of nurses for the challenges of the twenty-first century. Pre-learning or flipped classrooms can be offered online or virtually, which supports social distancing. VR can be used to familiarize not only student and novice nurses but also other student disciplines with perioperative workflows and team member roles. Most recently, the COVID-19 pandemic has required educators to meet many new challenges, including social distancing. This challenge was also an opportunity to introduce new learning modalities, such as recorded simulation scenarios which can be viewed via online platforms. Another innovative educational strategy that emerged was short 15-min in-person "snapshot" simulations or educational events.

Kaiser provides surgical residencies for doctors in podiatry and general surgery residencies as well as clinical placements for surgical technologist students and certified registered nurse anesthetist (CRNA) student clinicals. Students completing undergraduate nursing degrees and new graduate nurses are traditionally excluded from perioperative services and therefore have little to no experience caring for pre, intra, and post-operative patients. Due to the limited clinical experience in the OR as students, it is often hard to recruit nurses to the perioperative environment. Therefore, student nurses should be afforded the opportunity to complete an internship in the OR to learn about the unique environment and the nursing skills required to be successful. This would help fill the many vacancies being seen in the perioperative nursing community.

Applications (Apps) can be used to provide information about surgical patient care. VR can be a useful adjunct to clinical experience for not only the novice nurse but expert perioperative nurses as well. Nursing residences would provide the student and novice perioperative nurses, in conjunction with multimodal experiential learning techniques, important knowledge of surgical patient care.

Best Practices

There are several best practices that have led to the success of perioperative simulations in Kaiser Permanente and at the University of California San Francisco (UCSF). A few best practices include keeping it simple, garnering the support of leaders and creating champions for the program, inviting fellow educators and content experts to assist in simulations as facilitators, identifying clear goals for the scenario, and building on the success of prior simulations. Other best practices are to pilot test the experience before planning a full implementation, and involving clinicians as subject matter experts in the design of a low-fidelity experience is recommended because they will be able to identify crucial content that may be lacking in the experience. In-situ simulation is important when department workflows are being tested and when functioning OR equipment is part of the scenario, for example, an OR table or other large OR-specific equipment. In-situ simulation also encourages the participation of team members, including surgeons.

Finally, it is always good practice to ask the question, "Is simulation the best modality for the transfer of knowledge and achievement of the educational goals identified?"

Keeping it Simple

If the answer to the above question is yes, starting with a small participant group is more manageable for the novice educator who may not be experienced in facilitating simulation-based educational activities. These activities should include a pre-brief and debrief. Planning the experience with defined objectives is important for evaluating the success of the simulation exercise. In a mock code simulation, the objective can range from obtaining the crash cart, pushing the alarm, placing the defibrillator pads on the patient, or successfully performing closed-loop communication. All these outcomes should be clearly defined so that the facilitator can evaluate the team's performance. The initial group of participants can be other educators or team members who can provide honest feedback to improve the experience. Provide all participants in the pilot or "dress rehearsal" simulation with the opportunity to evaluate all aspects of the exercise, including the pre-brief and the debrief, through an immediate discussion of the exercise or a review of the recorded session, if possible. Recording can be easily done with a cell phone and tripod and viewed later to determine areas that may need improvement.

Ideally, experienced perioperative teams practice for critical events in pre-op, OR, and PACU during education or skills days. Simulation equipment is only sometimes needed to engage participants in the simulation. One example of a simple scenario in which no special equipment is required is the scenario of a fire drill and the evacuation of a patient from the OR. The potential for fire is increased in the OR. The three components of the fire triangle, oxidizer, fuel, and ignition source, are present during most surgeries. Oxidizers include oxygen and carbon dioxide. Sources of fuel include the patient's hair, surgical sponges, and alcohol-based skin antisepsis solutions. Ignition sources include electrosurgical cautery, laser, and fiber optic light sources. Annually 90–100 fires occur in the OR and can cause permanent injury or even death [5].

For expert nurses and perioperative teams, simulation of potentially real events, such as a fire in the perioperative setting, can reinforce existing knowledge by providing an opportunity to practice rare situations and emergencies. For example, perioperative nurses may have seen videos of surgical fires, but few have practiced the recommended steps to evacuate a patient, on the operating room table, from the OR. All that is needed for this simulation scenario is an empty operating room and an OR bed. Although this simulation is simple to set up, the learnings can be profound without needing to purchase expensive simulation equipment.

Both stable and ad hoc teams may not realize the value of this learning modality, but after participating in or even observing a simulation, most participants appreciate the value of this engaging learning environment. The engagement of the learner is facilitated by creating a psychologically safe space to reflect on practice. Simulation instructors gain insights into communication patterns and workflows by observing the simulation and facilitating the debriefing, especially if the debriefer takes the position of inquiry and respect for the knowledge experienced nurses already possess [6]. An example of this is the fire drill scenario outcome discussed below.

A fire drill goal can be as simple as moving a simulated patient quickly and safely out of a smoky operating room to the designated smoke compartment, per hospital policy and state regulations. In one case scenario, with a team of competent and experienced OR nurses new to simulation, the educator started by reviewing the functionality of an OR bed. When the expert nurses [7] realized they were being asked to move the bed from the OR to PACU, they pushed the competent nurses out of the way so they could experience the task first-hand. After achieving the goal of moving the "patient" to safety, the expert nurses hypothesized that there was a power outage, necessitating the use of manual bed controls, and moved the bed from OR to PACU again. These expert OR nurses, but neophyte simulation participants, not only built on the scenario, but they also taught their competent colleagues how to move a heavy OR bed quickly and efficiently from the OR and down a corridor to the PACU. Before this exercise, the nurses had not been enthusiastic about or understood simulation, but after this simple scenario, the nurses were enthusiastic about promoting this engaging learning modality to leaders and their colleagues.

Garnering Support and Creating Simulation Champions

Linking simulation-based education to organizational initiatives and regulatory requirements is helpful in garnering support from organization leadership and simulation champions. Since fire drills are a regulatory requirement, the fire drill scenario is a priority and will be supported by stakeholders who are required to conduct quarterly fire drills in patient care areas. By advocating for a simulation scenario that is a regulatory requirement, the nurse educator provides the rationale for support from engineering, nursing, and physician leadership.

Buy-in from nursing leadership, surgeons, and anesthesia are key. Many anesthesia providers and surgeons are familiar with simulation and appreciate the value of interdisciplinary critical event team training (CETT). In addition, it is helpful to identify frontline staff and practitioners and involve them in the development and ongoing support of simulation-based education. Do not hesitate to reach outside of the OR for simulation experts for situations in which simulation can be used to test, introduce, or educate on a new process or piece of equipment. An opportunity to introduce simulation as an educational modality and build champions presents itself when a surgeon needs to introduce a new procedure or a new patient population. The crisis checklist pilot discussed above was such an opportunity. Anesthesiologists wanted to know if a checklist would improve team responses during critical events; they needed nurses and surgical techs to test this theory. Permission was granted, and staff volunteered to participate because they were interested in the outcome, and this activity led to increased support among the staff for simulation activities.

Invite Fellow Educators and Content Experts

If you are an experienced simulation expert, invite novice educators and staff nurses to participate in simulation activities as facilitators. If you are a novice, invite simulation experts to assist you and provide feedback. Lessons learned in these collaborations will spread, and best practices be adopted. For example, having clear scenario goals and objectives can assist the subject matter expert address scenario workflow and fidelity (creating a facsimile of reality). Perioperative educators who have participated in the perioperative education days with other simulation educators from other locations have adopted best practices in their own perioperative departments, such as the importance of the information gathered from the debriefings. These insights can provide a working plan to address issues such as workflow and team communication, and learnings can be transferred to real life.

Build on the Success of Prior Simulations

The fire/evacuation scenario was incorporated into education days as the last scenario of the day. It worked well because the staff knew PACU was the smoke compartment because a review of the smoke compartments and possible exit routes identified had been completed prior to the simulation, an example of a flipped classroom. In this scenario, the learners were required to evacuate beyond the smoke compartment, per hospital policy, as this scenario was a general patient evacuation due to a large fire (or earthquake). The exit route through the Emergency Department (ED) was identified, and the paths from the four utilized operating rooms were mapped out. Pre-learning included the identification of exit routes from each operating room. After the fourth scenario and debriefing, facilitators were instructed to declare a fire on the floor or patient, which required the evacuation of the patient from the OR bed (see Appendix G). All four teams executed the goal well and met outside the ED for celebratory high-fives. The teams then returned the OR beds, complete with manikins, to the ORs, and a final group debriefing was conducted. Lessons learned: It was later noted that the ED was very impressed with the efficiency and energy of the OR teams. However, the ED team requested a heads-up prior to the next perioperative fire drill so they would be prepared to participate.

Sample Curriculum #1: A Perioperative Immersive Program for Senior Student and Novice Nurses

Training a nurse to work in the operating room is expensive, extensive, and labor-intensive. Costs include creating or buying curricula, developing experienced nurses to precept, the need for a clinical educator or faculty on-site, and upwards to 12 months of training before the nurse is competent and independent. The estimated costs of training an OR nurse are upwards of $59,000 [8]. Between 2017–2019, sixteen senior student nurses completed a 2-week immersive perioperative program at one Kaiser medical center. The program included classroom time with simulation of perioperative skills either in a classroom or operating room (see appendix H) and simple skills-based scenarios such as skin antisepsis (see appendix I). The 2-week immersion program was designed to expose the student to the patient's continuum of perioperative care from admission to discharge. Perioperative clinical experience, which includes time spent in the operating room, has been shown to increase "portable skills" and knowledge [9, 10]. The student nurse will retain the increased empathy, skills, and insights into the surgical patient experience that the student experiences with his or her surgical patients. These experiences became part of the novice nurses' practice and knowledge base (see Appendix J). A student nurse in a modern inpatient setting will gain little or no experience in the pre-op or post-operative care of patients receiving a new total joint, having a laparoscopic cholecystectomy, or even an aortic aneurysm repair, because these are outpatient surgeries after which these patients return to their home and communities. Participants had reported that nursing students, regardless of their interest, would benefit from a program in which they gained knowledge of and empathy for the patient's surgical experience as well as opportunities to practice and hone skills in a short period of time. This was the focus of the program, to give students hands-on experience, thereby increasing empathy for their patients and building the student's confidence through skill acquisition.

The following skills-based scenarios described are applicable to any nurse or student new to the operating room. The program provides a comprehensive introduction to the OR for either an immersion program, capstone preceptorship, or Peri-op 101 program. The Peri-op 101 training program takes a nurse 12 months to complete because American-trained nurses have no perioperative experience past 1 day of observation as a student. How much more cost-effective might the Peri-op 101 training program be if an elective program with simulation was included for interested students?

The 2-week immersive program introduces the student nurse to the three areas of perioperative nursing, pre, intra and postoperative care of the surgical patient. Prior to the first student immersion program in 2017, experienced perioperative nurses from all three areas were trained as preceptors, and the educator met with surgeons, anesthesia, and nursing leadership to garner support for the program. The 8-week student preceptorships focus on intra-operative care of the patient and reinforce the knowledge and skills learned during the immersion program. If a student has not completed the immersion program, the first 2 weeks of their preceptorship will mirror the immersion program curriculum. The 2020 immersion program was canceled due to the COVID pandemic; however, two applicants were able to complete the 8-week preceptorship prior to the winter surge.

Student nurses in the preceptor program add to their perioperative skill sets by participating in simulations. These simulations are also applicable to participants in the perioperative 101 training program as well. Activities include:

1. Simulation of anesthesia during intubation of adult and pediatric patients, with an introduction to airway adjuncts and bag mask techniques. An adult or intubation head, if available, appropriately lubricated, can be used for visualization of the vocal cords and for practice in assisting with intubation. Bag mask practice can be achieved with an adult or child manikin and the appropriate size mask and adult or Pediatric ambu bag.
2. Practice gowning, gloving, draping, and assisting with surgery in the scrub role.
3. Participation in briefings, time out, hand-offs between levels of care, and debriefings at the completion of the surgical procedure.

As a direct result of the perioperative immersion program, 18 students have completed 8-week perioperative preceptorships, and to date, nine, or 50% as new graduate nurses have completed or been accepted into perioperative 101 training programs.

Sample Curriculum #2: Peri-op 101 Training Programs

Facilities currently supporting a new nurse residency training program utilizing the Association of Operating Room Nurses (AORN) Peri-op 101 Program have many opportunities to incorporate low-fidelity simulation into the training sessions. Clinical scenarios that can be easily replicated in a low-fidelity manner include steps to reconcile a missing sponge at the end of a case or actions to take when the sterile field has been compromised. The course includes a skills lab validation checklist for each clinical topic which could easily be transformed into a simulation session. For example, in the skin antisepsis checklists, the student must demonstrate a surgical prep on an abdomen, extremity, and vaginal/perineum area (see Appendix K). Utilizing available manikins for this exercise is key to learning proper technique, especially when reviewing the concepts of moving from clean to contaminated areas of the body.

The simulation scenarios identified in the student immersion and perioperative preceptorship programs are applicable to Peri-op 101 [1], whether the nurse is a new graduate or an experienced nurse transitioning to perioperative services from other nursing disciplines. As illustrated, simulation and clinical experiences as a student are retained by the new grad, thereby decreasing the learning curve and decreasing the time required to achieve confidence, competence, and independence in an expensive Peri-op 101 training program. In the current climate of limited student exposure to perioperative nursing, neophyte nurses need to be socialized to the perioperative environment and introduced to workflows and patient care procedures specific to perioperative services. Students who participate in a 2-week immersive program adjust well to the perioperative environment and obtain skills and knowledge which are not only applicable to other nursing disciplines but also enhance their empathy and understanding of the patient's surgical experience. Training a nurse in the Operating Room (the focus of Peri-op 101) takes a year because the nurse has, coming into the program, no experience caring for intra-operative patients. Supported time spent in the OR increases student nursing skills levels, socialization, understanding of team dynamics, and reduces expensive training time as a new grad, and most importantly, increases, in the student's eyes, their confidence and ability to thrive in this challenging healthcare environment. Participants reported that nursing students solidified their desire to become operating room nurses by completing an immersion program and transitioning well to other peri-operative programs.

Sample Curriculum #3: Perioperative Team Education Day

A Perioperative Education Day includes simulation scenarios designed for 30 to 40 experienced perioperative participants. During a 4-h period, the simulation instructors facilitate the same scenario four times for four different teams of eight to ten participants. This allows each team to experience four different scenarios in the allotted time period. Participants should include a multidisciplinary team of nurses, anesthesia providers, surgeons, and allied health-care workers, including surgical technologists . Facilitators include simulation and content experts. A surgeon and anesthesia provider participate as standardized participants (SPs), who, in a simulation scenario, function within their scope of practice and are aware of the goals and objectives of the scenario. SPs may be essential or not, but including an SP adds fidelity and depth to a scenario. Each high-fidelity scenario requires three facilitators: a simulation expert, a content expert (experienced OR RN), and a debriefer with a manikin. Medium to low fidelity scenarios may be run by one or two content experts without a manikin.

The day starts with a welcome and introductions. Leadership involvement in this greeting provides an opportunity for leaders to demonstrate their commitment to good patient outcomes and their investment in the professional development of front-line staff and to meet and thank the facilitators for sharing their time and expertise. Participants are divided into four color-coded teams and receive a binder corresponding to their team color. Participants review the contents of the binder, agenda, and their team's first simulation location. For instance: red team, OR 1; blue team, OR 2; green Team, OR 3; yellow team, OR 4 (see appendices L, M). Each scenario is the same length of time and includes an introduction to the manikin, followed by the scenario and a debriefing. It is stressed that the participants will open supplies, the crash cart, give care just as in real life and give IV medications, per hospital policy, under the direct supervision of a provider. In the OR prior to the first scenario, the simulation facilitators in the OR or PACU introduce themselves, reiterate that the participants are expected to participate fully, and then introduce the team to the manikin. After the scenario, participants who participated in the simulation received a "sticker." This sticker provides visual confirmation that team members have already participated in a scenario. Facilitators can call on team members without stickers to participate in the next scenario.

A perioperative education day agenda should reflect issues identified from a staff needs assessment, input from leadership, and consideration of new policies and procedures. The educator should encourage suggestions for simulation scenarios based on real surgical cases from nurses who were involved in the patient's care. Word of caution, if a sentinel event has occurred with patient harm, simulation may not be the best modality for education because staff members may be traumatized by the original event, and a reflective discussion with a guided debriefing may be a better modality. Scenarios may be created based on chart review findings. An example of a scenario created from PACU staff feedback is available in (see Appendix N).

High-fidelity scenarios in the operating room and PACU may include:

- Sepsis, including undiagnosed sepsis (Adult manikin).
- Malignant Hyperthermia is an uncommon high-risk, time-sensitive event that may mimic other conditions. (Adult or pediatric manikin with simulation monitor).
- Pediatric respiratory failure leading to cardiac arrest (Pediatric manikin).
- Adult code secondary to local anesthesia systemic toxicity, pulmonary embolism (a risk factor in hip procedures), sepsis, or cardiac dysrhythmias.

When there is a challenge obtaining a manikin, a pediatric simulator can double as a small elderly adult if needed, or medium to low fidelity scenarios may be substituted.

Medium to low-fidelity scenarios in the OR may include:

- Incorrect surgical count, missing sponge, or another item. A manikin adds fidelity; however, a fake abdomen works well (see Appendix O).
- Fire in the OR to follow a previous scenario or standalone. No manikin is required.
- What's wrong with this room? Create an OR or another patient space with mistakes, such as the wrong blood type hung, heels not protected, etc. Participants identify the errors facilitated by a content expert. No manikin is required.

Prep Work: Leading up to the Education Day

The use of pre-learning or a flipped classroom is beneficial because the staff knows they will be called upon to perform during simulated events. When using this teaching method, each scenario should have corresponding didactic information, which is disseminated prior to the education day. A review of the crash cart, medications, and defibrillator should be conducted in the months prior to an adult code scenario. The days and weeks leading up to such an event provide the perfect opportunity for pre-work self-learning (the golden window). The educator should identify five or six possible scenarios, four of which will be on the agenda, and provide teaching modalities for all scenarios, such as handouts to promote engagement. A review of the crisis checklists or calculation of weight-based medications for pediatric patients can be done pre-work. Encourage participants to access online policies and other resources. Being prepared for the simulation experience can improve psychological safety. Emphasize simulation as an opportunity to not only hone skills but also improve teamwork and communication. If closed-loop communication is a goal during the scenario, make this a goal for the year because identifying a common goal allows for conversations about that goal and provides team members permission to use or request compliance of team members with the stated goal in real life, post-simulation. Provide examples of closed-loop communication and practice during huddles leading up to the event. An example of applying closed-loop communication in the OR is the surgical count process. For example, per AORN guidelines, both surgical technologists (ST) and RN count audibly and concurrently to identify the counted items. Closed loop communication occurs when both ST and RN concur, and the count is documented on the whiteboard in the OR.

Preparing for the Day

Identify and advertise the date as early as possible because people have busy lives outside of work and appreciate the time to plan their schedules. Include leadership, providers, and staff in deciding the educational content for the day because leaders and providers (surgeons and anesthesia) will have valuable insights, and staff when asked, will often suggest learning opportunities. Buy-in from stakeholders can be instrumental in allotting time and budget for education days to occur. Share the date and invite other simulation experts to join you. For example, if an expert is spearheading a project on sepsis, invite that expert to observe or facilitate the sepsis scenario. This provides an opportunity to introduce the expert to perioperative frontline staff and the staff to a leading expert in his or her field.

Send scenarios, goals, expectations, and agenda to the facilitators weeks prior to the education day to ensure facilitator engagement (see Appendix P). It is helpful to schedule one or two virtual meetings to identify goals, outcomes, and logistics ahead of time so everyone is on the same page and knows what to expect. Stress that action items from the debriefings are to be documented because concerns expressed during the debriefing should be addressed, which is easier to do if identified and written down. A cell phone picture of the debriefing notes can be sent to leadership, and leadership can address any issues or workflow challenges identified in the debriefing notes.

When planning simulation programs, consider inviting other professional development peers or content experts to assist with the planning and training. It is a great opportunity to mentor new simulation educators. Mentees can assist with gathering supplies such as gowns and gloves, as well as assist during the simulation and help with clean up afterward.

Canceling surgery to offer an education day may seem impossible, but seizing opportunities when they occur is a good idea. Consider times when a group of surgeons is out of town for a conference, resulting in "downtime" or offering simulation as part of an educational offering on a Saturday. Many operating room suites are underutilized on the weekend. Post a "save the date" months before the event so participants have time to plan. Make attending more fun than the "makeup package." Education is a regulatory requirement and therefore budgeted. Be sure to drive the education before an error or sentinel event.

Sample Curriculum #4: Using Simulation before Opening a New Hospital In 2014, Kaiser Hayward Hospital closed its doors after 58 years of service to the community. The staff and patients transitioned to a new hospital, Kaiser San Leandro, 15 miles away. Four educational activities were required of the staff prior to working in a new hospital environment. The four activities were:

1. Online orientation to the new hospital with regulatory and state requirements addressed
2. Physical orientation to the new hospital environment and patient flow through perioperative services.
3. Physical orientation to the department with a focus on new technology and new equipment
4. Workflow simulations in departments outside of perioperative services and two simple CETT scenarios (Sepsis and Malignant Hyperthermia).

The initial orientation with a patient focus was designed for staff to experience the new space first from a patient's perspective (see Appendix Q). This approach helped identify many of the staff workflows, such as the location of the admission department, operating rooms, and PACUs. Simulations using volunteer "patients" on the new motorized gurneys helped staff navigate patient workflows to departments outside of the OR, such as a trip to Radiology for a sentinel node biopsy. Ceiling lifts for patients with limited mobility were installed in some PACU bays, so a skills station was created in which the nurses and patient care technicians were required to move a patient from bed to chair using the ceiling lift. The "patient," a person of size, eloquently described her feelings of vulnerability and level of comfort during the transfer process. The nurses were appreciative of her insights and feedback. Two critical team training scenarios were chosen to help staff locate emergency equipment in this new space and test workflows focused on avoiding unnecessary stress and information overload. Lastly, two scavenger hunts were created to help orient staff to the new space. A fire safety scavenger hunt helped staff identify the location of fire exits, extinguishers, fire-pulls, and gas shut-off valves, and a supplies-focused scavenger hunt was run as a competition in which the fastest team to collect identified emergency supplies won a prize.

Use of Simulation to Validate Skills, Knowledge, and Attitudes of Experienced Perioperative Nurses New to an Organization

During times of crisis (such as a pandemic), experienced traveling nurses may need to be orientated and on-boarded in large numbers. Experienced nurses do not need extensive training; however, they do need to know hospital policies and new equipment, such as radio frequency (RF) technology for locating missing sponges, as well as institutional workflows. Simulation of skills can provide an opportunity to validate skills such as counting and communication modalities for time out, briefing, and hand, as well as assess the nurse's knowledge and attitudes (see Appendix R). Simulation of a patient scenario also provides the Travelers with the opportunity to ask questions about topics such as specimen collection, patient workflows, blood administration, medication administration, and the roles and responsibilities of other team members. Experienced nurses presented with a verbal scenario or case study can often "fill in the blanks." A simple patient scenario with a fake abdomen can be set up to demonstrate skin asepsis and practice RF sponge detection methods (see Appendix S). Filled with towels, a fake abdomen can be used to demonstrate effective chest compressions and demonstrate correct placement of defibrillator pads. Experienced nurses who are recognized for their expertise but are new to an organization are open to asking questions related to institutional policies, state regulations, the roles of co-workers, and workflows. The mental stimulation of thinking through a "case" prompts questions about specimen collection methods, count procedures, and more.

Integrating into Existing Education in the Clinical Setting

The process of integrating simulation into existing education can be a simple process when the steps of simulation best practices are analyzed and strategies are determined for assimilating simulation into current modalities of education and training. Having the appropriate team members involved is crucial for determining a successful strategy for education and ensuring all training needs are met, especially because of the interdisciplinary environment of the operating room. A nursing professional development specialist or clinical nurse educator experienced in leading education and training in multiple modalities and who understands adult learning principles is essential to ensure an effective teaching plan [11]. The strategy should encompass a needs assessment, determination of measurable outcomes, and assurance of support after training to evaluate the integration of training into clinical practice.

Incorporating Simulation into the Educational Design

The easiest way to start the simulation design process is to evaluate your existing education to determine if any simulation can be incorporated into the curriculum or educational program. Types of low-fidelity simulation include role-playing, which works well for practicing soft skills such as hand-over to another person and crucial or difficult conversations that often occur in the OR. Assigning roles to team members that differ from their own gives staff the opportunity to view a clinical situation from a different perspective and increase appreciation for teamwork and shared responsibilities for the patient outcome. Providing staff with detailed descriptions of the roles can help them to incorporate simulation into the culture where this modality may be new and uncomfortable. Providing a detailed script for staff to read can also provide a greater sense of comfort for those that may be unwilling to volunteer. Speaking out against lateral violence as a bystander is a great example of a common scenario that many staff face but are uncomfortable performing in an actual situation. This is a scenario where representation from all disciplines is crucial for training to be effective. Giving each participant an assigned role and script to read allows staff a safe space to practice dialogue that can be used in an actual situation. With each assigned role, each staff person either performs a task or reads a statement according to his or her script. This greatly relieves participants' level of stress during the simulation since they may not have pre-existing knowledge of the roles of each team member and aids in creating a safe learning environment. The existing perioperative environment serves as the ideal space to conduct these simulation exercises, as the goal is to replicate an actual scenario. Other examples of challenging scenarios in the operating room (OR) that are worth simulating include speaking up against witnessed unsafe practices or attempting to perform a time-out when team members refuse to engage in the process. Many examples such as these can be easily created in the existing space and prepared as a normal procedure. The great advantage of creating simulations in the OR (in situ) is the availability of supplies and equipment needed to recreate an actual surgery since many scenarios don't require a patient.

Conducting a practice run of a new procedure or orienting a new surgeon to a new facility is another opportunity for using simulation as a method to ensure smooth workflows and availability of all necessary supplies and equipment before the actual events are scheduled to take place. These mock procedures can be planned well in advance of a scheduled case and should involve the actual OR staff that will be scheduled in that case to provide them with increased preparation and can also aid in reducing anxiety that can accompany performing a new procedure or working with a new surgeon. For example, the implementation of robotic surgery in a surgery department presented multiple new workflows for the surgical team. These changes included complex room preparation, handling of robotic instrumentation, draping the robot, positioning the patient, and multiple technical demands placed on the team that was all new. Prior to actual surgery, it was beneficial for the whole team to practice the entire scenario to identify any needs and deficiencies. The more realistic the mock procedure, the more likely the team would closely identify actual practice gaps. A simulation of patient positioning, draping of the robot arms, opening the instrument sets, and having the surgeon review each step of the procedure was crucial in identifying where things were missing or needed for an actual patient case. And this can be done with a staff person volunteering to be placed in the surgical position in these situations.

Existing e-learning modules used to validate competency, such as sponge counting, can be assessed, evaluated, and revised if needed so the content includes a hands-on component. A combination of online learning and hands-on skills practice can provide the framework for a "flipped classroom," with the online module assigned as a pre-requisite for a hands-on component to reinforce the concept. An e-learning component can cover basic concepts, background, and rationale for content such as pressure injuries, fire safety, and malignant hyperthermia with a second educational modality that includes the hands-on component of training.

Case Example 1: Incorporating Simulation for Practicing Perioperative Patient Positioning

Patient positioning in the OR can be complicated due to the range of positions, devices, and prophylactic supplies available. Planning training for this topic over a longer period in smaller sessions may be more manageable both for staff and educators. The content can be focused on meeting one or two objectives rather than risking running out of time if staff have questions or want to engage in a discussion after the training. This method allows for more practice time using different devices during the simulation and better retention of the content specific to that position. For example, placing a patient in a prone position is challenging, and there are many patient variables that can be covered in a single session. Staff with varying heights and weights can act as patients to allow staff to determine the most appropriate positioning equipment and devices. After an increase in pressure injuries was reported in a pediatric OR with no trend in position type, it was determined that education and training in pressure injury (PI) prevention was needed. The injuries occurred in all areas of the body and correlated with surgeries over 4 h or more in length. The decision was made to conduct positioning training sessions for staff for specific surgical positions over a period of 6 weeks. The planning team consisted of anesthesia providers, OR nurses, OR management, equipment specialists, the clinical nurse educator, surgeons, and the wound and ostomy clinical nurse specialist (WOCNS), Training sessions included the use of infant and toddler manikins in various surgical positions on an OR table and placement of appropriate prophylactic devices and dressings on the correct high-risk areas of the body. The educator and WOCNS were available to provide staff with real-time feedback on positioning technique and demonstration of appropriate use of positioning devices. After the conclusion of the training sessions, the educator conducted weekly chart audits of PI prevention documentation, and the WOCNS tracked incidents of PI's. The incidence of PI's in pediatric surgery patients decreased significantly after training was completed. To promote the sustainability of PI prevention education, practice updates and reminders are displayed in the department and emailed to staff monthly.

Remember that clinical experts can be found in all areas of your facility and can provide invaluable support. These can include clinical nurse specialists, wound care nurses, pharmacists, anesthesia providers, and technicians. Specialty areas such as pediatrics have a variety of unique clinical experiences due to patient size and weight, and those hands-on activities can prove invaluable for training. Investing in basic manikins to serve as teaching aids for pediatric patients can be utilized in a multitude of simulation activities, including positioning, pressure injury prevention, prepping techniques, airway support, and CPR. High-fidelity simulator capabilities are not necessary to design effective simulation exercises.

Case Example 2: Incorporating Simulation for Testing New Procedures

A new procedure for adult patients was in the surgical specialty of head and neck; a surgery called Functional Endoscopic Sinus Surgery (FESS) with new imaging technology was tested in simulation with a new surgeon. Simulation of the surgery was conducted in the OR with the surgical team, who would assist with the first cases. Anesthesia was invited as the procedure included turning the OR table 180 degrees after the patient was intubated. This is not an uncommon practice in surgery, but it is important that anesthesia is aware of this step. Also important is the positioning of equipment in the room and the position of the team members in relation to the surgeon. Instrumental to the success of this simulation was the collaboration with the vendor, who supplied the instrumentation, a simulation head specific to the procedure, the expensive disposable imaging equipment required, and the purchased imaging unit. The surgeon took on the role of instructor and went through the procedure steps with her team, including setup, optimal positioning of the patient's head, the actual surgery with the disposable imagining instrumentation, and the order of non-disposable instrumentation. In addition to the surgery, the vendor reviewed the imagining unit with the circulating nurses to include the process for sending images to radiology. This simulation illustrates the collaboration between leadership, purchasing, the surgeon, and the vendor who was able to supply the equipment and needed (expensive) disposable supplies. Many surgical companies provide initial education for their products, including education of central sterile processing staff who will be cleaning and sterilizing non-disposable equipment. Leaders, when purchasing expensive surgical equipment, should consider agreements with the supplying company, which include education of front-line staff and the cost of disposable supplies to educate and provide hands-on practice in the final purchase agreement. The education plan should be discussed and agreed to prior to the purchase of new complex, expensive surgical equipment.

Challenges and Solutions

There is a paucity of literature that deals with the barriers to doing simulations in the operating room. The literature speaks of the advantages and benefits of including simulation training in formal education programs [12] and barriers to simulation in general. The barriers to general simulation in an operating room setting will be discussed.

As in most endeavors, the initial investment can be a significant barrier as high-fidelity manikins are often expensive [13], and the initial training on how to run the equipment can be time-consuming. Adamson [13], in her doctoral dissertation, surveyed Nursing school faculty who identified barriers to the use of simulation in nursing programs. The common themes identified were lack of time, lack of support, and lack of proper equipment. This, of course, was for nursing school programs. However, the same holds true in non-academic settings. One hospital facility has a high-fidelity (Hifi) manikin, another older, medium-fidelity manikin, and several low-fidelity basic life-support (BLS) type manikins available for education. There is, however, no dedicated space for simulation. There needs to be more funding for the maintenance of the equipment. The Hifi manikin is 9 years old and had not been updated until last year, only because the program and laptop being used had reached end-of-life and would no longer be supported by the vendor. Even then, only the minimum upgrade was purchased because of a lack of funding.

The equipment or lack thereof should not prevent the development of appropriate scenarios. For example, a tabletop simulation on paper works well to engage staff in discussions about care.

Time

Time is identified as a barrier in both academic settings and hospital settings. This is true of the perioperative setting as well. Many operating rooms are staffed at core levels and only have a few extra staff available to relieve others to attend classes or simulations. "Taking a room down" means the room cannot be used for actual surgeries, and, therefore, there is a loss of revenue for the facility, which could also mean the delay of critical surgery for patients. It has been found that in California, for example, 1 min of operating room (OR) time costs approximately $36 per minute [14]. Of the $36, $13–$14 are wages. The rest of the amount is related to direct costs (supplies). This cost is passed on to the patient in the form of charges which are usually marked up by a certain percentage. If a room is taken down, only some of the costs associated are eliminated. Staff wages still need to be paid, especially if the staff is attending training, although, in some budgets, training may be funded from a separate source.

The Kaiser organization requires simulation and mock events at least once annually. OR leadership must decide how much time to allot to these activities. For example, the OR at facility holds a Critical Events Teams Training (CETT) annually, alternating between the Ambulatory Surgery Unit (ASU) and the Main OR. During the CETT event, cases are delayed by 2 h so that all the staff can participate. The scenario is repeated in each room, and the entire OR staff, including some surgeons and anesthesia providers, participates. Unfortunately, this only occurs once a year. The rest of the time, there is 1 h allotted for education twice a month, which coincides with an anesthesia department meeting. This hour is used for staff meetings and more traditional education.

Staff Engagement

Staff engagement during the simulation scenario is very important for acquiring the full benefit of the experience. The simulation must be relevant to the participant's needs for adult learners to be engaged in the experience. Kharasch et al. [15], in developing their simulation programs, ensured that the learners were offered clinical information and learnings through simulation that were tailored to the discipline and training levels appropriate to everyone. They found that this encouraged learning, and learners gained more from the simulation experience. Kharasch et al. felt that a tailored approach contributed more to the expansion of their simulation program than the use of more advanced technology. If staff understand that simulation is a safe space to learn and share experiences, staff will be more engaged, and the culture may change to one of learning and development.

Having appropriately trained simulation personnel is important for staff engagement as well. If the simulation is running smoothly, engagement is likely to be higher. If the simulation personnel are struggling and the simulation is not running smoothly, the participants are more likely to lose interest quickly. Karasch et al. [15] speak of protected time for the physicians who were running the simulations. Eventually, a full-time nurse and simulation technician were hired to run the simulations, and they expect to be able to hire more staff as their program continues to expand. This refers to the previous section about time. If no time is allotted and protected, then it won't be easy to get the program off the ground, and expansion may not be feasible.

A meaningful experience relevant to the practice of experienced perioperative nurses may contribute to participant satisfaction. Johnston et al. [16] studied the elements of debriefing to include guiding questions from the facilitator to connect past clinical experiences with the training and bridge the simulation experience to potential future clinical situations. This was found to enhance critical thinking from the participants and increase the perceived value of the simulation experience to their practice [16].

Equipment

There are many types of simulation equipment on the market today. The limiting factors to purchasing equipment are space to store and securing funding. Funding will be discussed in its own section; space will be discussed here. High-fidelity simulators (HFS) require much storage space when not in use. The amount of space needed to adequately store the manikins when not in use can be significant if there is no dedicated simulation lab space. Any space where the manikins are to be stored must be large enough to accommodate the manikin and a gurney for storing the manikin. Of all the hospital departments, nowhere is storage more at a premium than in the OR. A tour of any OR will reveal equipment and supplies in hallways because all the storage areas are already full. There is simply no room for extraneous equipment that will not be used in patient care.

A simulation was planned for the OR, and due to storage constraints, the manikin was left on a gurney at the front desk of the OR. There was a sign placed on the manikin, so staff and visitors would not be startled by the "unattended patient" at the desk. There is no easy solution to equipment and storage space. As noted earlier, non-revenue generating space in most hospitals is at a premium, and storing the equipment in a non-environmentally controlled area is detrimental to the life of the manikin. Any space currently used for simulation or storage should be carefully guarded, and giving up that space should be avoided at all costs.

Funding

Funding is the biggest hurdle for non-academic centers to overcome. Manikins are not inexpensive, averaging about $250,000 each, not including maintenance and upgrades. This means a Sim family (2 adults, a child, and a baby) can cost about $one million dollars as an initial investment. An airtight business plan is required to secure funding. Grants are also a good source of funds to start the simulation program. The OR benefits from three possible sources of funding: the surgeons, the anesthesia group, and the hospital/nursing teams. Combining these three potential sources of funding may facilitate getting an OR-specific program up and running. It is critical that OR staff get training on emergency situations and rare events such as Malignant Hyperthermia (MH) [17]. It is worth the initial equipment investment so teams can practice and prepare for this rare event.

Simulation is often used so that staff can practice skills that are difficult or not ethical to practice on real patients. Without simulation, the lack of practice can lead to costly mistakes in administering care. These mistakes can be costly, potentially outweighing the cost of investing in simulation equipment.

Interface with Regulatory Bodies

Established elements of best practice can provide a framework for incorporating simulation into perioperative training and education. The International Nursing Association for Clinical Simulation and Learning. (INACSL) have established best practices to guide simulation practice for nursing. Standards of care from regulatory bodies or professional organizations such as the Association of Operating Room Nurses (AORN) should also be considered. High-risk, low-volume clinical situations are usually mandated by regulatory agencies for staff to demonstrate competency, and this is usually done through an annual competency validation or module requirement. Many facilities use these requirements as a basis for an annual education plan. Hospitals are required to report nurse-sensitive indicators data, such as catheter-acquired urinary tract infections (CAUTI) and hospital-acquired pressure injuries (HAPI), and this data can also be used to identify needs for increased education. An increase in patient safety incidents reflected through an incident reporting system or communication from the hospital quality and risk department may also identify areas of clinical practice deficiencies.

Conclusion

Leadership support is crucial for the success of simulation implementation in the perioperative arena because organizational leaders can ensure staff participation and accountability. Interdisciplinary collaboration is instrumental to a successful program since perioperative nursing practice takes place within a team environment consisting of anesthesia providers, surgeons, surgical technologists, and other allied healthcare professionals. Recruiting and identifying champions to promote successful perioperative education is an important early step to ensure consistent messaging amongst all team members and promote the importance of the training to their respective teams. Involving an interdisciplinary team that reflects the actual perioperative team helps to ensure that simulation will mimic an actual surgical environment and engagement in the process and reflects the value of the education for the team.

Simulation is a valuable modality for perioperative teams and, in the clinical setting, allows space for learning with knowledge gathering and sharing between peers. Surgery is increasingly complex, and although many surgical teams are "well-oiled machines," there are occasions when the surgeon or anesthesia provider and the team of RN and surgical technologists are strangers to one another. The simulation does not need to be complex or expensive; simple role-playing increases the willingness to speak up. Nowhere else in healthcare is patient advocacy more important; nowhere else does the patient so completely put themselves into the hands of strangers as in the operating room. Simulation of critical events and effective communication is not a nicety; it is a necessity. Increasingly medical and nursing institutions of learning have incorporated simulation and 'soft skills' into their curricula, so doctors and nurses are increasingly familiar with simulation and its benefits. It is not a question of whether we can afford simulation. It is a question of how we cannot afford the simulation of real events.

References

1. Association of Perioperative Registered Nurses (AORN) 2019. Perioperative 101: A core curriculum https://www.aorn.org/education/facility-solutions/periop-101.
2. Gaba DM, Howard SK, Fish KJ, Smith BE, Sowb YA. Simulation-based training in anesthesia crisis resource management (ACRM): a decade of experience. Simul Gaming. 2001;32(2):175–93.
3. Institute of Medicine. To Err Is Human: Building a Safer Health Care System. Washington, DC: National Academy Press; 1999.
4. Arriaga AF, et al. Simulation-based trial of surgical-crisis checklists. N Engl J Med. 2013;368:246–53.
5. Emergency Care Research Institute Solutions/accident-investigation-services/surgical-fire-prevention. Plymouth, Pennsylvania: Anesthesia Patient Safety Foundation; 2010. Prevention and Management of Operating Room Fires Video. www.ECRI.org.
6. Rudolph JW, Raemer DB, Simon R. Establishing a safe container for learning in simulation: the role of the pre-simulation briefing. J Soc Simul Healthc. 2014;9(6):339–49. https://doi.org/10.1097/SIH.0000000000000047.
7. Benner P. 2001 From novice to expert: excellence and power in clinical nursing practice. Prentice Hall Health. Commemorative edition.
8. Ball K, Doyle., D, Oocumma, N, I. Nursing shortages in the O.R: solutions for new models of education. AORN J. 2015;101(1):115–36. https://doi.org/10.1016/aorn.2014.03.015.
9. Crafoord M, Mattsson J, Fagerdahl A. Operating room nurses' perceptions of the clinical learning environment: a survey study. J Contin Educ Nurs. 2018;49(9):416–23. https://doi.org/10.3928/00220124-20180813-07.
10. Foran P. Effect of undergraduate perioperative education on recruiting novice RNs and retaining experienced RNs. AORN J. 2015;102(3):254–26.
11. Clinical Simulation in Nursing. Standards of Best Practice in Simulation, Vol. 12, Supplement, S5-S12; 2016. https://www.nursingsimulation.org/article/S1876-1399%2816%2930126-8/fulltext.
12. Reeves SA, Denault D, Huntington JT, Ogrinc G, Southard DR, Vebell R. Learning to overcome hierarchical pressures to achieve safer patient care: an Interprofessional simulation for nursing, medical, and physician assistant students. Nurse Educator. 2017;42(5S):S27–31. http://search.ebscohost.com.kaiserpermanente.idm.oclc.org/login.aspx?direct=true&db=c8h&AN=125761579&site=ehost-live.
13. Adamson K. Integrating human patient simulation into associate degree nursing curricula: faculty experiences, barriers, and facilitators. Clin Simul Nurs. 2010;6:e75–81. https://doi.org/10.1016/j.ecsns.2009.06.002.
14. Ely K. 2018. What are the implications of the costs of operating room time? AJMC from https://www.ajmc.com/view/what-are-the-implications-of-the-costs-of-operating-room-time.
15. Kharasch M, Aitchison P, Ochoa P, Menon S, Donlan S, Flaherty J, Wang EE. Growth of a simulation lab. Engaging the learner is key to success. 2011. Disease-a-month from https://www-clinicalkey-com.kaiserpermanente.idm.oclc.org/#!/content/1-s2.0-S001150291100232X.
16. Johnston S, Coyer F, Nash R. Simulation debriefing based on principles of transfer of learning: A pilot study. Nurse Educ Pract. 2017;26:102–8. https://doi.org/10.1016/j.nepr.2017.08.002.
17. Staff writer (2007). Simulation labs aid OR staff education. OR Management (23)1. http://web.a.ebscohost.com.kaiserpermanente.idm.oclc.org/ehost/pdfviewer/pdfviewer?vid=1&sid=e2bfed85-421a-4bcb-aaa2-2553c22147d7%40sdc-v-sessmgr01.

Part V

Simulation Operations and Administration

Simulation Operations

40

Rowena Saba and Leland Rockstraw

Introduction

The operations and management of a simulation center are critical to a successful experience for participants and facilitators and to the benefit of stakeholders, management, and staff. Operations consideration should include the effective management of resources within the context of the institution's mission and vision, the simulation center, and affiliates. In addition, understanding simulation resources such as personnel, supplies, equipment, technology and space associated with the delivery of simulation is part of the operations specialist role. This chapter will present strategies of operations and management to include simulation center roles, scheduling, the creation of scenarios workflow, review of the concierge model of high-fidelity scenario facilitation, skills center management, to include supply and inventory, equipment, staffing, use of technology, and the Healthcare Simulation Operations Specialist (CHSOS) certification.

A Standard for Operations: INACSL Standards of Best Practice

The operations of a simulation center require procedures and infrastructure to support and maintain day-to-day management. The interactions of procedures and infrastructure with the larger educational or healthcare systems will require knowledgeable and technically competent personnel to provide simulation-based education (SBE) activities [1]. Healthcare simulation supports learning in academic and clinical environments to aid in knowledge, skills development, critical thinking, and clinical reasoning. Basing operations on best practices standards specific to healthcare simulation will improve learner outcomes, reduce costs, improve efficiency, and allow effective use of technology. The International Nursing Association for Clinical Simulation and Learning (INACSL) created best practices standards in simulation operations [2] which defines areas operations including a strategic plan, personnel, resources, management, systems integration, and guidelines or policies and procedures. The six criteria required to meet the operations standards are:

- Implement a strategic plan that coordinates and aligns the resources of the SBE program to achieve its goals.
- Provide personnel with appropriate expertise to support and sustain the SBE program.
- Use a system to manage space, equipment, and personnel resources.
- Maintain and manage the financial resources to support the stability, sustainability, and growth of the SBE program's goals and outcomes.
- Use a formal process for effective systems integration.
- Create policies and procedures to support and sustain the SBE program [2].

Roles and Responsibilities

Job responsibilities are what simulation centers use to define work in a specific role and the functions the individual is accountable for accomplishing. Considering institutional goals, mission, vision, size, and diversity of learners will assist with determining the size of personnel and the given roles they will fill [3]. Andreatta [4] suggests three primary roles, which include administration (directors and managers), technical operations (coordinators, technologists, and technicians), and educational staff (instructors, facilitators,

R. Saba
School of Medicine, UNLV, Las Vegas, NV, USA
e-mail: rowena.saba@unlv.edu

L. Rockstraw (✉)
School of Nursing, University of Nevada, Las Vegas, Las Vegas, NV, USA
e-mail: leland.rockstraw@unlv.edu

J. M. Kutzin et al. (eds.), *Comprehensive Healthcare Simulation: Nursing*, Comprehensive Healthcare Simulation,
https://doi.org/10.1007/978-3-031-31090-4_40

and trainers). The following will explore the roles and responsibilities of these three primary areas.

The administration of a simulation center is responsible for the overall accountability and decision-making associated with the operations, funding, and attainment of goals. Communication, development, and management of policies and procedures, and meeting specific regulations, credentialing, and accreditations are also part of the administrative role. Assessment, development, implementation, and evaluation of simulation experiences, educational strategies, day-to-day operations, and financial management are critical aspects of the administrative role [5].

The technical operations and support of the functions provided in healthcare simulation require specialists with many functional roles, skill sets, and practice. Roles include director of operations, coordinators, information technologists, simulation specialists, skills specialists, and administrative assistants. The size of the simulation center and the population served will dictate and roles and number of staff.

The educational team would work collaboratively with key stakeholders to develop simulation scenarios to assist with the development of knowledge and practice of learners. The educational team should know adult learning practices and content specialists such as clinical, surgical, or other healthcare professionals. Roles can include education director, simulation facilitators, standardized patient coordinator, and simulation and debriefing facilitators. Healthcare content experts, such as nursing, physician, physical therapists, and behavioral health, must provide clinical knowledge and define expected behaviors [4].

Policy and Procedures

A policy and procedure manual helps a simulation center document the mission, vision, and standards of conduct, behavior, performance, day-to-day operations, regulations, financial processes, staff, governance, and educational and research information. This manual should describe how the simulation center will operationalize its mission and vision, list steps in how to implement various matters, and should be organized, indexed, complete, and coherent [5]. Policy and procedures will assist in maintaining standards, assuring consistency, and promoting effective operations of the simulation center. A simulation center policy and procedure manual should contain key components, which include general and administrative information, course educator's area, course and room scheduling, equipment and supplies, scenario information, operations, video recording and confidentiality, fiscal, customer relations, travel, research policy, safety and security [6]. Samples of policy and procedure manuals are available from several sources, including the Defining Excellence in Simulation Programs book (2015) published by the Society for Simulation in Healthcare.

Scheduling

The new sim center is built and ready to host incoming staff, students, and faculty at the start of the new semester. Where do the students go? When do the students go to the sim center? Are they practicing skills with task trainers or scenario-based simulations? How do they know where they are going and when? Although these questions seem easy to answer, getting there is something else. *Scheduling* is a skill that many need to appreciate. It is an art. Knowing how many students need to come for a skills center and following up with simulations is the majority of the work behind the scenes with a new cohort of nursing students. Each school and program have variations of cohort and clinical size as well as clinical hours determined by their board of nursing for hands-on practice in simulation. Those numbers, determined by state and institution, drive the curriculum, inevitably determining each nursing student's educational career down to the hour. The best way to start scheduling is to understand the curriculum, clinical hours, and clinical site placement hours needed and move on from there. There usually is a designated person to schedule, an administrative assistant, clinical placement staff, or faculty.

Software is an integral part of organizing and communicating the schedule to stakeholders, students, and colleagues. There are many types of scheduling software to choose from; depending on the institution, funding and simulation center can vary. Many major simulation vendors have a built-in scheduling platform to fully integrate the simulation center with that specific software. However, free scheduling software systems are available. Many institutions already have one, which could be a great starting point in understanding what system would work best for a simulation program. Creating policies and procedures to support and sustain the SBE program is crucial to the sustainability of the simulation program and, throughout this chapter, will be echoed frequently [2]. This policy and procedure will be the starting point of the foundation for determining deadlines to turn in requests, handling and managing conflicts between programs, and prioritizing scheduling requests. Creating policies and procedures to support and sustain the SBE program is crucial to the sustainability of the simulation program and, throughout this chapter, will be echoed frequently. Having this deadline for all programs is imperative when dealing with multiple programs or disciplines. For example, if the nursing program has an undergraduate and graduate program, both programs may request the exact dates, but the graduate program submitted the request first. Do they get that request fulfilled? Requesting exact dates and not having requests filled happens quite often within programs. One group would submit the request 1 year in advance while the other program still determines the dates. Is that fair to use the "first come, first serve" mentality? Working that specific issue out in a policy and procedure can alleviate that type of conflict. All parties are informed that deadlines are to be held and schedules only created after the deadline has passed, creating fairness for all programs using the simulation center. Another vital aspect of scheduling and policies is determining how much flexibility the sim center will give each program. Is there a 2-week or 1-month advance request needed for space? Will last-minute requests be allowed and considered? Can classrooms or non-center spaces flex into center spaces if needed? An example is if nursing faculty need check-off skills set up for IV but the only rooms available are debrief rooms, and can skills be practiced in all rooms that are non-centers and vice versa? As much as we try to prepare for scheduling issues and write policies for them, there will always be "hiccups" that occur. Sometimes, no matter how proactive one is, some policies and procedures will be born from a situation that unfolds during the natural day-to-day operations of running a simulation center.

Skills Centers

A simulation center may have at least one skills laboratory for students to practice their hands-on clinical skills. A skills center may be staffed by a full-time simulation operation specialist (SOS) or a full-time faculty member designated to the center for smaller simulation centers. Whatever the staffing role and designation, staffing the skills center is more than just having a body to be there for supplies, setting up, and breaking down the center. As with scheduling, starting with clear policies and procedures will assist the skills center in running smoothly for staff, students, and faculty.

Task Trainers

One major component is understanding what vendor has supplied the center's task trainers. If the simulation center is new, most vendors will assist with setting up and providing training for task trainers. This is an excellent introduction for those unaware of the different types of trainers available for specific skills. Also, every vendor will have specific care, maintenance, and troubleshooting instructions for a task trainer or simulator. At least one role of the sim center staff must have close knowledge of all the task trainers to maintain operational efficacy for the sim center and nursing program.

Supply and Inventory

This leads us to the management of storage and inventory of the supplies being used at the sim center. Each nursing course schedule and curriculum determine what supplies must be ordered and maintained. This is highly correlated to budget, so once this is determined, the skills center personnel can move forward with ordering, inventory, and distribution of supplies for each skills center. Another consideration for ordering supplies is fidelity. Fidelity is the level of realism associated with a particular simulation activity; fidelity can involve a variety of dimensions, including physical factors such as environment, equipment, and related tools (INACSL 2013).

The skill center SOS coordinates these related tools and equipment in conjunction with the faculty to ensure that the curriculum subject matter and outcomes can be met. An example is using actual medical-grade products versus simulated products. Some medical distributors produce medical-grade products at lower costs, which are great for simulation centers; however, some of those products may differ from those used at clinical sites. Some faculty may argue that having those products removes the fidelity of students learning those skills. This decision is left to the center's directors, course coordinators, and possibly the Deans.

Equipment and Repairs

Some repairs are simple and require little more than super glue or tape, while others require a significant overhaul of the manikin parts and pieces. Budget and warranty purchases are the main factors determining what, when, and how equipment can be repaired. For example, many vendors will offer extended warranties when purchasing an expensive piece of equipment, and purchasing the warranty gives administrators the peace of mind that their equipment will remain in working order for years to come. Many manufacturers include loaner equipment in their warranty purchases so facilities can continue courses if a piece of equipment fails. The warranty is not just "protection" for significant equipment repairs or failures but also a way to keep the SOS personnel responsible for the monthly inspections and maintenance. More minor repairs can often be found during monthly inspections, which are covered under the warranty. Catching these minimal repairs can aid in the longevity of the equipment. This subsequently leads to logging monthly inspections, repairs, and maintenance of equipment. There are several ways to do this; all are correct, but not logging and recording any of this is wrong! Cloud-based documents are easy to create and share with sim staff. Creating a log of the sim center's equipment, serial number, purchase date, and monthly maintenance may seem tedious; however, it will prove helpful in the long run. Consider discussing some of the "plans" task trainer vendors offer to replace consumable tissues regularly.

Technology Learning

Learning the technology for a simulation center may seem intuitive however is like learning a whole new language. Training simulation staff is time-consuming and will take time to happen. It takes anywhere between 6 months to 1 year to feel comfortable with the technology if the SOS is fully immersed with it daily—technology in the simulation center branches from low-fidelity task trainers to high-fidelity mannequins. Within the past 10 years, we've seen manikins go from no movements to full head turns and facial expressions. As clinical simulation progresses, technology shifts its gears to stay ahead. There are virtual reality simulators, mixed-reality, and augmented reality technology to aid clinicians in using simulations as a learning method. Attending webinars and joining simulation committees and forums is one way to stay abreast of all this new technology.

Staffing and Support

As technology advances in clinical simulation, understanding the demand to support that technology is vital for sustaining a simulation program. The need to support the technology aspect of simulation has created a need for SOS personnel. Depending on the number of simulations, the program dramatically changes the demands for personnel to support it. Faculty roles are teaching. SOS personnel's role is to support and maintain the simulation learning platform for the learners. Therefore, building a team is one of the most critical aspects of an efficient operational simulation center (Medical Simulation Design, Inc. 2010). Supporting technology is one aspect many faculty members have the time or knowledge to do. Software updates, upgrades, and new equipment models are time-consuming and specific tasks that many SOS personnel do. Supporting the sim center technology is similar to other institutions with a whole department to assist faculty with online platforms. There are specialized skills that make clinical simulation its department and entity.

Certified Healthcare Simulation Operations Specialist (CHSOS)

The CHSOS certification emphasizes everything brought up regarding SOS staffing and support. As clinical simulation gained momentum and the "sim tech" no longer just sat in front of the manikin to control it, the simulation technology specialist or SOS was born. What exactly does an SOS do? A person is defined as someone "with a diverse set of skills and expertise, both technical and administrative, related to the operation, support, and delivery of healthcare simulation" ([7]: p 148). This designation has grown worldwide throughout the simulation community, validating the contributions of the SOS personnel in simulation centers. We are seeing a new niche in the simulation community that belongs to the SOS staff members. This new niche is a non-student-facing, non-faculty, non-teaching group whose primary goal is to push technology and innovation to its limit. This innovation and creativity benefit the SOS, solidifying this specialized niche, and creating a learning platform that is revolutionizing technology, education, and healthcare.

Summary

The rules of a simulation center are shared within the policy and procedure manual and are an essential part of the center's operations. Policies and procedures provide direction or a roadmap for day-to-day processes and a way to communicate and apply standards and practices within the simulation center. They ensure compliance with laws and regulations, provide for decision-making, and assist with streamlining the business of the simulation center. Regardless of the program's operations size, and policies and procedures, time spent developing effective policies and procedures will benefit the simulation center stakeholders, learners, and staff.

References

1. Huang YM, Rice J, Spain A, Palagans J. Terms of reference. In: Palaganas JC, Maxworthy JC, Epps CA, Mancini ME, editors. Defining excellence in simulation programs. Philadelphia: Wolters Kluwer; 2014. p. 21–3.
2. The INACSL Standards Committee. INACSL standards of best practice: SimulationSM: operations. Clin Simul Nurs. 2017;13(12):681–7. https://doi.org/10.1016/j.ecns.2017.10.005.
3. Huang GC, Sacks H, DeVita M, Reynolds R, Gammon W, Saleh M, et al. Characteristics of simulation activities at North American medical schools and teaching hospitals: an AAMC-SSH-ASPE-AACN collaboration. Simul Healthc. 2012;7(6):329–33.
4. Andreatta P. Simulation center personnel. In: Crawford SB, Baily LW, Monks SM, editors. Comprehensive healthcare simulation: operations, technology, and innovative practice. Cham: Springer; 2019.
5. Herrington A, Gupta V. Roles and responsibilities of a medical simulation center manager. Treasure Island (FL): StatPearls Publishing; 2021.
6. Dongilli TA, Shekhter I, Gilavanes JS. In: Palaganas JC, Maxworthy JC, Epps CA, Mancini ME, editors. Defining excellence in simulation programs. Philadelphia: Wolters Kluwer; 2014.
7. Crawford SB, Baily LW, Monks SM, editors. Comprehensive healthcare simulation: operations, technology, and innovative practice. Cham: Springer; 2019.

41 Research in Nursing Simulation

Jill Sanko

Background

Simulation has been part of nursing education for over a century [1]. We find some of the earliest published examples of simulation-enhanced nursing education written in the mid to late 1800s by none other than Florence Nightingale [2] and a lesser-known Florence, Florence Lees (1874). Nightingale used simulation to teach proper hand hygiene (1969), while Lees, with co-author Henry Acland wrote about the use of "mechanical dummies" and models of arms and legs to teach bandaging techniques [3]. Little is known about whether Lees and Ackland, conducted research on their use of manikins, but Nightingale in contrast, is considered by many, the first nurse researcher.

Upon Nightingale's return from the Crimean War, she worked to improve hospitals; these efforts by many estimations, made her a pioneer in hospital reformation [4]. In her efforts to improve hospitals, she also established herself as a significant research methodologist and, in 1858, was elected as the first female Fellow of the Royal Statistical Society [4]. While there is no direct evidence of Nightingale having conducted simulation research specifically, given her focus on improving hospitals, patient safety, and the training of nurses and midwives, as well as her focus on research for application, it is not out of the realm of possibility that she was, in fact, the first simulation nurse researcher [4, 5]; indeed, she can be considered the first nurse researcher and her seminal work, the 'Nightingale method', used for conducting and disseminating research remains good advice for any student or novice researcher [5].

While there is evidence of the use of simulation in nursing education since the days of the two Florence's, we see the first efforts to coalesce a body of knowledge in this area in the 1970s. In the middle of the 1970s, we see the emergence of the first nursing group of thought leaders focused on using simulation in nursing education. This inaugural cohort of nursing educators met at the Health Education Media Association conference. It paved the way for developing the initial nursing organization focused on simulation—the International Nursing Association for Clinical Simulation and Learning [6]. Since the 1970s, INACSL has continued to be the leading nursing-based organization focused on the use and quality of simulation in nursing education. Noteworthy contributions from this organization include the publication of simulation standards, the development of a peer-reviewed indexed journal, an annual conference, the development of education and training programs, and other resources for nurse educators, healthcare providers, researchers, and students.

Although INACSL is the primary nursing organization focused on simulation-based education, many other nursing and non-nursing organizations now have specific content and foci in simulation as well. Examples of these organizational simulation-focused enterprises include the National League of Nursing (NLN) and their Simulation Innovation Resource Center (SIRC), which offers courses in simulation, fosters simulation research, and provides other resources related to the use or study of simulation-based education, the National Council of State Boards of Nursing (NCSBN) which offers guidelines for the use of simulation in nursing education, has an expert panel dedicated to its use, as well as other simulation focused resources. Likewise, the Society for Simulation

Supplementary Information The online version contains supplementary material available at https://doi.org/10.1007/978-3-031-31090-4_41.

J. Sanko (✉)
MGH Institute of Health Professions, Boston, MA, USA

Nova Southeastern University, Davie, FL, USA

Walden University, Minneapolis, MN, USA
e-mail: Jsanko@mghihp.edu; Jsanko@nova.edu; jill.sanko@mail.waldenu.edu

J. M. Kutzin et al. (eds.), *Comprehensive Healthcare Simulation: Nursing*, Comprehensive Healthcare Simulation,
https://doi.org/10.1007/978-3-031-31090-4_41

in Healthcare has a robust interprofessional membership, including a thriving extensively nursing-focused section.

With the growth of simulation, the professional and expert base has acted as a significant driver for careers in nursing focused on the use of simulation in education and for the conduction of research. Most nursing schools employ dedicated faculty and staff to run simulation and simulation research centers. Simulation has created a new sub-discipline of nursing where nurses use a combination of skills to carry out high-quality simulation-based education focused on developing nursing knowledge, skills, and attitudes. More and more, we are seeing nurse faculty researchers who have dedicated their careers to studying the impacts and outcomes of simulation-based education on nursing knowledge and skills. Most of these nurse faculty carry out this work as clinical or educator-track academicians. However, we have recently seen nurse scientists begin to do this work as part of tenured and tenure-track positions. Each shift in the nursing education/academic environment demonstrates the depth and growth of the simulation field on the whole, but more specifically within the nursing context. A 2018 article published in American Nurse Today (a publication of the American Nurses Association) outlines a career as a healthcare simulation educator [7]. This article speaks to the broader roles—but also highlights the researcher as a professional who conducts "studies using simulation as a tool to investigate clinical practice questions or identify the most effective uses of simulation, designing optimal healthcare processes and equipment" ([7]: p 59).

As more nurses find success with simulation as a research focus, we will likely see more interest in this area and, consequently, more demand for nurses with this expertise and the need to train researchers in it. Only some academic centers consider this line of research for tenure, but the landscape changes as the definition of impact and expectations for scholarly output broaden [8]. Moreover, simulation research is undoubtedly an area welcomed within the clinical track positions, so while simulation viewpoints as a tenure-line focus broaden, quality research is being conducted and carried out by nurse scientists pursuing careers on non-tenure track lines of scholarship and will continue to be pursued.

As a nurse scientist who has dedicated her career to the study of simulation to improve healthcare safety and teams, we need this work done regardless of who does it. However, for the discipline to continue to grow, we need to see more acceptance of simulation as a line of research widely accepted as part of tenure track work [8]. The future of simulation as a scientific discipline depends on the community to push higher education institutions to be more accepting of these pursuits [8].

Starting a Career—Educational Requirements

For those wondering where to start, below will outline some considerations for obtaining an educational foundation aligned for success as a nurse scientist interested in a simulation research focus. There are many ways to get to this baseline-specific simulation education that will bolster the chances of realizing a simulation-focused research career. Indeed, if asked, colleagues in the field for more than 10 years will agree that the career path looks much different to someone starting today, as compared to those who started a decade or longer ago. With the growth of simulation, there has also been explosive growth in educational opportunities accessible to launch careers.

A degree in nursing is the first step for those seeking to have nursing as their foundational degree. Given that simulation is a multidisciplinary field, one will find a variety of foundational degree types, including medicine, human factors, IT, physical therapy, biomedical engineering, and many more. For most nursing institutions, a bachelor's degree in nursing (BSN) will be the minimum required degree to work as a simulation specialist. A BSN should be coupled with a secondary certificate in simulation education, allowing one to demonstrate their qualifications to work as a simulation specialist and assist in research. However, there may still be very qualified individuals with years of experience who still need this formalized proof of qualification due to lack of availability earlier in their careers. Formal certification as a simulation educator or operations specialist through the Society for Simulation in Healthcare also demonstrates qualifications to work in simulation. However, these certifications require a few years of experience and location to sit for the certification exam.

Currently, the following are the available certifications for healthcare simulation [the first three offered through The Society for Simulation in Healthcare (SSH)]:

- The Certified Healthcare Simulation Education Specialist® (advanced or basic) CHSE (A)
- The Certified Healthcare Simulation Operations Specialist® (advanced or basic) CHSOS (A)
  - The Interdisciplinary Post-Bachelor's Certificate, from University of Central Florida
  - The Online Healthcare Simulation Certificate, from University of Central Florida
  - The Simulation in Healthcare Education Certificate of Professional Preparation, from Seminole State College of Florida

- The Graduate Certificate in Healthcare Simulation Online Program, from University of Michigan - Flint
- The Certificate in Simulation, from Drexel University
- The Healthcare Simulation, Graduate Certificate, from University of Alabama Birmingham
- The Healthcare Simulation Certificate, from Carolinas College of Health Science
- The HPEd Simulation Professionals Certificate, from MGH-Institute of Health Professions
- Healthcare Simulation Certificate, from Georgia College and State University[1].

While the certifications more limited, there are other many options for obtaining education on simulation-based education. A few examples include (certainly not an extensive list): The Center for Medical Simulation's instructor training courses, WISER's Simulation training, Mayo Clinic's simulation instructor development course, Mass General Hospital's Institute for Health Professions' Simulation-based education and Sim Ops (master's degree), University of Alabama at Birmingham's Master of Science in Healthcare Simulation, and Stanford Medicine's Simulation Instructor Course (see list at the end of the chapter). Organizations and websites also list simulation-focused degrees ranging from master's and doctorates in simulation to operations specialist-focused programs [9].

In addition to specific stand-alone certification courses and degree awarding programs, there are numerous other ways to broaden one's knowledge base. These include attending international, national, and regional conferences, taking a single course offered by any number of nursing organizations, and taking advantage of the free offerings several of the simulation companies put on. Many of these options come with the option of obtaining Continuing Education Units (CEU) that can be used at the time of renewal of nursing licenses and or simulation certification [CHSE® (A); CHSOS® (A)].

Obtaining a master's degree in nursing will allow one to teach outside of simulation within a Bachelor of Science Nursing program [10]. Many, if not all, nursing schools require those delivering didactic or clinical education to have a master's degree at a minimum. However, this is not a universal requirement. This degree level will likely be required of the simulation specialists at many institutions in the not-too-distant future but currently is not a widely supported requirement. It is advisable to investigate obtaining a certification or degree if the desire is to take on more substantial roles in simulation research or simulation-based education. Outside the specific simulation educational opportunities mentioned above, other terminal degree options are also worth exploring, especially for those interested in heading up research and publishing.

The decision to pursue a doctorate level degree, e.g., Doctor of Nursing Practice (DNP), Doctor of Nursing Science (DNS/DNSc), Education Doctorate (EdD), or a Ph.D. will allow, at most institutions, for one to carry out research as a primary investigator (PI). Outside of academia, there may be more variability regarding the minimum degree needed to conduct research as a PI. Thus, one would need to check specific policies.

It is important to note that one can carry out high-quality, impactful research without a doctorate. One of the leading landmark simulation studies was led by a nurse who did not have a doctorate [11]. Despite this example, regardless of the bachelor's or master's degree, it would be important for a non-doctorally prepared nurse to obtain additional education focused on research methods or seek the mentorship of a more knowledgeable or experienced researcher. There are many ways to find quality mentors through professional organizations focused on research. The Society for Simulation in Healthcare also has a virtual scholar's program where participants are paired with a mentor and participate in a year-long program focused on simulation-based research. Other programs with a similar goal include INACSL's research fellowship, CMS's research fellowship, and many other program-specific opportunities. One caution is that with the recent rapid expansion of simulation fellowships, a lack of standardization within the curricula has emerged [12]. It is prudent to vet the curriculum, program, and quality before investing in one.

Having addressed the basics of getting started as a nurse researcher focused on healthcare simulation research, the chapter will pivot and speak to other considerations related to research focused on simulation-based education and utilizing simulation as a data collection tool.

Best Practices

A quality and well-run simulation program is at the heart of any meritorious research program. Before engaging in research, one should ensure that the ability to carry out a study successfully can be achieved in the selected program. The first step of this task is assessing the environment and assessing if this setting is conducive to carrying out research. Generally, this begins with a foundation of quality programming in simulation nursing education. If not the one creating

[1]The aim is to present a complete list of certifications offered, however it is possible a program may have been omitted unintentionally.

the environment or running the program—it is recommended to have an interview with the program point of contact and ask pointed questions about their qualifications. Questions might include inquiries about their accreditation status, policies and procedures, and the quality and characteristics of their staff, equipment, and support.

Simulation research often does not originate solely from within a simulation program or center itself, but rather in concert with a simulation program, alongside its simulation faculty and staff. One is, however, apt to find considerable variation in who and how research is carried out from center to center. For programs with an established research arm, much of their output in terms of research will be generated from within this departmental entity. In other programs, the simulation program will support research queries brought by researchers who may or may not be formal members of the simulation team who run the program's day-to-day operations. In this scenario, the research is usually conducted in a partnership-like structure instead of as part of the aims of the research arm of the specific program.

Prior to beginning any study, a thorough understanding of the policies and procedures for conducting research should be undertaken. In addition, as a primary step, it is advisable to consult with the head of the simulation program or research arm to discuss restrictions for using space, software, equipment, consumables, and support persons. In many cases, fees will be assessed for using any or all these previously mentioned items. Many simulation programs' costs for carrying out simulation, which is part of courses, are absorbed by nursing schools as part of their overhead costing structure. This is often not the case with research, and it is rarely absorbed as part of overhead.

Due to the difficulty of generating revenue when a program is primarily in existence to provide simulation-enhanced curricula for a school's degree programs, many develop ways to offset this revenue "loss" by renting out space, equipment, or support personnel. Regardless of the specific structure, it will be important to know ahead of time if costs are associated with using the simulation space, equipment, and personnel. Do not assume that using a simulation center will be free for the department or university even if the entity who owns it, is the same one employing the researcher. It is common for fees to be assessed even for researchers who work within the same institution. Many times, the fees are at a discounted rate if employed there, but not always. Additionally, this information will be vital when creating a budget for grant applications if this is part of the research plan.

Other recommended topics to discuss with the point person of the simulation program are unique or specific needs to ensure the study's integrity. This includes, but are not limited to, a dialogue about who will complete the data collection, will recording of the scenarios and simulation learners be required, if so, where will recordings will be stored, for how long, and who will pay (if required) for storage costs, are there limitations related to the use of equipment, how will variances in how simulation is carried out be handled, alterations in the usual format or structure of pre-briefing, scenarios, and debriefing should also be settled early in the discussions. Additionally, a discourse on whether specific training of simulation personnel is required for the study. If so, who will train them, when will training occur, and will this occur during or outside regular business hours?

Researchers may need to catch up on the fact that most simulation programs' primary purpose is to support education rather than research. In programs with a primary focus on education support, engaging in the 'dance' of when and where research can take place is often necessary. Often there needs to be more space or human bandwidth to conduct studies during peak times when the simulation space and staff are running regular educational courses and programming. This means that research that does not overlap with a specific course will likely need to be carried out at an off-peak time, which often means evenings, weekends or term breaks. This may seem like no big deal, but it can impact recruiting research participants that may not be willing to show up on an evening, weekend or term break.

The most adept programs have formalized structures for research. Certainly, those who are accredited in research will have well-developed structures for conducting simulation research. If an institution or organization does not have a simulation program, look for programs that have achieved accreditation of their program, specifically one accredited in research. These programs are most likely to have high-quality structures that follow the established standards of practice.

When determining where, when, with whom, and how to operate research, also consider whether to research simulation as an outcome variable, as a manipulated variable, as a comparison, or will the study focus on something difficult to study in an actual setting, making simulation the tool for research, not the focus of the research. The skeleton of a simulation study will look very much like any other study in that it will have specific aims, research questions, and hypotheses. These "bones" of the study will inform study design and provide a basis for figuring out a needed sample size to reach power, statistical analysis approach, and measures needed to collect data. Simulation research differs due to multiple potential confounding variables not usual in studies that can hold steady conditions more precisely. As much as we standardize scenarios, pre-briefing, and debriefing for education, this is often only imperfectly executed. There needs to be no more than a slight deviation from perfect standardization for most educational goals to meet the learning outcomes. However, in the case of research, standardization becomes critical to reliably compare outcomes across groups or participants when running scenarios (often the intervention or place where intervention outcomes are measured) multiple times to collect the necessary data. It is infrequent that a large enough sample can be captured running a scenario a single time. Therefore from scenario run to scenario run, standardization of all elements of the simulation encounter must occur.

This standardization is easier said than done and requires strict adherence to small details, scrupulous faithfulness by all team members to plans, training goals, and rehearsal schedules, and probably most importantly, having all members of the team on the same page at all times during the simulation encounters where data capture is done. This author can share numerous times when miscommunication caused data loss and, in some cases, study loss. With the expense (time and capital) that research and research involving simulation takes, it is crucial to ensure you can do this efficiently and effectively. It is highly encouraged that a specific research manual or protocol is created for the team of people involved in the simulation aspects of the study. This is different but will become a part of the study-specific manual or protocol created as part of the study itself. This section of the study manual or protocol should consist of very detailed information, including scripts for standardized patients (SPs) or manikin voice actors, the timing of scenarios, timing of changes within scenarios, information shared in pre-briefing, pre-practice allowances, information for debriefing, specific inclusion of debriefing points, prop lists, manikin, task trainer lists, and room set up. It cannot be stressed enough that *ALL* details need to be spelled out. Further, each time a scenario is run (assuming you need to run multiple to have enough data), all aspects of the scenario need to be identical to the prior. This often means holding role players, pre-briefers, debriefers, and voice actor's constant across all scenarios. If this personnel constancy is not feasible, there must be very tight adherence among the various players to run an identical simulation experience continuously. Think about how Broadway does this. While the cast and location of a Broadway show may change, the show itself is reliably the same, such that Hamilton in Miami is much the same as if seen in New York.

Resources for Success

Every research program requires excellent loyalty to published research standards and reporting of simulation-based research [13]. Anyone conducting research should be familiar with ensuring that one can conduct research soundly and appropriately. One way to do this is to participate in a course if needed. Courses offered by one's university or institution can be tremendous and accessible sources of information specific to conducting research at that institution. These courses or informational sessions will provide an overview of the steps necessary to adhere to the university and institution's requirements.

Some universities and institutions require their researchers to become certified by an outside body in the ethical conduct of research. One such program that is widely used to meet this standard is the Collaborative Institutional Training Initiative Program (CITI). This certification program offers a comprehensive suite of courses on conducting research, from ethics to compliance. CITI courses additionally offer a history of the current regulatory body, explanations of conflict of interest, and best practices for researchers. There are many other types of programs, including those that are 'homegrown.' The critical thing to know is what is required and what is needed from both an institutional standpoint and a personal one.

As a simulation researcher, other resources may be uniquely crucial for guiding research endeavors and activities. To start, utilizing the simulation standards of best practices by INACSL and the Association for Standardized Patient Educators (ASPE) are wonderfully helpful resources for simulation and simulation research. INACSL includes the following standards:

(a) simulation design,
(b) outcomes and objectives,
(c) facilitation,
(d) debriefing,
(e) participant evaluation,
(f) professional integrity,
(g) simulation enhanced IPE
(h) operations.

ASPE has one standard around the best practice standards for standardized patients [14].

States of Being as a Simulation Researcher

Inquiry Versus Translational Approaches to Simulation Research

Many need to realize that research is bi-faceted, meaning that investigation requires both query and translational efforts to make the outputs of the work clinically or educationally relevant and practically impactful. While initial research to demonstrate and test a proof of concept or beginning to develop an understanding of the problem is essential, the ability to translate findings into consumable applicatory approaches is equally important. Creating a team of research-minded simulation nurses with expertise in both query and translation phases of research represents a well-balanced team with greater abilities to make significant impacts; this takes a little forethought and an understanding the nuances of degree structures and research processes.

In terms of degrees—it is crucial to understand the fundamental differences between a DNP and a PhD-prepared nurse scientist (degrees such as EdD, DNSc are not discussed—but are worth understanding as there may be instances in which having an EdD or DNSc on your team acts as an additional benefit). Because of the differences in their training and foci DNPs and PhDs serve in complementary roles within the structure of a well-balanced research team.

Doctor of Nursing Practice

A DNP-prepared nurse represents the highest level of preparation within the ladder of education for nursing practice for those individuals focused on the scholarship of nursing practice and application or integration of such practices into clinical settings [15]. DNP nurses are taught to consider the challenges, approaches, and appropriateness of applying research findings as a practice discipline to improve clinical practice, influence policy, inform science or educate nurse peers, clinicians, scholars, and other leaders [15]. In addition to these skills and knowledge sets, DNP-prepared nurses find themselves more often in roles focused on applying implementation and improvement science to advance the quality of healthcare and healthcare delivery [15]. It is not uncommon to find DNPs in leadership roles that are clinically based or educationally positioned. Many of these individuals wear two hats—one as a clinician and one as an administrator. Because their degree is practice-based, many DNPs continue to practice clinically alongside other non-clinical role such as professor (educator) or hospital administrator.

Doctor of Philosophy

A PhD-prepared nurse represents the most outstanding level of formal education for a career in research and in the quest to discover new information [15]. You will find these nurse scientists serving in any number of leadership roles both within and outside of academia. They are well-versed in research methods, and many can execute complex data analyses and interpret data to understand phenomena under investigation [15]. While the majority specialize in either quantitative or qualitative approaches to answering questions, they are educated, in most instances, to carry out both research methodologies; a growing minority are equally capable in both approaches or mixed methods.

Academic Versus Hospital-Based Settings and Research Considerations

Another important consideration is the differences between conducting research within, or for an academic setting instead of within, or for a clinical or hospital-based setting. In many healthcare systems, there are opportunities to bridge the two settings through partnerships or within the organizational structure. Many healthcare systems have clinical facilities that are part of larger academic endeavors and allow for the ease of research to be carried out in cooperative arrangements. Often these collaborations are mutually beneficial to both the clinical and academic arena. They also allow for systems integration work to be carried out for quality improvement.

Academic Areas

Research carried out in academic areas can take the form of a ubiquitous number of research topics; often, this research is driven by the interests of the simulation program and the scholars that are part of the faculty—thus, these interests vary. For example, research was completed at the author's institution using or focused on simulation in patient safety, end of life, teams and teamwork, medication safety, systems thinking, and IPE. These projects aim to improve healthcare and healthcare delivery and find new and effective paths to successfully use simulation to improve the education and clinical preparedness of pre-licensure and graduate healthcare students.

Systems integration research can often be an integral quality measure for organizations composed of both clinical and educational enterprises. In these organizations, systems integration research is used to identify areas needing improvement (often within the clinical arm of the organization), and the academic arm is tasked with carrying out the intervention (usually education). Outcome data may be collected on either side. However, the key to this research relationship is the relationship itself, and the sharing of data such that a synergistic data-driven feedback loop is formed between the two for the benefit of the research and the goals of both arms of the organization. Research that is part of systems integration endeavors may take the form of many topics, including patient safety, efficiency improvements, patient satisfaction betterment, or in response to a sentinel or never event.

The discussion of systems integration research here is relatively superficial, but it is worth noting because it can be a cornerstone of a simulation program. Additionally, it is one of the areas in which a simulation program can earn accreditation of their programs. If one is interested in learning more, a recommended resource is the chapter titled Systems Integration by Dunn et al. in The Comprehensive Textbook of Healthcare Simulation by Levine et al. [16]. An excellent example of a study done utilizing a systems integration approach was a study conducted by an interdisciplinary team of simulation researchers from the Winter Institute for Simulation Education and Research in partnership with the University of Pittsburgh, University of Pittsburgh Medical Center, School of Nursing, school of medicine and their Center for Quality, Safety, and Innovation. This study addressed the urgent need to ready medical teams in the wake of the Ebola epidemic occurring in 2014. This study described the central role that a simulation program can play in partnering with mission-critical areas of a healthcare system from a systems perspective [17]. The publication provides readers with a template for conducting and successfully implementing a simulation-based educational training program to address a critical clinical need.

Challenges and Solutions

Conducting research is full of challenges and rewards. However, if one loves simulation and can learn to love the challenge of asking a questions and then designing a way to answer them, research can become a second love, and the challenges are worth the 'sometimes headaches.' The most helpful advice is to be patient and know that each step in the process gets easier as one learns to navigate the places where hiccups are most apt to occur. Utilize resources wisely and avoid doing it alone if one can do it with others. Ask if there are standard language libraries for studies, i.e., many places have a standard language library to describe resources and environment, protections of human subjects, and data storage. These are nearly ubiquitous aspect of grant applications and IRB submissions. Do not reinvent the wheel if possible. If a standard language library does not exist, work to build one. It will be beneficial for future programs.

Funding research may be the greatest challenge for simulation researchers. There are only a few simulation-specific grants available. However, there are a few available to novice simulation researchers. These tend to be smaller but often can be used for seed funding for larger grants—more about larger grants in a second. The following organizations have offered simulation-specific grants yearly: SSH, INACSL, the National League of Nursing, Sigma Theta Tau, and the Academy of Society for Academic Emergency Medicine.

Larger grants may be found through government mechanisms as well as foundational grants. In this area—however, one will need to fit project ideas with the goals and alignments of the granting organization/governmental request for proposal. When considering funding for simulation research, several foundations, including the Josiah Macy Foundation, The Doctors Company Foundation, the National League of Nursing, and the National Patient Safety Foundation, come to mind. Many insurance companies have RFPs for projects to improve healthcare outcomes, the Robert Wood Johnson Foundation, and others. Foundational grants have a fair amount of variability regarding available funds and priorities from year to year—keep this in mind when planning to write these.

Governmental grants can be more significant sources of funds to carry out projects. When writing this chapter, few government RFPs could support simulation research—but they were specific regarding the request. When looking for a project aimed at improving medication safety, the author was looking for improving safety in the context of perinatal, neonatal, and pediatric care, and sought projects with goals to use simulators to improve providers' skill acquisition, and projects using simulation modeling and systems science to address health disparities. Beyond the specific examples of grants found supported by a government agency, there are a few other general government-sponsored grants where the investigator can propose their idea—these are generally advertised as investigator-initiated and are in the R families of grants. Government grants are complex. Therefore it is recommended to find a mentor who has had experience submitting, thus gaining support through a team to help one become familiar with the myriad of forms required when submitting them.

Other sound advice is not to get discouraged by "failure," so many of the grants you will apply for will be competitive, and few will receive them. A decision not to fund is not necessarily a judgment of the idea or writing but rather just a reflection of the highly competitive nature of the process and priorties of the cycle. Request and read feedback; feedback can help gain a stronger position for the next attempt. While the grant writing process is often filled with trepidation, it can also be rewarding when funding occurs, but know that it can often take many attempts to secure grant funding. Getting grants is like getting a first credit card; with demonstrated funding and good stewardship, it is easier to get additional ones. Start with small seed funding grants and plan to build upon the work completed with the help of grants for proof of concept or studies that aim to collect baseline data. Grant applications are much more robust with preliminary data and proof of concept already worked out.

Summary

Careers centered on simulation are in their adolescence. Therefore, much of the road remains unpaved. As an early adventurer in this field, help pave the way; and recognize there is more than one path or way. When engaging in a career, find places and supportive people. Careers that lack these can make for a long and lonely trek.

References

1. Sanko J. Simulation as a teaching technology: a brief history of its use in nursing education. Distance Learn. 2017;14(1):21–9.
2. Nightingale F. Notes on nursing: what it is, and what it is not. New York: Dover Publications; 1969.
3. Lees FS, Acland HW. Handbook for hospital sisters. London: W. Isbister; 1874.

4. McDonald L. Florence Nightingale: the making of a hospital reformer. Health Environ Res Des J. 2020;13(2):25–31. https://doi.org/10.1177/1937586720918239.
5. McDonald L. Florence Nightingale a hundred years on: who she was and what she was not. Womens Hist Rev. 2010;19(5):721–40. https://doi.org/10.1080/09612025.2010.509934.
6. International Nursing Association for Clinical Simulation and Learning. History. In: INACSL.org. 2015. https://www.inacsl.org/about/history/.
7. Lindell D, Poindexter K, Hagler D. Consider a career as a healthcare simulation educator. Am Nurse Today. 2018;11(5):58–9.
8. Sanko JS, Calhoun AW, Issenberg B, Kelly M, Battista A. Reflections on career pathways of simulation focused experts in the field. Simul Healthc. 2020;15(6):432–7.
9. Baily L. Healthcare simulation degree programs: comprehensive list. Healthy Simulation. 2019. https://www.healthysimulation.com/20183/healthcare-simulation-degree/.
10. Institute of Medicine (IOM) (US). Committee on the Robert Wood Johnson Foundation Initiative on the Future of Nursing, at the Institute of Medicine. The future of nursing: leading change, advancing health. Washington, DC: National Academies Press; 2011.
11. Hayden JK, Smiley RA, Alexander M, Kardong-Edgren S, Jeffries P. The NCSBN National Simulation Study: a longitudinal, randomized, controlled study replacing clinical hours with simulation in Prelicensure Nursing Education. J Nurs Regul. 2014;5(2):S3–S40.
12. Hughes KE, Hughes PG. Medical simulation fellowships. Treasure Island (FL): StatPearls Publishing; 2020.
13. Cheng A, Kessler D, Mackinnon R, Chang TP, Auerbach M. Reporting guidelines for healthcare simulation research: extensions to the CONSORT and STROBE statements. Adv Simul. 2016;1:25. https://doi.org/10.1186/s41077-016-0025-y.
14. Lewis K, Bohnert CA, Gammon WL, Holzer H, Gliva-McConvey G. The Association of Standardized Patient Educators (ASPE) Standards of Best Practice (SOBP). Adv Simul. 2017;2(10):1–8. https://doi.org/10.1186/s41077-017-0043-4.
15. Trautman DE, Idzik S, Hammersia M, Rosseter R. Advancing scholarship through translational research: the role of PhD and DNP prepared nurses. Online J Issues Nurs. 2018;23(2):1–8. http://ojin.nursingworld.org/MainMenuCategories/ANAMarketplace/ANAPeriodicals/OJIN/TableofContents/Vol-23-2018/No2-May-2018/Advancing-Scholarship-through-Translational-Research.html
16. Levine AI, DeMaria S Jr, Schwartz AD, Sim AJ. The comprehensive textbook of healthcare simulation. New York: Springer Science & Business Media; 2013.
17. Phrampus PE, O'Donnell J, Farkas D, Abernethy D, Brownlee K, Dongilli T, Martin S. Rapid development and deployment of Ebola readiness training across an academic health system, simulation in healthcare. J Soc Simul Healthc. 2014;11(2):82–8. https://doi.org/10.1097/SIH.0000000000000137.

Seeking Excellence in Simulation for Nursing Education and Practice: Accreditation, Certification, and Standards of Best Practice

42

Penni I. Watts, Tedra Smith, Beth Hallmark, and Becky Damazo

Introduction

A simulationist is a professional involved in providing simulation activities, products and services [1, 2]. A nurse educator who fulfills the role of a simulationist may work in many different settings, such as an acute care hospital or a school of nursing. Regardless of the setting, the simulationist and their institution in which they work should continually seek excellence and quality in their simulation programs. Through the modality of simulation and the integration of accreditation, certification and standards, a quality learning platform can be established for nursing education.

Accreditation for simulation programs defines and sets the framework and administrative backdrop that will create an environment where simulationists can excel. Accreditation shows a commitment to quality and encourages implementation of rigorous evidence-based practices. Certification validates the individual effort to understand and meet established simulation methods. The certified instructor demonstrates the principles that promote teaching excellence.

The Healthcare Simulation Standards of Best Practice™ are tools to measure the value of the simulationists efforts against recognized norms in simulation education. Standards provide a detailed process for evaluating and improving simulation operations and delivery methods that benefit simulation programs, teams, educators, and learners [3]. Using standards to guide practice demonstrates a commitment to evidence-based practices. These three elements—Accreditation, Certification and Standards—work together to create a masterpiece of simulation-based learning (Fig. 42.1).

As simulation programs reflect on their practices, they should ask themselves a few questions: Does the program have policies and procedures specific to simulation education? Would the program stand up to defined simulation standards? Do program educators understand simulation methods and work toward simulation excellence? If so, have these educators become certified? In short, is the program built on a strong, evidence-based foundation that promotes excellence in simulation education and practice? Accreditation, certification, and standards are the three components of a strong simulation program. These are tools that can be used to determine the quality of existing programs and guidelines to use for program development.

Simulation in healthcare has expanded dramatically over the last 10 years. With the decrease in clinical sites and patient experiences simulation has become a mainstay for those involved in any area of nursing education. Due to the increased focus on systems integration and patient safety in hospitals and programs simulation practice has become the educational backbone of quality patient care. Currently there is an increased demand for understanding what constitutes "best practice" in simulation and assurance that programs are offering quality and excellence in the application of simulation across the curriculum.

Simulationists are avidly seeking not only quality and excellence in simulation experiences, but recognition and validation for the work of simulation education. Nursing programs and clinical facilities are at a pivotal time to truly excel in simulation education. With the increased focus on patient safety, simulation provides the important bridge to assure students can interact professionally with other healthcare workers and can be an important voice in the healthcare team.

P. I. Watts (✉) · T. Smith · B. Hallmark
School of Nursing, University of Alabama at Birmingham, Birmingham, AL, USA
e-mail: piwatts@uab.edu; tedraka@uab.edu; beth.hallmark@belmont.edu

B. Damazo
Belmont University, Nashville, TN, USA

Rural Northern California Simulation Center, California State University, Chico, USA

J. M. Kutzin et al. (eds.), *Comprehensive Healthcare Simulation: Nursing*, Comprehensive Healthcare Simulation,
https://doi.org/10.1007/978-3-031-31090-4_42

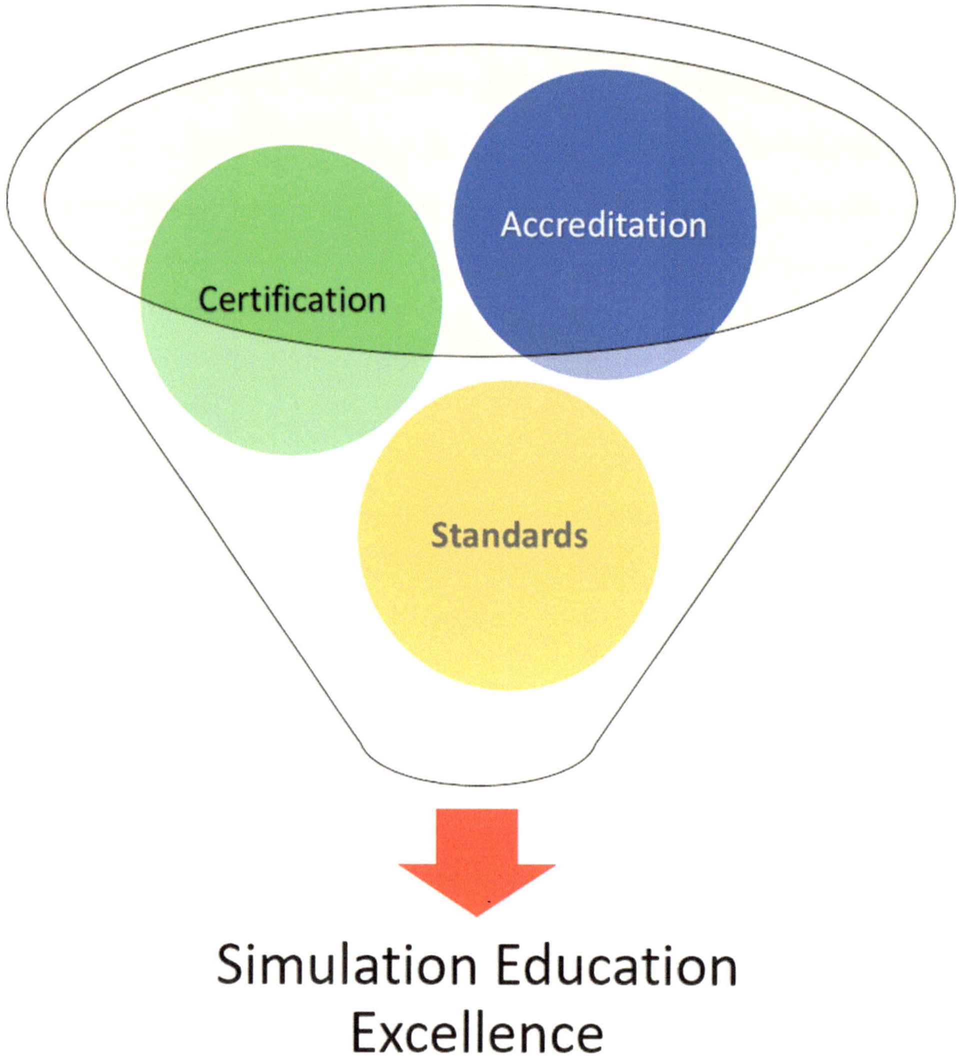

Fig. 42.1 The formula for assuring quality simulation

Nursing programs-in both academic and hospital settings—should recognize and embrace the idea that there are evidence-based approaches to conducting simulation education. Accreditation assures that programs meet international standards that will support simulation methods. Nurses have a strong history of recognizing excellence through participating in certification and have received certifications in a myriad of specialties, such as Critical Care Registered Nurse (CCRN), Certified Nurse Educator (CNE), etc. Simulation Certification provides recognition for the educator and verifies they have the knowledge and expertise needed to conduct quality simulation experiences. To advance one's personal and professional growth, educators should seek validation and recognition for their simulation expertise through certification. The quality of simulation experiences should be measured against the evidence that supports the standards of best practice for simulation. In this chapter, the value of accreditation, certification, and standards of best practice for individuals, programs and institutions seeking quality educational experiences will be discussed.

Accreditation

Currently, the Society for Simulation in Healthcare (SSH) as an internationally recognized simulation society, is the only group offering peer-reviewed simulation accreditation. The Society for Simulation in Healthcare is an organizational member of the Institute for Credentialing Excellence. Accreditation of simulation programs by the Society for Simulation in Healthcare (SSH) began in 2010 with several select programs recognized for their excellence in simulation education. To be accredited a program is defined as an organization that has dedicated resources, whose goal is to specifically target improving patient safety and outcomes through assessment, research, advocacy, and education using simulation methodologies [4]. Since the initial programs were accredited, the SSH has developed a rigorous process that focuses on program expertise in the areas of Assessment, Research and Teaching/Education. The SSH uses a peer-review system that examines "processes and outcomes" in each of these areas. Programs are not limited to academic settings but include medical centers, stand-alone simulation facilities, and other qualifying educational institutions.

Accreditation in general demonstrates that said program follows rigorous standards and best practices in the development and growth of a simulation program [4]. The SSH accreditation uses a modular approach to accreditation entailing a series of core standards that serve as the foundation of the simulation program. Programs can then define one or more of the above standards (assessment, research, teaching/education) to focus on specific program expertise. If a program then feels confident that they meet core and applied standards they can then apply for additional recognition in simulation integration and patient safety and/or simulation fellowship.

Nursing program accreditation provides a quality measurement tool to determine if programs meets or exceeds minimum quality standards. Accreditation helps institutions create goals for self-improvement and heightens faculty members' and administrators' awareness and responsiveness to areas needing improvement. While nursing programs are familiar with overall program accreditation, simulation program accreditation takes a unique view of how the program is meeting simulation education standards. Simulation Accreditation is not specific to nursing but is designed to take a broad view of institutions that engage in simulation education such as hospitals, academic settings, medical associations, stand-alone facilities, and other settings. Table 42.1 is a brief overview of each area of accreditation by SSH and the associated standards [5].

Table 42.1 Society for Simulation in Healthcare Accreditation Standards [5]

Area of accreditation	Standard categories
Core—all programs must include	1. Mission and governance 2. Program management 3. Resource management 4. Human resources 5. Program improvement 6. Integrity 7. Expanding the field
Accredited programs must choose at least one:	
1. Assessment	1. Resources and technology 2. Assessors 3. Assessment tools 4. Assessment support
2. Research	1. Mission 2. Research oversight 3. Research activity 4. Researchers 5. Research collaboration 6. Compliance
3. Teaching/education	1. Educational activities 2. Educational activity design 3. Qualified educators 4. Evaluation and improvement
Additional (optional) recognition areas	
• Systems integration	1. Mission and scope 2. Integration activities
• Fellowship	1. Program infrastructure 2. Program resources 3. Educational activities 4. Scholarship 5. Program evaluation and improvement

Programs may initially apply for provisional accreditation. This allows programs to gain important feedback on their program and processes. Programs that apply for provisional accreditation typically do not have the required 2 years of data needed for full accreditation but seek to experience the peer review process to prepare for full accreditation through feedback and review.

The process of full accreditation requires two full years of data that are submitted via a self-study prior to a visit by members of the accreditation team. The team will review the documents prior to their visit and seek clarification related to any questions from the documentation submitted. The process is collegial and seeks to help all programs be programs of excellence, providing education using simulation that meets or exceeds the standards set forth in the requested documentation.

Nursing programs filing for SSH accreditation need to make a clear distinction between the academic accreditations such as the Commission on Collegiate Nursing Education (CCNE) and the National League for Nursing Center of Excellence (NLN COE). CCNE focuses on ensuring the quality of baccalaureate, graduate programs in nursing focusing on the effectiveness of educational practices. The NLN Center of Excellence (COE) in Nursing Education provides a designation for schools of nursing and health care organizations that have achieved excellence in a specific area and is recognized for outstanding innovations with program acknowledgements on commitment and sustainability. While academic accreditation can be documented as a part of program evidence—all policies, procedures and standards used for SSH accreditation need to be simulation specific. Simulation Accreditation provides a program internal validation and demonstrates to stakeholders and the general public that a program strives to be a program of excellence and that the processes, courses and resources used for simulation meet international standards.

Certification

While accreditation defines the standards for programs, certification is an individual pursuit. Defining simulation excellence in a group of individuals who may already hold advanced degrees and certifications in their health care specialties has been challenging. Because of the many career

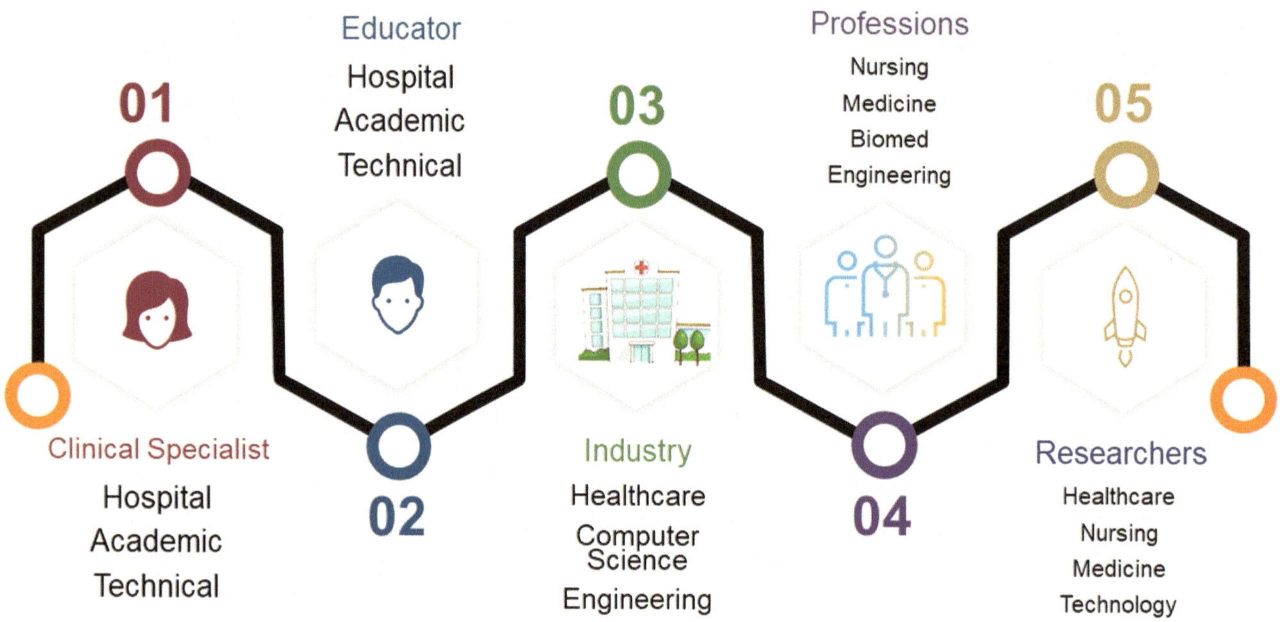

Fig. 42.2 There are many pathways to certification

pathways that lead to simulation, validation of expertise and knowledge that defines the field must apply to the many different job environments where healthcare simulation is found [6]. Simulation Certification represents the needs of a diverse and growing community of simulation experts from around the world. The SSH has developed a strong simulation program that is fully accredited by the National Commission on Credentialing Agencies (NCCA) (Fig. 42.2).

As simulation is increasingly relied upon in medical education, the need for standardization and adherence to best practice has become more important. A best evidence in medical education systematic review of high-fidelity medical simulations found that learning is facilitated under the right conditions, including a controlled environment, simulator validity, defined outcomes, and providing feedback [7]. The National Council of State Boards of Nursing landmark study concluded that one of the conditions for simulation success included faculty members who are formally trained in simulation pedagogy [2]. Those who are certified conducts simulation-based experiences with clear evidence of an understanding of simulation education and/or operations methods.

Benefits of Simulation Certification

- Simulation is a formal recognition of the specialized knowledge in simulation education or technology.
- By participating in the process of simulation you confirm your commitment to excellence in a developing area of healthcare expertise.
- Participation in certification supports the development of standardization and a pool of knowledge of best practices.
- Certification is recognized internationally as a standard for either simulation education or technology that strengthens organizational, community, and learner confidence in the quality of education.
- Encourages individual performance improvement and knowledge development.

Types of Certifications

There are four certifications available through the Society for Simulation in Healthcare [8]:

Two Basic (Entry) Certifications

Professionals who desire to become certified as either Certified Healthcare Simulation Educators (CHSE) or Certified Simulation Operations Specialists (CHSOS) are required to meet application criteria through SSH and complete a standardized examination. A Bachelor's degree or equivalent combination of education and experience is necessary for eligibility.

Applicants are eligible for CHSE if they serve a role in healthcare simulation education and can verify 2 years of involvement with healthcare simulation education, research, or administration. Similarly, CHSOS applicants must demonstrate 2 years of continuous involvement in the role of healthcare simulation operations (Fig. 42.3).

Two Advanced Certifications

CHSE-A and CHSOS-A are reserved for professionals that have proven to be experts in healthcare simulation education or technology as well as leaders and mentors to others in the simulation community. The application is portfolio-based and awarded to high performing leaders in healthcare simulation. Requirements include basic certification, a minimum of 5 years of experience in healthcare simulation, and a master's degree or equivalent experience.

Continuing Education Requirement

Simulation is evolving and changing to reflect new demands, education methods and technologies. Certification is a commitment to lifelong learning and has a continuing education requirement for certification maintenance. The original certification is granted for a 3-year period. After that time, applicants may apply for renewal by completing professional development requirements or retaking the examination. Additional information about SSH certification and requirements for each level of certification can be found on the SSH website at www.ssih.org.

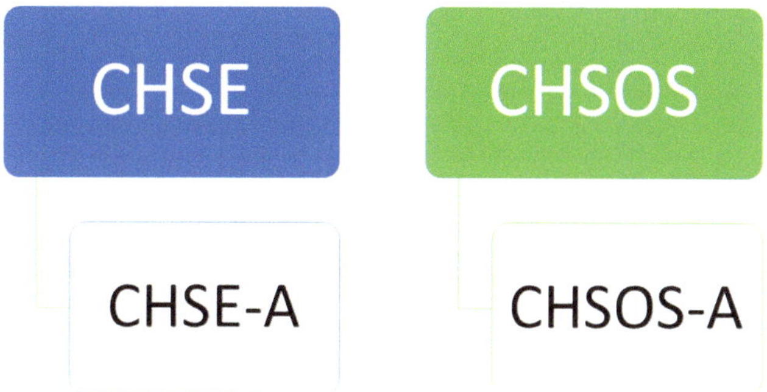

Fig. 42.3 The many pathways to certification

Simulation Certification vs Certificate in Simulation Education or Technology

There are a growing number of academic programs offering certificates that provide a curriculum that will result in a certificate or degree in either simulation education or technology. These programs can provide a foundation for an applicant's knowledge base. The certificate is not the same as becoming certified. Though certificate courses can provide information and experience that will support simulation certification they are not requirements or replacements for completing the certification exams (Fig. 42.4).

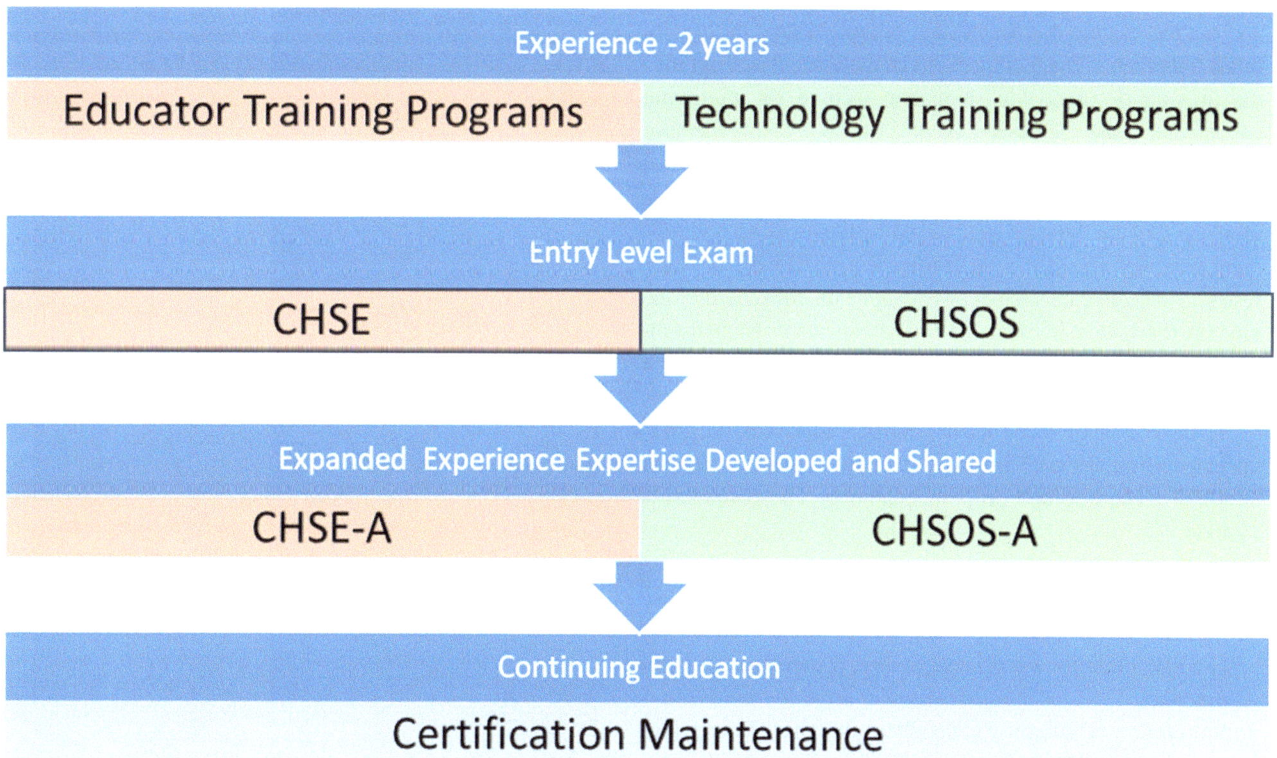
Experience -2 years
Educator Training Programs
Technology Training Programs
Entry Level Exam
CHSE
CHSOS
Expanded Experience Expertise Developed and Shared
CHSE-A
CHSOS-A
Continuing Education
Certification Maintenance

Fig. 42.4 Steps to certification

Simulation Education Standards

Simulation standards provide guidelines for nursing faculty and hospital educators to design and facilitate a successful simulation. These standards are based on evidence derived through structured research to promote optimal learner outcomes and achievement of identified objectives. Nursing educators are tasked with encouraging the use of evidence in patient care, so it is essential that best practices are also used to educate. The NCSBN (2014) report states that the most important way to ensure high-quality simulation is to incorporate best practices into a simulation program; these best practices include simulation design, outcomes and objectives, facilitation, debriefing, participant evaluation, professional integrity, simulation enhanced interprofessional education (IPE), and operations [2].

INACSL initiated development of standards of best practice in 2011. Over the years there have been revisions and additions, and in 2021 the standards were rebranded as the Healthcare Simulation Standards of Best Practice™ (HSSOBP™) by INACSL with the support and of the global community [3]. By rebranding the standards, the focus shifted to an interprofessional and international application of the standards in simulation practice. These standards were created to be used independent of each other to support the design and implementation of simulation. Each standard has criteria necessary to meet the standard and outlines required elements that provide details on how to fulfill the criteria. The incorporation of these standards signifies the importance of quality simulation focused on improving patient outcomes. The HSSOBP™ provide a comprehensive picture of the process educators can use to evaluate and improve simulation and its delivery methods. The standards were developed through the rigorous work of professionals with a commitment to quality who provided extensive review of evidence-based research in healthcare simulation education. In 2021, each of the nine standards were revised with two new standards being developed. Table 42.2 provides the standards and summary for each HSSOBP™ standard [3].

There are other recognized standards that provide guidance for simulation education that may also be useful for simulation training and program planning. These standards include:

- Standards of Best Practice on Standardized Patients published by Association of Standardized Patient Educators (ASPE) https://www.aspeducators.org/standards-of-best-practice
- Simulation Dictionary published by the Society for Simulation in Healthcare https://www.ssih.org/Dictionary
- Capability Framework published by The Gathering of Healthcare Simulation Technology Specialists https://simghosts.org/page/capability_framework

Table 42.2 The Healthcare Simulation Standards of Best Practice™ by INACSL with the support and input of the global community

Standard	Summary
Simulation design [9]	This standard describes the basic elements of designing a simulation-based experience (SBE). This includes consultation with content and simulation experts, using appropriate modality and fidelity for realism, creating a prebrief and debrief plan, developing an evaluation plan, and completing a run-through prior to implementation
Outcomes and objectives [10]	In this standard, elements included are determining learner outcomes and creating objectives, identifying appropriate simulation modality and fidelity, and establishing level of facilitation in the meeting objectives
Facilitation [11]	In this standard, the facilitative approach is determined by the level of learning, experience, and competency of the participants, and should be conducted by a trained individual applying cues at an appropriate level
Prebriefing: preparation and prebriefing [12]	This standard includes elements of developing a prebriefing plan considering the level of learner and learning outcomes. This entails preparation and briefing for the SBE. The simulationist should be knowledgeable in prebriefing and the scenario
The debriefing process [13]	This standard outlines the process in developing a debriefing plan including being conducted by a trained person, debriefing style based on a theoretical framework, encourages reflection and identification of performance deficits, and ensures psychological safety and confidentiality
Evaluation of learning and performance [14]	In this standard, evaluation of the learner is considered and developed based upon whether the experience is formative, summative or high-stakes
Professional integrity [15]	This standard outlines element of professional integrity to include the Healthcare Simulationist Code of Ethics, ensuring a safe learning environment, and confidentiality of performance and scenario. Respect of diversity, equity, and inclusivity is necessary of all those involved in the SBE
Simulation Enhanced Interprofessional Education (Sim-IPE) [16]	This standard describes how to conduct Sim-IPE including being based on a theoretical or a conceptual framework and utilizing best practices in the design, implementation, and evaluation of the experience
Operations [17]	This standard outlines overall operations of the SBE program. It entails several elements including maintaining a strategic plan to achieve the programs goals, providing personnel with appropriate expertise, managing all available resources, and creating policies and procedures to support the SBE program
Professional development [18]	This standard outlines professional development for the simulationist. It includes performing an needs assessment of the simulationist and developing a plan that addresses learning outcomes and continual reevaluation of the plan based on feedback

https://www.inacsl.org/inacsl-standards-of-best-practice-simulation/

- Healthcare Simulationists Code of Ethics published by the Society for Simulation in Healthcare https://www.ssih.org/SSH-Resources/Code-of-Ethics
- International Simulation Data Registry (ISDR) https://www.ssih.org/SSH-Resources/International-Simulation-Data-Registry-ISDR

As simulation continues to evolve and as the research surrounding simulation education develops, it is important for nursing leaders to continue to monitor and implement the best educational practices using simulation education.

Summary

Overall, nursing programs—whether academic or hospital based—can benefit from participation in credentialing and promoting simulation standards. Though challenging, programs can distinguish themselves and make a statement to the quality of their simulation education activities through program accreditation, educator certification and the documented use of evidence-based standards. Accreditation can provide a means to assemble educational and quality benchmarking data to improve programmatic performance. As organizations strive to ensure greater patient safety, accreditation is a way to assure high quality simulation experiences that translate to practitioners who are skilled and reduce the risk of harm to patients. Though simulation accreditation will complement academic program accreditation, such as AACN or NLN, it should be considered a separate process and the competencies and standards are unique.

Simulation professionals can achieve recognition by completing Certification in Healthcare Simulation Education or Certification in Simulation Operation Specialist. Certification is rapidly becoming a benchmark for instructor quality and is listed as a qualification for hiring in many institutions. Certification is a way to ensure educators are qualified and have demonstrated their ability to meet certification standards. Those individuals who have become simulation leaders can move forward with advanced certification.

Establishing standards for simulation education and practice is necessary to create the foundational structure on which to build simulation experiences. With recognized, evidence-based standards, programs can access an established series of guidelines assure quality in simulation-based education. The Healthcare Simulation Standards of Best Practice™ in simulation education provide detailed guidance in quality simulation education. There are other recognized standards for guidance in specific aspects of program development. Nurses have the responsibility for programs that will lead to quality education that will result in safe patient practices. Accreditation, certification, and the use of evidence-based standards are tools that help assure educational program excellence.

References

1. Hardie L, Lioce LA. Scoping review and analysis of simulation facilitator essential elements. Nurs Prim Care. 2020;4(5):1–13.
2. Hayden JK, Smiley RA, Alexander M, Kardong-Edgren S, Jeffries PR. The NCSBN national simulation study: a longitudinal, randomized, controlled study replacing clinical hours with simulation in prelicensure nursing education. J Nurs Regul. 2014;5(2):s4–s41.
3. INACSL Standards Committee. Healthcare Simulation Standards of Best Practice™. Clin Simul Nurs. 2021;58:33–9.
4. Khan M, Sasso RA. Obtaining medical simulation center accreditation. Treasure Island (FL): StatPearls Publishing; 2021.
5. Society for Simulation in Healthcare, Committee for Accreditation of Programs HS. CORE standards and measurement criteria. 2016. https://www.ssih.org/Credentialing/Accreditation.
6. Whitworth KA, Long JP. Certification in medical simulation. Treasure Island (FL): StatPearls Publishing; 2020.
7. Issenberg SB, McGaghie WC, Petrusa ER, Lee Gordon D, Scalese RJ. Features and uses of high-fidelity medical simulations that lead to effective learning: a BEME systematic review. Med Teach. 2005;27(1):10–28.
8. Society for Simulation in Healthcare. Credentialing and Certification. 2021. https://www.ssih.org/Credentialing/Certification.
9. INACSL Standards Committee, Watts PI, McDermott DS, Alinier G, Charnetski M, Ludlow J, Horsley E, Meakim C, Nawathe P. Healthcare Simulation Standards of Best Practice™ simulation design. Clin Simul Nurs. 2021;58:14–21.
10. INACSL Standards Committee, Miller C, Deckers C, Jones M, Wells-Beede E, McGee E. Healthcare Simulation Standards of Best Practice™ outcomes and objectives. Clin Simul Nurs. 2021;58:40–4.
11. INACSL Standards Committee, Persico L, Belle A, DiGregorio H, Wilson-Keates B, Shelton C. Healthcare Simulation Standards of Best Practice™ facilitation. Clin Simul Nurs. 2021;58:22–6.
12. INACSL Standards Committee, McDermott DS, Ludlow J, Horsley E, Meakim C. Healthcare Simulation Standards of Best Practice™ prebriefing: preparation and briefing. Clin Simul Nurs. 2021;58:9–13.
13. INACSL Standards Committee, Decker S, Alinier G, Crawford SB, Gordon RM, Jenkins D, Wilson C. Healthcare Simulation Standards of Best Practice™ the debriefing process. Clin Simul Nurs. 2021;58:27–32.
14. INACSL Standards Committee, McMahon E, Jimenez FA, Lawrence K, Victor J. Healthcare Simulation Standards of Best Practice™ evaluation of learning and performance. Clin Simul Nurs. 2021;58:54–6.
15. INACSL Standards Committee, Bowler F, Klein M, Wilford A. Healthcare Simulation Standards of Best Practice™ professional integrity. Clin Simul Nurs. 2021;58:45–8.
16. INACSL Standards Committee, Rossler K, Molloy M, Pastva A, Brown M, Xavier N. Healthcare Simulation Standards of Best Practice™ simulation-enhanced interprofessional education. Clin Simul Nurs. 2021;58:49–53.
17. INACSL Standards Committee, Charnetski M, Jarvill M. Healthcare Simulation Standards of Best Practice™ operations. Clin Simul Nurs. 2021;58:33–9.
18. INACSL Standards Committee, Hallmark B, Brown M, Peterson D, Fey M, Decker S, Wells-Beede E, Britt T, Hardie L, Shum C, Arantes H, Charnetski M, Morse C. Healthcare Simulation Standards of Best Practice™ professional development. Clin Simul Nurs. 2021;58:5–8.

Assessment/Regulation of Nurses Using Simulation (UG, GRAD, CPD)

43

KT Waxman and Marie Gilbert

There are many ways to assess simulation programs, simulations themselves, and faculty performing the simulation. In the United States academia, regulation occurs through the governing bodies that include Boards of Nursing, Commission on Collegiate Nursing Education (CCNE), Western Association of Schools and Colleges (WASC), National League for Nursing (NLN), and government regulations. In the service sector (hospitals, clinics, etc.) the regulations may not be as strict but things are changing as we speak. Governing bodies include The Joint Commission, American Nurses Credentialing Center (ANCC) Magnet, American Society of Anesthesiologists, Departments of Health, and more. It is important for simulation to be regulated and specifically, have faculty and educators follow standards of practice. The International Nursing Association for Clinical Simulation and Learning (INACSL) published the first set of standards in 2011, and the organization has continued to develop new standards as evidence comes available. INACSL created INACSL Standards of Best Practice: Simulation^{SM} for the following domains:

Simulation design; outcomes and objectives; facilitation; debriefing; participant evaluation; professional integrity; simulation enhanced IPE; and operations. It is highly recommended that anyone teaching in simulation follow these standards. When regulatory bodies assess the effectiveness of simulation programs, having evidence that these standards are followed is helpful. The Society for Simulation in Healthcare (SSH) has developed standards for accreditation of simulation centers and programs. The domains are: Assessment, Research, Teaching/Education, Systems Integration, and Fellowship. Following the SSH and INACSL standards are important as programs are built, whether or not they eventually become accredited or not.

This chapter will review the types of regulations one may encounter while working in simulation whether it be in an academic institution, hospital, or other.

Academia

The National Council of State Boards of Nursing (NCSBN) is comprised of nursing regulatory bodies from the 50 U.S. states, District of Columbia, and four U.S. territories [1]. The purpose of each state Board of Nursing (BON) is to ensure nursing programs comprehensively cover the knowledge and skills that students will need to be licensed and to practice safely and competently as new graduate nurses [2]. Although each state has their own regulations around the amount of simulation that can be used to replace clinical hours, the NCSBN is influential. The NCSBN Simulation Study [3] provided data that up to 50% of traditional clinical practice hour across the prelicensure curriculum could be substituted with simulation. Furthermore, to mitigate concern that nursing programs might begin to substitute simulation for traditional clinical experience without the appropriate environment, administrative support, or faculty preparation, the NCSBN convened an expert panel who developed national guidelines for use of simulation in the undergraduate nursing curriculum [4]. However, despite data from the NCSBN Simulation study and recommended guidelines, there is great variability in how BONs are defining and regulating the use of simulation in prelicensure nursing education including the amount of traditional clinical hours that can be replaced with simulation [5].

INACSL completed a survey of all states regarding the simulation regulations in 2016 and keeps updated data, of each state's BON and the full results are on their website at www.inacsl.org. At the time of this writing, the website reports that 17 states now allow schools of nursing to utilize

KT. Waxman (✉)
UCSF School of Nursing, San Francisco, CA, USA
e-mail: kt.waxman@ucsf.edu

M. Gilbert
Central California Center for Excellence in Nursing, California State University, Fresno, CA, USA
e-mail: mgilbert@mail.fresnostate.edu

J. M. Kutzin et al. (eds.), *Comprehensive Healthcare Simulation: Nursing*, Comprehensive Healthcare Simulation,
https://doi.org/10.1007/978-3-031-31090-4_43

Table 43.1 The National Council of State Boards of Nursing (NCSBN) Data of % of allowed Simulation by State

Up to 50%: (17 states)		Up to 30% (2 states)	Up to 25% (7 states)
Arkansas	North Carolina	Washington DC	California
Florida	South Carolina	Oklahoma	Illinois
Iowa	South Dakota		Indiana
Kentucky	Tennessee		Mississippi
Louisiana	Texas		Nevada
Minnesota	Washington		Vermont
New Hampshire	West Virginia		Virginia
New Mexico	Wisconsin		California
Michigan			

As of September, 2020-excluding COVID-19 waivers

simulation as a substitute for up to 50% of the required clinical hours, with an additional 11 states allowing for 25–35% of clinical hours to be replaced with simulation. Simulation has forced states to relook at the entire clinical experience and its effectiveness [6] (Table 43.1).

The remaining 25 states have no regulation about the use of simulation as part of the required clinical hours. While each state has a description about clinical hours, some with simulation and some without, they also have a required minimum number of clinical hours per program. Recently (2023), New York state joined Washington DC and Oklahoma by allowing up to 1/3 of the clinical hours in nursing education to be replaced with simulation, as long as it is conducted by an instructor with relevant training, certification, or accreditation.

Percentages of simulation use are unequal when one looks at schools within the state. Some schools of nursing require the minimal number of clinical hours based on the overall regulation, while some require more than what is required. That being said, 25% of 1000 hours is different than 25% of 800 hours which can impact the school significantly while trying to stay compliant. Other regulatory bodies do not allow simulation to substitute for clinical hours. In New Zealand, simulation hours may not be included in calculating clinical experience hours [7]. However, the use of simulation is valued and all students are required to have access to simulation learning resources to appropriately prepare them for clinical experiences to ensure the safety of health consumers, students, and staff [7]. Australia also does not allow simulation hours to be included in the minimum requirement of 800 hours of workplace experience [8].

In the United Kingdom, the standards for pre-registration nursing programs do no discuss the number of clinical hours required or the substitution of clinical hours with simulation. It does, however, require that approved education institutions, together with practice learning partners, ensure simulation-based learning is used effectively and proportionately to support learning and assessment and pre-registration nursing programs [9].

An over-reliance on simulation to replace clinical experiences was identified as a warning sign that a nursing program could be falling below the standard to graduate safe and competent nurses was an over-reliance on simulation to replace clinical experiences [10]. This is an interesting finding from the NCSBN report "Regulatory Guidelines and Evidence-Based Quality Indicators for Nursing Education Program" and warrants further discussion. NCSBN authors identified that this item could be affected by a number of intervening variables, such as the program having a lack of sufficient hands-on clinical experiences or increasing the use of simulation without adhering to accepted simulation guidelines [4, 10].

Although regulatory bodies across the globe vary on the use of simulation to substitute for clinical hours, there appears to be agreement that simulation experiences and simulation programs should adhere to best practices and where applicable national standards. Standards, guidelines, and best practices have been published by the International Nursing Association for Clinical Simulation and Learning (INACSL) [11–18], the National Council of State Boards of Nursing [19], the Society for Simulation in Healthcare [20], Canadian Association of Schools of Nursing [21], and The Association of Standardized Patient Educators (ASPE) [22].

Hours of Simulation Versus Hours of Clinical

In addition to the ongoing debate regarding how much clinical learning can be substituted in simulation is the discussion regarding the ratio of clinical hours to simulation hours. In simulation, all four levels Millers Pyramid can be addressed: knows, knows how, shows how, and does [6]. Emerging evidence suggests that, through the completion of more activities in higher levels, learners can become competent/proficient in significantly less time. Higher levels of performance occurred in much less time in simulation as compared the clinical environment [23]. This is likely due to the deliberate attention placed on specific learning objectives and through the careful planning associated with simulation. When incorporating simulation into the curriculum, it is important to follow local regulations regarding simulation hours versus clinical hours.

The deliberation regarding how much simulation and the ratio of hours of simulation to clinical hours frequently omit an important consideration regarding which environments facilitate specific learning outcomes most effectively. More research and consideration needs to focus on "what learning objectives can only be met in traditional supervised clinical experiences," "what learning objectives can only be met in simulation," and "when given the option between traditional clinical and various types of simulation, which option(s) most effectively and efficiently achieves learning objectives?" [24].

COVID-19 Pandemic

Recently, during the COVID-19 pandemic, schools of nursing were forced to move to an online, screen-based method of teaching with and without simulation. Many hospitals around the US topped allowing clinical placements while in the midst of caring for COVID-19 patients. Faculty needed to be trained in the simulation methodology quickly. Several state's governments issued waivers to the current BON simulation regulations in an effort for students to meet their clinical hour requirement by substituting simulation. Most states loosened their regulations while other states stuck to their original regulations creating discourse between schools and hospitals. The NCSBN's website was continuously updated for recent waiver information. An example of a policy change was the enaction of Assembly Bill 2288 in California. This bill, signed by the Governor September 29, 2020, focused on the state of emergency (COVID-19) and allowed schools of nursing to request that the approved nursing program be allowed to reduce the required number of direct patient care hours to 50% in geriatrics and medical-surgical and 25% in mental health-psychiatric nursing, obstetrics, and pediatrics if certain requirements are met. Requirements included: evidence that no alternate agency or facility was available and accessible; the alternate learning experience is at least equivalent to the learning experience provided by the direct patient care clinical practice hours; and upon termination of the state of emergency, the temporary reduction provided shall cease as soon as practicable or by the end of the academic term, whichever is sooner. Furthermore, the bill requires that any substitute clinical practice hours not in direct patient care that are simulation experiences are based on the best practices published by the International Nursing Association for Clinical Simulation and Learning, the National Council of State Boards of Nursing, the Society for Simulation in Healthcare, or equivalent standards approved by the board [25].

Despite opposition from the California Board of Registered Nursing, pursuant to the Governor's Executive Order 39-20, the Department of Consumer Affairs directed the Board of Registered Nurses (BRN) to waive the 75% direct patient care experience requirement during the COVID-19 pandemic [26], and with the passage of AB 2288, Chapter 282, Statues of 2020, the percentage of simulation can increase during a state of emergency [25].

Service

The Joint Commission, an important accrediting body for hospitals and health systems has incorporated key standards into their work. The mission of The Joint Commission is to continuously improve health care for the public, in collaboration with other stakeholders, by evaluating health care organizations and inspiring them to excel in providing safe and effective care of the highest quality and value. Its vision is that all people always experience the safest, highest quality, best-value health care across all settings [27].

In response to critical patient safety issues, effective January 1, 2021, The Joint Commission introduced two new standards to address complications in maternal hemorrhage and severe hypertension/preeclampsia. These standards include hosting in-situ drills to identify system issues at least once a year for each condition. These drills must include a post event debrief with all disciplines as part of the process [28]. Drills require scenarios and environments that represent real events in hospital environments and therefore healthcare simulation is a valid strategy to use.

Simulation Accreditation and Certification

Globally there appears to be limited consistency in simulation regulation, however, professional organizations such as the American College of Surgeons (ACS), American Society of Anesthesiologists (ASA), Society for Simulation in Healthcare (SSH), Society for Simulation in Europe (SESAM), and the United Kingdom based Association for Simulated Practice in Healthcare (ASPiH) have procedures to accredit simulation programs. Although regulatory bodies do not generally mandate accreditation, receiving it demonstrates programs have been independently reviewed and adhere to high standards, providing quality simulation education.

The Veterans Health Administration (VHA) Simulation Learning, Education and Research Network (SimLEARN) awards simulation certification at three levels (Basic, Intermediate, and Advanced Tier) to VHA Simulation Programs that meet strict criteria for implementation of simulation practice at their facility and externally to meet the healthcare needs of our nation's Veterans [29]. VHA Simulation Programs voluntarily apply to SimLEARN for one of the three levels based on their own self-evaluation and submit narratives and other supporting documents describing the work of their program, including educational offerings, systems probing, process improvement, research, dissemination efforts through publications and presentations, mentorship, faculty development, and quality improvement initiatives. Additionally, SimLEARN staff lead a site visit for any program that applies for Advanced Tier certification. By achieving SimLEARN certification, a VHA facility Simulation Program is recognized for its expertise and commitment to furthering the mission, vision, and values of the VHA.

Return to Practice

A final consideration in this chapter is regulations regarding the use of simulation when a provider is returning to practice. Certified Registered Nurse Anesthetists (CRNAs) who have been out of practice for 4 years or longer or who fail to comply with the Continued Professional Certification Program must recertify with the National Board of Certification and Recertification for Nurse Anesthetists (NBCRNA) to demonstrate clinical competency before returning to practice anesthesia [30].

A requirement to complete a set number of clinical hours was identified as the greatest barrier for recertification and reentry to practice. Securing a hospital that allowed non-certified clinicians to practice anesthesia was a significant barrier to completing the clinical hours required to return to practice as a CRNA due to liability concerns [31]. NBCRNA addressed this barrier by reviewing the requirements in the then NBCRNA Refresher Program, and on August 1, 2016, the NBCRNA transitioned from the Refresher Program to the Reentry Program. The Reentry Program requires the completion of continuing education credits, including four topic-focused modules critical to nurse anesthesia care, a standardized examination, and high-fidelity patient simulation as a substitute for direct patient care clinical hour requirements [32]. The standardized examination requires successful completion of high-fidelity simulated anesthesia scenarios demonstrating adequate and appropriate identification of and intervention for the 20 Step 2 activities required by the NBCRNA [31].

Summary

Every state in the US and countries around the world have regulations of some type although there is no consistency. It is critical to check local and regional board of nursing's regulations to ensure what you are doing is compliant. We hope that 1 day, there will be more standardization with simulation which is why we, as nurses, need to continue to advocate with our boards and regulators as we move forward to ensure quality care and patient safety.

Testimonial

"The Durham, North Carolina VA Health Care System (DVA HCS) Simulation Program is one of the original VA facilities that earned SimEARN Certification at the Advanced Tier Level in 2015. DVA HCS recertified in 2017 and again in 2020. As Simulation Educator Coordinator and Co-Director of the Interprofessional Advanced Fellowship in Clinical Simulation at DVA HCS, I am honored that our Simulation Program has earned this Certification by meeting the high SimLEARN standards for delivering simulation education for interprofessional staff and trainees, probing systems and processes for latent threats, engaging in research and quality improvement initiatives, disseminating work through publications and presentations, mentoring and developing interprofessional team members to employ simulation methodologies in their clinical sphere, and serving in leadership capacities locally, regionally, and nationally to further the use of simulation for optimizing Veteran care. As a Simulation Program, we are privileged to have the support of our facility and regional leadership, along with support from the national SimLEARN office. This outstanding VA leadership is integral to our success as a Simulation Program and our work in serving our nation's Veterans."

Mary E. Holtschneider, MEd, MPA, BSN, RN, NPD-BC, NREMT-P, CPTD

Co-Director, Interprofessional Advanced Fellowship in Clinical Simulation

Simulation Education Coordinator, Nursing Professional Development Specialist, VISN 6 Simulation Champion Durham, North Carolina VA Health Care System

Nursing Program Manager, Duke Area Health Education Center (AHEC) Durham, North Carolina

References

1. National Council of State Boards of Nursing (NCSBN). U.S Members. https://ncsbn.org/member-boards.htm. Accessed Oct 2020.
2. Spector N, Hooper J, Silvestre J, Qian H. Board of nursing approval of registered nurse education programs. J Nurs Regul. 2018;8(4):23–9.
3. Hayden JK, Smiley RA, Alexander M, Kardong-Edgren S, Jeffries PR. The NCSBN National Simulation Study: a longitudinal, randomized, controlled study replacing clinical hours with simulation in prelicensure nursing education. J Nurs Regul. 2014;5(2):S1–S64.
4. Alexander M, Durham CF, Hooper JI, et al. NCSBN simulation guidelines for prelicensure nursing programs. J Nurs Regul. 2015;6(3):39–42.
5. Bradley CS, Johnson BK, Dreifuerst KT, et al. Regulation of simulation use in United States Prelicensure Nursing Programs. Clin Simul Nurs. 2019;33:17–25.
6. Waxman KT, Bowler F, Forneris S, Kardong-Edgren S, Rizzolo M. Simulation as a nursing education disrupter. Nurs Admin Q. 2019;43(4):300–5.
7. Nursing Council of New Zealand. Handbook for pre-registration nursing programmes. Wellington: Nursing Council of New Zealand; 2020.
8. Australia Nursing and Midwifery Accreditation Council. Registered Nurse Accreditation Standards. 2012.
9. Nursing and Midwifery Council. Realising professionalism: standards for education and training. Part 3: Standards for pre-registration nursing programmes. 2018.
10. Spector N, Silvestre J, Alexander M, et al. NCSBN regulatory guidelines and evidence-based quality indicators for nursing education program. J Nurs Regul. 2020;11(2):S1–S62.
11. International Nursing Association for Clinical Simulation and Learning. INACSL standards of best practice: Simulation[SM] simulation glossary. Clin Simul Nurs. 2016;12:S39–47.
12. International Nursing Association for Clinical Simulation and Learning. INACSL standards of best practice: Simulation[SM] simulation design. Clin Simul Nurs. 2016;12:S5–12.
13. International Nursing Association for Clinical Simulation and Learning. INACSL standards of best practice: Simulation[SM] outcomes and objectives. Clin Simul Nurs. 2016;12:S13–5.

14. International Nursing Association for Clinical Simulation and Learning. INACSL standards of best practice: Simulation^{SM} facilitation. Clin Simul Nurs. 2016;12:S16–20.
15. International Nursing Association for Clinical Simulation and Learning. INACSL standards of best practice: Simulation^{SM} debriefing. Clin Simul Nurs. 2016;12:S21–5.
16. International Nursing Association for Clinical Simulation and Learning. INACSL standards of best practice: Simulation^{SM} participant evaluation. Clin Simul Nurs. 2016;12:S26–9.
17. International Nursing Association for Clinical Simulation and Learning. INACSL standards of best practice: Simulation^{SM} professional integrity. Clin Simul Nurs. 2016;12:S30–3.
18. International Nursing Association for Clinical Simulation and Learning. INACSL Standards of Best Practice: Simulation^{SM} simulation-enhanced interprofessional education (SIM-IPE). Clin Simul Nurs. 2016;12:S39–47.
19. National Council of State Boards of Nursing (NCSBN). NCSBN Modern Rules 2017. https://www.ncsbn.org/3863.htm. Accessed 1 Mar 2021.
20. Society for Simulation in Healthcare (SSH). Teaching/Education Accreditation Standards. https://www.ssih.org/Credentialing/Accreditation/Full-Accreditation. Accessed 1 Mar 2021.
21. Canadian Association of Schools of Nursing. Practice domain for baccalaureate nursing education: guidelines for clinical placements and simulation. Ottawa: Canadian Association of Schools of Nursing; 2015.
22. Lewis KL, Bohnert CA, Gammon WL, et al. The association of standardized patient educators (ASPE) standards of best practice (SOBP). Adv Simul. 2017;2:10.
23. Sullivan N, Swoboda SM, Breymier T, et al. Emerging evidence toward a 2:1 clinical to simulation ratio: a study comparing the traditional clinical and simulation settings. Clin Simul Nurs. 2019;30:34–41.
24. Haerling K, Prion S. Questions regarding substitution of simulation for clinical. Clin Simul Nurs. 2020;50:79–80.
25. Low. AB-2288 Nursing programs: state of emergency. 2020. https://leginfo.legislature.ca.gov/faces/billTextClient.xhtml?bill_id=201920200AB2288. Accessed 1 Mar 2021.
26. Office of Governor Newsom. Executive Order N-39-20. https://www.gov.ca.gov/wp-content/uploads/2020/03/3.30.20-EO-N-39-20.pdf. Accessed 11 May 2020.
27. Commission TJ. About The Joint Commission. https://www.jointcommission.org/about-us/. Accessed 7 Mar 2021.
28. Commission TJ. Prepublication requirements: new standards for perinatal safety. https://www.jointcommission.org/-/media/tjc/documents/standards/prepublications/new_perinatal_standards_prepub_report_pdf. Accessed 4 Apr 2021.
29. Sonnenberg G. VHA facilities earn simulation certifications. https://www.simlearn.va.gov/SIMLEARN/FA_2015_21_Simulation_Certifications_2015.asp. Accessed 7 Mar 2021.
30. National Board of Certification and Recertification for Nurse Anesthetists. NBCRNA reentry handbook. https://www.nbcrna.com/docs/default-source/continued-certification/reentry/reentry_hb.pdf?sfvrsn=8f404db3_8. Accessed 1 Mar 2021.
31. Collins RM, Svoboda CJ, Vacchiano CA, Titch JF, Muckler VC. Recertification and reentry to practice for nurse anesthetists, phase II: evaluating reentry to anesthesia practice using high-fidelity simulation technology. J Nurs Regul. 2019;10(2):21–30.
32. Heyes ME, Schnitzen L, Starr DG, et al. Recertification and reentry to practice for nurse anesthetists: determining core competencies and evaluating performance via high-fidelity simulation technology. J Nurs Regul. 2018;8(4):43–55.

Part VI

The Future of Nursing Simulation

The Future of Simulation

44

Ann Russell, Jordan Holmes, Nancy McNaughton, Kerry Knickle, and Juanita Richardson

Introduction

Attempting to forecast simulation's future, especially amid a global pandemic, is a fool's game. However, as educators and researchers in the field of simulation; analyzing, understanding, and sharing learnings are essential for future planning. Reflection, learning, anticipation, and adaptation are fundamentals of human cognition, performance, and evolution—and core principles of simulation. By sharing simulation experiences (stories) that emerged in response to COVID-19, others may garnish ideas and reflections on how local solutions might generalize across institutional and geographical borders and assist with future planning during these uncertain yet exciting times for the field of simulation.

COVID-19 initiated the rapid transition from traditional well-established simulation-based education methods in health professions education to online and virtual solutions. An estimated 22 million learners worldwide transitioned to online learning in spring 2020 [1]. The impact on health professions education has been profound. Faculty and Institutions have grappled with how best to meet the needs of the learners without the benefit of tried and true face-to-face and hands-on simulation. Colleges and universities became ghost towns, and simulation centers, typically highly sought-after learning, and professional development spaces, remained empty and unused. While valuable low to high-tech simulators collected dust, schools continued to try to figure out how to re-open with reduced numbers of students, faculty, and staff to ensure social distancing measures were in place while providing the best education possible to prepare our future healthcare workforce.

More specifically, programs like the applied health sciences, nursing, and medicine, to name a few, that rely on simulation to develop technical and professional skills and competencies were greatly affected by the pivot to online and virtual learning. This chapter explores the future of simulation in the context of performance-based learning through case studies in the applied health sciences during COVID-19 and beyond. We will explore educational and simulation solutions that facilitated the migration to online and virtual learning and highlight the advantages and disadvantages afforded by this shift. We will consider mid-to long-term simulation solutions vis à vis the pandemic and the global "new normal" in health sciences education. Although the future of simulation is uncertain, the best predictor of the future is past behavior. Given this, the only thing known for sure is that there will be constant change in simulation and health professions education.

The Context

This chapter uses a case-study approach to explore curricular adaptations in simulation-based education at The Michener Institute (Michener) in Toronto, Canada. The Michener is a post-secondary institute in the city center adjacent to Toronto's Discovery District—a world-class science and discovery research park inhabiting 2-square kilometers of con-

A. Russell
The Michener Institute for Applied Health Sciences,
Toronto, ON, Canada
e-mail: arussell@michener.ca

J. Holmes · J. Richardson (✉)
The Michener Institute of Education at UHN,
Toronto, ON, Canada
e-mail: jholmes@michener.ca; jrichardson@michener.ca

N. McNaughton
The Michener Institute of Education at UHN,
Toronto, ON, Canada

Institute of Health Policy, Management and Evaluation (IHPME),
University of Toronto, Toronto, ON, Canada
e-mail: nmcnaughton@michener.ca

K. Knickle
Centre for Learning Innovation and Simulation, The Michener
Institute of Education at UHN, Toronto, ON, Canada
e-mail: kknickle@michener.ca

J. M. Kutzin et al. (eds.), *Comprehensive Healthcare Simulation: Nursing*, Comprehensive Healthcare Simulation,
https://doi.org/10.1007/978-3-031-31090-4_44

centrated brain power, employing more than 50,000 people, of whom almost half work in the medical and research-related fields [2]. The Discovery District has nine teaching hospitals affiliated with the University of Toronto and more than 30 specialized medical and scientific research centres [2]. The Michener is a school of applied health sciences with approximately 1000 full-time students and 13 academic programs including but not limited to the imaging sciences (radiological technology, nuclear medicine, molecular imaging, ultrasound), primary care, and acute care (respiratory therapy, cardiovascular perfusion, anesthesia assistant, chiropody/podiatry) and the medical laboratory sciences (diagnostic cytology, medical laboratory sciences, genetics technology). All of Michener's academic programs commonly use advanced computer technologies and software for professional practice. Machine learning and artificial intelligence are embedded in many essential applied health technologies (podiatry and radiation therapy). Simulation in Michener's context is embedded in the technology and used to build professional and patient care competencies using the Simulated Participant Program.

The benefits of simulation include allowing learners to develop situated cognition. Situated cognition is the idea that learning takes place when the person is doing something. Learning is created through activities and the social constructs developed through the learning process. However, being able to translate learning into practice is often the missing link. Simulation allows for learners to bridge this gap. Cognition in the wild, is the idea that human cognition adapts to the surroundings. But, without practice, healthcare practitioners are not able to develop and adapt their understanding of situations. This is where simulation can fill the void and help practitioners advance their understanding of complex topics and clinical scenarios.

Case Studies

Three case studies are presented in this chapter.

Case Study 1 Virtual simulation: explores the potential for using VR.

Case Study 2 Simulated participants: explores the use of SPs in an online course.

Case Study 3 Integrated library sciences: explores the intersection of the library with clinical learning.

The chapter concludes with reflections and considerations on the future of simulation, including advancing the state of simulation research by collaborating with library scientists essential to finding "just in time" evidence for rapid curriculum design, creation of new research-based resources, and participating in the co-creation of research and evaluation on new simulation methods.

Case Study—Virtual Reality

Introduction

Telesimulation has established a tradition of removing access barriers to delivering simulation and has provided a glimpse into what the future could hold for effective simulation at scale. Virtual reality (VR) simulation will complement and expand the evolution towards reach and scale that telesimulation began while preserving aspects of physical and environmental fidelity that may be lost with conventional telesimulation. This chapter will describe examples at the Michener Institute with VR simulation and reflect on both its current limitations and future potential. This section will also focus on the key areas of differentiation related to the science of learning for skills development, which has roots in cognitive psychology, motor learning, and theories of expertise.

Virtual reality simulation is computer technology used to create an immersive three-dimensional environment where objects have a sense of presence, and users' interface with the environment using speech recognition and haptic devices [3]. VR has demonstrated early success as a therapeutic intervention, including in mental health [4, 5] and rehab sciences [6, 7]. Examples of VR for training have been developed in some clinical contexts, most notably in critical care, patient assessment skills, and surgical skills [8–10]. However, VR remains arguably on the fringes of simulation-based training. PPE training via VR was developed due to a need for training and a lack of supplies; will this continue in the future?

Key design principles that leverage the unique characteristics of VR will be discussed as will the concepts that are supported by a recent meta-analysis of instructional design features in simulation [11]:

Deliberate Practice

"It takes 10,000 h of practice to become an expert in a field". This truism, often associated with Malcolm Gladwell's 2008 bestseller 'Outliers,' is an oversimplification of Anders Ericsson's theory of deliberate practice. Deliberate practice states that it is not so much the *amount* of practice that is important but the *quality* of practice. Specifically, deliberate practice entails:

(a) Repetitive performance of skills, coupled with
(b) Rigorous skills assessment that provides learners with
(c) Specific, informative feedback that results in increasingly
(d) Better skills performance [12]

This cycle of deliberate practice has been operationalized into countless successful skills development programs, though it has been remarkably underutilized in computer-based training. VR has the distinct advantage of collecting and synthesizing precise performance data to support deliberate practice, as factors such as time on task, sequence of action, and relative hand position can be tracked, compared to gold-standard, and communicated to learners in real time. When coupled with motivational feedback and goal setting (badging and gamification in the VR context), this performance feedback has consistently positive effects on learning [13].

Mastery Learning

Mastery learning is a relatively simple concept—knowledge and skills development is maximized when tasks are broken down into 'chunks' that increase in difficulty, where learners must master simple steps before progressing to more difficult ones. There must be clear objectives defining mastery outcomes at each stage so that learners and educators are clear on progression. For example, a course on conflict de-escalation should require learners to master fundamental principles of active listening before progressing to managing an emotionally escalated situation. Mastery learning is also highly related to the concept of *distributed practice*, where it has been demonstrated that knowledge and skill retention is much greater with multiple "inoculations" of training over a period versus one-shot training programs (e.g., as with typical weekend courses taken by medical professionals). VR, especially self-directed learning modules, have the distinct advantage of distributing practice over time with clear mastery objectives.

Learning Through Observation

Observation of others, particularly when it is combined with physical practice, can make important contributions to learning [13]. This is true for motor learning and complex behavioral skills. Being able to model expert practice is a key determinant of how novices improve. In a VR context, 4D motion capture can model and demonstrate precise movements and networked VR allows learners to leverage the observational and social nature of learning. Further, lines of sight for observers in VR do not suffer from any limitations that apply to in-person simulation, as observers can take any perspective they wish without impeding the sightlines of others.

Situated Cognition

Despite many efforts to develop generalized skills such as critical thinking and problem-solving, years of education evidence point to the fact that learning is highly contextual. It is rare for training to extend beyond the context in which it is learned [14]—for example, learners are unlikely to take what they learn about performing a complex medical procedure and transfer those skills to another procedure without contextualized practice. This is one of the greatest potentials of VR—the environment is so easily changed that it can be tailored to the unique requirements of the activity, culture, and social context. Precisely matching the learning environment to the required context is often cost-prohibitive in real-life simulation.

VR at Michener

At the Michener Institute, VR as a simulation modality has been used in two different contexts, de-escalation of responsive behaviors and radiation therapy:

Deescalation of Responsive Behaviours

Providing experiential opportunities for caregivers of persons with dementia (PWD) to develop skills that maximize safe, compassionate care is a key priority in healthcare. The Michener Institute has collaborated with clinical educators for several years to develop in-person simulation sessions for nurses and other healthcare providers who encounter PWD with responsive behaviors. However, in-person simulation has limitations. The full expression of behaviors must be limited to ensure that both learners and simulated patients (SPs) are not physically harmed. This compromises the authenticity of the simulations and limits the effectiveness of training, as learners cannot fully experience the management of complex behaviors that risk progressing to physical threats. Further, learners in live simulation sessions do not have the opportunity to fully experience the patient's perspective, limiting the potential for developing empathy and compassionate care.

To address these limitations, a collaboration with the Ottawa Hospital Research Institute (OHRI) was developed to create a VR platform where simulations are delivered in a risk-free environment that fully leverage opportunities for de-escalation training, situational awareness, and empathy building through literal perspective-taking (see Fig. 44.1). Subject matter experts from Baycrest, a Toronto hospital specializing in senior care, were brought in to refine and scale the VR platform and simulation curriculum to maximize opportunities for effective education for formal and informal caregivers.

While a formal mixed-methods research study regarding the efficacy of this platform is underway, there is great potential in VR as a medium through which to teach de-escalation skills. In particular, VR allows for the safe incorporation of the environment in de-escalation scenarios,

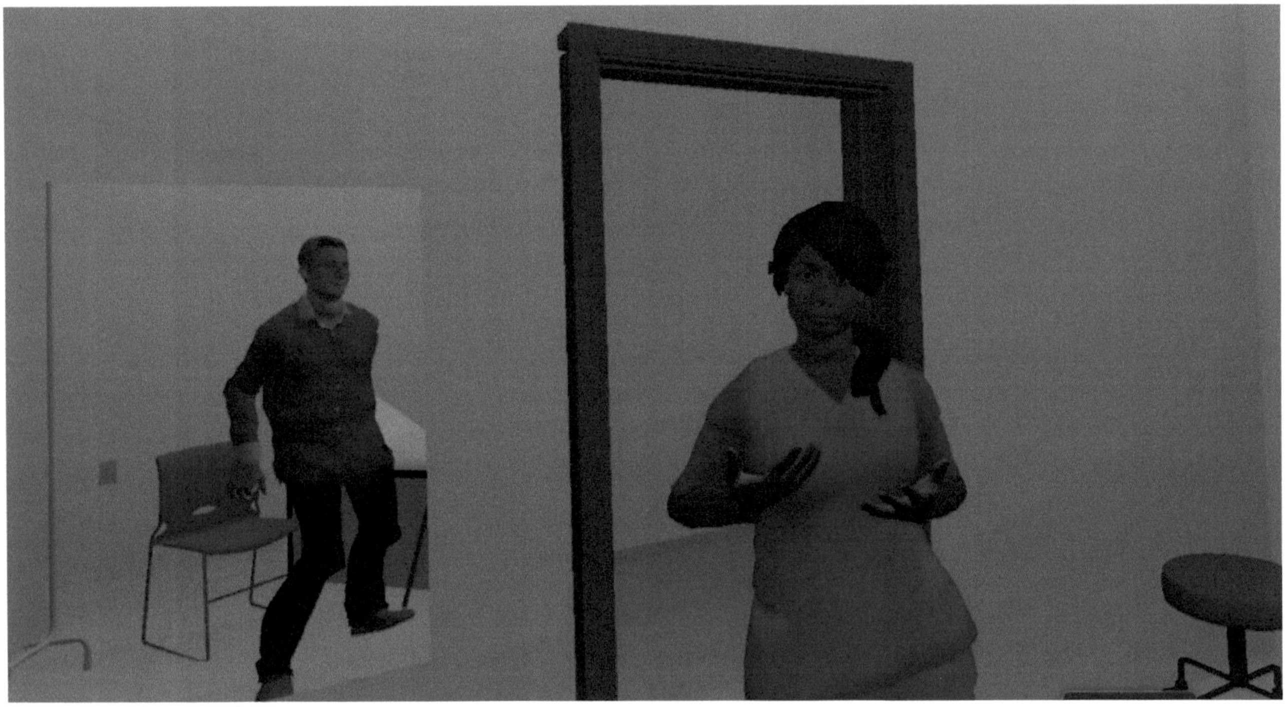

Fig. 44.1 VR de-escalation of responsive behaviors using the platform developed by OHRI, Michener, and Baycrest

such as when the SP, who is portraying the patient, chooses to use an IV pole or a chair to threaten or attempt to harm the caregiver. Escalating to this degree is not possible during in-person simulations and allows participants to explore the boundaries of de-escalation versus getting more assistance.

Radiation Therapy

The COVID-19 pandemic greatly affected in-person simulation for all of the programs at the Michener Institute, including Radiation Therapy. Radiation Therapy was fortunate because it had access to a very sophisticated virtual reality software package that mimics the operation of a real linear accelerator for the treatment of cancer.

Usually, over the summer, students practice with a physical linear accelerator, different than the real thing only in that the high energy beam is disabled. Students position simulated patients on the treatment bed and make sure that the mega-electron volt energy beam is going to target the right location in the body. In the VR version, students have the ability to cover cross-sectional anatomy, review and critique the treatment volumes in 3D, and display doses to each of the volumes displayed, leading to a discussion of target coverage and optimal dose (see Fig. 44.2).

This would be impossible to do using the "almost-real" linear accelerator on-site. Interestingly, faculty reported that the pandemic year's students became very adept at problem-solving and clinical reasoning.

Though anecdotal, this relates to a study Jeff Cheung and colleagues published from the Wilson Centre in Toronto [15]. It was found that integrating conceptual knowledge and procedural skills training was associated with improved skill retention and transfer. Jeff called it blending knowing how with knowing why. Perhaps a happy accident of the pandemic, with a move to online simulation with a heavy focus on the cognitive domain, has led to a relative de-emphasis on knowing how and a greater emphasis on knowing why. Moving forward, it is important to uncover the optimal balance of knowing how and why and determining when students must attend training in the sim lab to perform essential clinical skills versus when alternative educational technologies can be used.

Further Areas of Training

In addition to the above examples, the following training areas hold promise for VR-based health professions education. These recommendations reflect the current strengths and limitations of VR platforms and some key priorities in the health sector.

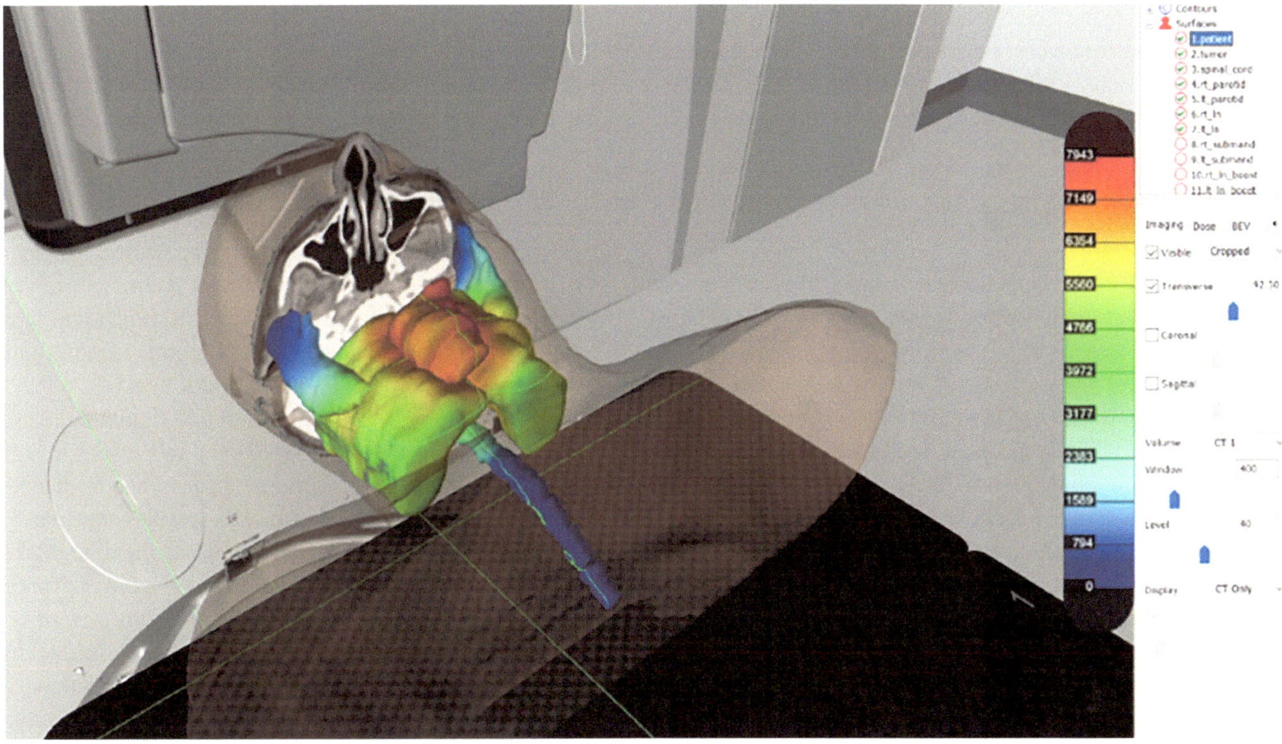

Fig. 44.2 Linear accelerator VR using virtual VERT

Personal Protective Equipment

Countless videos exist on how to safely don and doff personal protective equipment (PPE). While these videos can be helpful from a knowledge perspective, donning and doffing are highly psychomotor and situated in stressful environments. However, there are more effective ways to teach the life-saving skills of proper PPE donning and doffing than simply a video and static, decontextualized practice in a sterile lab. Further, as the COVID-19 pandemic demonstrated, real PPE must be prioritized for clinical use. VR is the ideal teaching environment, as supplies are limitless, and learners can engage in deliberate practice without regard for waste. Importantly, PPE donning and doffing is an example of a procedure with a single set of best practice guidelines. There is one best way to do it, and learners can be assessed against that gold standard. As with any computerized simulation that models a finite number of choices, this greatly helps to manage the complexity and validity of the simulation.

Hospital Acquired Conditions (HACs)

Most hospitals have identified a list of hospital-acquired conditions (HACs) that are a high priority to target to improve patient outcomes, many of which directly involve nursing care and expertise. For example, the following HACs could benefit from immersive VR training:

- Central line infections (training on standardized central line insertion to avoid infection)
- Pressure injuries (training on procedures to rotate patients—body mechanics, lifts, etc.)
- C. difficile infection (room disinfectant training for cleaning staff, nurses)
- Falls (training on identifying patients at risk for falls and what to do post-fall)
- Adverse drug events (training on medication dispensing units, e.g., Pyxis)

Like the PPE example, the best HACs to target with VR training are likely those with an established best-practice guideline that can be realistically modeled in VR.

Emergency Response

When an emergency response is called in a hospital, health professionals have precious few minutes to act and perform life-saving interventions. Cardiac arrest response is a team activity: where there is usually a group of different individuals from physicians, nursing, and respiratory therapists who converge on the scene and practice principles of crisis resource management (CRM), a complex set of non-technical skills, to coordinate and prioritize care. Cardiac arrest in VR is an excellent application of highly contextualized social learning that comprises procedural and communication skills. Ideally, it could be structured as either a self-directed learning experience with the learner taking the role of any health professional with accompanying bots/AI or a networked experience with other human participants. Learners would be given feedback about the accuracy of key decisions and the effectiveness and timeliness of interventions (e.g., time to defibrillation).

Human Factors Testing

Every time a new clinical space is built, clinicians spend countless hours with architects and designers envisioning how the new space will work. How will new equipment fill the space? How will traffic flow? Will the medication cabinet be reachable by the pharmacist? Many forward-thinking organizations take time to build either tabletop or full-scale models of new clinical spaces to perform robust use-case testing of new clinical areas before they are built. VR presents a unique opportunity to leverage the power of a networked environment where multiple clinicians can virtually live in a space and work out the design kinks before any ground is broken. While some architectural firms offer aspects of this service, they are generally static and do not incorporate any education or testing principles—it is used as a sales pitch or a crude model. Future VR development could pair the 'what' with the 'how'—what would the space look like, and how would clinicians live in it? Clinical space transformations are multi-million dollar projects, and VR allows organizations to spend some money up-front to ensure that their investment will meet their clinical needs.

Limitations to VR

While VR has the potential to be a transformational medium for simulation-based education, it does come with several current limitations:

1. VR is expensive. Most VR solutions require a powerful PC with a dedicated graphics processing unit (GPU) to render immersive 3D environments. In 2021, a typical PC powerful enough to drive VR starts in the $1000 range, and a dedicated VR headset adds between $300 and $1000, depending on the unit's capabilities. However, the trend in VR for education is certainly tending towards mobile: an all-in-one wireless VR unit such as the Oculus Quest 2 can be had for as low as $299, and many VR companies are now developing for mobile VR exclusively. All-in-one units significantly reduce cost and complexity, and future iterations will be better and cheaper. It is within the realm of possibility to imagine a future where every health science student would be issued VR goggles at the beginning of their program.
2. Limited hand function and haptic feedback. For consumer-grade VR equipment, touch controls are rudimentary, with the hand range of function limited to grabbing and pointing by pressing a trigger button. This rules out most VR applications for complex psychomotor skills. Further, haptic feedback is limited to subtle buzzing. However, progress is being made in this area every year. For example, some VR systems can detect a user's precise hand position using cameras, eliminating the need for hand controllers. Pre-production hardware is also in development for complex haptic feedback mechanisms. It is worth noting that some custom VR solutions use very sophisticated control and haptic systems, such as for laparoscopic surgery. However, these solutions tend to run in the tens or hundreds of thousands of dollars.
3. Cybersickness. VR tricks the brain into thinking the user is moving, and scenarios that employ movement in a 3D space can often lead to nausea, dizziness, and headaches, especially for people new to VR. It takes a while for learners to get their "VR legs," similar to the time it takes to be comfortable with motion at sea. However, advances in technology and scenario design limit the severity of cybersickness. For example, newer high-refresh-rate displays (i.e., 90 Hz or greater) are much easier on the eyes than older units, limiting headaches and choppy, nausea-inducing motion.

Conclusion

VR represents a significant path forward for simulation, allowing students to learn in environmentally authentic and contextually appropriate scenarios at a distance. The opportunity for the democratization of learning is enormous, as proximity to a simulation center is a current rate-limiting step for many forms of training. However, it is also clear that simulation centers will not disappear any time soon: VR, like most computer-based simulations, is effective and scalable for acquiring cognitive and behavioral skills: most psychomotor skills will require time with physical and procedural trainers. However, this will not always be true. There will likely come a time when training on a physical model in a brick-and-mortar building will seem passe.

Case Study—Simulated Participants

Introduction

Simulated participant (SP) based education involves live simulation professionals in its delivery. It is an experiential pedagogy that, at its core, invites learners to engage deeply when learning and practicing a range of communication and technical competencies. SP-based education is recognized within the larger healthcare simulation field as a methodology with attendant accountabilities, outlined in ASPE (Association of Standardized Patient Educators) and INACSL (International Nursing

Association for Clinical Simulation and Nursing) International Simulation Standards of Practice. There is an established literature within the health professions regarding the value of human simulation in enhancing communication and technical proficiency. Elements that ensure quality in SP-based educational offerings include thoughtful case design, collaboration with stakeholders, appropriate pitching expectations, and case content to the student's skill level.

In the following section, the planning, development, and delivery of an online course for applied health science students that engages human simulation as a featured learning approach will be reviewed. The benefits, challenges, and discoveries for students, faculty, and SPs, along with considerations for building community across online platforms will be discussed.

Although online technologies have been engaged for applied health professions learning for decades, the global pandemic has reinforced the online approach, as experienced SP educators and course leads modified their perceptions regarding the value of online versus face-to-face human simulation-based methods for learning.

The SP (Simulated Participant)

During in-person encounters SPs require significant training before being allowed to interact with learners. SPs must arrive to any session fully trained, clearly understanding the session learning objectives, and prepared to fully engage and accurately portray their role. The adherence to the case materials and an accurate portrayal of the patient is always the key priority for the SP. The SP's consistent focus is on the experience and feedback provided to the student. The adept SP calibrates their behavior and effects within the portrayal, to challenge the unique skill level of the learner, especially if the case is for teaching and learning purposes as opposed to assessment. During an encounter, the SP can "earmark" key moments of the interaction that will inform their feedback. In an online environment, many of the same requirements for SPs remain. However, an SP may attempt to make visible, through their feedback, the impact of a student response that might not be as apparent as in a live face-to-face encounter. For example, the effects of behaviors like eye contact or proximity between interactants in person will differ in an online encounter. Training that addresses online particularities is necessary for the SP prior to the case and can enhance the experience for both learners and faculty in successful teaching and learning outcomes.

The Learner

The need for clarity and transparency for the learner is key when conducting SP encounters. The transition to online experiences due to the pandemic affected the confidence and equilibrium of many SP encounters due to the unfamiliar environment and distance between learner, SP, and faculty member. For every learner, performance and subsequent evaluation are of utmost concern. Students in applied health disciplines and other health professional trainees require hands-on opportunities to integrate knowledge into practice for which simulation is ideally suited. Rethinking how problem-solving, clinical decision-making, and skills not requiring physical contact were to be integrated led to innovative design solutions.

The principles driving gold standard simulation education include unconditional positive regard for the learner, empathic respect for learner anxiety, detailed case scenarios with clear learning objectives, and creating a supportive climate for "practice through performance" exploration and risk-taking. A well-designed curriculum with clear information regarding the class processes and expectations further evidence this.

Faculty

Faculty educators can be excited and unnerved delivering simulation sessions in person, let alone online. Preparing and determining the focus for the session; what the students will experience and understand as a result, are critical considerations. The SP-faculty alliance cannot be overstated here. This collaborative relationship fosters safety, encourages confidence, and builds professional competencies with students.

COMM700: Entry to Practice Communication Course

Target Disciplines

The COMM 700 case study is an example of a professional communication skills course delivered for students transitioning to clinical placements. The course took place in one-and-a-half-hour blocks over 4 days. It was attended by 144 students across Podiatry, Radiation Therapy, Radiation Technology, and Respiratory Therapy who were in their summer simulation semester before transitioning to clinical placements in the fall.

The faculty was a combination of invited clinical subject matter experts, library resource scholars, student service counselors, health professionals, and simulation educators. The team included educators and technology support staff who took responsibility for behind-the-scenes management of the student chat and any problems with internet access to the course. It was a true collaborative effort.

Background

With no indication of imminent change to physical distancing measures, the Centre for the Advancement of Simulation Education (CASE), in collaboration with the Centre for Learning Innovation and Simulation (CLIS) at the Michener Institute of Education at UHN, created an innovative online COMM700, a 4-day summer semester communication skills course, dedicated to simulation in preparation for students entering clinical placements in the fall.

The summer semester is traditionally a 13-week hands-on offering from early May to the end of July. With approval and support from faculty and program Chairs, the 4-day interactive online course for "Entry to Practice Communication" was conceived and designed, drawing in part from existing content expertise while eliciting involvement from opinion leaders and professionals on the front lines of clinical practice as presenters.

The goals for this course included: an increased understanding of the current COVID-19 clinical environments, greater comfort and competence employing a wide range of communication and feedback techniques, broader awareness of bias, judgment, and assumption, and enhanced interpersonal skills capacity toward entry to practice fluency. It cannot be overstated here how essential the collaboration with our institutional team was in supporting the course organization, administration, and technology requirements.

Across the concurrent 4-day program, course content included (1) Coping in a COVID World, (2) The Essential Skills of Communication, (3) The Stories We Tell Ourselves, and (4) Connecting the Dots.

- Day 1: *"Coping in a COVID World"* included an array of speakers addressing (1) Managing fear and anxiety, (2) Reflecting on the Patient Experience, (3) The Challenges of Empathy and PPE (Personal Protective Equipment, (4) Gaining knowledge of COVID-19: Information and Discussion (5) Systems stories of resilience (adaptive capacity) and (6) Simulation (Meet A Stressed and Exhausted Colleague from the Front Lines)
- Day 2: *"The Essential Skills of Communication"* focused on (1) Communication and Active Listening, (2) Conflict, (3) Discussion, reflection, and debriefing of an angry patient-clinician in a two-part simulated interaction, (4) Tools of Analysis in Raising A Concern and (5) Hands-on Practice in Responding to Challenging Statements
- Day 3: *"The Stories We Tell Ourselves"* The key content here included (1) Assumption and Judgment of Others, (2) The Tenets of Effective Feedback, (3) Giving and Receiving Feedback, (4) Providing Feedback, and (5) A Case Study: Feedback as a Conversation.
- Day 4: *"Connecting the Dots"* The final session was intended to consolidate learning. A simulation involving a family member was designed to be portrayed life online in real-time by four different simulated participants (SPs), each playing the same role. The learning objectives captured the essential themes across the entire course materials.

The SPs were prepared for their roles and the technical requirements, adjusting to the new requirements with relative ease and skill.

SP Innovation

In preparation for COMM700 course simulations, several videotaped high-affect scenarios were required as part of a reflective exercise for Day One. Due to pandemic restrictions, the SPs could not engage in any live or online face-to-face interaction. Portraying the case scenarios and creating a videotaped monologue seemed an insurmountable challenge without access to the digital media department.

However, the SPs were astonishing and with their own capability and creative innovation created a fully realized video production complete with sound, lighting, and set décor, all created and self-produced by themselves. Video links were created and the feedback was overwhelmingly positive. Without this urgent dilemma, the subsequent discovery of SP's prowess and ingenuity in contributing to online simulation education would likely not have been made visible.

Large Group Simulation

An alternative to the SP created video was a large group simulation. In this use case, students volunteered to turn on their cameras and engage with the SP. Students were scheduled into three different time slots allowing three smaller groups to engage in the simulations. The lead facilitators were available to support and coach each student during their interaction, allowing for time-outs to reflect on what was happening and think about their next steps before going back into the interaction.

Students observing their colleagues actively provided peer feedback through the chat link and then in live discussion after each student/SP encounter. Student observers actively participated, and created a community of practice, supporting each other, and visibly demonstrating the communication skills, feedback, and compassionate behaviors they acquired through the course.

Building Community-Discussion

Facilitation of each interaction occurred with unexpected similarity to the live process. As instructors, we developed a palpable sense of our audience, something that we could never have imagined, given that we came from a face-to-face experiential teaching and learning culture.

We were surprised at the level of interactivity and our ability as facilitators to access the thinking of the students during the sessions. With few exceptions, the student engaging with the SP online was remarkably similar to the face-to-face interaction. They listened and noticed verbal and nonverbal cues; we were able to pause during "timeouts" to discuss their concerns, and explore different strategies before returning to the interaction with the SP.

In both live and online simulation teaching and learning, observers often do not have enough time to express their views or are shy to do so in front of their peers. As facilitators, we do not always hear what the students are worried about, thinking about, or questioning. While face-to-face sessions allow a more informed "reading of the room" opportunity, to visually discern a lack of participation or disinterest. However, the online environment allows for alternative means of engaging learners. Although observers were restricted from posting chats during the online encounter, the feedback and questions following each encounter were far-reaching. These covered substantive and process issues, situational ethics, professional responsibility, issues of power, scope of practice, and questions about other communication skills and techniques they might employ to better support the patient/client.

Learning from our colleagues in practice is one of the privileges that simulation learning allows. We found that as a result of the community bond the students created over the 4 days, the learning was deeper than we imagined possible, evident in their reflections and evaluations.

Publication

Nightly assignments inviting students to reflect on their learning from the day, focusing on core themes, allowed us to hear from the students about what they were taking away. It had the added benefit of allowing us to evaluate the effectiveness of the course methods and design as we delivered it, allowing greater responsiveness to students' interests and needs. An added benefit of collecting the thoughtful reflections students submitted as part of their grades was an offer from our Learning Resource Centre to help interested students publish their reflections on learning from the course. This led to the publication of a special edition in the Michener Institute's open-access student journal. A link to the publication is below.

Link: https://journals.publicknowledgeproject.org/michener-student/index.php/michener-student/issue/current

Our challenges involved the technological support required to carry out the course. The number of students in class meant we needed dedicated people to manage the chat and ensure students were not engaging in side conversations. Course facilitators could not manage delivering the materials while also observing the side chats. Recounting one experience, we had a student type a comment into the chat that light-heartedly mocked another student. The comment was close to calling someone out for a private experience. We were concerned with the comment that was posted, but before we had a chance to respond, another student stepped into the chat and chided the first student for their comment. The student who initially posted the comment subsequently apologized. This accountability was amazing to witness. Would we have had knowledge of the exchange if we had been in a face-to-face environment? The students were creating their community rules of engagement.

As with all online learning, there were connectivity issues for some students. In addition, limitations of our platform prevented us from seeing more than four people simultaneously. The complexity of creating and moving people between break-out rooms required that we adjust our format to simplify the number of possible points of breakdown. The rule of thumb became one of simplifying and adapting to balance delivering material with the technology platform. Our relationship as teachers with technology has changed dramatically, acknowledging that it is the essential partner in making online learning work effectively.

Student Evaluation

Another collaboration for our online program was with the Applied Education Research team who evaluated the feedback from the students. The majority of feedback was positive and included comments such as:

> "...the simulations were very impactful.... It was amazing to see the different approaches and responses to one situation that may occur in a clinical setting."

> "Humanizing yourself to the patient through your ways of communicating is key..."

Student feedback included responses to the question: Which aspect(s) of the course do you think will impact your practice the most?

> "I think the COVID lesson and the final connecting the dots lesson will impact me the most... enjoyed seeing the skills that were taught in the first three classes being applied to a real-life situation."

> "...empathetic communication and being able to connect with not only the patient but their family as well".

> "How to give and receive feedback, and how to communicate effectively in a demanding situation seem most applicable to my future practice."

> "...the simulations were very impactful.... It was amazing to see the different approaches and responses to one situation that may occur in a clinical setting."

> "Humanizing yourself to the patient through your ways of communicating is key..."

Future Directions

There are now numerous resources to assist educators in navigating online education platforms to ensure student interactivity and engagement. What we can add to the discussion is our acknowledgment of the need for adaptability as educators now working across different platforms. Recognition of the need to be a "lifelong learner" was never more relevant for professionals working in simulation-based education. Of interest to us is that regardless of the plethora of online platforms, all offering something slightly different from each other, the educational principles we discovered in the development implementation of the Comm 700 are foundational and transferable whether working face-to-face or at a distance.

These include preserving the communication gestures with students that inspire connection.

Working to notice individual learners' unique skills and characteristics is not lost on the observer participant, who may hesitate to participate in a "throng." We would like to think as educators, we can interrupt the "what's the use" attitude related to reluctant participation by stimulating audible responses or chat ideas. This may require a sometimes forgiving nod to timing and scheduling within reason. Attention paid matters.

Case Study—Integrated Library Sciences

As the academic library for the Michener School of Applied Health Sciences, the Learning Resource Centre (LRC) has a history of collaboration with the team from the Centre for Learning, Innovation, and Simulation (CLIS). The LRC's primary goal is to contribute to improved learner experiences and outcomes, and we have worked with our partners from the Simulation team to provide various opportunities to our students, including:

- Dry lab models and resources: The LRC's collection of models and other resources enables the students to practice technical clinical skills as well as "soft" skills such as communication, leadership, and collaboration through the on-site, on-demand creation of "pop-up clinics". The students use the LRC spaces to simulate a clinical environment with students role-playing the various participants—practitioner, patient, observer, evaluator—in a scenario. This simulated activity helps students develop clinical competencies while modeling professional interpersonal skills.
- 3D printing: The LRC partnered with CLIS to acquire and deploy a 3D printer to allow students to have hands-on experiences of discovery and creation—including building anatomical models, understanding anatomical structures, and envisioning future applications of such devices.
- iPads at the simulated bedside: Enabling "just in time" knowledge transfer through integrating learning resources directly into the students' environment is a key strategy of the LRC. The CLIS and LRC staff have observed best practices in simulation settings where iPads loaded with relevant apps are positioned at the bedside. Easy access to knowledge in context and available in the moment allow students to have a robust learning experience and lock in the learning by experiencing knowledge transfer in practical application.

When the global pandemic changed education, all of these hands-on, in-person experiences were disrupted. At that time, to ensure the safety of our students, faculty, and staff, the physical library at Michener was closed and access to LRC staff, services, tools, and resources went exclusively online via our virtual library website and Teams consultations. Collaboration between the LRC, CLIS, and the broader Learning, Innovation, and Research (LIR) team went from being an opportunity and being an imperative.

For the LRC, the first impact of the Big Pandemic Pivot was to move into rapid development mode to support knowledge synthesis and knowledge transfer. There were two immediate challenges:

1. The volume of information—scientific and otherwise—on the virus was overwhelming. It was difficult for healthcare professionals to easily ascertain the veracity, authority, and authenticity of any "science" being presented.
2. All teachers were required—very suddenly and unexpectedly—to halt face-to-face instruction and rapidly transition to an alternate delivery in academic and clinical settings.

To answer these challenges, we partnered with CLIS and the broader LIR teams, as well as the University Health Network (UHN) Health Sciences Libraries, UHN Clinical Education, and The Institute for Education Research (TIER). Our shared goals were to develop two knowledge portals: The Science of COVID-19 (https://guides.hsict.library.utoronto.ca/covid19) to facilitate knowledge mobilization, curating high-level resources related to the latest science on COVID-19 as well as resources to support "upskilling" healthcare professionals in critical care; and,

- Teaching and Learning in the Time of COVID-19 (https://guides.hsict.library.utoronto.ca/teachlearnCOVID) to curate the volume of information on online pedagogy—relevant, reliable sources of information to facilitate knowledge synthesis and knowledge mobilization to enable all our teachers and learners to realize the best education and the best teaching and learning experience.

The disruption in face-to-face learning at Michener provided another opportunity for the LRC to partner again with LIR and CLIS in the delivery of Communications 700 (also known as "Week 3" as it was delivered in the third week of the Summer term—the first term which Michener students started exclusively online).

For Michener students, faculty, and staff, the start of the Summer term was a time of heightened anxiety, greater uncertainty, and enormous stress. In programs that had been historically very hands-on, what would teaching and learning look and feel like—being virtual, remote, distanced? One clear opportunity was to develop a unique simulation course focused on communications skills and emotional intelligence competencies in the context of a global pandemic when the patients and healthcare practitioners were experiencing different emotions.

The LRC participated in the Communications 700 course to reassure our students that they have access to all the resources, services, and tools developed by the LRC staff via our website and through consultation with our professional librarians to enable not only their immediate academic success but also to develop the digital information literacy skills to ensure their future success as healthcare professionals and as life-long learners. The commitment to the course on the students' side focused on their reflections on the presented learnings. Could these reflections be dual purposed—and provide another simulation experience for our students by inviting them to submit their reflections to MICH: The Student Journal of the Michener Institute (https://journals.publicknowledgeproject.org/michener-student/index.php/michener-student/issue/view/39)—the open access journal managed by the LRC.

MICH was launched in September 2019 with the view of providing our students with a forum to share their voices and for them to experience scholarly communication in a "safe" environment, simulating the publishing process and the thrill of seeing their articles in print without the stress of submitting to a name-brand journal. Leading up to September 2019, the librarians in the LRC had been working with faculty to fully develop our students' digital information literacy competencies. Having a critical approach, understanding the value of information creation and dissemination, recognizing authoritative sources, and approaching literature searches like strategic exploration are all elements of the framework for the conversation of scholarship and are all competencies we seek to instill in our students through our digital information literacy workshops and consultations. It was in the course of this work that a faculty member came to us, commenting on the increased quality of the assignments being submitted by her students as a result of the LRC workshops and lamenting the lack of venue where our students writing and other works could be showcased. We had also been discussing our students' research capacity—and how to help prepare them for their roles in furthering their professions through scholarly communications. Why not develop an open-access journal, shepherded by the LRC and focused on the contributions of Michener students to showcase their work? Thus, MICH: The Student Journal of the Michener Institute was born with Vol. 1 Issue 1, released September 13, 2019.

In April 2020, in the new Communications 700 course, the LRC asked the students participating in the course to share their reflections for publication in our student open-access journal. The students' motivation was threefold:

1. Take advantage of a professional outlet for the roller-coaster emotions all were experiencing and the chance to reflect on what it means to be an empathetic healthcare professional during a global pandemic crisis;
2. Realize the goal of contributing to the professional literature by joining the scholarly conversation—and having a good story (with published evidence) for a future employer when asked: "What did you do during the pandemic?";
3. Experience the publishing process via simulation—all the rigor of contributing an article to a journal without the fear of rejection.

The students of the Communications 700 course embraced the opportunity. Their candid reflections and unvarnished voices are available in MICH Volume 2 Issue 1 (https://journals.publicknowledgeproject.org/michener-student/index.php/michener-student/index). Their stories are moving—and speak to the commitment of the Michener students to their future careers as healthcare professionals. The LRC remains committed to supporting our students in developing a capacity for scholarship and competencies related to furthering the scholarly conversation of all the applied healthcare professions. This simulated publishing opportunity opens the door to a lifetime of scholarship.

Some selected reflections from our students published in MICH:

"I discovered that validating, appropriate questioning, and empathy are some of the most effective communication skills. As healthcare practitioners, we see multiple patients a day. We hear multiple stories daily, and sometimes it becomes easier to not let ourselves emote and feel what the patient and their family feel. I believe this desensitizes us as people. Hence, validating their emotions allows us to remind ourselves of situations where we may have experienced similar emotions. By asking the right questions, open-ended and kind, we facilitate conversation."

"Leaders and decision-makers in businesses and governments are working hard for our safety and well-being. I have also seen the tears, frustration, anger, disappointment, exhaustion, and bravery of the frontline healthcare workers, who symbolize courage and self-sacrifice. I recognize the importance of a friendly smile, eye contact, and human touch and its impact on the patient's trust and confidence… While the pandemic tests our adaptive capacity, we will continue to educate ourselves in knowledge and values to stay strong and create a healthy world."

"In retrospection, the Canadian government's response to mitigate and manage the Covid-19 outbreak was slow, given the delayed explicit specifications on enforcing safety measures to minimize deaths, it consequentially allowed the escalation of Covid-19 cases to burden the healthcare system, which also resulted in a national quarantine inflicting economic damage… Canada appears to struggle in implementing its own version of local/regional protocols to efficiently re-open the economy. Continuous delays in revising restrictions and implementing protocols will ultimately bring a cycling effect to negatively impact the Canadian economy, its population health, and government debt."

"This is new to all of us, including the faculty, administration staff, and technology moguls that run our school. They have gone above and beyond to make things work and give us the best possible clinical skills training in these unexpected times. We've been thrown into this new era with uncertainty with extra camera setups in labs and learning new platforms like GoTo Meetings and Blackboard Collaborate for online simulations. There is little chance of returning to how the world bustled just 3 months ago. It might never be the same as it was. The schools may have to alter their curriculums just like the governments are scrambling for stability. Future graduates must keep their heads up for what is to become of in-lab, hands-on, applied health sciences."

"We are all working together to reach a common goal: to stop the pandemic that has gripped our nation and the world. As a society, we have adapted to our current situation, and I am pleased to see people helping whenever they can. For example, a nearby distillery has begun producing hand sanitizers rather than beer, medical students have gathered forces to collect personal protective equipment (PPE), people are distributing masks... the list is exhaustive. It is the kindness of these people whom I appreciate during the new COVID climate we are navigating together."

Conclusion

Technology innovations that began because of the pandemic will only serve to accelerate the pace of adoption in health professions education. The continued adoption of Extended Reality (XR) and alternative educational methods, such as smartphone apps, will continue to be incorporated into the educational landscape both virtually and physically. Artificial intelligence will add additional layers of complexity over the next decade. But, regardless of the technology that is implemented, the most important development is the continued collaboration between departments and programs. Reducing duplication of services, increasing access to services, and sharing of courses is necessary to continue to foster the work that was started because of the pandemic. In Canada, collaborations between the Maple League of schools in Atlantic Canada, the Tri-University Group in southern Ontario, and through Education City in Ottawa already exists which allows for sharing of online courses and maximizing student experiences. However, we must remain vigilant that the technological divide does not proliferate inequalities. COVID has been a great equalizer and divider with the more educated and more funded being able to work from home or obtaining access to computer simulations. Ensuring that there is equality and inclusiveness in advanced technological educational programs is essential as we continue to develop new methods of education. Nursing education needs to continue to incorpoate simulation into the myriad of educational opportunities for students and staff. Educators should look outside of the traditional simulation methodologies and techniques commonly used in nursing and collaborate with interprofessional teams and other health professions to take cues from innovative programs both within and outside of nursing. This chapter aims to shed the light on opportunities for nursing education to branch out and engage with other, often less thought about, professions and techniques.

References

1. Muñoz-Najar A, Gilberto A, Hasan A, Cobo C, Azevedo JP, Akmal M. Remote Learning during COVID-19: Lessons from Today, Principles for Tomorrow. Washington, D.C.: World Bank Group; 2021. Retrieved from: https://documents1.worldbank.org/curated/en/160271637074230077/pdf/Remote-Learning-During-COVID-19-Lessons-from-Today-Principles-for-Tomorrow.pdf.
2. https://torontodiscoverydistrict.ca.
3. Lioce L. Healthcare Simulation Dictionary. Second. Agency for Healthcare Research and Quality. 2020. https://www.ahrq.gov/patient-safety/resources/simulation/terms.html. Accessed 22 Nov 2020.
4. Wechsler TF, Kümpers F, Mühlberger A. Inferiority or even superiority of virtual reality exposure therapy in phobias?—a systematic review and quantitative meta-analysis on randomized controlled trials specifically comparing the efficacy of virtual reality exposure to gold standard in vivo exposure in agoraphobia, specific phobia, and social phobia. Front Psychol. 2019;10:1758.
5. Donker T, Cornelisz I, van Klaveren C, van Straten A, Carlbring P, Cuijpers P, et al. Effectiveness of self-guided app-based virtual reality cognitive behavior therapy for acrophobia: a randomized clinical trial. JAMA Psychiatry. 2019;76(7):682.
6. Laver KE, George S, Thomas S, Deutsch JE, Crotty M. Virtual reality for stroke rehabilitation. Cochrane Database Syst Rev. 2015;2015(2):CD008349. https://doi.org/10.1002/14651858.CD008349.pub3.

7. Cano Porras D, Siemonsma P, Inselberg R, Zeilig G, Plotnik M. Advantages of virtual reality in the rehabilitation of balance and gait: systematic review. Neurology. 2018;90(22): 1017–25.
8. Mohamadipanah H, Perrone KH, Nathwani J, Parthiban C, Peterson K, Wise B, et al. Screening surgical residents' laparoscopic skills using virtual reality tasks: who needs more time in the sim lab? Surgery. 2019;166(2):218–22.
9. Pulijala Y, Ma M, Pears M, Peebles D, Ayoub A. Effectiveness of immersive virtual reality in surgical training—a randomized control trial. J Oral Maxillofac Surg. 2018;76(5):1065–72.
10. Nickel F, Brzoska JA, Gondan M, Rangnick HM, Chu J, Kenngott HG, et al. Virtual reality training versus blended learning of laparoscopic cholecystectomy: a randomized controlled trial with laparoscopic novices. Medicine. 2015;94(20):e764.
11. Cook DA, Hamstra SJ, Brydges R, Zendejas B, Szostek JH, Wang AT, et al. Comparative effectiveness of instructional design features in simulation-based education: systematic review and meta-analysis. Med Teach. 2013;35(1):e867–98.
12. Issenberg SB, Mcgaghie WC, Petrusa ER, Lee Gordon D, Scalese RJ. Features and uses of high-fidelity medical simulations that lead to effective learning: a BEME systematic review. Med Teach. 2005;27(1):10–28.
13. Wulf G, Shea C, Lewthwaite R. Motor skill learning and performance: a review of influential factors. Med Educ. 2010;44(1):75–84.
14. Monteiro S, Sherbino J, Sibbald M, Norman G. Critical thinking, biases and dual processing: the enduring myth of generalizable skills. Med Educ. 2020;54(1):66–73.
15. Cheung JJH, Kulasegaram KM, Woods NN, Moulton C, Ringsted CV, Brydges R. Knowing how and knowing why: testing the effect of instruction designed for cognitive integration on procedural skills transfer. Adv Health Sci Educ. 2018;23(1):61–74.
16. Patel T. To the uncertain future clinical practitioner. MICH Stud J Michener Inst Educ. 2020;2(1):5738.
17. Shaikh J. COVID-19—the new 'normal'. MICH Stud J Michener Inst Educ. 2020;2(1).
18. Chan JWY.. Covid-19 impact on Canadian economy and population health. MICH Stud J Michener Inst Educ. 2020;2(1).
19. Zafar SF. COVID, respiratory therapists and our future. MICH Stud J Michener Inst Educ. 2020;2(1).
20. Mah K. Coping in a COVID world. MICH Stud J Michener Inst Educ. 2020;2(1).

Index

J. M. Kutzin et al. (eds.), *Comprehensive Healthcare Simulation: Nursing*, Comprehensive Healthcare Simulation,
https://doi.org/10.1007/978-3-031-31090-4